DOCTOR, PATIENT AND THE LAW

A selection of practical issues

THIRD EDITION

S A STRAUSS

SC BA (STELL) LLB (OFS) LLD (UNISA)
Professor of Law in the University of South Africa
Advocate of the Supreme Court of South Africa

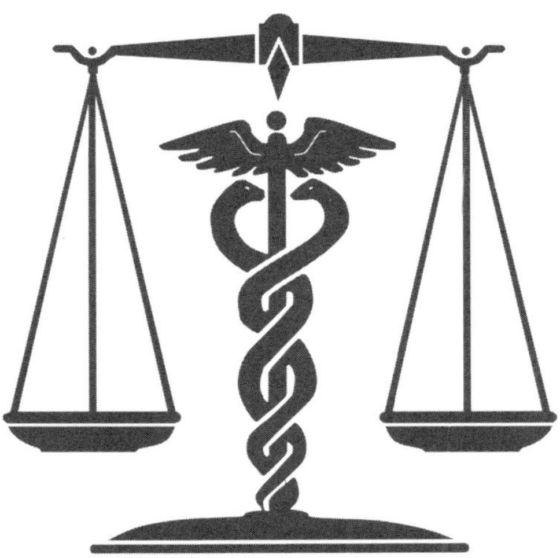

J L van Schaik

Published by J L van Schaik (Pty) Ltd,
1064 Arcadia Street, Hatfield, Pretoria

First edition 1980
Second, revised edition 1984
Third, revised edition 1991
ISBN 0 627 01777 0

Cover illustration by Alida Carpenter
Cover design by Barrett Joubert and Linette Downes
Typeset in 10/11 Century Old Style by ORBiT CC, Pretoria
Printed and bound by National Book Printers, Goodwood, Cape

For Rosanna, Ben,
Marita and Sybrand

Acknowledgements

This book is not offered as a textbook on medical law. Rather, as the subtitle suggests, a selection of practical legal issues relating to the doctor-patient relationship has been made.

The *causa causans* of this book is to be found in an invitation extended to me, a number of years ago, by the editor of the *South African Medical Post* to contribute a regular column on "Medicine and the Law" to his journal.

The pharmaceutical company Scherag (Pty) Ltd was the first organisation in South Africa to publish a journal devoted exclusively to medical law and finance, appropriately called *Medical Law & Finance*, and I was asked to contribute articles to that publication on a regular basis. In 1980 its scope was broadened and its name changed to *S A Practice Management/S A Praktykbestuur.*

Through the years readers of these journals have submitted many interesting medico-legal questions, and a number of these have formed the subject of my articles. From time to time I was asked by readers whether it was not possible for these articles to be published in book form, and this book – the first edition of which appeared in 1980 – is a response to that request.

First and foremost therefore, thanks are due to the readers of the journals mentioned, for their sustained interest in my articles over the years. I am grateful to the various publishers for agreeing to these articles being reproduced in this form.

A very special word of thanks is due to those members of the personnel of the Scherag and Essex divisions of Scherag (Pty) Ltd with whom I have had the privilege of collaborating over the years.

Unless otherwise stated, chapters of this book have previously appeared as articles in the *South African Medical Post, Medical Law & Finance,* or *S A Practice Management/S A Praktykbestuur.* Where necessary, chapters have been updated.

I should further like to express my gratitude to the publishers and editors of the following journals or publications for kind permission to reproduce, mostly in amended form, articles that appeared in these: the *South African Medical Journal* (South African Medical Association); *De Rebus* (the Association of Law Societies of the Republic of South Africa); the *South African Journal of Criminal Law and Criminology* (Messrs Butterworth & Co); the *Comparative and International Law Journal of Southern Africa* (Institute of Foreign and Comparative Law, University of South Africa); the *South African Cancer Bulletin* (the National Cancer Association of South Africa); and *Medicine and Law* (International Centre of Medicine and Law).

I wish to thank the South African Broadcasting Corporation for kindly allowing me to reproduce an amended version of the text of a talk by me which was broadcast as part of their 1978 series, "University of the Air", and published in a booklet styled *Alcoholism.*

My interest in medical law has brought me into contact with many doctors and lawyers in this country and abroad who share this interest. To them I owe a great debt of gratitude for their friendship and the insight they have given me into medicine and its relationship with the law. They are too numerous to mention by name, but amongst my overseas friends two must be singled out: Judge Amnon Carmi of Haifa, Israel, and Professor Erwin Deutsch of Göttingen, Germany.

A special word of thanks is due to the Human Sciences Research Council and the

Association of Law Societies, whose generous financial grants have enabled me to attend international conferences on medical law, as I have indicated in the text.

I am grateful to Mrs Marian Odendaal and Mrs Frieda Haussler for valuable linguistic advice given to me in the preparation of the first and second editions, respectively, of this book. Mrs Ann Shiel and Mrs Ina Dörfling were of great help to me in this respect in the preparation of the third edition. It goes without saying, however, that I bear sole responsibility for the text as published in its final form.

Last but not least, I wish to express my sincerest appreciation to the publishers of this book, Messrs J L van Schaik (Pty) Ltd, and in particular Mr Helgaard Raubenheimer, for their sustained interest in this publication. I owe a great debt of gratitude to Mrs Linette Downes of J L van Schaik Publishers who was responsible for the technical side of this edition, for her enthusiasm, competent services and constructive suggestions.

I have incorporated in the text statutory and case law up to the end of February 1991.

THE AUTHOR

Contents

Acknowledgements vi

Table of cases xi

I Contract between doctor and patient, and issues of consent

1. Some practical legal problems pertaining to consent to treatment 3
2. Truth-telling in medicine: a legal perspective 14
3. May the doctor refuse to attend a patient? 23
4. Refusal of blood transfusion by Jehovah's Witness 29
5. Informed consent and the unwilling ophthalmological patient 35
6. Consent to an operation on a mental patient 37
7. Does the doctor guarantee that the patient will be cured? 40

II Medical and dental fees

8. Medical fees: basic principles 45
9. Medical schemes and the doctor's fees: some legal aspects 49
10. Discounting ("cession") of doctors' accounts and factoring 57
11. Collection of debts : the perennial headache 59
12. Is "blacklisting" of patients who have a record of bad debts permissible? ... 63
13. Doctor requested by third party to attend patient: who must pay doctor's fees? 66
14. May a dentist claim a fee for a denture from a dissatisfied patient? 69

III Contracts between doctors

15. Drawing up a partnership agreement: some points to bear in mind 73
16. Sharing of consulting rooms 77
17. Contracts of employment entered into by general practitioners 79
18. Covenant restraining ex-partner or ex-employee from practising in same neighbourhood 82

IV Emergency treatment

19. Rescue, emergency medical treatment and the law 89

V Professional secrecy, patient records and medical certificates

20. Professional secrecy in relation to spouses 103
21. Medical certificates and professional secrecy: some legal issues 106
22. The keeping of medical records and the rights of doctor and patient to these 110

VI Mental patients, psychiatry and the law

23. Criminal responsibility and mental abnormality 121
24. Epilepsy and the law 136

VII Organ and tissue transplantation; rights to tissue

25. The law relating to organ and tissue transplantation 147
26. The patient's rights to tissue removed during an operation 160
27. May a hospital destroy the remains of a still-born foetus? 163

VIII Contraception, sterilisation, artificial insemination and related topics

28. Legal problems connected with contraception and sterilisation 169
29. Failed sterilisation: liability for "wrongful conception" 175
30. Artificial insemination 181
31. In vitro fertilisation and surrogate motherhood: some issues 187
32. Genetic manipulation: the potential legal liability of the practitioner 191

IX Abortion

33. The Abortion and Sterilisation Act 207
34. The Abortion and Sterilisation Act and the drama of Miss X 219
35. Can the use of an intra-uterine device amount to illegal abortion? 222

X Transsexualism

36. Transsexualism and the law 227

XI Medical negligence, malpractice liability

37. Medical malpractice liability: doctor, insure thyself! 243
38. "Mere" error of judgment may constitute negligence 249
39. Legal liability for a wrong diagnosis 252
40. The doctor's liability for dangerous side-effects of penicillin 254
41. Volkmann has yet another sequel in court 257
42. Compartment syndrome resulting in loss of leg: hospital held liable for premature discharge of patient 262
43. Patient burnt by earth plate of cautery: who is liable? 264
44. Can a failure to adequately inform the patient constitute negligence? 267
45. The missing swab and the theatre nurse's legal liability 270
46. Radiological mishaps 272
47. Anaesthetic mishaps 276
48. Failure of general practitioner to call in specialist gynaecologist to assist in problem case 280
49. Superior vena cava torn during mediastinoscopy 282
50. Plastic surgery: medico-legal aspects 285
51. Legal liability for defective drugs 292

XII Hospital liability, superintendents and employees

52. Hospital liability for delicts committed by professional personnel 299
53. The legal liability of a hospital superintendent 306
54. Patient insists on leaving hospital too soon after operation 308
55. Liability of hospital or staff for loss of patient's property 310
56. Suspension of a hospital doctor for misconduct 312
57. Handling of hospital strikes 314

XIII Death, death certification, dying and euthanasia

58. Death and the moment of death: some reflections by a lawyer 321
59. "DOA" (dead on arrival) certificates 329
60. Certification of death in cases of sudden cot-death 334
61. The euthanasia debate: a South African view 336
62. The "Living Will" and the "right to die" 344

XIV Alcohol abuse and drunken driving

63. The alcoholic and the law 351
64. The taking of blood samples in drunken driving cases 357
65. Blood-alcohol: must the specimen taken be representative of the driver's blood generally? 359
66. Drunken driving and "breathalyser" tests: some legal problems 361
67. Some problems of proof relating to excessive blood-alcohol concentration 364

XV Disciplinary proceedings

68. Medical Council disciplinary inquiries: some do's and don'ts 369
69. The duties of the Medical Council in disciplinary cases 376
70. Medical practitioner suspended from practice: legal implications for his partners 378
71. What legal action can a doctor take against a person who has lodged a complaint against him with the Medical Council? 381
72. Pharmaceutical gifts to doctors: legal and ethical implications 384
73. May a private hospital pay a commission to doctors who refer patients? 387

XVI Medical care of prisoners and detainees

74. The legal rights of prisoners and detainees to medical treatment 391
75. Medical care of prisoners and detainees 402
76. Legal questions surrounding hunger-strikes by detainees and prisoners 409

XVII Miscellany

77. Child abuse: some legal issues 417
78. Medical experimentation involving children 420
79. Presence of "outsiders" at post mortem examination, and disclosure of findings 424

80. Patient consults another doctor without informing first doctor 427
81. Medical strikes outlawed by Parliament 429
82. Company not entitled to run a dispensary in a private clinic 431
83. Giving expert evidence in court: is the doctor entitled to be remunerated?. 433
84. Inquests and the doctor 436
85. Medical practice in company form 439
86. Acts specially pertaining to the medical profession 441
87. Doctor practising from his home: legal issues 444

Annexure

SAMDC rules of conduct 449

Index 459

Table of cases

A

Adams v Uys (1929) 14 PH J26 (C) 421
Administrateur, Natal v Trust Bank van Afrika Beperk 1979 (3) SA 824 (A) 21
Administrator, Natal v Edouard 1990 (3) SA 581 (A) 170, 179, 193, 197, 243
Administrator, Transvaal and Others v Traub and Others 1989 (4) SA 731 (A) 316
Albrighton v Royal Prince Alfred Hospital [1980] 2 NSWLR 542 (CA) 304
Anonymous v Weiner 270 NYS 2d 319 (NY) 229
Application of North Shore University Hospital (Bland) (reference not available) 34
Argus P & P Co v Van Niekerk (1895) 2 OR 40 67

B

B, (a minor), Re [1981] WLR 1421 199
Baiki v Pretoria Municipality 1921 TPD 376 52
Barker v T E Hopkins Ltd (1959) 1 WLR 966 98
Bayer South Africa (Pty) Ltd and Another v Viljoen 1990 (2) SA 647 (A) 292
Behr v Minister of Health 1961 (1) SA 629 (SR) 68
Behrmann and Another v Klugman 1988 WLD, unreported 41, 176
Bester v Commercial Union Versekeringsmaatskappy van SA Bpk
1973 (1) SA 169 (A) 20
BK Tooling (Edms) Bpk v Scope Precision Engineering (Edms) Bpk 1979 (1) SA 391 (A) 69
Blore v Standard and General Insurance Co 1972 (2) SA 89 (0) 265
Blyth v Van den Heever 1980 (1) SA 191 (A) 21, 246, 253, 257, 369
Bonner v Moran 126 F 2d 121 (DC Cir 1941) 421
Boswell v Minister of Police and Another 1978 (3) SA 268 (E) 199
Botha v Botha 1972 (2) SA 559 (N) 104
Boyce v Petrovsky WD, Mo September 1981 411
Bozzoli v Station Commander John Vorster Square, Johannesburg 1972 (3) SA 934 (T) ... 202
Broadway v Jeffers 194 SE 642 (South Carolina, 1938) 68
Brudo v Chamberlain 1912 TPD 131 290
Buls and Another v Tsatsarolakis 1976 (2) SA 891 (T) 40, 252, 288
Byrne v East London Hospital Board 1926 EDL 128 301

C

Campos v Weeks 53 Cal Rptr 915 (Cal 1966) 256
Canterbury v Spence (1972) 150 App DC 263, 464 F 2d 772 18
Cassidy v Minister of Health [1951] 2 KB 343 300
Chatterton v Gerson and Another [1981] QB 432 .... 9, 13, 268
Chrisafogeorgis v Brandenburg 55I11 2d 368, 304 NE 2d 88 (1973) 197
Christian League of Southern Africa v Rall 1981 (2) SA 821 (0) 202, 210, 219, 220
Clair v Port Elizabeth Harbour Board, Kennedy v The Same 5 EDC 311 (1887) 264
Cobbs v Grant (1972) 8 Cal 3d 229, 104 Cal Rptr 505, 502 P 2d 1 .... 18, 20
Conroy, Re 486 A 2d 1209 (1985) 347
Corbett v Corbett (otherwise Ashley) [1970] 2 All ER 33 .... 234, 235, 237
Corbin v Philadelphia 195 Pa 461 (1900) 98
Correira v Berwind 1986 (4) SA 60 (Z) 3, 27
Cox v Cartwright 121 NE 2d 673 (Ohio) 70
Crivon v Barnett Group Hospital Management Committee, *London Times* 19 Nov 1959... 253
Crook v Griqualand West DM Co (1886) 4 HCG 16 66

D

Dale v Hamilton 1924 WLD 184 265
David Wuhl (Pty) Ltd and Others v Badler and Another 1984 (3) SA 427 (W) 84
De'Ath (substituted by Tiley) v Additional Magistrate, Cape Town 1988 (4) SA 763 (C) . 436
De la Rey's Transport (Edms) Bpk v Lewis 1978 (1) SA 797 (A) 60
De la Rouviere v S A Medical and Dental Council 1977 (1) SA 85 (N) 376
Director of Hospital Services v Mistry 1979 (1) SA 626 (A) 312
Divisional Commissioner of SA Police, Witwatersrand Area, and Others v SA Associated Newspapers Ltd and Another 1966 (2) SA 503 (A) 372, 375
Dixie, Ex parte 1950 (4) SA 748 (W) 37
Dube v Administrator, Transvaal 1963 (4) SA 260 (T) 257, 301, 304
Durham v United States 214 F 2d 862 (1954) 123
Dyanti and Another, Ex parte, 1989 (4) SA (CKGD) 110

E

Economic Data Processing (Pty) Ltd and Others v Pentreath 1984 (2) SA 605 (W) 110
Edouard v Administrator, Natal 1989 (2) SA 368 (D) 170, 177
E G Electric Co (Pty) Ltd v Franklin 1979 (2) SA 702 (E) 21
Eggeling and Another v Law Union and Rock Insurance Co Ltd 1955 (3) SA 592 (D) 421
Emeh v Kensington, Chelsea and Fulham Area Health Authority and Others, [1984] 3 All ER 1044 (CA) 175
Essa v Divaris 1947 (1) SA 753 (A) 310
Estate Mathews v Redelinghuis 1927 WLD 307 84
Esterhuizen v Administrator, Transvaal 1957 (3) SA 710 (T) 10, 18, 31, 93, 250, 268, 310
Eyre v Measday [1986] 1 All ER 497 (CA) 176

F

Forman v Barnett 1941 WLD 54 83
Freeman v Home Office [1983] 3 All ER 589 (QB) 4
Fulls v Mollentz (1896) 13 SC 369 67

G

Gillick v West Norfolk and Wisbeck Area Health Authority and Another [1985] 2 All ER 402 (HL) 173, 422
Gleitman v Cosgrove 49 NJ 22, 227 A 2d 689 (1976) 196
Gold v Essex County Council [1942] 2 KB 293 300
Goldberg v Minister of Prisons 1979 (1) SA 14 (A) 391, 394
Gordon v Barnard 1977 (1) SA 887 (C) 172
Greaves & Co (Contractors) Ltd v Baynham Mickle and Partners [1975] 3 All ER 99 (CA) 40
Greenman v Yuba Power Products Inc (1963) 59 Cal 2d 57, 13 ALR 3d 1049 293

H

Harris v Commissioner of Prisons 1965 (2) SA 645 (T) 393
Hartl v Pretoria Hospital Committee 1915 TPD 336 301
Hatcher v Black (QB), *London Times* 2 July 1954 250
Hauman v Nortje 1914 AD 293 69
Hawker v Life Offices Association of South Africa and Another 1987 (3) SA 777 (C) 64
Hermer v Fisher and Others 1960 (2) SA 650 (T) 84
Hewatt v Rendel 1925 TPD 679 302
Hillyer v Governor of St Bartholomew's Hospital [1909] 2 KB 820 300
Holloway v Hauver 322 A 2d 890 (Maryland, 1974) 266
Honey v Minister of Police 1980 (3) SA 700 (Tk) 394
Hughes v Fletcher 1967 (1) SA 326 (SR) 245
Hurley v Eddingfield 145 Ind 416, 59 NE 1058 (1901) 24

J

Jackovach v Yocom 212 Iowa 914 (1931) ... 93
Jacobs v Theimer 519 SW 2d 846 (1975) ... 196
James, Ex parte 1954 (3) SA 270 (SR) ... 104
Jehovah's Witnesses in the State of Washington et al v King County Hospital Unit No 1 (Harbourview) et al 278 E Supp 488 (1967) ... 34
Johannesburg City Council v Venter 1936 TPD 287 ... 421
John F Kennedy Memorial Hospital v Heston 279 A 2d 670 (NJ 1971) ... 24
Johnston v Powell (1909) 19 CTR 86 ... 290
Jonker v Jonker 1970, TPD, unreported ... 236
Jorgensen v Meade-Johnson Laboratories Inc 483 F 2d 237 (10th Cir, 1973) ... 197

K

Klingenberg's Exor v Lademan (1898) 5 OR 105 ... 164
Kroonstad Westelike Boere Koöperatiewe Vereniging Bpk v Botha and Another 1964 (3) SA 561 (A) ... 295
Kruger v Boltman 1933 PH A3 (E) ... 70

L

L v J 1985 (4) SA 371 (C) ... 184
Landman v Mienie 1944 OPD 59 ... 422
Langeni and Others v Minister of Health and Welfare and Others 1988 (4) SA 93 (W) ... 316
Langley Fox Building Partnership (Pty) Ltd v De Valence 1991 (1) SA 1 (A) ... 305
Liassou v Pretoria City Council 1979 (3) SA 217 (T) ... 373
Lindsay and Others v Stofberg NO 1988 (2) SA 462 (C) ... 73, 299
Lourens NO v Colonial Mutual Life Assurance Society Ltd 1986 (3) SA 373 (A) ... 247
Lower Umfolosi District War Memorial Hospital v Lowe 1937 NPD 31 ... 301
Ludlow v Swindon Health Authority 1989 QBD, unreported ... 277
Luka v Lowrie 136 NW 1106 (1912) ... 93
Lutzkie v South African Railways and Harbours and Another 1974 (4) SA 396 (W) ... 199
Lymbery v Jefferies 1925 AD 236 ... 269

M

Magna Alloys and Research (SA) (Pty) Ltd v Ellis 1977 (4) SA 494 (N) ... 83
Magware v Minister of Health NO 1981 (4) SA 472 (Z) ... 24, 26
Mail Newspapers plc v Express Newspapers plc [1987] FSR 90 ... 322
Malan en Andere v Van Jaarsveld en 'n Ander 1972 (2) SA 243 (C) ... 84
Malette v Shulman and Others [1988] 47 DLR 18 ... 34
Marais v Pilkington 1905 TS 650 ... 434
MAWU v Hart 1985 (6) ILJ 478 ... 50
May v Broun 492 P 2d 776 (Oregon, 1972) ... 265
McConnel v Williams 65 A 2d (1949) ... 302
McGarry v J A Mercier Co 262 NW 296 (Mich, 1935) ... 114
McIvor v Southern Health and Social Services Board (Northern Ireland) [1978] 1 WLR 757 ... 111
McKay and Another v Essex Area Health Authority and Another [1982] 2 All ER 770 (CA) ... 198
McLoughlin v South African Medical and Dental Council 1947 (2) SA 377 (W) ... 376
Meaker NO v Roup, Wacks, Kaminger & Kriger and Another 1987 (2) SA 54 (C) ... 51, 56
Meyer v SA Medical and Dental Council 1982 (4) SA 450 (T) ... 373
Mhlongo and Another NO v Minister of Police 1978 (2) SA 551 (A) ... 303, 395
Minister of Community Development and Another v Koch 1991 (3) SA 751 (A) ... 305
Minister of Police v Rabie 1986 (1) SA 117 (A) ... 304
Minister of Police v Skosana 1977 (1) SA 31 (A) ... 399
Minister van Justisie, Ex parte: In re S v Grotjohn 1970(2) SA 355 (A) ... 409
Minister van Polisie v Ewels 1975 (3) SA 590 (A) ... 24, 90, 412
Minister van Polisie v Gamble 1979 (4) SA 759 (A) ... 395

Mitchell v Dixon 1914 AD 519 .... 252, 265
Mitchell v Maison Libson 1937 TPD 13 264
Mokoena and Others v Administrator, Transvaal 1988 (4) SA 912 (W) 317
Monk v Doctor's Hospital 403 F 2d 580 (CA, DC 1968) 266
Mulloy v Hop Sang 2 Western Weekly Law Reports 714 (1935) 94
MT v JT 355 A2d 204 (NJ 1976) 237
Mtetwa v Minister of Health 1989 (3) SA 600 (D) 302, 303
Muzik v Canzone del Mare 1980 (3) SA 470 (C) 20

N

National Union of Textile Workers and Others v Stag Packings (Pty) Ltd and Another 1982 (4) SA 151 (T) 16
Ngxale v Minister of Justice of the Ciskei 1981 (2) SA 554 (E) 396
Nishi v Hartwell 52 Hawaii 188, 473 P 2d 116 (1970) 22
Noll and Others v Alberton Frames (Pty) Ltd and Others 1989 (1) SA 730 (T) 51

O

Oats v Niland 1914 CPD 976 70

P

Palmer v Palmer 1955 (3) SA 56 (0) 5, 33 169, 170
Parkes v Parkes 1916 CPD 702 104
Paton v Trustees of British Pregnancy Advisory Service [1978] 2 All ER 987 211
Pearce v Fine and Another 1986 DC & LD, unreported 273
People v Labrentz 104 NE 2d 769 (1952) 34
Peri-Urban Areas Health Board v Munarin 1965 (3) SA 367 (A) 23
Pest Control (Central Africa) Ltd v Martin 1955 (3) SA 609 (SR) 85
Phillips v De Klerk 1983 TPD, unreported 29, 94
Pickering v Standard General Insurance Co Ltd 1980 (4) SA 326 (ZAD) 142
Pilkington Brothers (SA) Ltd v Lillicrap, Wassenaar and Partners 1983 (2) SA 157 (W) .. 21
Pinchin NO v Santam Insurance Co Ltd 1963 (2) SA 254 (W) 199
Polpark Dispensary (Pty) Ltd v SA Pharmacy Board 1977 (1) SA 115 (7) 431
Polpark Dispensary (Pty) Ltd v SA Pharmacy Board 1978 (2) SA 816 (A) 431
Poser v Petit, unreported 434
Pratt v Davis 118 Ill App 167 (1905) 170
Preller and Others v Jordaan 1956 (1) SA 483 (A) 311
Pretorius v SA Geneeskundige en Tandheelkundige Raad 1980 (2) SA 354 (T) 373
Prince v Massachusetts 321 US 158 421
Pupu, In re, 1959 (3) SA 480 (SR) 126

Q

Quinlan, In re 70 NJ 10, 355 A 2d 647, 429 US 922 (1976) 343

R

R v Ahmed 1959 (3) SA 776 (W) 129, 132
R v Arthur, unreported 198
R v Bethlehem Municipality 1941 OPD 277 55
R v Botha 1959 (1) SA 574 (0) 129, 132
R v Bourke 1916 TPD 303 128
R v Cawood 1950 (4) SA 91 (E) 358
R v Davidow 1955 WLD, unreported 339
R v Dhlamini 1955 (1) SA 120 (T) 129, 137
R v Du Plessis 1950 (1) SA 297 (0) 129, 137
R v Hosiosky 1961 (1) SA 84 (W) 294
R v Kaukakani 1947 (2) SA 807 132
R v Kemp [1957] 1 QBD 399; [1956] All ER 249 128

R v Kennedy 1951 (4) SA 431 (A) 128
R v Koortz 1953 (1) SA 371 (A) 131
R v Kruger 1958 (2) SA 320 (T) 128
R v Kumalo 1956 (3) SA 238 (N) 132, 138, 139
R v Lloyd 1929 EDL 270 358
R v Makali 1950 (1) SA 340 (N) 323, 345
R v Malcharek, R v Steel [1981] 2 All ER 422 (CA) 322
R v Matthews 1943 CPD 8 165
R v Mbete 1954 (4) SA 491 (E) 50
R v Mkize 1959 (2) SA 340 (N) 138
R v M'Naghten (1843) 10 Cl Fin 200, 8 ER 718 .... 123, 130
R v Mokwanazi 1959 (3) SA 782 (W) 130, 132, 138, 139
R v Ngema, R v Cele 1960 (1) SA 137 (A) 132, 138
R v Peverett 1940 AD 213 339
R v Pratt 1960 (4) SA 243 (T) 141
R v Roberts 1957 (4) SA 265 (A) 128, 134
R v Schoonwinkel 1953 (3) SA 136 (C) 129, 136, 138
R v Smit 1906 TS 783 .... 131, 139
R v Spicer 1945 AD 433 358
R v Stapelton (1952) 86 CLR 358 131
R v Stone [1977] QB 354 410
R v Sullivan [1983] 2 All ER 673 (HL) 140
R v Van der Merwe 1953 (2) PH H124 (W) 294
R v Van Schoor 1948 (4) SA 349 (C) 294
R v Victor 1943 TPD 77 138
R v Von Zell 1953 (3) SA 301 (A) 128, 131, 134
R v Westrich 1927 CPD 455 131
Rall NO v Landdros vir die Distrik Heilbron 1980 (3) SA 287 (O) 210, 220
Rautenbach, Ex parte 1938 SR 150 252
Re P (a minor) (1982) 80 LGR 301 212
Reyneke v Mutual and Federal Insurance Co Ltd 1991 (3) SA 412 (W) 343
Riback v Riback, 1984, unreported 184
Richter and Another v Estate Hamman 1976 (3) SA 226 (C) 9, 11, 18, 19, 267, 289
Robson v Theron 1978 (1) SA 841 (A) 75, 76
Roffey v Catterall, Edwards & Goudré (Pty) Ltd 1977 (4) SA 494 (N) 83
Rogaly v Weingartz 1954 (2) SA 791 (D) 84
Rompel v Botha 1953 TPD, unreported 10

S

S v Aandeweg 1986 (1) SA 211 (C) 443
S v Adams 1986 (4) SA 482 (A) 127
S v Arnold 1985 (3) SA 256 (C) 135
S v Bezuidenhout 1964 (2) SA 651 (A) 128, 132
S v Bezuidenhout 1985 AD, unreported 272
S v Burger 1980 (3) SA 1219 (T) 365
S v Campher 1987 (1) SA 490 (A) 135
S v Chretien 1981 (1) SA 1097 (A) 129, 134, 252
S v Collop 1979 (4) SA 381 (C), 1981 (1) SA 150 (A) 208, 222, 223
S v De Bellocq 1975 (3) SA 548 (T), 1969 THRHR 385 .... 200, 339
S v De Bruyn 1976 (1) SA 496 (A) 134
S v De Waal 1976 (2) SA 289 (O) 360
S v Dickenson 1982 (2) SA 84 (A) 365
S v Du Preez 1972 (2) SA 519 (SWA) 131
S v Ebrahim 1973 (1) SA 868 (A) 125
S v Eyden 1982 (4) SA 141 (T) 125
S v Francis 1977 (1) SA 643 (A) 360
S v Fraser 1987 (1) SA 399 (E) 355
S v Gaba 1981 (3) SA 745 (O) 357

S v Goliath 1972 (3) SA 1 (A) 98, 324
S v Graham 1975 (3) SA 569 (A) 53
S v Harris 1965 (2) SA 340 (A) 127, 131
S v Hartmann 1975 (3) SA 532 (C) 340, 346
S v Heyns 1978 (1) SA 399 (E) 355
S v Hibbert 1979 (4) SA 717 (D) 409
S v Iveson 1975 (3) SA 90 (0) 359
S v J 1975 (3) SA 343 (T) 134
S v Johnson 1969 (1) SA 201 (A) 129, 138, 352
S v Jubelius 1976 (2) SA 295 (T) 360
S v Kahita 1983 (4) SA 618 (C) 125
S v Kavin 1977 (2) SA 731 (W) 131
S v Kelder 1967 (2) SA 644 (T) 352
S v Khoza 1982 (3) SA 1019 (A) 322
S v Kosztur 1988 (3) SA 926 (A) 128, 134
S v King 1971 (2) PH H103 (T) 207
S v Kramer and Another 1987 (1) SA 96 (W) 96, 276
S v Kruger 1976 (3) SA 290 (0) 208, 209
S v Laubscher 1988 (1) SA 157 (A) 135
S v Leeuw 1980 (3) SA 815 (A) 125
S v Lehnberg 1975 (4) SA 553 (A) 133
S v Lombard and Another, Pretoria Magistrate's Court 1979 265
S v M 1985 (1) SA 1 (A) 134
S v Majola and Others 1980 (3) SA 705 (W) 125
S v Mahlinza 1976 (1) SA 408 (A) 123, 128, 132, 140
S v Mamyila 1913 TPD 464 126
S v Marengo 1990 WLD, unreported 341
S v Matjhesa 1981 (3) SA 854 (O) 126
S v McBride 1979 (4) SA 421 (O) 364
S v Melamu 1978 (1) SA 421 (O) 364
S v Mkwetshana 1965 (2) SA 493 (N) 294
S v Mnyanda 1976 (2) SA 751 (A) 126, 127, 128, 133, 134, 141
S v Mogale, AD June 1981, unreported 403
S v Mogorosi 1979 (2) SA 938 (A) 125
S v Motaung and Others 1990 (4) SA 463 (A) 322
S v Nagel 1978 (1) SA 363 (C) 442
S v Naidoo 1971 (3) SA 605 (N) 137
S v Ncube 1978 (1) SA 1178 (R) 137, 140
S v Nel 1987 TPD, unreported 280
S v Nell 1968 (2) SA 576 (A) 134
S v Ngang 1960 (3) SA 363 (A) 137
S v Oberbacher 1975 (3) SA 81 (SWA) 357
S v Patel 1973 (2) SA 208 (NC) 443
S v Pieterse 1982 (3) SA 678 (A) 134
S v Piccione 1967 (2) SA 334 (N) 129
S v Popo 1978 (1) SA 476 (A) 354
S v Posel 1977 (4) SA 476 (A) 441
S v Pretorius 1978 (4) SA 197 (T) 364
S v Progress Dental Laboratory (Pty) Ltd and Another 1965 (3) SA 192 (T) 69
S v Robinson and Others 1968 (1) SA 66 (A) 339
S v Sibanda 1978 (3) SA 217 (R) 442
S v Sibiya 1984 (1) SA 91 (A) 133
S v Skeyi 1981 (4) SA 191 (N) 125
S v Smith 1984 (1) SA 583 (A) 133, 140
S v Stellmacher 1983 (2) SA 381 (SWA) 127, 352
S v Steyn 1963 (1) SA 797 (W) 128
S v Strydom 1978 (4) SA 748 (E) 364
S v Terblanche 1981 (1) SA 791 (T) 365

S v Thomo and Others 1969 (1) SA 385 (A) 322
S v Tricket 1973 (3) SA 526 (T) 129, 130, 132, 139
S v Tsafendas, 1966 CPD, unreported 121
S v V 1984 (1) SA 44 (T) 132
S v Van As 1967 (4) SA 594 (A) 395
S v Van den Berg 1975 (3) SA 354 (0) 360
S v Van der Merwe 1977 (3) SA 747 (T) 286, 441
S v Van der Merwe 1982 (1) SA 313 (O) 365
S v Van Druten, regional court, Tvl 1971 207
S v Vis 1974 (2) SA 437 (0) 207
S v Webb (2) 1971 (2) SA 343 (T) 134
S v Wiid 1990 (1) SACR 561 (A) 135
S v Williams 1986 (4) SA 1188 (A) 151, 322
S v Yengeni and Others 1990 (1) SA 639 (C) 397
SA Geneeskundige en Tandheelkundige Raad v Van Rensburg 1982 (2) SA 745 (T) 375
SA Medical and Dental Council v McLoughlin 1948 (2) SA 355 (A) 10, 19
SA Wood Turning Mills (Pty) Ltd v Price Bros Ltd 1962 (4) SA 263 (T) 69
Sabi-Limpopo Authority v Triangle Ltd 1978 (4) SA 313 (RA) 51
Sasfin (Pty) Ltd v Beukes 1989 (1) SA 1 (A) 56, 57
Saunders, Re, 492 NYS 2d 510 (1985) 347
Savage and Pugh v Knox 1955 (3) SA 149 (C) 84
Seetal v Pravitha and Another NO 1983 (3) SA 827 (D) 11
Shaheen v Knight 11 D & C 2d 41 (1957) 175, 196
Shidiack v Union Government 1912 AD 642 .... 375, 393
Shiels v Minister of Health 1974 (3) SA 276 (RAD) 70
Sidaway v Bethlem Royal Hospital Governors and Others [1984] 1 All ER 1018 (CA), [1985] 1 All ER 635 (HL) 9
Sigaba v Minister of Defence and Police 1980 (3) SA 535 (Tk) 394
Simms v Simms 1981 (4) SA 186 (D) 236
Silva's Fishing Corporation (Pty) Ltd v Maweza 1957 (2) SA 256 (A) 23, 25
Smit v Van Niekerk 1976 (4) SA 293 (A) 104
Sorell v Smith [1925] AC 700 64
Soumbasis and Another v Administrator of the Orange Free State and Another 1989 OPD, unreported 262, 308
South African Mutual Aid Society v Cape Town Chamber of Commerce 1962 (1) SA 598 (A) 53
South African Optometric Association v Frames Distributors (Pty) Ltd t/a Frames Unlimited 1985 (3) SA 100 (O) 51
Stadsraad van Vanderbijlpark v Uys 1989 (3) SA 528 (A) 445
State of Kansas v Ronald Shaffer 574 P 2d 205 (Kan 1977) 322
St Augustine's Hospital (Pty) Ltd v Le Breton 1975 (2) SA 530 (D) 301
Stoffberg v Elliot 1923 CPD 148 31
Sutherland v White 1911 EDL 407 .... 70, 289

T

Thake and Another v Maurice [1986] 1 All ER 497 (CA) 41, 176
Times Media Ltd v South African Broadcasting Corporation 1990 (4) SA 604 (W) 63
Tothill v Gordon 1930 WLD 99 63
Triangle Ltd v Sabi-Limpopo Authority 1978 (1) SA 724 (R) 51
Troppi v Scarf 31 Mich App 240, 187 NW 2d 511 (1971) 196
Tshabalala v Minister of Health 1987 (1) SA 513 (T) 314
Tucker and Another v SA Medical and Dental Council and Others 1980 (2) SA 207 (T) 370
Tulloch v Marsh 1910 TPD 453 69

U

Udale v Bloomsbury Area Health Authority [1983] 2 All ER 522 (QB) 175

Union Government (Minister of Mines and Industries) v Union Steel Corporation (SA) Ltd 1928 AD 220 51
US v Freeman 257 F2d 606 (1966) 130

V

V v R 1979 (3) SA 1006 (T) 183, 193, 194
Van Aswegen v Lombard 1965 (3) SA 613 (A) 433
Van Wyk v Lewis 1924 AD 438 ..... 244, 270, 276, 284, 302
Verhoef v Meyer 1976 AD, unreported 35
Veriava and Others v President, SA Medical and Dental Council and Others 1985 (2) SA 293 (T) 372
Vincent v Long 1988 (3) SA 45 (C) 381, 382
Volschenk v President, SA Geneeskundige en Tandheelkundige Raad 1985 (3) SA 124 (A) 374

W

W v H 1965 (3) SA 740 (O) 169
W v W 1976 (2) SA 308 (W) 237
Wagner v International Railway Co 232 NY 176, 133 NE 437 (1921) 99
Weinberg v Mervis 1953 (3) SA 863 (C) 82
Weir-Mason v Minister of Justice 1958 (3) SA 299 (N) 395
White v Narick 292 SE 2d 54 (WVa 1982) 411
Whitehouse v Jordan and Another [1981] All ER (HL) 249
Wilsher v Essex AHA [1986] 3 All ER 801 (CA) 304

Y

Yorston v Pennell 153 A 2d 255 (1959) 255

Z

Zant v Prevatte 248 Ga 832, 286 SE 2d 715 411

PART I

Contract between doctor and patient, and issues of consent

1 Some practical legal problems pertaining to consent to medical treatment

General considerations

At the outset it must be stated that, independent from any contract between doctor and patient, the doctor owes the patient a duty of care: when performing an operation or treating a patient, the procedure should be executed with such professional skill as to avoid injuring the patient. Failure to do so amounts to a delict (civil wrong), entitling the patient to claim damages. Liability of a doctor to a patient is, therefore, not dependent on the existence of a contract between the parties or on the patient having given consent to undergo treatment.[1]

One sometimes hears the view that the legal relationship between doctor and patient is based upon a professional right of the doctor. But this is only half the truth. Ordinarily their legal relationship is a consensual one entered into on an *ad hoc* basis. As a general rule, the independently practising doctor is under no obligation to treat any person requesting his services. As a so-called "independent contractor", he is at liberty to select or refuse patients at will.[2] This freedom is qualified in two respects only: First, a doctor who arbitrarily and unreasonably refuses to attend to a seriously ill or injured person, may be held liable if the patient cannot manage to get another doctor and suffers harm.[3] Secondly, once a doctor has accepted a patient and has embarked upon a specific course of treatment, he may not unilaterally abandon the patient if abandonment might be harmful to the patient (unless the patient makes it impossible for the doctor to continue treating him).[4] He must either carry on with the treatment to its conclusion or, with the consent of the patient, transfer the latter to another doctor.

There being no legal duty in general upon a doctor to accept a patient, it is also true that the doctor has no general right to treat any person. Legally the doctor's right to operate or treat is based entirely on the patient's consent – apart from emergency cases[5] where a patient is brought to a doctor in an unconscious or semi-conscious state, and apart from instances where the patient is under a statutory duty to submit to e g vaccination, medical examination or treatment in his own interest or for the purposes of public health. Thus statutory provision is made for medical officers of health to require persons suspected, on reasonable grounds, of being carriers of communicable diseases (such as AIDS) to undergo a medical examination and to submit to treatment.[6] Immigration officers have comparable powers in respect of aliens on South African soil.[7] Likewise, in the case of mental patients institutionalised under the Mental Health Act[8] by virtue of a compulsory detention order, the consent of the

1 *Correira v Berwind* 1986 (4) SA 60 (Z).
2 This is the traditional point of departure – see S A Strauss & M J Strydom *Die Suid-Afrikaanse Geneeskundige Reg* (1967) 175 *et seq* – but in the light of subsequent developments in our law, this statement is now subject to the qualifications stated in the text.
3 See below 23.
4 See Strauss & Strydom *op cit* 112.
5 See below 89 *et seq*.
6 Government Notice R2438 of 30 October 1987 (*GG* 11014) promulgated under the Health Act 63 of 1977, sections 32, 33 and 34.
7 Government Notice R2439 of 30 October 1987 (*GG* 11014) promulgated under the Admission of Persons to the Republic Regulation Act 59 of 1972, section 54 (1) (*g*).
8 Act 18 of 1973.

patient is not required for "standard" psychiatric treatment.[9] The provisions of the Abuse of Dependence-producing Substances and Rehabilitation Centres Act,[10] pertaining to investigations with a view to eventual institutionalisation of suspected alcoholics or drug addicts, also clearly authorise medical and psychiatric examination – and rehabilitative treatment in the event of a detention order being made – without the consent of the patient.[11] In terms of the Prison Regulations[12] every prisoner must, as soon as possible after reception in a prison, be examined by the medical officer.

In those cases where the consent of the patient is required, an ailing person may stubbornly or stupidly refuse to submit to medical treatment which is absolutely essential in order to preserve his life or even to save his life. All that the doctor may do is to prevail upon the patient to undergo treatment. If the patient is an adult of sound mind and yet persists, there is nothing the doctor can do. In this respect our law recognises a qualified "right to die".[13] The doctor must respect the patient's wishes. There are numerous cases on record in which doctors were held legally liable for failure to do so. Subjecting a patient to medical treatment against his express will may legally be tantamount to assault, and in certain circumstances even to what lawyers term *crimen iniuria* (a serious impairment of the dignity of another). There are special considerations, however, regarding prisoners who resort to a hunger-strike; this subject is discussed elsewhere.[14]

In the normal course of events, obtaining a legal consent does not present practical difficulties. By calling out or consulting a doctor for his complaint, the patient tacitly consents to such treatment as in the doctor's opinion is medically indicated. But there are several legal "snags". A few simple common-sense rules may save the doctor unpleasant legal complications, especially where the patient is a potentially "difficult" person. The four golden rules are:

- Obtain consent from the person legally competent to give consent.
- Obtain an informed consent.
- Obtain a clear and unequivocal consent.
- Obtain a comprehensive consent.

I shall now deal in some detail with each of these rules.

Consent must be obtained from the person legally capable of giving it

(a) In the case of adults

Here this will normally be the patient himself. He must, of course, be in his sound and sober senses in order to give a valid consent. If he is intoxicated, strongly under the influence of drugs or premedication, unconscious or in a complete state of shock,

9 Section 9 (3) of the Act authorises a magistrate to issue an order "authorising the patient to be received, detained and *treated* at an institution ..." (my emphasis). It would appear that the magistrate's order is sufficient to authorise psychiatric treatment without consent of any other person. The same would seem to apply to urgent cases in terms of section 12. Regulation 6(5) under the Act (see Government Notice R565 of 27 March 1975) supports the view that no consent by another person is required. See also the definition of "patient" in section 1 of the Act. See also J L Snyman *Die Siviele Opneming van Geestesongesteldes: Regte en Regsbeskerming van die Betrokkene* (1981, LLD thesis, Univ of S Africa) 369-642. The position in English law appears to be similar. See *Freeman v Home Office* [1983] 3 All ER 589 (QB) at 597 *d – f*. As Snyman correctly points out, these considerations do not apply to drastic or irreversible procedures, such as the performance of a leucotomy. Mental Health regulation 7 contains detailed requirements to be complied with before a leucotomy may be performed, including the consent of the next of kin or the official *curator ad litem*. See also below 38.

10 Act 41 of 1971, see e g sections 30(4) (6), 34, 35 and 36.

11 See section 30(4) (*b*).

12 Prison regulation 93 contained in GN R2080 of 31 December 1965 as amended.

13 See below 29.

14 See below 409.

he is legally incapable of giving consent. Before a serious operation is undertaken, the patient must first be restored to a more or less normal state of mind. It goes without saying, however, that where it is an emergency, the operation may take place without consent.

In the case of medical treatment of, or operations on, mentally ill patients, the consent of one of the following persons must be sought in this order of precedence: the curator, appointed by the court to the person or property of the patient; the patient's spouse, parent, major child or brother or sister.[15] If a patient is in a mental institution, the superintendent of the institution may, in serious cases as defined in the Mental Health Act,[16] give consent where none of the relatives or other persons mentioned can be found. As mentioned above, consent for "standard" psychiatric treatment of mental patients received in institutions under a compulsory detention order, is not required.

As far as married couples are concerned, the general rule is that each spouse, either husband or wife, is fully entitled to consent independently to any medical treatment. What is more, a husband may not compel his wife to undergo treatment against her will.[17] A husband or wife does not require the consent of the other spouse for sterilisation or for the application of contraceptive measures.[18] As far as the termination of pregnancy is concerned, a woman likewise does not require the consent of her husband, except (possibly) where termination is desired on the ground that the child will be irreparably seriously handicapped.[19]

(b) Juvenile patients

Obtaining a legally "safe" consent where the patient is a minor, i e an unmarried person below the age of 21 years, is a matter of general concern to medical practitioners.

Where a parent or guardian is available to give consent, there are no problems. The doctor will, as a rule, be perfectly safe in relying upon the consent of either the father or the mother or, in case of orphans or adopted children, of the person who is the legal guardian of the child. In the event of a direct conflict between the father and the mother of the child, the doctor would be safe to give effect to the father's views, except where these are manifestly against the medical interests of the child. Where the parents request an operation which is medically indicated, but the minor refuses to submit to it, the doctor would, of course, be quite safe in relying upon parental consent. The minor is, after all, subject to parental power. There may, however, be special considerations concerning contraceptive measures, sterilisation and abortion; these are discussed below.[20]

It is to be noted that a parent may by common law delegate various incidents of his parental power to a person who acts *in loco parentis*[21] (on behalf of the parent) such as a teacher, a youth leader or a relative in whose care the child is temporarily. Where a parent has expressly or tacitly authorised such a person to consent to medical treatment on his behalf, that person may lawfully do so.[22]

A difficulty may present itself where the child is in need of an operation or medical treatment, but the parents on religious or other grounds refuse to consent. However, Section 39(1) of the Child Care Act[23] offers a solution. The subsection provides that where a doctor is of the opinion that it is necessary to perform the operation or to

15 Mental Health Act 18 of 1973, section 60A, and see discussion below 38.
16 *Ibid.* For a fuller discussion of the position of the superintendent, see below 38.
17 *Palmer v Palmer* 1955 (3) SA 56 (0), 59.
18 See below 169.
19 See below 211.
20 See below 169, 211.
21 P Q R Boberg *The Law of Persons and Family* (1977) 316, n 9.
22 On proxy consent, see also Mason & McCall Smith *Law and Medical Ethics* (1983) 115, and my note in 1985 *SAPM* No 3, 12.
23 Act 74 of 1983.

submit the child to treatment, and the parent or guardian refuses his consent, the doctor must report the matter to the Minister of Health and Welfare,[24] who may then consent in lieu of the parent or guardian. The same provision applies to the situation where the parent cannot be found, or is by reason of mental illness unable to consent, or is deceased. Significantly the Child Care Act declares the parent or guardian liable for the costs of the medical treatment involved.[25]

The Child Care Act also makes provision for consent to be given by the medical superintendent of a hospital in emergency cases, without consulting the parent or guardian of a child.[26] The superintendent must satisfy himself on two points: first, that the operation (or treatment) is necessary to preserve the life of the child, or to save him from serious and lasting physical injury or disability; secondly, that the treatment indicated is so urgent that it ought not to be deferred for the purpose of consulting the parent or guardian of the child. The parent or guardian is liable for the costs of the operation or treatment thus authorised. Cases of absolute emergency may occur where it would be altogether impracticable or dangerous to defer action in order to request the medical superintendent to give consent. An example would be cardiac arrest where cardiopulmonary resuscitation (CPR) must be resorted to without any delay. Without a doubt the doctor, nurse or paramedic can take immediate action without first seeking consent or official authorisation of any kind. In such a case the rescuer can rely on the common-law doctrine of necessity.[27]

The Child Care Act further vests heads of institutions (namely reform schools, schools of industries and children's homes) with powers of authorising medical operations on, or treatment of, children who are inmates.[28] The same criteria apply as in the case of medical superintendents. It is to be noted, however, that where the operation or treatment is not of such an urgent kind, the head of the institution must first consult the parent or guardian, or the Minister of Health and Welfare.[29] The Child Care Act specifically provides that the powers of the management of an institution do not include the power to consent to medical treatment or operations attended by serious danger to life.[30]

What has been said in the preceding paragraph is of equal application to persons in whose custody a child has formally been placed under the Child Care Act or the Criminal Procedure Act.[31]

An operation may be performed on a minor prisoner without the consent of his parents or guardians if the prison's medical officer is of the opinion that it is in the interest of the prisoner's health or life, and it is not possible or practicable to obtain the parent's or guardian's consent.[32]

The statutory provisions discussed do not detract from the rule that the Supreme Court is the upper guardian of minors and may be approached to authorise a medical procedure, particularly where there is a dispute between parent and child, or between parent and doctor. This may be necessary, for example, where a parent at-

24 This section of the Act is presently administered by the various "own affairs" departments. The Minister of Health Services and Welfare, Administration House of Assembly, has delegated her power under section 39(1) to the following officials: (a) the director of social services (or a deputy director or assistant director); (b) regional director of the Department (or a deputy regional director or the assistant director of a service office).

25 Section 39(3).

26 Section 39(2).

27 On emergency treatment generally, see below *et seq.*

28 Section 53(3).

29 *Ibid.* As was mentioned in note 24 the Act is currently administered by the "own affairs" departments (except for chapter 1 and section 60 thereof, which are administered by the Minister of National Health and Population Development).

30 Section 53(3).

31 Act 51 of 1977, section 290. And see Child Care Act, section 53(1).

32 Government Notice R2080 of 13/12/1965 (as amended from time to time), regulation 111(3)(6) in terms of the Prisons Act 8 of 1959.

tempts to compel an unwilling minor daughter to have her pregnancy terminated[33] or to apply contraceptive measures.[34]

Can a minor independently consent to an operation or treatment? This question becomes of paramount importance where it is not a case of dire emergency and where the minor is not a neglected child or the inmate of an institution. Take the example of a scholar, university student, or office employee in his late teens who consults a doctor or a dentist. His parents live in a distant town or are on an overseas tour. His ailment is not such that there is an imminent threat to his life, but there is a clear indication for medical treatment, which might involve surgery, without undue delay. The patient is obviously a responsible individual who can make an intelligent assessment of the situation after having been informed of the diagnosis. It would seem grossly unrealistic, if not unprofessional, for the doctor to defer treatment for several days or weeks until the parents can be reached and asked whether they consent to the treatment indicated. In these cases, section 39(4) of the Child Care Act makes it possible for a minor who is 18 years of age or older, to independently consent to medical treatment or to the performance of an operation upon himself.

It is submitted that a child of 18 years or older may refuse medical treatment, unless he is compelled by his parent or guardian (or any of the persons authorised in the Child Care Act to exercise *quasi* parental power) to submit to treatment, which is reasonably required.

Must the provisions of section 39(4) of the Child Care Act be interpreted in such a manner as to prohibit a minor below the age of 18 from consenting independently? This question is controversial. My submission is that the Legislature did not intend the subsection to embody such a prohibition and that an intellectually mature minor may consent independently to any medical procedure properly understood by him or her. (This becomes particularly relevant in regard to contraceptive treatment given to girls below the age of 18, a matter which is discussed in greater detail below.)[35] It goes without saying that the more drastic the envisaged medical treatment and the younger the minor, the wiser it would be for a doctor to obtain parental consent or substituted consent in terms of the statutory provisions required. (*It is to be noted that a Bill published in 1991 envisages lowering the statutory age of consent to medical* treatment – *as opposed to an operation – to 14 years.*)

It is submitted that in regard to medical or dental treatment for minor ailments – such as consultations for colds, flu, minor stomach conditions or filling of cavities – parental consent need not be *ad hoc* but can be given in general. The consent can even be conveyed by the minor to the doctor on behalf of his or her parent. Take the example of a parent whose 17-year-old child goes to school in a distant town. The parent tells the child to consult a doctor or dentist whenever he needs medical or dental care. In my opinion it is not necessary for the practitioner to obtain specific consent from the parent for administering to minor ailments. What is more, the minor, on behalf of the parent, in these cases concludes a contract with the doctor entitling the doctor to hold the parent liable for payment of his fees for attendances. Settlement of accounts rendered in respect of previous attendances will constitute proof of the existence of such a contract. Naturally, where the doctor has reason to doubt whether the parent has authorised the child to act as his "agent" in concluding a contract with the doctor, the latter should insist on express parental authorisation before attending to the child.

The legal position regarding parental consent to medical treatment of a minor has been somewhat compounded by section 3 of the Children's Status Act of 1987,[36] which

33 See below 211.
34 See below 171.
35 See below 171.
36 Act 82 of 1987.

laid down that where an unmarried minor has an illegitimate child, her (the mother's) guardian shall be vested with the guardianship of the illegitimate child (unless a competent court makes an order to the contrary). This provision would lead to the inevitable conclusion that the unmarried mother herself may not give consent to the medical treatment of her own child. This could lead to serious practical difficulties where the mother's guardian cannot be traced, which can only be resolved by resorting to the statutory provisions of the Child Care Act discussed above. The question has particularly arisen whether the unmarried mother is legally unable to consent to blood testing of the baby (with a view to its adoption) for communicable diseases such as syphilis or AIDS. A fact of life is that unmarried mothers frequently hide the birth of an unwanted child from their parents. I would submit that the taking of a blood sample for this purpose can hardly be regarded as a "medical operation" or "medical treatment" and that the unmarried mother can consent to the taking of a specimen of *her own* blood, provided she understands what the procedure entails and voluntarily agrees to it. This, however, would not solve the dilemma of obtaining consent for taking a blood specimen from *the infant;* consent is required for that and legally it is only the unmarried mother's parent or guardian who can give that consent.[37] (*It is to be noted that a Bill published early in 1991 envisages that the right will be given to a person who is 14 years or older to consent to medical treatment of his or her child. If the Bill were to become law, the problem which I have described would largely be remedied.*)

Obtaining an informed consent: must the doctor tell?

Knowledge and appreciation – these are two of the basic elements of consent. In our time, patient autonomy – the right to self-determination as opposed to the traditional attitude of medical paternalism – is increasingly emphasised by lawyers and doctors alike.[38] As a general rule there is no question of legal consent unless the party concerned is fully au fait with what he is consenting to. In the medical field this requirement is not without problems: there may be some doubts in the doctor's mind on the correctness of the diagnosis; there may be alternative methods of treatment for a particular case; many medical procedures involve a certain amount of risk; the effects of the treatment undertaken may not be altogether predictable; a successful outcome cannot always be guaranteed; there is the possibility of an idiosyncratic reaction in the patient to be reckoned with. The question is, considering these difficulties, to what extent the patient should be apprised of the diagnosis, the nature of the treatment proposed, and the inherent risks of such treatment.

Dealing with the diagnosis first: legally there would ordinarily be no duty upon the doctor to inform the patient fully of the diagnosis.[39] The diagnosis concerns the question *Why?* It may be based on a complexity of symptoms and it involves scientific assessment of the case on the basis of the doctor's knowledge, skill and experience. It may be impractical to attempt giving the patient, in layman's language, a general indication of the diagnosis. The full diagnosis must generally be given only where the patient stipulates this as a condition to giving his consent to an operation or treatment. It goes without saying that where medical intervention is necessary to make a diagnosis, for example exploratory surgery, the patient must give his consent for such.[40] Disclosure of the diagnosis is also necessary where the information is material to the patient's decision to undergo or refuse the treatment.[41] Finally, there

37 See my remarks in *SA Practice Management* 1989(3) 5.

38 See e g D Giesen "From paternalism to self-determination to shared decision making" in *Law and Medicine* (eds Bennett *et al*, 1988) 107 *et seq*, F F W van Oosten *The Doctrine of Informed Consent in Medical Law* (LLD thesis, Univ of S Africa, 1989) 144, 269, 414, 446.

39 Strauss & Strydom 198.

40 Van Oosten 443.

41 *Ibid* 433-4.

would be a therapeutic duty to inform the patient of the diagnosis where failure to do so may cause him physical or mental harm.[42]

Of considerable legal significance is the necessity to inform the patient on the question *What?* i e the treatment which will be given and the expected results thereof. The nature of the proposed medical procedures should be described in simple terms and in such detail that the patient may apply his mind intelligently. Where a final diagnosis is impossible in the absence of an exploratory operation, or where there is the possibility of extension of the operation agreed upon, the patient should be so informed. The patient should, in unequivocal terms, be informed of those results that are inevitable, e g where a colostomy will be undertaken, the patient must be told that he will be fitted with an artificial opening of the colon on the surface of the body; where a hysterectomy is undertaken, the woman should be told in simple terms that she will be unable to bear children. Civil cases have been brought against doctors who failed to give express information on such inevitable results of surgery. In informing the patient it is wise for the doctor to underestimate rather than to overestimate the former's intelligence.

In medico-legal literature, considerable attention has been paid to the question of the extent to which the patient should be informed of uncertain, potential hazards. It has been suggested that there is no duty upon the doctor to inform the patient of remotely possible consequences. It has also been suggested that the duty to inform of a particular risk should be based upon empirical, statistical knowledge of the percentage of cases in which it will ensue, e g where it exceeds 7% or 10%. The feasibility of the latter criterion is doubtful, however. A court is more likely to leave the duty to inform to sound medical judgment, and to limit it to such disclosures as a reasonable medical practitioner would make in the same or similar circumstances.[43]

In certain American jurisdictions, the "doctrine of informed consent" has been interpreted as requiring the doctor to furnish the patient with all the material details of the proposed treatment, including the inherent risks. The criterion by which the materiality is to be judged is not according to the medical standard, but what – in the judgment of the court – the doctor knows or should know would influence the patient in deciding whether or not to undergo the procedure. The standard is therefore not so much that of the reasonable doctor but rather the reasonable (or prudent) patient.[44]

The English courts have so far refused to follow the American standpoint and still uphold the view – apart from a minority judgment in the landmark *Sidaway* case[45] – that all that is required of a doctor in informing a patient, is to act in accordance with a practice accepted as proper by a body of reasonable, skilled medical practitioners.[46] The "doctrine of informed consent" accordingly forms no part of English law. In *Sidaway's* case a woman was severely disabled after damage to her spinal cord during a laminectomy and foraminectomy. Her claim for damages was based on the allegation that the surgeon had never mentioned the possibility of danger to the spinal cord. The court held, on expert evidence adduced at the trial, that it was in accordance with accepted medical practice in England not to give a specific warning of such risk because it was so remote. The judgment has drawn considerable critical comment in England.[47]

After a thorough critical analysis of South African, English and West German law, Van Oosten[48] comes to the conclusion that "patient consent as a requirement of lawful

42 *Ibid* 435.

43 See *Richter and Another v Estate Hamman* 1976 (3) SA 226 (C) 232H. Compare *Chatterton v Gerson and Another* [1981] QB 432. The two cases are discussed in detail below 267-8.

44 A landmark case was *Canterbury v Spence* (1972) 464 F2d 772.

45 *Sidaway v Bethlem Royal Hospital Governors and Others* [1984] 1 All ER 1018(CA), [1985] 1 All ER 635 (HL).

46 See e g *Chatterton's* case *supra*, *Hills v Potter* [1983] 3 All ER 716(QB), *Sidaway's* case *supra*.

47 Van Oosten 137. On *Sidaway's* case and informed consent in general, see also J M Burchell "Informed Consent' – Variations on a Familiar Theme" 5 *Med Law* 293 (1986).

48 *The Doctrine of Informed Consent in Medical Law* (*supra*, note 37) 447.

medical interventions embodies the fundamental principle of patient autonomy". He maintains that "to enable the patient to come to a rational decision he must be given a general idea of the nature, scope, administration, importance, consequences, risks, dangers, benefits, disadvantages and prognosis as well as of the alternatives to the proposed intervention". To achieve that, says Van Oosten,[49] "the doctor must proceed from the basis of the information which the prudent patient in the individual patient's position as a medical layman, would require to reach a rational decision".

In South African case law the duty of the doctor to inform the patient has not received much attention as yet. It has been held that where there are "serious risks" involved in shock therapy for neurosis, the patient must be apprised of these.[50] Another leading South African judgment (1957) deals with an action for damages brought as a result of disfigurement and the loss of extremities resulting from irradiation.[51] The court ruled as follows:

"[A] therapist not called upon to act in an emergency involving a matter of life and death, who decides to administer a dosage of such an order and to employ a particular technique for that purpose, which he knows beforehand will cause disfigurement, cosmetic changes and result in severe irradiation of the tissues to an extent that the possibility of necrosis and a risk of amputation of the limbs cannot be excluded, must explain the situation and the resultant dangers to the patient ... and should he act without having done so and without having secured the patient's consent, he does so at his own peril." (In this case there had been a diagnosis of Kaposi's haemangiosarcoma. This was first treated by superficial irradiation under the Chaoul unit and then followed by deep therapy under the Maximar unit. The patient was awarded R20 000 damages by the Supreme Court.)

But where the possibility of an adverse reaction following upon medical treatment is very remote – such as incontinence and a loss of power in the patient's foot following a phenol block administered for coccygeal pain – it is not necessary to forewarn the patient thereof.[52] The court indicated that in informing a patient, a doctor's conduct must in principle be judged by reference to the standard of the reasonable doctor: "In reaching a conclusion [as to the giving of information to the patient regarding the dangers attached to the operation] a Court should be guided by medical opinion as to what a reasonable doctor, having regard to all the circumstances of the particular case, should or should not do."

To the general rule that a patient in a non-emergency case must be informed of the nature of the treatment and the substantial risks it holds for him, there is one exception, it is submitted, viz that there is no such duty upon the doctor where the patient's state of mind is such that full awareness of the severity of his condition or of the drastic nature of the treatment indicated, would be therapeutically detrimental, e g where cancer is diagnosed. Although a South African court has never been called upon to decide this issue, it may safely be assumed that this common-sense view (which is widely supported in medico-legal literature and has become known as the doctrine of therapeutic privilege)[53] will be upheld by our courts in a suitable case.[54] In a 1948 judgment of our Appeal Court,[55] the Chief Justice, Mr Justice Watermeyer, observed *obiter:* "It may sometimes be advisable for a medical man to keep secret from his patient the form of treatment which he is giving him."

It may perhaps be argued that the requirement of an informed consent need not

49 *Ibid* 448.
50 *Rompel v Botha*, TPD 1953, unreported, referred to in *Esterhuizen's* case 1957 (3) SA 710 (T) at 719.
51 *Esterhuizen v Administrator, Transvaal* 1957 (3) SA 710 (T).
52 See *Richter's* case, *supra*, and compare *Chatterton's* case, *supra*.
53 For a fuller discussion of this doctrine, see below 15.
54 See also the judge's remarks in *Richter's* case *supra* at 232G quoted below 267, and see Strauss & Strydom *op cit* 210 *et seq*. See further Annas *The Rights of Hospital Patients* (1975) 67-68.
55 *South African Medical and Dental Council v McLoughlin* 1948 (2) SA 355 (A), 366.

be insisted upon in cancer cases or in cases where AIDS is diagnosed at all, because every cancer or AIDS diagnosis involves an "emergency" in the sense that the sufferer is faced with certain death sooner or later. It is extremely doubtful, however, whether a court would be prepared to uphold this contention. The emergency doctrine is generally restricted to situations where measures must be taken immediately to save the life of a patient at death's door, and who (on account of being unconscious or semi-conscious) is incapable of expressing his will. There is no reason to assume that courts will in general condone a deliberate omission on the part of a medical practitioner to obtain the consent of a patient who is perfectly capable of expressing his will, or where the consent of a parent or guardian may readily be obtained in the case of a minor. This clearly, was also the view of the court in the 1957 judgment referred to above.

Must a person who is ill and consults a doctor, who then takes a blood sample, be informed that the sample will be tested for HIV?

Legal opinion is divided. On the one hand there is the view – which appears to command the support of the majority of lawyers internationally who have commented on the issue – that there is no valid consent if a doctor carries out a test for HIV, having told the patient that a blood sample was being taken "for tests", because there is an implied representation on the part of the doctor that the tests to be carried out are merely routine.[56] This view rests on the assumption that a test for HIV would not, in the light of current medical opinion, be regarded as routine. On the other hand there is the view that because there is no risk inherent in the blood test itself, there is no need to inform the patient. A positive result may produce grave social consequences, but there is no risk of grave physical consequences in the blood test as such.[57]

In my opinion the latter view is the correct one. As I have mentioned above, according to our law, a doctor is required to inform the patient of the general nature of a medical procedure proposed, as well as any substantial risk attached to it. The procedure in question is the taking of blood and there is no substantial risk involved. It goes without saying that the patient must consent to the procedure as such, i e the taking of a blood sample. In the past doctors have routinely taken blood samples without informing the patient of all (or any) conditions for which it would be tested. Why should possible HIV-positivity be singled out as a condition of which the patient must be informed beforehand?

This opinion is perhaps of academic interest only to South African doctors in view of the guidelines on matters pertaining to the management of patients with HIV infection formulated by the SA Medical and Dental Council (SAMDC) in April 1989. The council made the following ruling, *inter alia:* "With regard to routine screening for HIV, the informed consent of the patient is required, prior to such a test being performed. In the case of a public health surveillance programme, where anonymity can be assured, and the patient cannot be identified, informed consent for the performance of this test is not required. (Consent for the taking of the specimen obviously remains imperative.)"[58] The SAMDC statement is indicative of what the attitude of reasonable doctors is.

It should be stated that, legally speaking, a patient would be entitled to be informed of the positive outcome of an HIV test even where he has not been informed beforehand that his blood would be tested for HIV.[59] It goes without saying that if he went to the doctor specifically with the request that his blood be tested for HIV, he would be entitled to be informed of the outcome of the test whatever it might be. The duty to inform would arise out of the contract entered into by the parties and would be

56 See e g M Sherrard, quoted by C Dyer in 296 *BMJ* 1791 (25/6/88).
57 See e g L Charles, also cited by Dyer.
58 See *SA Practice Management* 1989 (3) 21. Cf *Seetal's* case 1983 (3) SA 827 (D) 861.
59 See further below 16.

legally enforceable. Even if a person merely donates blood and tests positive, he should be informed forthwith.[60]

A discussion of informed consent would be incomplete without mentioning the modern view that "over-informing" of a patient may be tantamount to not informing the patient at all. A doctor would err by furnishing the patient with such a massive amount of technical, medical information about his condition that the latter is unable to digest it.[61] "Consent" given by the patient in these circumstances would therefore not be a real consent. It has been suggested that a doctor can be held delictually liable if over-informing the patient has the effect of causing him psychological or physical harm.[62]

Obtaining a clear, unequivocal and comprehensive consent

Although the legal relationship between doctor and patient is essentially a consensual one, the law does not require the parties to go about it as though they were drawing up a deed of sale. Ordinarily the contract between doctor and patient is established tacitly when the doctor, being consulted, commences to examine the patient. As far as the doctor's legal position is concerned, however, it is crucial for him to ensure that there should subsequently be no question about what exactly the patient has consented to. Often medical treatment entails a certain amount of risk. Upon the assumption that the patient has been adequately apprised of the risks, the next step is to ensure that the patient has left no doubt that he is prepared to undergo the suggested treatment notwithstanding the risk.

Where the treatment is very drastic or unusual, it may be to the advantage of the doctor to take a written and signed consent in which the nature of the treatment is described in detail. This is very seldom done in actual practice, but can be of the utmost importance in safeguarding the doctor against unwarranted legal proceedings. Thus I have personally advised doctors undertaking conversive surgery in cases of transsexualism to obtain a full and clearly formulated written consent from the patient in which the proposed procedures (e g castration and amputation of the penis), as well as the expected and potential consequences thereof, including psychiatric sequelae, are fully outlined.

I have said that the consent should be unequivocal. This brings me to the problem of the patient who, on the basis of his own medical "wisdom", or perhaps on account of his personal anxieties, stipulates definite conditions for the treatment: he refuses to take medicines prescribed by the doctor; he refuses to submit to some of the examinations necessary to make a proper diagnosis; he objects to a specific type of anaesthetic; he stipulates that surgery proposed by a doctor must not result in impotence of infertility; he may on religious grounds prohibit a necessary incidental procedure such as a blood transfusion. Where the conditions imposed by the patient are such that the doctor is precluded from practising "good medicine", there is legally only one safe thing for him to do, viz to refuse the case. However, in proper circumstances the doctor may resort to alternative medical procedures which, although not the best, are nevertheless scientifically approved. The important thing is for the doctor to realise that he may not simply ignore the conditions imposed by the patient. If he does so, he may not be dealing with a consenting party any longer, thus exposing himself to a civil action for damages.

In general the law does not require consent to treatment or an operation to be in writing. It goes without saying, though, that the taking of a written consent may be advisable to avoid arguments at a later stage over what exactly the patient has con-

60 Cf CW van Wyk *Aspekte van Regsproblematiek rakende VIGS* (LLD thesis, Univ of S Africa,1991).

61 See E Deutsch *Arztrecht und Arzneimittelrecht* (1983) 53.

62 *Ibid,* and see H-H Jescheck *Lehrbuch des Strafrechts* (4th ed, 1988) 255, who cites the case of a doctor who informed a patient who suspected cancer, to such an extent that she became mentally ill.

sented to, should a dispute arise. A proper written consent, signed by the patient (or his or her parent, guardian, etc) and signed by a witness attesting to the authenticity of the patient's signature, and dated, may therefore be of considerable evidential importance. Only in exceptional cases, however, does the law *require* a consent to be in writing. Examples: consent to a leucotomy under the Mental Health Act;[63] consent to sterilisation under the Abortion and Sterilisation Act;[64] consent to medical treatment of, or an operation performed on, a mental patient under the Mental Health Act.[65]

In South African hospitals the usual procedure with admission of patients is for the clerical staff to make an entry on the admission form (which also serves as a consent form) of the type of treatment or operation to be undertaken. This is almost always done on the basis of the information supplied by the patient who fills in this part of the form himself. The information supplied by the patient is sometimes incomplete or even incorrect.[66] Doctors are not always aware of the legal risks inherent in this practice. Hospital staff should be trained and cautioned to question the patient adequately in order to record the correct information. A simple precaution for the doctor undertaking the treatment or surgery would be to make a prior check on the accuracy of the information supplied by the patient on the admission form. In actual practice this is apparently done very seldom – an omission which may have unfortunate legal consequences for the doctor.

Getting the patient to sign a *pro forma* expressing consent to undergo an operation "the effect and nature of which have been explained to me", should be a valuable reminder to everyone of the need for explanation and consent. But it would be no defence to an action based upon assault, if no explanation had in fact been given. The consent would have been expressed in form only, not in reality.[67]

The consent given by a patient on the admission form should be reasonably specific and comprehensive. A consent to submit to any unspecified operation or to any treatment within the doctor's discretion would undoubtedly be ruled invalid by our courts on account of vagueness. If a dispute were to arise in such a case, a court would probably rely exclusively on the prior verbal negotiations between doctor and patient. This may mean a protracted trial involving judicial rulings on credibility.

In the hospital form the operation or treatment should be mentioned by name. The medical practitioners involved, e g the surgeon and anaesthetist, should likewise be mentioned by name. Any limitations insisted upon by the patient should be stated expressly and the form should contain a general clause by which the patient agrees to incidental procedures, such as premedication, anaesthesia, exploratory surgery and alternative surgical procedures. I have seen hospital admission forms in South Africa which are deficient in regard to particularity. It goes without saying that a check should be kept on any deletions the patient makes on the admission form.

63 See below 37.
64 See below 215.
65 See below 38.
66 Sometimes the patient is embarrassed by the nature of the operation proposed and deliberately gives a false description of the operation he will undergo. See the cases quoted by M DeMere in 1975 *Legal Medicine Annual* 293, at 295-6.
67 *Chatterton v Gerson* [1981] Q B 432 at 443 D-E.

2 Truth-telling in medicine: a legal perspective

Introduction

Death has always been an event of crucial significance in religion, and in the practical application of the law it is an important juristic fact. Yet in Western society, death as such, and in particular dying as the final act or process in the human existence, has virtually been a taboo until very recently.

But in the last decade or so there has been an unprecedented interest in the moral, ethical and legal issues surrounding death and the dying human. The current debate was sparked by advances in medical technology, and special impetus was given by the first human heart transplants in the late sixties. Organ transplantation highlighted the extremely difficult decisions doctors must make on resuscitation of moribund persons and artificial maintenance of life. The debate goes far beyond the narrow – and ancient – issue of euthanasia.[1]

A number of major books on death and its implications have been published in recent years. To mention a few only: In *Death, Dying and the Biological Revolution* (1976), Robert M Veatch, a specialist on medical ethics, explores issues such as the following: Is death moral? How is death defined? Dying morally. The patient's right and obligation to have the truth. *The Dying Human* (1979)[2] contains the proceedings of an international symposium on the subject, held in Israel in 1978. It covers a wide range of topics, from a philosophical consideration of death and suicide to the legal rights of the dying. In *Medico-Legal Implications of Death and Dying* (1981), David W Meyers embarked upon a detailed discussion, on the basis essentially of American positive law, of the medical and legal implications involved in death and/or care of the dying and terminal patient. His book bears ample testimony to the wide practical reach of a modern legal system in relation to death and dying.

Truth-telling: Biblical references

As De Vries[3] has pointed out, there is conflicting behaviour in the Old Testament with respect to the telling or withholding of truth when confronted with a terminal patient. Indeed, in one and the same Biblical book, the Second Book of Kings, there are two different patterns of behaviour.

In 2 Kings 8:7-11 it is related that the prophet Elisha came to Damascus at a time when Ben-Hadad, king of Aram, was ill. When the king was told of the prophet's arrival, he sent Hazael to him to enquire of the Lord through him whether he would recover from his illness. The prophet told Hazael: "Go and tell him that he will recover, but the Lord has revealed to me in fact he will die." Here, the truth was withheld.

In 2 Kings 20:1-6, again, the story is related of Hezekiah's serious illness and his

1 The euthanasia debate continues unabatedly. In this country a symposium was held in 1978. Its proceedings were published in a book bearing the title *Euthanasia* (1978, eds G C Oosthuizen, H A Shapiro and S A Strauss). In 1980 Professor Christian N Barnard published his controversial book *Good Life Good Death* (subtitled *A Doctor's Case for Euthanasia and Suicide*).

2 Eds André de Vries and Amnon Carmi.

3 *The Dying Human*, viii-ix.

sorrow when the prophet Isaiah told him that it was the word of the Lord that he was a dying man and would not recover. But before the prophet left the citadel, the word of the Lord came to him to go back to Hezekiah and to tell him that his prayer had been heard and that he would be healed, with the prospect of another fifteen years of life. Here the truth was told, "with a remarkable change of truth content", in the words of De Vries.

The duty to inform

The question whether there is a duty on a doctor who has diagnosed a serious illness in a patient which will in all likelihood result in the latter's death, to inform him of the seriousness of his condition, is a much discussed one. There are many sides to this question.

Should the patient be told at all? If so, how much should he be told? Should the patient be spared most of the details, the doctor rather taking the next of kin in his confidence and informing them fully? Should the patient only be informed if he insists upon being told? What is the doctor's position where the patient insists that he should not be told?

Can the patient contractually bind the doctor to tell him the truth? Is it improper for the doctor to refuse to comply with such an undertaking – or to be more specific, can the doctor be sued for breach of contract if he fails to honour such an undertaking? Is there any basis for a delictual claim for damages in this situation?

What about the interests of others who may be affected by the patient's sickness? Can they be informed by the doctor without the patient knowing or consenting? Apart from a right to inform others who have a material interest in the information, can it be said that in special circumstances there may even be a duty on the part of the doctor to inform them?

In endeavouring to answer these questions I am confining myself strictly to the legal issues relating to truth-telling, in the knowledge that from a practical point of view the problem is not primarily legal, but rather one of professional ethics. Yet, as the emergence of the doctrine of "therapeutic privilege" in American law has demonstrated, there is a definite legal dimension to the subject of truth-telling in medicine.

As a point of departure it may be stated that the doctor's legal duty of disclosure to the patient is a relative one only. On the basis of case law as it has evolved in a number of countries, including South Africa, it can be said that there is no absolute duty on the doctor to inform the patient on all aspects of his examination, the findings made in the course of the examination, the doctor's diagnosis, the treatment given or envisaged and the general prognosis.

Disclosing diagnosis

As far as the diagnosis is concerned, it is submitted that in the absence of an express or implied agreement to the effect that the patient must be informed of it, there is in general no duty on the doctor to do so.

Lawyers who operate mainly in the hard world of economics and commerce, and who seek to establish cold facts to which the law must apply, may be inclined to overlook the problems confronting a doctor in making a diagnosis.

I often heard Hillel Shapiro warning students that "the language of the body is limited". And as William F Finn[4] has remarked, there is an inherent fallibility in all biological events: The physician cannot be sure; a pain in the chest may be indigestion, or a coronary heart attack, or a cancer of the oesophagus or a nervous spasm.

4 In his thought-provoking paper, "Do you really want to know that you are dying and will your doctor tell you?" in *The Dying Human*, 171 and 172.

All the physician can say initially is: "I cannot be sure." The physician, by nature a conservative, does not want to make a diagnosis unless he is sure. He avoids prophecy, prognostication and predictions.[5] Moreover, the concept of a "differential diagnosis" is well known to every physician.

Rosoff[6] is undoubtedly right when he cautions doctors not to represent the diagnosis as a precise and sure identification of the problem. "Where such is not the case," he says, "there is danger to the physician in not making this clear, since knowledge of what is wrong is a crucial factor in the patient's decision to accept the proposed treatment."

On the other hand, once the doctor has established the diagnosis with reasonable certainty, there would in my opinion be nothing to prevent him from informing the patient thereof. The doctor clearly has a wide discretion. He may judge it in the manifest interest of the patient to know the seriousness of his condition to enable him to bring his earthly affairs in order and to prepare to meet his Maker – and no court of law, I think, would find fault with the doctor being motivated by these considerations. Moreover, as Veatch[7] has forcefully argued, to many patients the anxiety of not knowing their diagnosis accurately must be at least as great as that of knowing the terrible truth.

If there is a firm agreement that the doctor should tell the patient of the diagnosis, the latter may probably, by way of an action for specific performance, compel the doctor to disclose. I am not aware, though, of any case of this kind that has ever come before a South African court. In any event, it should be mentioned that our courts have traditionally been reluctant to order specific performance in cases involving obligations of a personal nature and prefer to allow the plaintiff to sue for damages in the alternative.[8] But it may be impossible for a patient to show that he has suffered any damage as a result of the breach of a contractual duty by the doctor to inform him.

As Deutsch[9] has indicated, a firm undertaking on the part of the doctor to disclose the diagnosis to the patient will usually be implied where the patient went to him with the express desire of seeking a second opinion.

Special considerations relating to AIDS

Special considerations apply to a condition such as AIDS because it is an extremely serious communicable disease and, as yet, incurable. Moreover, unlike a disease such as Hepatitis B, it cannot be prevented by way of immunisation. These factors also bring the interests of persons other than the patient to the fore.

There can be no question that the doctor is legally bound to inform a patient if the latter has been positively tested and diagnosed as an HIV carrier. First, the patient himself has a vital interest in being informed of the seriousness of his condition. Secondly, and of no less importance, there are the interests of the patient's sexual partner or partners and of medical personnel who will be attending to him in taking steps to avoid being infected. The duty to inform arises also where the patient has not consulted the doctor with a view to being diagnosed, but where routine testing is done, for instance where a blood donor's blood is tested.

In my opinion, the doctor would be entitled to inform the patient of a positive HIV test even if the latter has expressed the wish – as has already occurred – not to be

5 *Ibid.*
6 Arnold J Rosoff *Informed Consent* (1981) 42.
7 *Death, Dying and the Biological Revolution*, 212.
8 But see the decision in *National Union of Textile Workers and Others v Stag Packing (Pty) Ltd and Another* 1982 (4) SA 151 (T) which involved an application for reinstatement of servants who had allegedly been dismissed wrongfully.
9 Erwin Deutsch *Arztrecht und Arzneimittelrecht* (1983) 43.

told if the test is positive. When a patient has contracted such a serious disease, the public interest – i e the interest of other members of society who might be infected by the patient – must certainly outweigh the patient's desire not to receive bad news.

The public interest is also of decisive importance in answering the question whether the doctor who has made the diagnosis, may inform other persons who may possibly be harmed by the patient's condition. In my view there can be no doubt that a doctor would be legally entitled to inform the known sexual partner(s) of an infected person and other medical and nursing personnel who will attend to him, even if the patient does not consent to their being informed.

Is there a legal *duty* on the doctor to do so? According to our law there is a qualified duty on a person to come to the rescue of another.[10] It is unlikely though that in the present context the duty would be interpreted by a court of law as requiring a doctor to take active steps to directly inform the sexual partner(s) of the patient. The decision of this issue will depend on what is regarded as reasonable in all the circumstances of the case. It is submitted that ordinarily the doctor who has made the AIDS diagnosis will be regarded as having acquitted himself of his duty to society once he has informed the patient of the diagnosis and has warned him of the potentially dire consequences for his or her sexual partners and potential offspring unless "safe sex" is practised. A doctor can hardly be expected to cast himself in the role of a private investigator/information officer seeking out and warning the sexual partners of the patient. If, however, it were to come to the knowledge of a doctor who has properly counselled a patient, that the latter refuses to practise "safe sex", and the identity of a regular sexual partner – such as the patient's husband or wife – is known to the doctor, it may conceivably be regarded as reasonable for the doctor to act.

The SA Medical and Dental Council in 1989 formulated the following important guidelines regarding information being given to parties other than the patient:

"Confidentiality

"The health care professions are fully aware of the general rules governing confidentiality.

"Council is confident that if doctors fully discuss with patients the need for other health care professionals to know of their condition, in order to offer them optimal treatment and also to take precautions when dealing with them, the reasonable person of sound mind, will not withhold his consent regarding divulgence to other health care workers.

"If having considered the matter carefully in the light of such counselling, the patient still refuses to have other health care workers informed, the patient should be told that the doctor is duty bound to divulge this information to the other health care workers concerned with the patient. All persons receiving such information must of course consider themselves under the same general obligation of confidentiality as the doctor principally responsible for the patient's care.

"If it were found that an act or omission on the part of a medical practitioner or dentist had lead to the unnecessary exposure to HIV infection of another health care worker, the Council would see this in a very serious light and would consider disciplinary action against the practitioner concerned.

"Informing the patient's spouse or other sexual partners:

"Questions of conflicting obligations also arise when a doctor is faced with the decision whether the fact that a patient is HIV positive or suffering from AIDS should be disclosed to a third party, other than another health care professional, without the consent of the patient. The Council has reached the view that there are grounds for

10 See below 24. Compare J Taitz 78 *S Afr Med J* 29 (1990).

such a disclosure only where there is a serious and identifiable risk to a specific individual who, if not so informed, would be exposed to infection. Therefore, when a person is found to be infected in this way, the doctor must discuss with the patient the question of informing a spouse or other sexual partner. The Council believes that most such patients will agree to disclosure in these circumstances, but where such consent is withheld, the doctor shall consider it a duty to seek to ensure that any sexual partner is informed in order to safeguard such a person from a possibly fatal infection."

The need for adequate counselling of a patient prior to the performance of an HIV test and after the test has turned out to be positive, has been stressed by a number of ethicists and other commentators. Legally speaking, it is particularly important to alert the patient to the risks his condition brings about for others, *after* a positive test.

Medical treatment

It is in relation to the treatment envisaged by the doctor – i e the *what* as opposed to the *why* – that the duty to inform has been emphasised in medico-legal literature and the judgments of courts. In principle medical intervention is lawful only if the patient has consented to it, and consent is legally possible only if it is based on adequate knowledge and appreciation, on the part of the patient, of the nature of the procedure and the substantial risks it involves.[11] It goes without saying that this principle does not only apply to medical treatment in the strict sense of the word, i e therapeutic procedures, but also to medical examinations accompanied by a risk to the patient's health or life, such as exploratory surgery, myelography, angiography and pyelography, to mention only a few of many diagnostic techniques.

Therapeutic privilege

Jurists' rigid insistence in the past upon informed consent has in recent years made room for a more realistic approach. Today it is realised that to insist that the patient be fully informed at all times, is not always in his interest. Full knowledge of what lies medically in store for him may cause despondency and a serious depression, and may have the effect of discouraging the patient from submitting to surgery or other treatment which may cure him, or at the very least, relieve his suffering. An Israeli judge, J Türkel,[12] bluntly says that "in the majority of cases, it is our duty to lie to the terminal cancer patient ... In principle I cannot see any difference between giving an analgesic drug, or other drugs to such a patient and the giving of a drug named illusion".[13]

In the USA the courts have recognised that there are situations where a full disclosure to the patient is not medically sound, and thus should not be legally required. The term "therapeutic privilege" was attached to this situation, which has featured largely as a defence in cases where an action for damages was brought against doctors on the basis of a lack of informed consent.[14]

The parameters of the doctrine of therapeutic privilege are as yet undefined in American law.[15] In fact, so far it is perhaps no more than "a theme running through

11 See e g *Esterhuizen v Administrator, Transvaal* 1957 (3) SA 710 (T); *Richter and Another v Estate Hamman* 1976 (3) SA 266 (C).

12 "Remarks on Telling the Truth or Lying" 4 *Med Law* 91 (1985).

13 In 1984 *S Afr Med J* 157 it is reported that 98% of doctors would reveal a diagnosis of cancer to the patient; 20 years ago only 12% would do so.

14 On therapeutic privilege in general see Rosoff *op cit* 54-56; Meyers *op cit* 83. Two leading cases quoted by these authors are *Canterbury v Spencer* (1972) 150 App DC 263, 464 F2d 772 and *Cobbs v Grant* (1972) 8 Cal 3d 229, 104 Cal Rptr 505, 502 P2d 1.

15 Meyers *op cit* 83.

minority decisions",[16] and there is some indication that American juries may not be so quick to accept it as a defence.[17] Rosoff[18] points out that a doctor would be well advised not to rely on this defence unless it is clearly documented that the patient's sensitivity was well above the norm. He advises that to document a patient's high susceptibility to anxiety, confirmation of the doctor's observation by another doctor and/or relative or close friend of the patient should be sought and entered on the patient's treatment record.

In German law, therapeutic privilege has also been recognised within narrow limitations, although not by that name. Laufs[19] refers to it as "Kontraindikationen der Aufklärungspflicht" (contra-indications to the duty to inform). The German courts have clearly moved away from the older and very rigid standpoint on the doctor's duty to disclose, although it cannot be said that the juristic view has become fully reconciled with the medical view.[20]

At a symposium on medical law and ethics held in Heidelberg in 1981, I heard prominent jurists and doctors emphasising that there may in a given situation even be a *duty* not to inform the patient.

So far therapeutic privilege has received virtually no attention in the judgments of our courts, except for a single *obiter dictum* in a disciplinary case *(South African Medical and Dental Council v McLoughlin)*[21] in which the then Chief Justice, Mr Justice Watermeyer, observed that "it may sometimes be advisable for a medical man to keep secret from his patient the form of treatment which he is giving him".

I would submit that if a case were to come before a South African court in which it appears that it would undoubtedly have been detrimental to the patient had he been informed in precise terms of the nature of the treatment, and the doctor – after serious consideration of all the implications – deliberately decided not to tell the patient, the doctor should in the absence of any ill consequence to the patient not be held liable for assault. In such a case the doctrine of necessity ought to be applied, in any event where the patient has not expressly refused medical treatment.[22] In a careful analysis of therapeutic privilege, Deutsch[23] has drawn attention to the fact that non-disclosure to the patient may be justified not only in the interest of the patient himself, but also where a substantial danger may be created for third parties if the doctor were to inform the patient.

Patient refuses treatment

What is the position if the patient, after being told that he is dying or that his condition is very serious, refuses further drugs or treatment? Can the doctor in any way be held legally liable if the patient's death is accelerated or he suffers some other ill effect in consequence of his refusal?

I can think of no principle of our law whereby a doctor who in good faith tells a patient what his condition is, can be held liable for a refusal on the part of the patient to undergo further treatment.

Our law is still fundamentally individualistic and to a large extent the individual is the master of his own fate. It is part of the reality of life that we all suffer the conse-

16 Burton A Johnson "An Overview of Informed Consent" in A Everette James *Legal Medicine with Special Reference to Diagnostic Imaging* (1980) 281 and 290.
17 Rosoff *op cit* 54.
18 *Op cit* 55.
19 Adolf Laufs *Arztrecht* (2nd ed, 1978) par 81.
20 *Ibid* par 66, 67. On German law see also F F W van Oosten *The Doctrine of Informed Consent in Medical Law* (LLD thesis, Univ of SA, 1989) 278, 386.
21 1948 (2) SA 355 (A) at 366. Compare the remarks made by the judge in *Richter and Another v Estate Hamman* 1976 (3) SA 226 (C) at 232G, quoted below 267.
22 Compare Van Oosten 423-8.
23 *Op cit* 51-52.

quences of our own personalities. The law protects the individual only against *wrongful* infringements upon his private sphere. There is nothing unlawful in the action of a doctor who, in attending to a patient at the latter's request, tells him exactly what is wrong with him – even if the doctor could be accused of a lack of professional tact or a bad bedside manner.

In modern Western society the right to patient autonomy, as opposed to medical paternalism of an earlier era, characterises the doctor-patient relationship.[24]

Emotional shock

What has been said in the preceding section will likewise apply to a patient who suffers a severe emotional shock or depression in consequence of being told the truth. Our law recognises the principle that a person is entitled to claim damages where he was wrongfully caused nervous shock or psychiatric injury.[25]

In order to recover damages, the defendant must prove that the emotional shock was not merely insignificant and of short duration. Moreover, he must convince the court that it was attributable to the fault of the perpetrator. This means that at the very least there must have been negligence, which in practical terms means that the consequences of the act would have been foreseen by the notional reasonable person who would have found himself in the position of the wrongdoer.

It goes without saying that where a doctor is consulted by a patient it is ordinarily on the understanding that the patient wants to find out what is wrong with him, and if possible to be cured. There is no question either of wrongfulness or of fault on the part of the doctor if he does exactly what is required of him, namely to inform the patient. Obviously some doctors have a better style than others in communicating with the patient, but if the patient cannot "take it", that seems to be his problem and not the doctor's.

Liability for nervous shock is perhaps conceivable only where the patient expressly forbade the doctor from telling him if he found a serious condition, such as cancer, and the doctor disregarded this request. It is difficult to be categorical on this, for the simple reason that it may be in the best interest of the patient to inform him, at least by implication, of the diagnosis despite his refusal to be informed. Let us take the example of a female patient who has consulted a doctor about a lump in her breast. After a thorough examination, including a biopsy and pathological tests, it is established that the growth is malignant. The woman's life can be saved by means of a mastectomy. Even if the doctor were to avoid using the words "cancer" or "malignancy", the patient would undoubtedly know what was wrong with her if the doctor were to suggest a mastectomy. If the doctor were to disregard the woman's prohibition against her being informed of her condition, it may be argued that he would be able to rely on the defence of necessity.[26]

As stated above,[27] a doctor would in my view be entitled to disregard the wish of

24 S R Benatar "Introduction to Medical Ethics" in *Ethical and Moral Issues in Contemporary Medical Practice* (ed S R Benatar, 1985) 5 *et seq*. Compare L Moutsopoulos "Truth-Telling to Patients" 3 *Med Law* 237 (1984).

25 *Bester v Commercial Union Versekeringsmaatskappy van SA Bpk* 1973 (1) SA 769(A); *Muzik v Canzone del Mare* 1980 (3) SA 470 (C). Compare J C van der Walt "Skoktoediening: 'Wie sal die aftreksom maak?'" in *Huldigingsbundel vir W A Joubert* (1988) 247 *et seq*; J Neethling, J M Potgieter and P J Visser *Law of Delict* (1990) 243-6.

26 With the sources at my disposal I could find nothing in American case law – where there is an abundance of material on medical malpractice liability – indicating that a court may be prepared to hold a doctor liable in such a situation. (In *Cobbs v Grant supra* it was held *inter alia* that the doctor's *duty* to disclose information material to the patient's decision to undergo treatment falls away where the patient requests that he not be informed of the risks connected with the treatment. But the decision does not seem to go beyond that. See Meyers *op cit* 82.) Bernard J Ficarra "Medical Negligence based on Bad Faith, Breach of Contract, or Mental Anguish" in 1980 *Legal Medicine Annual* 187, cites no case in which liability in this situation was considered.

27 Page 16.

a patient not to be told if his AIDS test turns out to be positive. Medical ethicists stress the importance of proper counselling of a patient who has been diagnosed HIV positive but this – in my opinion – is an ethical rather than a legal duty.

Negligent diagnosis

Naturally the situation will be different where the doctor has negligently made a wrong diagnosis and has come to the conclusion that the patient is suffering from a serious condition. Cousins[28] relates a case of a mistaken diagnosis of melanoma, made in one of the most prestigious cancer centres in the USA. The recommended surgery was only two days away when the patient's brother, an oncologist, performed a separate biopsy specimen evaluation that showed the growth to be benign. Apparently the records of two patients had been erroneously switched. Cousins does not say whether the mistake was caused by negligence.

An erroneous diagnosis is of course possible even where the highest degree of care has been observed in the examination of the patient. Assuming, however, that there was demonstrable negligence in the making of the diagnosis or, at the very least, in conveying the incorrect information to the patient, there is the possibility of legal liability. I have already referred to the action for culpable causation of nervous shock which has been given recognition in our law.[29] This possibility assumes special significance if an extremely serious condition such as HIV infection is negligently diagnosed.

Quite apart from that, our Appellate Division has upheld the principle that a person who makes a negligent misstatement to another, resulting in patrimonial damage – e g financial or economic loss – to the other, may be held liable. This applies even if the statement was not made in a contractual relationship.[30] It is clear that these forms of delictual liability may have wide ramifications in the medical field, in cases where there has been a lack of due care in imparting important information to patients. A case in point would be where a patient is subjected to a drastic and expensive operation which he was advised to undergo, and which was not necessary at all because of a wrong diagnosis, negligently made.

Quite apart from liability for giving the patient wrong information, there is the possibility of the doctor being held liable if the patient was not treated at all or was not treated correctly because of negligence involved in the making or conveying of a diagnosis. Thus in *Blyth v Van den Heever*[31] a doctor was held liable for damages for having failed to diagnose an impending ischemia in a patient's fractured arm upon which he had performed an operation. There have also been cases in which a doctor was held liable for failure to refer a patient to a specialist, in consequence of a negligent diagnosis.

Informing next of kin

One last point: I have already observed that the doctor ordinarily has a wide discretion as to whether he will inform the patient of the diagnosis, and if so, how much he will tell him. Is the doctor entitled to decide not to tell anything to the patient himself, but rather to take the latter's wife or children into his confidence?

Looking at it from a strictly legal or ethical perspective, one may perhaps assume the standpoint that where the patient is still mentally competent, his illness is his busi-

28 Norman Cousins "A Layman Looks at Truth Telling in Medicine" 244 (1980) *JAMA* 1929.

29 As to American law, see the cases cited by Ficarra *op cit* 198-199.

30 *Administrateur, Natal v Trust Bank van Afrika Beperk* 1979 (3) SA 824 (A); compare *E G Electric Co (Pty) Ltd v Franklin* 1979 (2) SA 702 (E) and *Pilkington Brothers (SA) Ltd v Lillicrap, Wassenaar and Partners* 1983 (2) SA 157 (W).

31 1980 (1) SA 191 (A). The case is discussed in detail below 257.

ness alone and not that of the next of kin.[32] After all, the duty to maintain professional secrecy is upheld both by the law and by an explicit ethical rule.[33]

But in regard to terminally ill patients, my submission is that this view is far too rigid and does not sufficiently acknowledge the need for ordinary human compassion and the realities of family life. I can see nothing wrong with the doctor deciding there would be no point in telling the patient he is at death's door, and that he should rather inform the immediate relatives whose duty it will be to give the patient loving care in the final days of his life, so that they can prepare themselves for it.[34] It is inconceivable to me that any professional body or a court of law would be so harsh as to condemn a doctor in these circumstances for a breach of professional secrecy.

In the case of a serious communicable disease, such as AIDS, there may be an ethical and legal duty to inform the patient's husband or wife.[35]

Adapted from an article published in 1983 De Rebus *66.*

32 In *Nishi v Hartwell* 52 Hawaii 188, 473 P2d 116(1970), quoted by Rosoff *op cit* 95, it was held *inter alia* that a physician's duty of disclosure runs only to the patient and not to any member of his family.

33 Veatch *op cit* 240 *et seq* argues strongly that where the patient is still mentally competent, doctors should respect the patient's right to privacy and should not readily disclose to the next of kin.

34 As J Stolinova of Czechoslovakia has pointed out in his paper entitled "Ärztliche Aufklärung der Familie aus Juristischer Sicht: Pflicht, Zulässigkeit, Grenzen" delivered at the Fifth World Congress on Medical Law (Belgium, 1979), the juristic implications of the doctor informing a patient's next of kin has so far received very little attention. He argues that in some situations the necessity to inform the next of kin will become of paramount importance, even without the consent of the patient or against his will. He pleads for statutory regulation of the duty to inform in these cases.

35 See above 17.

3 May the doctor refuse to attend a patient?

Questions

The following question was put to me: "I am a general practitioner with a large number of patients on my records. I find it difficult to cope with my practice as it is, let alone accept new patients. Although I am not altogether unwilling to take in new patients, I feel that my primary duty is to attend my 'old' patients.

"My question is: may I refuse to attend a new patient who calls me out at night, or who presents in my consulting rooms? What is my position if I were required to attend a total stranger who has been injured in an accident or who has fallen ill in circumstances where I am the most 'convenient' doctor available?

"And what about my existing patients? Some of them are 'difficult' people. I am sometimes called out at odd hours by patients who turn out to be not really ill. It has on occasion transpired that a patient who calls me out in the early hours of a Sunday morning is suffering from nothing worse than a bad hangover. Some of these patients are bad payers when it comes to settlement of their accounts.

"Can I refuse to respond to a call, on the grounds, for example, that I am exhausted or that other patients may require my services? Can I be held legally liable if I refuse to respond to a call and the patient subsequently dies from an injury or the disease from which he suffers?"

Another question that has often been put to me in recent years is whether a medical practitioner may refuse to attend to a patient whom he suspects or knows to be HIV positive.

Yet another question is whether a doctor may refuse to attend to patients in a situation where, because of political unrest, rioting or civil disturbances it would be dangerous for him to enter a particular neighbourhood or area.

My answer to these questions is as follows:

Liability for "mere omission"?

The traditional view of our law was that failure on the part of someone to act "positively" to ward off danger from another (or to protect the latter's interests otherwise) generally could not lead to any liability on the part of the former.[1]

As far as the doctor is concerned, one of our most eminent Roman-Dutch jurists, Johannes Voet,[2] writing by the turn of the 17th century, expressly stated that a doctor who refuses to attend a patient cannot be held liable under the Aquilian law (i e for damages), "although", adds Voet, "it would suit the duty of the good man to come to help the imperilled fortunes of his neighbour, if he can do it without hurt to himself".

1 The textbook example given to generations of law students – and cited by the Appellate Division in *Silva's Fishing Corporation (Pty) Ltd v Maweza* 1957 (2) SA 256 (A) 260H, and again as recently as 1965 in *Peri-Urban Areas Health Board v Munarin* 1965 (3) SA 367 (A) 373E – is that if I happen to see someone else's child about to drown in a pool, I do not owe a legal duty to anyone to try and save it. From what follows in the text it is clear that this statement is no longer of universal validity. Compare Neethling, Potgieter & Visser *Law of Delict* (1990) 59.

2 *Commentarius ad Pandectas* 9.2.3 The translation quoted is that of P Gane *The Selective Voet being the Commentary on the Pandects* (1955-1958).

Voet hastens to point out, however, that a doctor who performs a good operation but then abandons the curative treatment, will not escape liability.

In the USA, incidentally, the Indiana Supreme Court in 1901 in the *Hurley* case,[3] expressly held that "the state does not require and the doctor does not engage that he will practice at all or on other terms than he may choose to accept". In this case a doctor refused to attend an ailing man, although there were no other patients demanding his services at the time. He failed to give any reasons for his refusal. The patient died subsequently, but the doctor was exonerated from any liability. The right of a doctor arbitrarily to refuse to accept any person as a patient – even in a dire emergency – has subsequently been reaffirmed by numerous American authorities.[4] These authorities also emphasise that the mere fact that a doctor on previous occasions rendered a patient services does not affect the right of the doctor to subsequently refuse to attend that patient.[5]

In our law the doctor's right of refusal was traditionally justified on the ground that no one could be held liable for a so-called "mere omission". (It was in this context that Voet made his general statement on the right of a doctor to refuse a patient.) According to the customary view, liability for an omission could only be incurred in special circumstances such as the following:

- Where the defendant has by a "positive" act created a potentially dangerous situation and refrains from taking steps to avoid the danger. In the medical situation an example would be where a doctor spontaneously commences treatment of the victim of a traffic accident and then, when the patient is still in need of continued treatment, "abandons" him.[6]
- Where the defendant has assumed control over a dangerous object and then neglects to exercise proper care over it. A possible medical example would perhaps be where Dr A has commenced a blood transfusion; his attendance elsewhere is required urgently and he requests his colleague, Dr B, to carry on with the transfusion; B fails to exercise proper care over the apparatus or the procedure.
- Where the defendant is under a statutory duty to act and neglects to do so, e g a district surgeon or medical officer of health fails to vaccinate patients who present for compulsory vaccination.
- Where the defendant has by contract assumed certain duties and fails to carry these out, e g a casualty officer in the employ of a hospital authority fails to attend an injured patient brought into his ward.[7]

(In all these cases, the plaintiff will of course have to prove that the doctor's omission was either intentional or accompanied by negligence.)

Rescue duty

At this point it is important to note that the traditional view that no liability will lie for a mere omission, came under attack in our law by the middle of this century. In a series of cases the Appellate Division intimated that delictual liability may indeed be founded on "pure" omission.

This was conclusively decided in the case of *Minister van Polisie v Ewels*[8] (1975). The facts were simple enough: a policeman who was off duty, unlawfully assaulted the plaintiff in the presence of other policemen who were on duty; these policemen

3 *Hurley v Eddingfield* 156 Ind 416, 59 NE 1058 (1901).
4 See Stetler & Moritz *Doctor and Patient and the Law* (4th ed, 1962) 121 *et seq*: A R Holder *Medical Malpractice Law* (2nd ed, 1978) 7 *et seq*.
5 *Ibid.*
6 Compare Holder *op cit* 8.
7 *Ibid* 10. Compare *Magware v Minister of Health N O* 1981 (4) SA 472 (Z), discussed in the text.
8 1975 (3) SA 590 (A). On the *Ewels* case see also J Taitz 78 *S Afr Med J* 29 (1990), 30.

failed to come to the plaintiff's aid. The question to be decided was whether the state could vicariously be held liable for such omission, on the basis that there was a legal duty on the policemen to protect the plaintiff.

Chief Justice Rumpff held that the state could indeed be held liable, and he stated the law as follows: As point of departure it is accepted that in general there is no legal duty upon a person to prevent someone else from suffering damage, even if the former could easily have prevented the damage and even if it could be expected from such a person, on purely moral grounds, to act positively in order to prevent the damage. There are nevertheless circumstances in which a legal duty to act positively may arise. These circumstances are not confined to cases where there has been "prior conduct" on the part of the defendant. "It appears that the stage of development has been reached where an omission may be regarded as wrongful conduct also where the circumstances are of such a nature that the omission would not only evoke moral indignation, but also that the juristic convictions of society would require that the omission ought to be regarded as wrongful and that the damage suffered ought to be made good by the person who failed to act positively."[9]

The Chief Justice referred to an earlier decision of the court in which the principle had been enunciated that a duty to rescue another "is simply a duty to act reasonably and such a duty may arise out of the circumstances of the case" (*Silva's case*,[10] 1957). To this he added: "Just as the duty to rescue may in certain circumstances be a legal duty, so a duty to protect may be a legal duty."[11] Every case, he said, must be assessed on its own facts.

It is therefore clear that our law has evolved from its older, highly individualistic stance, to a viewpoint reflecting a healthy social responsibility.[12] A court may now well hold a doctor liable for harm suffered by an injured or ailing person, where the doctor was aware of his condition and unreasonably refused or failed to attend. The word "unreasonably" must be emphasised.

In establishing whether or not a failure to act was unreasonable, the court will undoubtedly be guided by factors such as: (1) The doctor's actual knowledge of the patient's condition; (2) the seriousness of the patient's condition; (3) the professional ability of the doctor to do what is asked of him; (4) the physical state of the doctor himself (he is a human being and if he is completely exhausted, superhuman efforts will not be demanded of him); (5) the availability of other doctors, or even of nurses and paramedics; (6) the interests of other patients; (7) whether attending to the patient would expose the doctor to danger; (8) whether the patient is desirous or not to be treated; (9) professional ethical considerations.

Professional ethical considerations cannot be underrated. The ethical standards set by the medical profession are extremely high. Although the South African Medical and Dental Council's code of ethics does not explicitly prescribe to doctors not to refuse calls, it can hardly be doubted that an unreasonable refusal to attend would be regarded as improper conduct.

A number of years ago, the SAMDC made the following ruling: "A medical practitioner is free to decide whomever he will serve. A practitioner may, however, be required to justify his actions should unnecessary suffering or death result from his refusal to attend a patient; in cases of emergency, a practitioner is obliged to render assistance under all circumstances." According to Levenstein[13] this ruling can be interpreted broadly to mean that a doctor may not deliberately ignore an emergency situation such as a road accident. The Council has also ruled that it is unacceptable

9 At 597A (my translation).
10 *Silva's Fishing Corporation (Pty) Ltd v Maweza supra* 263D.
11 At 597E (my translation).
12 Compare P Boberg "Liability for Omissions" (1982) 11 *BML* 194.
13 *SA Medical Post*, 28 September 1978.

for a general practitioner to state in advance that he will not attend to patients in their homes. The Council may require a practitioner to justify his conduct should unnecessary suffering or death occur in consequence of his refusal to make a house call.

International codes of ethics have repeatedly underlined the duty of the doctor to respect and protect human life.

As was to be expected, the *Ewels* ruling soon made itself felt in the field of medical liability. In the Zimbabwean case, *Magware v Minister of Health NO*,[14] (1981) the Supreme Court of Zimbabwe gave direct effect to the decision in *Ewels* in relation to the legal duties of casualty staff of a hospital.

In this case the patient sustained an unstable bimallelar fracture dislocation of his right ankle as a result of an accident. He was treated by the casualty staff of a State hospital over a period of about three months. Later he brought a claim against the State on the basis of an alleged breach of the implied agreement between him and the defendant, whereby the defendant undertook through his employees to treat him and to conscientiously employ reasonable care and skill.

The patient alleged that the casualty staff had applied a plaster of Paris cast to his ankle without ensuring that it was moulded appropriately to stabilise and prevent slippage of the fracture dislocation. They also failed to check the dislocation at any early stage by means of X-rays after the plaster cast had been applied. When an X-ray was ultimately taken, the patient averred, it revealed that the fracture was in an unacceptable position and required immediate correction, but the staff failed to take the appropriate action necessary to correct it. As an alternative ground of action, the plaintiff alleged that the staff members were negligent in their treatment of him. As a result his injury did not heal as it would otherwise have done, and he claimed 5 000 dollars as damages.

The defendant, the Minister of Health, denied any contractual relationship between the parties. He admitted the alleged negligence, but averred "that such negligence consisted only of acts of omission" and accordingly did not give rise to delictual liability (i e liability for wrongful conduct) on the part of the State. The defence was therefore based on the traditional view – which formerly also held sway in South Africa – that there can be no delictual liability for a so-called "mere omission" in the absence of prior conduct on the part of the defendant or a special relationship between the parties.

The patient's counsel cited English authority in support of the proposition that doctors and hospital authorities, whenever they accept a patient for treatment, are under a duty to use reasonable care and skill to cure him of his ailment.

Mr Justice Smith based his judgment in favour of the patient largely on the *Ewels* ruling. The judge held that it was clear that there was a moral and professional duty on the part of the casualty staff to act reasonably towards the patient. Once the staff had undertaken treatment and engaged in applying a plaster cast, there was set up a special relationship between them and the patient, different from the relationship between the patient and a disinterested stranger. The patient was in the care of the medical staff.

"In my judgement," the judge concluded, "on a consideration of the facts and what could be expected of the casualty medical staff as compared with the consequences of inaction, and having regard to the conceptions prevailing in this country, there was a legal duty to act reasonably."

It is respectfully submitted that in *Magware* it was not necessary for the court to rely on the *Ewels* doctrine, for the simple reason that where a patient is admitted to a casualty ward of a hospital, the ultimate accountability of the hospital need not be based on a so-called "mere omission". Apart from other considerations, a casualty of-

14 1981 (4) SA 472 (Z).

ficer in the employ of a hospital authority undeniably assumes a duty towards patients brought into the casualty ward, in terms of his contract of employment.[15]

There can, in my opinion, nevertheless be no doubt that in effect the judgment in *Magware* will be followed by the South African courts.

Patients with AIDS

May a doctor in private practice or employed by a hospital refuse to attend to an identified AIDS patient or a patient suspected of having AIDS?

As a general rule a doctor in private practice may refuse to accept any particular patient or class of patients at will. Legally the doctor is an "independent contractor". But, as I have stated, an exception to the rule is an emergency situation where it is a matter of life and death.

Because the typical AIDS case does not present itself as a life-and-death situation, a privately practising doctor may therefore refuse to accept such cases.

In its 1989 guidelines on the management of AIDS patients, the SAMDC conceded that – except in an emergency "or where no other treatment facility is available" – the medical practitioner or dentist is not legally obliged to accept a particular patient in his private practice. However, the Council endorsed the view "that ethical medical and dental practice will be conducted in a spirit of compassion which transcends the letter of the law".

The legal position of the hospital doctor is quite different from that of the private practitioner. The obligations of such a doctor depend on his conditions of employment, which would ordinarily entail the duty to treat all patients admitted to the hospital, irrespective of their illness. A hospital doctor who refuses to attend to certain types of patients in need of medical care, may therefore make himself guilty of a breach of contract, which might entitle the employer to dismiss him. Apart from that, a hospital doctor who refuses to perform his duties, may make himself guilty of an illegal strike. Strikes by doctors and nurses are prohibited in absolute terms and constitute a criminal offence. It is highly doubtful, however, that a refusal to attend to a single patient or a few patients of a certain type would be regarded as a strike in terms of section 55A of the Medical, Dental and Supplementary Health Service Professions Act.[16]

A rider must be added to the statement concerning the employer's right of dismissal: By common law it is an implicit term of a contract of employment that the employer undertakes to provide reasonably safe working conditions. A hospital authority will, therefore, be obliged to ensure, first, that employees are properly trained in safe methods of handling high-risk patients, and, secondly, that they are equipped with proper facilities to ensure reasonable safety, e g rubber gloves. Although there may be only a minimal risk involved in the handling of patients with AIDS, several tragic cases from all over the world have been reported of health-care workers who were infected with HIV in the course of their occupational duties. This fact imposes a special responsibility on hospital authorities. Apart from providing protective equipment, a hospital authority should also ensure its health-care personnel are informed that a particular patient has been diagnosed as HIV positive.

From the ethical point of view, the SAMDC has adopted the following position in relation to AIDS patients admitted to public hospitals: "In the public sector, or in other situations, where the patient has little or no choice regarding his medical or dental attendant, the doctor or dentist is obliged to attend to all patients who consult him

15 It is also possible that in the regulations governing State hospitals there is a provision imposing a duty upon doctors employed by the hospital to attend to casualty cases. Note that there need not even be an explicit or tacit agreement between the hospital and the patient that the latter will be admitted and treated. See *Correira v Berwind* 1986 (4) SA 60 (Z) and see above 1.

16 Act 56 of 1974.

or are referred to him in the course of his duty. Such attention will, as always, be given to the best of the practitioner's ability and with respect and compassion towards the patient."

Civil unrest: doctor's attendance required

A difficult situation may arise when serious and violent unrest occurs, resulting in people being severely injured or killed. A medical practitioner is telephonically requested to enter the area to attend to a victim in dire need of medical treatment. The doctor cannot be guaranteed police protection.

Clearly the law does not require a doctor to risk his own safety even if it is a life-and-death emergency for the patient. We are not dealing with the situation where someone is employed to perform an intrinsically dangerous task, as is the case with a soldier, policeman or fireman. A privately practising doctor is a free agent and may decide freely whether or not he is prepared to expose himself to the risk. The position may be different in the case of an Army doctor or medic, acting under military orders. Bravery on the part of civilians is deserving of praise. But the law – and the SAMDC, it is submitted – will not sanction a doctor who refuses to imperil his own life to save another's.

Conclusion

As our law stands today, a doctor who arbitrarily and unreasonably refuses or fails to respond to a request to attend a seriously ill or injured person, may be held legally liable for damage suffered by the patient. Should the patient die and it transpires that the doctor could have saved his life, the doctor might be held accountable to his dependants. But where medical intervention would have exposed the doctor to danger, the law will not visit him with any sanction.

4 Refusal of blood transfusion by Jehovah's Witness

The case of *Phillips v De Klerk* (1983)[1] is of special significance in relation to the refusal of medical treatment by a patient. The facts of the case were as follows:

Mr P, an electrical engineer of Johannesburg, was travelling in the Northern Transvaal when he was seriously injured in a car collision near Pietersburg. He was trapped in the driver's seat of his wrecked car. After he was freed, he was taken to a hospital in Pietersburg. It appeared that he had sustained several fractures. At a later stage he also contracted a lung infection.

Ten days later, while P was still in hospital, Dr D, an orthopaedic surgeon who attended to P, approached the Supreme Court in Pretoria with an urgent *ex parte* application for an order authorising him or another doctor to give P a blood transfusion. In the papers submitted to the court, it was stated that the patient's wife who was present in the hospital, had refused on religious grounds to consent to a blood transfusion.

It was alleged that the condition of the patient, who found himself in the hospital's intensive care unit, was deteriorating by the minute. The patient had suffered a serious loss of blood as a result of his earlier injuries with the result – so it was stated – that there was not enough blood to carry oxygen to his important bodily organs and in particular to his brain. The doctor stated that if a blood transfusion was not done within six hours, the patient would die.

On the same day the application was lodged, the judge granted the order applied for and the registrar of the court was authorised to convey the contents thereof to Dr D and the hospital.

Some seven months later the patient brought an application to the Supreme Court for the order to be set aside. In his supporting affidavit he mentioned that he was a member of the Jehovah's Witness Faith. It is a fundamental tenet of that faith, the patient stated, that "in accordance with God's Law we do not accept blood transfusions".[2]

The patient explained that members of his faith "are not actuated by an attitude of defiance of death or desire to commit suicide, nor are we reconciled with the idea that we will necessarily die if no blood is administered". "Our sincere belief is," he said, "that by the grace of God we shall survive, and we hope and pray that it will be God's will that we shall live."

Mr P further stated that he had been conscious after the accident. He could remember that he had asked the Police on their arrival at the scene of the accident why they had lighted flares in close proximity to the vehicles, in view of the obvious danger of a petrol fire while he (Mr P) was still trapped in his car.

On arrival at the hospital and admission thereto, P stated, he was fully conscious. He requested staff members to telephone his wife in Johannesburg to inform her of the accident. He also told the staff that under no circumstances was he to be given a blood transfusion. He offered to furnish the hospital and the doctor treating him

1 TPD March 1983 (unreported).
2 For an interesting survey on the attitudes of medical practitioners in South Africa towards Jehovah's Witnesses who refuse blood transfusions, see J H Cloete *Jehovah's Witnesses in South African Medical Practice* (unpublished M Fam Med thesis, Univ of the Orange Free State, 1983).

with a written absolution from any possible claim against them resulting from his refusal to permit a blood transfusion.

P said that at no stage had he been notified by Dr D of any intention to apply for a court order. Nor was his wife informed although she was in the hospital on the day D approached the court.

In actual fact, P stated, the blood transfusion authorised by the court was never administered. Later he was transferred to a hospital in Johannesburg. It was of particular significance that he recovered from his injuries without the necessity of a blood transfusion. "This has demonstrated that apart from my beliefs, the administration of a blood transfusion was not essential to my recovery," he said.

In an affidavit by Dr B, a physician who had been called in as consultant to the hospital in which P was initially treated, it was stated that he (Dr B) had also strongly recommended a blood transfusion. However, Dr B was prepared to respect P's refusal to receive blood. Dr B further stated that it had appeared in the course of several conversations he had had with the patient, that the latter was *compos mentis*. "Notwithstanding the fact that he spoke with difficulty," Dr B said, "it was clear to me that he was fully conscious and that he followed and understood the nature and drift of all conversations. There was nothing wrong with his judicative faculty."

When P's application for the previous court order to be set aside was heard by the Supreme Court, it was not contested by Dr D. Mr P's counsel informed the judge that he had been requested by Dr D's counsel to convey to the court that although there was no opposition on the part of Dr D, the latter's attitude was that the matter had become "academic" and that Dr D wanted to avoid further legal costs to run up, but that Dr D did not concede anything in regard to the merits of the application. However, it was argued by counsel for Mr P that as far as the latter was concerned, the case had not become "academic" at all; Mr P contended that his rights of personality had been affected by the previous court order – which was still in existence – and that he had become involved in legal expenses to apply for that order to be rescinded.

Mr Justice Esselen, who heard the case, said he was dealing with the case on the basis that it was unopposed. On the papers before him he was satisfied that Mr P was *compos mentis* at the relevant time and that he was entitled to refuse to be given blood. The order previously made was erroneous, the judge said, and accordingly he ordered that the previous order be set aside and that Dr D pay costs on an unopposed basis.

As far as is known, the case was the first in South Africa in which a court, after a substantive application, delivered a judgment on the right of an adult person of sound mind to refuse a blood transfusion on religious grounds. According to press reports a case had previously occurred in Johannesburg (in February 1982) in which an urgent court order was sought in an *ex parte* application late one Friday night to authorise hospital personnel to give a blood transfusion to a Jehovah's Witness who had refused blood. The patient (a Mr *Dyson*) had also been seriously injured in a road accident. The application for a court order was apparently based on the contention that the patient, on account of his condition, was incapable of validly expressing his will. According to the reports the judge (Mr Justice Margo) telephonically gave the order applied for.

It is respectfully submitted that the judgment for rescission of the previous court order given in the *Phillips* case is fully in accordance with the general principles of our law, and must be welcomed as underlining the right of the individual in a free society to dispose over his own body in so far as that right is not in conflict with the overriding social interest.

In this case the patient, although seriously injured, was fully capable of expressing his will and of assessing the possible consequences of his refusal to be given a blood transfusion. In my opinion there is no principle in our law whereby a court can overrule a patient's will in these circumstances. I have never understood the Roman-Dutch standpoint that a person is not *dominus membrorum suorum*[3] – master of his own bodily members – to mean that the doctor has a professional right to treat a patient against his will. It is submitted that legally there are only three possible grounds of justification for a medical intervention, viz –

- the patient's consent (or the consent of someone legally capable of consenting on his behalf);
- *negotiorum gestio*, which entitles a doctor to administer emergency medical treatment in those cases where on account of the patient's condition he is unable to consent;
- necessity, i e where the interests of society are at stake (which would entitle a doctor to treat the patient even against his will), for example where medical intervention is necessary to prevent the spreading of a contagious disease.[4]

More than half a century ago, in the Cape case of *Stoffberg v Elliot*,[5] the law was stated as follows: "In the eyes of the law every person has certain absolute rights which the law protects. They are not dependent on statute or upon contract, but they are rights to be respected, and one of the rights is absolute security to the person ... Any bodily interference with or restraint of a man's person which is not justified, or excused or consented to is a wrong ... [A] man by entering a hospital does not submit himself to such surgical treatment as the doctors in attendance upon him may think necessary ... He remains a human being, and he retains his rights of control and disposal of his own body; he still has the right to say what operation he will submit to, and ... any operation performed upon him without his consent is an unlawful interference with his right of security and control of his own body and is a wrong entitling him to damages if he suffers any."

It follows that to perform a medical operation upon or to administer treatment to a person against his will, or even without his consent, amounts to an assault, for which the doctor may be held liable in a civil action for damages and be criminally prosecuted.[6] As far as a claim for damages is concerned, a South African court will probably not award more than a nominal amount where it appears that the doctor has in fact saved the patient's life.[7] If, however, the patient has suffered harm in consequence of the blood transfusion, such as an infection with a serious disease on account of the blood having been contaminated, substantial damages may conceivably be awarded.

In the absence of an overriding social interest, or an interest such as that of a minor child who is dependent upon the person concerned, the mentally competent individual's right to control his own destiny in accordance with his own value system, his *selfbeskikkingsreg*, must be rated even higher than his health and life. To put it in slightly different terms: if there is a conflict between the desire of a person to go his own way, to forego medical treatment and to expire in his own manner, on the one hand, and the desire of the doctor to cure him of his disease or to secure his health, on the other, the former should be accorded preference. There is neither a general right nor a general duty on the part of a person to protect another against himself.

In his famous book *On Liberty* (1859), John Stuart Mill[8] gave eloquent expression

3 See e g Matthaeus *De Criminibus* (1644) prol 3.3; Van Leeuwen *Het Rooms-Hollands Recht* (1708) 4.3, 5.9; Moorman *Verhandelinge over de Misdaden en der selver Straffen* (1770) inl 3.4; 2.11.5.
4 This ground of justification has been given express statutory recognition *inter alia* in those provisions (section 33(*j*) of the Health Act 63 of 1977) relating to compulsory immunisation.
5 1923 CPD 148.
6 Cf *Esterhuizen v Administrator, Transvaal* 1957 (3) SA 710 (T).
7 Compare the note by D Brahams *The Lancet* 9.12.89, p 1407.
8 John Stuart Mill *On Liberty* (1859) Cambridge Univ Press edition (1989) 13.

to the idea of personal autonomy: "[T]he only purpose for which power can rightfully be exercised over any member of a civilised community, against his will, is to prevent harm to others. His own good, either physical or moral, is not a sufficient warrant. He cannot rightfully be compelled to do or forbear because it will be better for him to do so, because it will make him happier, because in the opinions of others, to do so would be wise or even right." Added Mill: "It is, perhaps, hardly necessary to say that this doctrine is meant to apply only to human beings in the maturity of their faculties."

It is submitted that our law allows a person to refuse medical treatment or a particular form of treatment, even if that may result in the patient's health deteriorating or in his death. If a doctor is of the opinion that any particular condition imposed by a patient is medically unsound (e g to refuse to receive blood) the doctor would be entitled to refuse to treat the patient at all. If the doctor were to decide to perform the procedure without giving the patient blood, it is advisable that the doctor insist on the patient giving him a prior undertaking in writing to the effect that the patient waives any claim he might have had in consequence of any ill effect flowing from the operation being performed in this manner.

In a situation where the patient is physically, mentally or psychologically in such a state that he cannot express his will at the crucial time and it is a life-or-death situation, a doctor may unquestionably act upon his own, without the consent of the patient or without the consent of any other person. The situation would be different, however, if the patient had previously, when he was still of sound mind and in full control of his senses, refused to be treated or to be given a particular form of treatment. If a man in a concrete situation, where it is proposed that he be subjected to a particular form of treatment immediately, is entitled to refuse that treatment, there is in my opinion no reason why he would not be entitled to express a "standing" refusal at an earlier stage. Such a refusal, if properly recorded – e g in the form of the so-called "Living Will"[9] – would then stand until revoked by the person who has made it. It should be seen as nothing but a statement to the following effect: "I am stating here and now that I am not consenting to medical procedure X being performed upon me, should this at any stage be proposed." Naturally such a statement remains freely revocable, but unless revoked, remains legally effective.

In principle the motive upon which a refusal of medical treatment, or a specific form of treatment, is based, should be legally irrelevant. It does not matter whether it is upon religious grounds, out of fear, or out of a desire to die an early death. Thus it is inconceivable that a doctor can claim any legal basis for forcing a patient diagnosed to be suffering from cancer, to undergo chemotherapy or X-ray treatment against his (the patient's) will, where the latter would prefer to take the chance of dying an earlier and even a more painful death.

As far as a refusal on religious grounds is concerned, it is true that South African law shows a definite preference for Christian principles[10] but except in so far as specific legislative measures promote or protect Christian values to the exclusion of other values, other religions may of course be practised. In this sense freedom of religion applies in South Africa. At any rate, differential views *within* Christianity are accepted in principle.

The fact that suicide is regarded as sinful or evil and contrary to Christian principles – or the tenets of any other faith – seems to be irrelevant in the present context, for the simple reason that a refusal to undergo medical treatment *per se* cannot be equated to a desire or attempt to bring about one's own death. The patient may be all too keen to live, but may nevertheless fear to "go under the knife", or may believe that he will live, despite his refusal to submit to treatment – as was so vividly illus-

9 On the "Living Will" see also below 344.
10 See J D van der Vyver *Die Beskerming van Menseregte in Suid-Afrika* (1975) 74 *et seq.*

trated by the *Phillips* case. Apart from these considerations, the mere refusal to be medically treated will ordinarily not constitute an immediate threat to the life of the patient, his position would thus not be comparable to that of the man who has announced his intent to commit suicide and is pointing a gun at his head or is standing on the edge of a window of a tall building, ready to jump. It is not denied that in these clear-cut cases of impending suicide through an act of violence on the part of the person who wants to kill himself, an outsider may rely on the defence of necessity in interceding and saving the person.[11]

It is therefore submitted that once the doctor has reasonable grounds for believing that the patient is a Jehovah's Witness and has at an earlier stage expressed a firm refusal to be given a blood transfusion should this be contemplated at a future stage, the doctor has no right to override the will of the patient, nor, with respect, would a court of law be entitled to do so. It should be emphasised that it is the will of *the patient* that must be established. The relatives as such do not have the right to veto emergency treatment, or conversely, to veto any consent given by the patient.[12]

With due respect, the view of Grobler and Verschoor[13] that a doctor is entitled to ignore a refusal to undergo a life-saving blood transfusion, expressed by a patient of sound mind and sober sense, is untenable.

As Smit[14] has argued on persuasive grounds, such a view would open the door to a professional right *(beroepsreg)* to treat being accorded to the medical practitioner and a denial of the individual's *selfbeskikkingsreg*.[15]

To hold that a mentally competent, adult patient may validly refuse a blood transfusion would in no way affect the rights of a minor. It is not disputed that a parent does not have the right to veto medical treatment indicated as necessary to save the life or health of his minor child. The provisions of the Child Care Act[16] vest the Ministers involved in the administration of the Act, with wide powers to give consent to medical treatment of children in the absence of parental consent, and, within certain limitations, even to override an explicit parental refusal. As is widely known, the Minister of Health and Welfare has delegated his powers in terms of these provisions to certain officials of his Department.[17]

It is to be noted that where a patient refuses to undergo any form of medical treatment proposed by the doctor, it would be advisable for the latter to insist upon the patient signing a proper "refusal and waiver" form.[18]

What is the position in other countries? In England, as far as could be ascertained, there have been no cases so far on refusal of medical treatment by a patient on religious grounds. As far as adults are concerned, authoritative writers have intimated that where an adult patient refuses a blood transfusion on religious grounds, his refusal should be respected.[19] The position is different in regard to minor patients.[20]

11 See my remarks below 91. In my opinion the legal position of the hunger-striker in prison who manifests an intent to starve to death is comparable to that of the suicide, so that intervention in the form of medical treatment would be justifiable on the basis of necessity. See below 409 *et seq*.

12 Compare *Palmer v Palmer* 1955 (3) SA 56 (O).

13 N J Grobler & T Verschoor "Bloedoortapping op Jehova-getuies" 1982 (March) *Geneeskunde* 141.

14 P C Smit "'n Beroepsreg om te Genees!" 1983 (19 February) *SA Medical Journal* 282.

15 In this survey (see note 2 *supra*) Cloete has found that the notion of a professional duty to heal was rejected by 80 per cent of doctors in South Africa who responded to his questionnaire (see his thesis, p 98).

16 Act 74 of 1983, section 39(1). It is to be noted that the medical procedures envisaged by this subsection are restricted to procedures that are attended with serious danger to life, and that the factor of immediacy, or absolute urgency, is not a prerequisite. See also *supra* 5.

17 See *supra* 5.

18 A good example of such a form is to be found in the Appendix to the article by H Z Schaub & R S Chabon 1 *Med Law* 273 (1982) 287.

19 J Leahy Taylor (ed) *Medical Malpractice* (1980) 74; C R A Martin *Law relating to Medical Practice* (2nd ed, 1979) 296.

20 *Ibid.*

Martin[21] has suggested that American case law be followed, i e that a parent may not on religious grounds veto medical treatment vital to the health and life of the child.

In the USA the general rule that has emerged from decisions of the courts is that a conscious, competent adult patient may refuse permission for the performance of any medical or surgical procedure, even if the ultimate result of the refusal is the patient's death.[22] Where the patient is a minor, however, the courts have had no hesitation in overriding a parental refusal made on religious grounds.[23]

Likewise, where an adult patient was mentally incompetent on account of serious injury when brought to hospital, and was unable to consent to or refuse treatment, courts were sometimes prepared to order a blood transfusion to be given despite the refusal of relatives.[24]

But in Canada a doctor was held liable for damages for giving an unconscious patient a blood transfusion despite the fact that she carried a card stating that she was a Jehovah's Witness. The doctor had seen the card before deciding to give her blood. The fact that the doctor saved the woman's life was of no avail to him.[25]

There have been several cases in the USA in which a blood transfusion was authorised by a court despite refusal on the part of a mentally competent adult. In all of these cases the interests of minor children or unborn children were at stake.[26] In one of these cases[27] a young mother who had just given birth to a child developed a severe haemorrhage. Here, clearly, the interest of her infant in her survival was at stake, although this was not the basis of the court's decision. As Roth and Wild[28] have pointed out, the court's ruling was nevertheless not unequivocal.

In Germany it has been held that a father may not on religious grounds veto the giving of a blood transfusion which is necessary to save the life of his minor child.[29]

Adapted from a paper read in the Senate Lecture series of Witwatersrand University, Johannesburg, August 1983. It was first published in Ellison Kahn (ed) The Sanctity of Human Life *(1984), and is published in this form by kind courtesy of Professor Kahn.*

21 *Op cit*, 296.

22 93 ALR 3d (1979) 67 *et seq*, particularly 77-80; A B Roth & R A Wild "When the Patient Refuses Treatment: Some Observations and Proposals for Handling the Difficult Case" (1979) 23 *St Louis Univ L J* 329; A J Rosoff *Informed Consent* (1981) 265 *et seq*; H Z Shaub & R S Chabon "When the Patient Refuses Treatment: Legal, Ethical and Practical Considerations" (1982) *Med Law* 273. See in particular also *In re Brook's Estate* 205 NE 2d 435 (1965).

23 Rosoff *op cit* 198-99, 201-202; Shaub & Shabon *op cit*; *Jehovah's Witnesses in the State of Washington et al v King County Hospital Unit No 1 (Harborview) et al* 278 E Supp 488 (1967); *People v Labrentz* 104 NE 2d 769 (1952).

24 See e g *John F Kennedy Memorial Hospital v Heston* 279 A 2d 670 (NJ 1971) quoted by Roth & Wild *op cit* 437-438. Compare 93 ALR 3d 67, 80 *et seq*.

25 *Malette v Shulman and Others* [1988] 47 DLR 18. The case is discussed and criticised by D Brahams in *The Lancet* 9.12.89, p 1407.

26 See 93 ALR 3d 67, *et seq*; for cases dealing specifically with refusal on religious grounds, see 93 ALR 3d 67, 83 *et seq*; *Application of North Shore University Hospital (Bland)* (reference not available) quoted by Roth & Wild *op cit* 435; Shaub & Chabon *op cit* 274.

27 *Application of North Shore University Hospital (Bland)* (see preceding footnote).

28 *Op cit* 435.

29 1968 *Neue Juristische Wochenschrift* 212.

5 Informed consent and the unwilling ophthalmological patient

Legal principles regarding the requirement of informed consent to surgery were brought to the fore in the 1976 judgment of the Appellate Division in the case of *Verhoef v Meyer.*[1]

In the case, tried in the Pretoria Supreme Court, a 65-year-old female patient made a series of allegations against the defendant doctor, an ophthalmologist who also filled a university chair.

The patient contended that she had consulted the doctor in connection with a condition in her right eye, diagnosed as a retinal detachment. The doctor allegedly assured her that the condition could easily be "fixed up" by means of an operation.

She claimed that the operation subsequently conducted, was a failure. She did not regain her sight as the doctor had allegedly assured her.

In the alternative the patient averred that the doctor had failed to adequately inform her of the fact that such an operation could possibly not be successful, and that she consented to the operation in ignorance of such fact.

In the course of the trial it transpired that the patient had also accused the doctor of not having in fact himself performed the operation but having left it to another medical practitioner who at the time was a "student" ophthalmologist. The patient at one stage also accused the doctors involved of having surgically interfered with the left eye without her consent.

The defendant doctor raised the defence that he had properly informed the patient of the nature of the operation and that she had fully consented. He alleged that he had warned her of the possibility of the operation not being successful. He denied that he had "guaranteed" a successful outcome, adding that if he had done so, his two assistants (who were present) "would have thought their professor was going crazy".

The doctor claimed that the operation was successful in that the retina became properly fixed to the choroid. He further claimed that the patient regained her peripheral eyesight, which had been absent prior to the operation.

At the trial it was common cause that the patient had signed a hospital admission form in which she consented to an operation. Shortly after her admission to the hospital she intimated that she was no longer willing to undergo the operation. The doctor alleged that subsequently, a day or two afterwards, she nevertheless gave oral consent to the operation.

During the trial the patient contended that because the doctor had not properly informed her, she had not realised her consent to an operation would authorise a *surgical* operation.

The trial involved a good deal of conflicting evidence as to the parties' respective versions of what had transpired. The trial judge, Mr Justice Joubert, had to make a finding on the credibility of the various witnesses.

In his judgment the judge remarked that he approached the patient's evidence with caution because her demeanour in the witness box indicated "that she can become very excited and agitated about anything with which she is confronted which

1 Transvaal Provincial Division, 12 September 1975, unreported.

is contrary to her preconceived notions". Thus she believed in nature-healing and not in surgical treatment. She also believed "that the ethics of doctors compel them to keep each other's mistakes secret".

The defendant doctor, on the other hand, made "a very good impression" upon the trial judge. "He was modest, calm, polite and replied clearly and relevantly to questions without hesitating or avoiding."

The judge held that where the patient's evidence conflicted with that of the medical witnesses, he accepted the latter. He ruled that the patient had failed to establish her case on a preponderance of probabilities and that the doctor succeeded in proving his defence.

In the course of his judgment the judge – ostensibly with his tongue in his cheek – quoted Groenewegen, a famous 17th century Roman-Dutch legal authority, to the effect that "the earth covers the inadequacies of doctors and for that reason they are not brought before the courts or otherwise they are often excused".[2]

The patient took the judgment on appeal to the Appellate Division where it came before five judges. The Appeal Court confirmed the judgment.[3] Mr Justice Wessels wrote the court's judgment to which unanimous concurrence was given by his brethren.

The case demonstrated the advisability in cases of drastic or unusual surgery, of a medical practitioner setting forth in writing the essential nature of an operation and the risks involved, and the taking of a detailed written consent – in so far as this is practicable. The case further indicates that where a patient who has given consent to an operation becomes unwilling, great caution should be exercised in ensuring the fullest documentation of a subsequent consent. By such caution a suit for malpractice may well be avoided.

2 My translation of Groenewegen's *De Legibus Abrogatis, ad Inst* 4.3.7, quoted by the judge.
3 Appellate Division, 23 November 1976.

6 Consent to an operation on a mental patient

In 1978 an amendment to the Mental Health Act[1] largely clarified the legal position regarding consent to medical treatment of or an operation on mental patients. But not all difficulties have been solved.

Prior to that amendment, the relationship doctor and mental patient was not without problems as regards the question of consent. From a strictly legal point of view, a person suffering from a severe mental disability (a "lunatic" or "insane" person, in the older terminology of our courts) cannot enter into contracts. From the point of view of criminal or delictual liability he cannot validly consent to actions which, if it were not for his consent, would constitute a criminal offence or a civil wrong (delict).

The test applied in practice is whether the person concerned was or was not capable of appreciating and understanding the nature of the transaction into which he purported to enter.

In the field of medical treatment, the answer whether or not a mentally disabled patient himself can validly consent, would depend on an inquiry along the following lines: Are the patient's mental abilities such that he can take cognisance of the type of treatment? Can he appreciate the nature and consequences of the treatment? Can he form the desire to undergo the treatment or at least reconcile himself with the fact that he will undergo the treatment? In this context it is the mental abilities of the patient that are decisive and not necessarily the exact classification or diagnosis of the type of mental disability from which he is suffering.

In the case of a minor patient who is mentally unable to consent, a parent or guardian can by common law give the necessary consent. As far as the major patient is concerned (i e the patient 21 years or older), from a strictly legal point of view only the personal curator could in common law consent. This was confirmed in the 1950 Transvaal case of *Dixie*.[2]

In that case the doctors had recommended a leucotomy. The court ruled, in general terms, that a non-emergency operation cannot lawfully be performed without the consent of the patient. If he is not competent to give it, consent must be given by "some person in authority over his person". "The fact that he is a patient in a hospital," the court ruled, "does not entitle those in charge of it to perform any surgical operation upon him which they may consider beneficial." A curator for the person of the patient was accordingly appointed by the court to consider whether an operation was to be performed and to consent thereto if it were so decided.

From the *Dixie* judgment it is clear that in the case of a serious non-emergency operation, a parent or relative of a mental patient was not legally entitled to simply give the necessary consent. Even if a relative were legally entitled to give consent, the sad fact is that mental patients, detained in institutions, are sometimes abandoned by their relatives. The appointment of a personal curator, again, would involve a costly application to the Supreme Court.

Subsequently, special consent provisions were framed in the regulations under

1 Act 18 of 1973.

2 *Ex parte Dixie* 1950 (4) SA 748 (W).

the Mental Health Act for leucotomies but these were of specific application to that type of operation only.[3]

In 1978, a new section (section 60A) was inserted into the Mental Health Act[4] making explicit provision, in general terms, for consent to medical treatment of, or operations performed on, mental patients to be given on behalf of such patients. This was a welcome improvement to our law. The section refers to a "patient" and "patient" is defined in the Act[5] as "a person mentally ill to such a degree that it is necessary that he be detained, supervised, controlled and treated ..."

Section 60A sets up a priority list of persons who may consent on behalf of the patient: the curator, appointed by the court to the person or property of the patient; the patient's spouse, parent, major child or brother or sister. It is provided that the persons enumerated will have precedence in that order, unless the consent is being withheld unreasonably, or the operation or treatment is urgent and the person having precedence cannot be found timeously. In that event the person following in precedence may consent.

If there are none of the persons enumerated, or if such persons cannot be found after reasonable enquiry, the superintendent of the institution "where the patient finds himself" can consent. The superintendent is required to hold the opinion, on reasonable grounds, that the life of the patient is endangered or that his health is seriously threatened. Consent must be given in writing.

A shortcoming of the new section is that as far as consent by a superintendent is concerned, it would seem to apply only to patients in mental institutions, either because of formal admission as a voluntary patient for treatment, a patient by consent or an out-patient,[6] or in consequence of a formal reception order.[7]

The section refers to an institution "where the patient finds himself" and this would indicate in my opinion something more than the patient being "casually" brought to an institution, or by coincidence "finding himself" there; ostensibly a formal act of admission or reception in the institution is required by the Legislature.

What about the patient who is in private care and has neither a curator nor relatives, or who was deserted by his relatives? It is suggested that to obviate the necessity of an application to court for a special curator to be appointed, the Legislature should make provision for the superintendent of the hospital in which the operation will be performed or treatment will be given, to give consent in special circumstances (similar to the power given by section 39(2) of the Child Care Act[8] to medical superintendents in respect of children).

Note that section 60A clearly does not authorise a superintendent to consent to a

3 Regulation 7, Government Notice R565 of 27 March 1975. A practitioner who intends performing a leucotomy upon a mentally ill person must give at least 30 days prior notice to the Director-General, Department of National Health and Population Development. At the same time he must furnish the Director-General with a medical report by a panel of at least three psychiatrists that all other methods of treatment previously applied, have failed. No such report may be furnished unless the patient has been admitted to a provincial hospital department of psychiatry, or a State psychiatric hospital, for observation and investigation to enable such report to be furnished. The Director-General must also be provided with evidence that consent has been given by the following persons: (a) in the case of a person received under section 3 of the Act, the written consent of such person given by himself; (b) in the case of a person received under section 4 or 9 of the Act, the consent in writing of a near relative of such person; (c) where no such near relative is available, the consent in writing of the official *curator ad litem*. The leucotomy may only be performed by a registered neurosurgeon who has been nominated by the panel which recommended the leucotomy. No leucotomy may be performed without the approval of the Director-General.

4 By Act 10 of 1978.

5 Section 1.

6 In terms of chapter 2 of the Act.

7 In terms of chapter 3 of the Act.

8 Act 74 of 1983. See *supra* 6.

sterilisation merely for convenience, or to an abortion in circumstances where the life of the woman is not endangered or her health seriously threatened.

It is further to be noted that the section obviously deals with medical treatment and operations other than "standard" psychiatric treatment. It is submitted that a reception order issued by a magistrate in terms of section 9 of the Mental Health Act, is sufficient to authorise psychiatric treatment without the necessity of obtaining consent from any other person. The same would seem to apply to urgent cases dealt with under section 12.[9]

9 See *supra* 4, note 9.

7 Does the doctor guarantee that the patient will be cured?

The standard of care required of a medical practitioner who undertakes the treatment of a patient is not the highest possible degree of professional skill, but reasonable skill and care. This principle was reaffirmed by the Transvaal court in the 1976 case of *Buls and Another v Tsatsarolakis*.[1] The plaintiff, a bricklayer, had tried to start the engine of a concrete mixer. The engine backfired and the starting handle struck his right wrist. He went to the hospital where he was examined by the casualty officer on duty, Dr B. X-rays were taken but Dr B found no evidence of a fracture.

On a second visit to the hospital, Dr B communicated to the plaintiff the fact that since his first visit the hospital's part-time radiologist had examined the X-ray plates but had not found any fracture. Subsequently the plaintiff consulted a private specialist orthopaedic surgeon, who referred him for X-rays, and these revealed a fracture of the scaphoid bone of the right wrist. At the trial, the specialist testified that in his opinion Dr B was negligent in that at the second visit Dr B had failed to immobilise the plaintiff's wrist. Another specialist testified, however, that there was no neglect of duty by Dr B. His conduct was that which he would have expected from an ordinary casualty officer. Dr B was not an expert in problems of the type which arose, and he gave it the attention of a general practitioner.

The court held that the plaintiff had failed to establish negligence. A factor in the decision was the finding of the trial court that at the second visit, Dr B had told the plaintiff that he should come back if he continued to experience pain. This the plaintiff did not do.

In the course of his judgment, Mr Justice Nicholas raised the following question: "Every man has a legal right not to be harmed; but is there, apart from a contract, a legal right to be healed? It is no doubt the professional duty of a medical practitioner to treat his patient with due care and skill, but does he, merely by undertaking a case, become subject to a legal duty, a breach of which founds an action for damages, to take due and proper steps to heal the patient?"

As far as he could ascertain, the judge observed, the cases of medical negligence in the South African law reports have all arisen out of physical injury or harm sustained by the plaintiff. In the present case, however, the plaintiff alleged, not that he had suffered personal injury or harm as a result of the negligence of Dr B, but that he suffered pecuniary loss as a result of the delay in the treatment of the injury which he had sustained.

The judge observed that although the question he posed was an interesting one, it was not argued and it was not necessary for the purpose of the decision to answer it.

I would respectfully submit that the answer to the question is as follows: where a patient consults a doctor who undertakes to treat him, the doctor assumes no greater duty than to treat the patient with due care and skill, unless the doctor has expressly guaranteed that the patient will be healed by his treatment – something which the prudent doctor will generally not do.

This is also the view of the English courts. In the case of *Greaves*[2] Lord Denning

1 1976 (2) SA 891 (T).
2 *Greaves & Co (Contractors) Ltd v Baynham Mickle & Partners* [1975] 3 All ER 99(CA).

had the following to say about the employment of a professional man: "The law does not usually imply a warranty that he will achieve the desired result, but only a term that he will use reasonable care and skill. The surgeon does not warrant that he will cure the patient. Nor does the solicitor warrant that he will win the case."

In *Eyre v Measday*[3] the English Court of Appeal, in rejecting a woman's claim for damages following an unsuccessful sterilisation, supported that view. The doctor had told the woman the operation he intended to perform "must be regarded as a permanent procedure", but he did not inform her there was a small risk of pregnancy occurring after the operation. She contended in court that the doctor, by necessary implication, had committed himself to an unqualified guarantee as to the success of the operation. The court held, however, that "in the absence of any express warranty, the court should be slow to imply against a medical man an unqualified warranty as to the results of an intended operation, for the simple reason that it is most unlikely that a responsible medical man would intend to give a warranty of this nature".

In a comparable case, *Thake and Another v Maurice*,[4] the English Court of Appeal likewise refused to come to the conclusion that there had been a guarantee of success. The doctor had performed an unsuccessful vasectomy on a married man. One of the judges conceded that there may be cases where, because of the claims made by a doctor for his method of treatment, the court is driven to the conclusion that the result of the treatment is guaranteed. "But in the present case I do not regard the statements made by the [doctor] as to the effect of his treatment as passing beyond the realm of expectation and assumption. ... [W]hat he said was spoken partly by way of warning and partly by way of what is sometimes called 'therapeutic reassurance' ... Furthermore, I do not consider that a reasonable person would have expected a responsible medical man to be giving a guarantee. Medicine, though a highly skilled profession, is not, and is not generally regarded as being, an exact science. The reasonable man would have expected the defendant to exercise all the proper skill of a surgeon in that speciality: he would not in my view have expected the defendant to give a guarantee of 100 % success." Another judge made the following observation: "Of all sciences medicine is one of the least exact. In my view a doctor cannot be objectively regarded as guaranteeing the success of any operation or treatment unless he says as much in clear and unequivocal terms." (The court nevertheless ordered the doctor to pay damages to the woman and her husband because he had been negligent in failing to warn that a vasectomy could be followed by naturally regaining of fertility.)

A South African court, in the case of *Behrmann and Another v Klugman*,[5] found that the reasoning by the English judges was "very persuasive". The case was also one of an unsuccessful vasectomy. Mr Justice Melamet held that even if the doctor had used the phrase "end of the road" or "you will not father a child", it was not intended in the context as "irreversible" other than to describe the nature of the operation and was not intended to give a guarantee as to the permanent success of the operation. The court accordingly found that no claim for breach of contract by the doctor was established.

The refusal of the courts to regard "therapeutic reassurance" as constituting a guarantee that the patient will be cured, is sensible. I am reminded of a saying attributed to the Afrikaans sage, Langenhoven: If you need a doctor, look for one who will encourage you; if you need a lawyer, look for one who will discourage you.

3 [1986] 1 All ER 488 (CA).
4 [1986] 1 All ER 497 (CA).
5 1988 WLD unreported.

PART II

Medical and dental fees

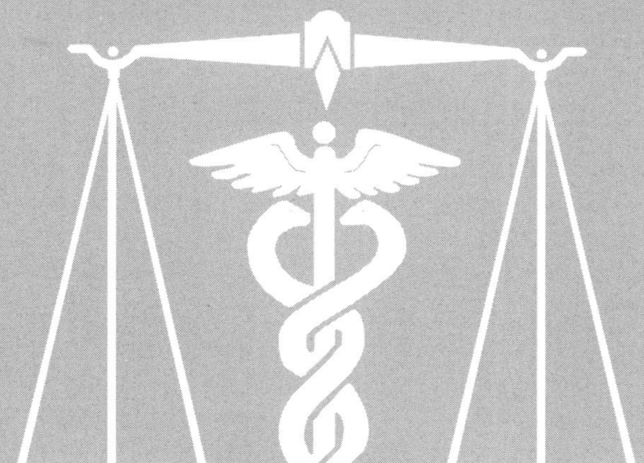

8 Medical fees: basic principles

Introduction

In essence the South African system of health care is a non-socialised system. Generally speaking, medical practitioners are not employed by the State but practise independently. The patient who consults a doctor enters into a direct relationship with him and must remunerate him privately for his services. (The patient may, of course, belong to a medical scheme which will pay the doctor on his behalf.) It is therefore a free-enterprise system in the sense that the relationship between the parties depends on the agreement entered into and that the State is not a party to the relationship, nor does the State undertake to provide medical services to all.

As far as the terms of their agreement are concerned, the relationship between doctor and patient is nevertheless not a free-enterprise type of relationship in the fullest sense of that expression. The law has placed important limitations upon the terms of the contract between doctor and patient. Thus a doctor is not at liberty to charge the patient any fee he wishes or the patient is willing to pay. The Medical, Dental and Supplementary Health Service Professions Act[1] makes provision for disciplinary control by the South African Medical and Dental Council to ensure that doctors' fees are reasonable. Another legal limitation upon the contents of the contract between doctor and patient is that a doctor may not enter into an agreement whereby the patient undertakes to assume the risk for negligent treatment.[2]

Although there is no national health service in South Africa, similar to that operative in England, provision has been made for free or semi-free medical and hospital services for the lower income groups and indigent persons, in State and provincial hospitals. In the rural areas the district surgeon, who is a medical practitioner in the full-time or part-time employ of the State, plays an important role in this regard.

State and provincial hospitals also admit private patients, i e paying patients treated by private practitioners. These hospitals offer special facilities usually not provided by private institutions, e g casualty departments and intensive care units.

Fees must be reasonable

The Medical etc Act[3] provides that unless the circumstances render it impossible, a medical practitioner must, before rendering a professional service, inform the patient or a person responsible for his maintenance (e g a father) of the fee he intends to charge. But this must be done only where the doctor is so requested, or where the fee exceeds that usually charged for such service. In the latter instance, the doctor must also inform the person concerned of the usual fee.

The doctor must furnish the patient with a detailed account within a reasonable period. A patient may within three months after receiving an account, apply in writing to the Medical Council to determine what a reasonable fee would be. A claim referred to the Council is not recoverable until a determination has been made, and then only

1 Act 56 of 1974.
2 Cf S A Strauss & M J Strydom *Die Suid-Afrikaanse Geneeskundige Reg* (1967) 317.
3 Section 53.

to the extent of the determination. Apart from such action, the Council may still take disciplinary action against the practitioner. It is to be noted that for the purposes of these statutory provisions, "professional services" include the supply and fitting of any artificial part of the human body.

The Council may from time to time determine and publish the fees as norm for the determination of a reasonable fee. As yet the Council has not done so. The Medical Association of South Africa (MASA), however, publishes a tariff list of recommended fees on an annual basis and its views on what constitutes a reasonable fee for a particular service will no doubt serve as a guideline for the Medical Council in settling a dispute between a doctor and his patient.

In terms of the Medical Schemes Act[4] the Representative Association of Medical Schemes (RAMS) may, by means of notice in the *Government Gazette,* determine a scale of benefits in respect of services rendered to members of medical schemes. Before such a scale is determined, the Association must consult representative professional associations, such as the MASA. So far, determinations have been made on an annual basis.[5]

A doctor who renders a service to a member of a medical scheme must, within 30 days and monthly thereafter, furnish the patient with an account. If the doctor's account does not exceed the scale of benefits, he may within two months after delivery of the first account, send the account – if it is still unpaid – to the patient's medical scheme. The scheme must then pay the account direct to the doctor. Apart from these statutory provisions, a number of medical schemes are willing to receive an account, which is in accordance with the scale of benefits, direct from the doctor and to settle it direct with the doctor. This system is known as "guaranteed payment".

The significance of these provisions is that a doctor whose fees exceed the RAMS scale of benefits must look to the patient for payment. The scheme will not pay the doctor direct. Such an account must be sent to the patient, who will then claim the scheme's contribution in accordance with the official scale. The patient must then settle the doctor's account by paying the doctor in full, i e also that part of the fees which is in excess of the official scale. Regrettably, some patients fail to pay the doctor's account despite the fact that they have received the scheme's contribution. The majority of medical practitioners prefer "guaranteed payment" and charge fees in accordance with the scale of benefits.

The old system of "contracting out" by doctors was abolished by the 1984 amendments to the Medical Schemes Act. The phrase "contracted out" is nevertheless still used by doctors who prefer to charge fees higher than the official scale of benefits. There is general dissatisfaction among medical practitioners regarding the fees provided for in the scale of benefits. Doctors who charge fees higher than the latter, are guided by the MASA's recommended fees, determined on an annual basis. The MASA fees are considerably higher than those listed in the scale of benefits.

What has been said here regarding the scale of benefits and accounts, applies in equal measure to hospitals, clinics, nursing services and services rendered by members of supplementary health services.[6]

Dispensing of medicine by doctor

Since we are on the subject of medical fees, a few comments should also be made on dispensing of medicine by doctors.

4 76 of 1967, section 29.

5 The determinations currently (February 1991) in force are the following: for medical practitioners, Notice 1049 of 14.12.90 (*GG* 12896); for dentists Notice 989 of 30.11.90 (*GG* 12868).

6 As far as other professionals are concerned, a scale of benefits has been determined for physiotherapists (see Notice 987 of 30.11.90, *GG* 12868) and private hospitals (see Notice 988 of 30.11.90, *GG* 12868).

Provided that his name has been entered in a special register kept by the Medical Council, a medical practitioner or dentist may personally compound or dispense medicines prescribed by himself or by another practitioner with whom he is in partnership or with whom he is associated as principal or assistant or *locum tenens*, for use by patients under treatment of such practitioners. However, medical practitioners or dentists are not entitled to keep an open shop or pharmacy.[7] It is considered unethical for doctors to make an excessive profit on medicines so dispensed.

A doctor or dentist who desires to exercise this right of independent compounding or dispensing of medicine, must apply to the Council to have his name entered in the special register. The Council may impose conditions that must be complied with. The Council may also, after an investigation, remove the doctor's name from this register, or suspend his right to dispense for a specified period.

The Council is vested with wide powers of investigation, to establish whether malpractices in this respect (or involving other ethical aspects of the medical profession) are taking place.[8]

If the Council is of the opinion that a dispensing doctor's consulting rooms are not situated within a reasonable distance of a retail pharmacy, it may authorise a nurse employed by the doctor to supply medicine to a patient. Only medicines mentioned in the first four schedules to the Medicines etc Control Act may thus be supplied. Such supply must take place in accordance with the doctor's directions.[9]

A medical practitioner or dentist may not accept or obtain from a pharmacist any commission or other reward in connection with any prescription given by such medical practitioner or dentist. Contravention of this prohibition constitutes a criminal offence (involving a maximum fine of R200) and may lead to disciplinary action by the Medical Council.[10]

Discount to patients for cash payment

It is certainly not *illegal* for a medical practitioner to grant a patient a discount on his fees for cash payment or for payment of his account within a specified time, in the sense that a law of the land will be contravened.

The *ethical* aspect of a cash discount, however, is something which has been somewhat controversial and which should be carefully considered. Ethical Rule 1 of the Medical Council which deals with advertising, contains no express prohibition on a doctor informing his patients of the fact that he will grant a discount if his account is paid in cash. In the past the Council frowned upon doctors who printed a notification to that effect on their accounts or who put up a notice in their waiting rooms. However, there was apparently no objection to a doctor personally telling a patient who enquired whether he could get a discount.

Present economic policy is strongly against price collusion and free competition is encouraged. The Competition Board in 1987 even pronounced itself in favour of pharmacists being able to freely advertise their professional fees.[11]

It is difficult, in this atmosphere of free competition to lower the cost of health-care services, to envisage the Medical Council objecting to a medical practitioner *bona fide* informing his patients of his willingness to give a discount for cash payment of his account – be it by way of personal communication or a statement on patient accounts.[12] The SAMDC frowns upon consulting rooms notices, though.[13]

7 Act 56 of 1974, section 52.
8 *Ibid*, section 41A.
9 *Ibid*, section 52A.
10 *Ibid*, section 57.
11 See *SA Practice Management* 1988 (1) 26.
12 See *SA Practice Management* 1991 (1) 18. From the article by a prominent general practitioner, G Davie, published in *NAPG Bulletin* 1990 (2) 25, it is clear that doctors are also using newsletters to their patients to convey this information.
13 See *SA Practice Management* 1991 (1) 18.

In April 1989 the Medical Council passed the following resolution: "A recommendation that practitioners be allowed to grant rebates on direct payment of accounts was accepted by the Council. However, practitioners were warned not to fall prey to any form of advertising in the process of informing patients of such rebates."[14] In my opinion the conveying of information by the methods mentioned above, can certainly not be regarded as constituting advertising or touting for patients.[15]

Prepayment of doctors' accounts

From a purely legal point of view a provider of services is entitled to require a client to make a deposit prior to the service being rendered. This is commonly done by repairmen and merchants (taking lay-byes) and even by professional men such as attorneys.

The Medical Council, however, in principle regards the prepayment of medical fees as ethically impermissible. A doctor is entitled to insist on immediate settlement of his account once the service has been rendered, but he may not insist on advance payment. An exception is made in the case of a doctor or dentist who must purchase a prosthesis or artificial dentures for his patient.

The Council has also decided that plastic and reconstructive surgeons may enter into an arrangement in terms of which a financial institution, acting on behalf of the patient, may issue a guarantee for payment of the surgeon's eventual account. A plastic surgeon may, therefore, require a patient to make a deposit with a bank to enable the bank to issue such a guarantee.[16]

"Splitting" of accounts not permissible

Because of the system of guaranteed payment, direct to the doctor, by medical schemes of fees charged in accordance with the RAMS scale of benefits, the question arose whether it would be possible for a doctor to render two accounts: one for a fee in accordance with the scale and another for the balance of the fee which would be chargeable in terms of the MASA's recommended maximum. (The idea was that the first account would be sent to the medical scheme and that the doctor would look to the patient for settlement of the second.)

Not surprisingly, the SAMDC expressed its disapproval of such a practice. The Council resolved that it was not permissible for a practitioner to render two different accounts for one service rendered. But a rider was added: A doctor may claim the part of the account for which the patient is responsible by means of a cash payment after rendering the service. This is on condition that an account is rendered before payment, whereafter an account on which this payment is reflected as credit, may be rendered to the patient and the medical scheme. The Council also decided that there is no objection to dividing the account into different columns – such as one indicating the portion the patient would normally receive as a benefit from the medical scheme, the second indicating the portion for which the patient would be responsible and thirdly the total of the preceding – provided one account only was rendered to the patient.[17]

It is to be noted that the system of guaranteed payment is currently (1991) under review and it is possible that it may be statutorily abolished.

14 See 75 *S Afr Med J* (20/5/89) 466 and compare 74 *S Afr Med J* (17/9/88) 264.
15 See also my note in *SA Practice Management* 1990 (2).
16 See *SAMDC/SAGTR Bulletin* No 6 (Sept 1989) 9.
17 See article by N M Prinsloo in *SA Practice Management* 1989 (1) 21.

9 Medical schemes and the doctor's fees: some legal aspects

Introduction

In this chapter some legal aspects of medical schemes are addressed. It is, of course, not suggested that the issues raised are an exclusive list or that they are even representative of important legal aspects of medical schemes. This is no more than a discussion of some questions put to me from time to time.[1]

Medical schemes and medical insurance

Medical insurance, i e insurance against medical expenses that may be incurred by a person or his dependants at a future date, has come to the fore in recent years. In January 1989 the Department of National Health and Population Development issued a press release in which interested parties were invited to make submissions on the subject to the Registrar of Medical Schemes. It was pointed out in the press release that the Central Council for Medical Schemes and the government had already decided that amendments to legislation could be considered to allow medical insurance to develop within the framework of three criteria: negotiability had to be assured, the government was not to become involved in tariffs determination and the proposed legislation should not cause an escalation of State expenditure on health services.

To comply with these criteria it was required that insurance for medical expenses would have to include certain features, e g prescribed minimum benefits, continuity of insurance and interchangeability between insurance schemes.

It is clear that profound thought will have to go into the conceptualisation of full medical insurance before it will eventually materialise.

In the meantime, as is well known, certain insurance companies are already offering hospital insurance to the public for serious illness ("dread disease") such as heart attacks, cancer or strokes or any serious condition requiring hospitalisation. Some of these policies even cover pregnancy and offer additional lump sums in the event of accidental death. These policies are, therefore, a form of mixed medical and accident insurance.

Where exactly then does the distinction between insurance and medical schemes lie?

This question presupposes that there is in fact legally such a distinction. Looking at it from the point of economics, however, it must be stated that the benefits offered by our system of medical schemes is, of course, nothing other than a form of insurance.

But in legal terms the legislature has nevertheless drawn a distinction between insurance, as governed by the Insurance Act 27 of 1943, and medical schemes, as governed by the Medical Schemes Act 72 of 1967. In general terms, the Legislature has in section 33 of the latter Act reserved "the business of a medical scheme", i e medical "insurance" as provided for by the Act, exclusively for registered medical schemes. This reservation has nevertheless not been done in a watertight fashion.

Without going into the fine detail of the statutory provisions of the two Acts, it is

1 I am indebted to Dr J J du Toit of Port Elizabeth for directing my attention to a number of legal issues that have arisen in connection with medical schemes.

clear that "catastrophe" insurance in the form of personal accident policies is permissible despite section 33 of the Medical Schemes Act. And "personal accident policy" is defined in the Insurance Act, section 1, in such terms as to include death, injury or disability resulting from an accident, as well as, alternatively, "sickness causing ... disability".

As I understand the legal position resulting from the combined effect of the wording of the respective Acts – bearing in mind that insurance as such is governed by both the Insurance Act and the common law – a personal accident policy in the form of "sickness disability" is permissible, without the necessity of the scheme being registered as a medical scheme, provided it is not linked to any "services" as defined in the Medical Schemes Act. Some lawyers hold the opinion that the latter requirement is not even necessary because disability insurance taken out by individuals does not amount to a "scheme".[2]

The legal validity of "RAMS" action in terms of section 29 of the Act

A question which the lawyer is asked from time to time by doctors who are dissatisfied with the scale of benefits as determined by the Representative Association of Medical Schemes (RAMS) in terms of section 29 of the Medical Schemes Act, is whether a doctor or group of doctors or a medical association may approach the Supreme Court with an application for an order to set aside the gazetted scale of benefits or any item or items therein.

The answer to that question is a qualified "yes". First, the court will undoubtedly interfere if any of the requirements stated expressly in section 29 – pertaining to the steps RAMS must take prior to publication of the scale of benefits – has not been met. These are: complying with the conditions (if any) prescribed by the Minister in terms of subsection (1); consulting with the "majority" professional association concerned; maintaining the ratio between a "domestic" tariff and its (RAMS's) own tariff.

The requirement of consultation stated in subsection (1) (*c*) reaffirms the administrative-law principle of *audi alteram partem*, i e to hear the views of those who will be affected by an administrative decision, prior to the exercising thereof. The Legislature's use of the word "consult" in the subsection is significant. "Consult" clearly is not such a strong term as "negotiate". The ordinary meaning of the word "consult" in the present context is to have deliberations, or to take into consideration the feelings or interests of the other party. "Negotiate" means to confer with another with a view to a compromise or agreement. (I am quoting "Oxford" definitions.[3]) The Legislature clearly did not intend that RAMS and the "majority" medical association should reach an actual agreement before the scale of benefits was published. Thus in *R v Mbete*[4] it was held that where "consultation" was required in a statute, all that was necessary was that the scheme in question be put before the necessary parties and that they be given full opportunity to state their views; "consultation" in the section did not mean "agreement".

Apart from attacking RAMS's action under the section on the basis of alleged non-compliance with the express statutory requirements, there is the possibility of launching an attack on the basis of general (common-law) principles of administrative law. RAMS has been vested with an administrative discretion, and the manner in which such a discretion must be exercised, and the grounds upon which it may be attacked, have been mapped out well in court decisions. I shall endeavour to sum up the salient points briefly.

The first is that the result of the exercise of an administrative discretion need not necessarily be reasonable from the point of view of those affected by it. According

2 I have had the advantage of seeing an opinion by an esteemed colleague in which this standpoint was persuasively argued.

3 The *Concise Oxford Dictionary* s v "consult" and "negotiate".

4 1954 (4) SA 491 (E). Compare *MAWU v Hart* 1985 (6) ILJ 478.

to the prevailing majority judicial view, reasonableness is not *per se* a requirement of legally valid administrative action.[5] It is trite law that the court will interfere with the exercise of an administrative discretion on limited grounds only, such as proof that the body has acted *mala fide* or from ulterior or improper motives, that it has not applied its mind to the matter before it, that it has failed to exercise a discretion at all, that it has disregarded the express provisions of a statute, or has acted *ultra vires*, i e beyond its powers.[6] But the court would be unable to interfere with a due and honest exercise of discretion, even if it considered the decision itself, i e the end result of the administrative act, inequitable or wrong.

The unreasonableness of a decision will only be a factor in persuading the court that the manner in which the discretion was exercised was defective. As it was put by the Appellate Division many years ago in a classic judgment:[7] emphasis is laid on the necessity of the unreasonableness "being so gross that something else can be inferred from it, either that it is inexplicable except on the assumption of *mala fides* or ulterior motive, or that it amounts to proof that the person upon whom the discretion is conferred, has not applied his mind to the matter". Inability on the part of an administrative organ to give a rational explanation for its reasons to arrive at a particular result may be regarded as indicative of such a degree of unreasonableness as to invalidate its action.

The conclusion is that any interested party who has demonstrated the necessary *locus standi*,[8] will be unable to assail a RAMS determination of a scale of tariff honestly arrived at, after due consultation (as required by the Act), on the basis of a consideration of the general economic state of the country, what the organised medical profession regards as reasonable remuneration for medical services, the financial resources of the public in general and the proportion thereof that is reasonably affordable for medical services.[9] The fact that certain sophisticated medical services are becoming relatively more expensive because of their "high-tech" basis and that doctors would generally like to be better remunerated for their services, is a factor that must naturally be considered, but is certainly not the only factor in assessing the reasonableness of a determination.

The nature of the contract between a medical scheme and a member, and the rights of the doctor

The question about medical schemes doctors have asked me more frequently than any other, is whether a doctor can sue a scheme for payment (a) of the benefit due to a patient to whom the doctor has attended, or (b) of the benefit payable direct to the doctor. Practitioners sometimes complain that medical schemes generally are, or a particular medical scheme is, slow in paying out benefits.

As far as (a) is concerned, the answer is quite simply "no". Membership of a medical scheme gives rise to a contract[10] between a member and his scheme, the content

5 *Union Government (Minister of Mines and Industries) v Union Steel Corporation (SA) Ltd* 1928 AD 220, 236; compare M Wiechers *Administratiefreg* (2nd ed, 1984) 271.
6 Wiechers 271.
7 *Union Government* case, *supra* note 5.
8 Individual medical practitioners will undoubtedly have *locus standi*, but the *locus standi* of an association of doctors is doubtful (see e g *South African Optometric Association v Frames Distributors (Pty) Ltd t/a Frames Unlimited* 1985 (3) SA 100 (O); *Noll and Others v Alberton Frames (Pty) Ltd and Others* 1989 (1) SA 730 (T)) unless it is the "majority" association referred to in section 29(1) (*c*) of the Act, alleging non-compliance with the duty to consult.
9 In *Triangle Ltd v Sabi-Limpopo Authority* 1978 (1) SA 724 (R) a minister's determination of water rates was successfully attacked on the ground that they were unreasonable because they exceeded the economic objectives of the agreement between him and the body supplying the water. (The decision was upheld on appeal in *Sabi-Limpopo Authority v Triangle Ltd* 1978 (4) SA 313 (RA).)
10 *Meaker N O v Roup, Wacks, Kaminer & Kriger and Another* 1987 (2) SA 54 (C), at 61 G-H.

of which is determined by the provisions of the Medical Schemes Act, the regulations thereunder, the rules of the scheme and any special arrangement legally agreed upon between the member and his scheme. There are only two parties to that contract, the member and the scheme. The doctor is no party to that contract, although he may be the ultimate receiver of a benefit provided for by the scheme which will be paid out to the member.

As regards benefits to the member himself, the contract between the member and the scheme is not even a contract for the benefit of a third party, or *stipulatio alteri* as it is known in legal terminology. Such a contract occurs where two persons enter into an agreement whereby one of them promises to do something for a third party; if the third party knows of the promise and accepts it, he obtains a right of action to enforce it. It is not essential that the acceptance by the third party be formal; it may be inferred from his conduct in the circumstances.[11]

In terms of the Act, a medical scheme is a scheme established with the object of making provision for the obtaining, free of charge, by members of a service as defined, or the granting of assistance to members in defraying expenditure incurred by them in respect of a service.[12] As we know, the Act does not in general impose a duty upon medical schemes to pay direct to a supplier of service. That duty applies in terms of section 32 only in respect of services for which the fees claimed are in accordance with the scale of benefits (except for the situation envisaged in section 32(2)(*b*) which pertains to special Ministerial regulation).

In respect of fees not in accordance with the scale of benefits, medical scheme rules provide for payment of the benefits to the member direct and exclusively, for reasons that are well known and need not be stated now. Although the ultimate object is, of course, that the amount thus paid to the member should be used by him, in addition to the amount that must come from his own pocket to make up the balance of the doctor's fee, there is no question of an agreement whereby the medical scheme promises to "do something" for the doctor. There is, accordingly, no promise which may upon acceptance by the doctor constitute a contractual obligation on the part of the scheme towards the doctor. There is simply no *vinculum juris* ("regsband") between doctor and medical scheme. The only *vinculum juris* is one between member and medical scheme. To the extent that any suing may be called for, it is the member who will have to sue the medical scheme.

A comparison may be made with the situation in an old case on the *stipulatio alteri*, *Baikie v Pretoria Municipality*:[13] Land belonging to an assigned estate was sold by public auction, and it was a condition that arrear rates due to the municipality should be paid by the purchaser. The municipality thereafter attempted to sue the purchaser for the rates, but the court held that the condition was purely to regulate a right as between the purchaser and the seller and it was never intended by them for the benefit of the municipality.

As far as (b) is concerned, i e where the benefit is payable direct to the doctor in terms of section 32(3)(*b*), because his fee is in accordance with the scale of benefits, the situation is somewhat different, in my opinion. Here an obligation arises by statute and not solely by virtue of any contract to which the doctor is or may become a party. (It is not necessary for the doctor to rely on and prove a *stipulatio alteri*. But it would nevertheless appear that there is in fact also a *stipulatio alteri* here. The patient has agreed with the medical scheme that in terms of their contract – the content whereof is co-determined by the Act, the regulations and the scheme's rules – the scheme shall pay direct to the doctor.)

11 Wille and Millin's *Mercantile Law of South Africa* (18th ed (1984) by J F Coaker and D T Zeffertt) 75 *et seq.*

12 Act 72 of 1967, section 1.

13 1921 TPD 376.

In the event of the medical scheme failing to meet its obligation, the doctor will therefore be entitled to sue the scheme. Whether it will serve any useful purpose to issue summons, will of course depend on the circumstances. A scheme with a dilatory tendency will probably be quick to pay once a letter of demand is received, and thus "pre-empt" the service of summons. However, the right of the doctor to bring action against the scheme direct is clearly of practical significance whenever the circumstances are such that a judgment against the debtor, the medical scheme, is desirable for some or other reason.

I shall deal below with the question whether a doctor who obtains no satisfaction of his right to be paid direct by a medical scheme because of its financial inability, will be entitled to recoup his loss from the patient.

In connection with the nature of the agreement between a medical scheme and an employer generally, reference may also be made to the case of *South African Mutual Aid Society v Cape Town Chamber of Commerce*.[14] In that case a medical aid society was keen to limit membership to persons who had been employees of the employer concerned at the stage when the agreement was entered into, and to prevent new employees from becoming members because of an "adverse claims experience". The court held, however, that in terms of the agreement between the parties, the society was compelled to accept new employees as members. The decision turned on the interpretation of the terms of the agreement.

Payment by a scheme of benefit to a person not entitled thereto

The juristic nature of the doctor's right *vis-à-vis* the member of a medical scheme and/or the scheme itself is of practical importance also in cases where a medical scheme mistakenly pays a benefit to someone not entitled thereto.

There may be several reasons for the making of such an undue payment, e g (a) where there is a waiting period and payment is made prior to the person being registered as a member; (b) where a person's membership has terminated and payment is made to him or direct to a doctor before the fact of termination of membership has come to the attention of the scheme, or (c) where there has simply been an erroneous calculation on the part of the medical scheme's personnel and an amount in excess of what is actually due, is paid.

The question is whether the undue payments thus made can be recovered by the medical scheme from the payee, or – if this proves to be difficult for practical reasons – whether the amount paid can be set off by the scheme against future indebtedness that may arise in respect of the payee.

Reclaiming money which has been paid by mistake (liability on the *condictio indebiti*), is not without problems. Decisions of South African courts have stated that payments made under mistake of law are not recoverable. This view has been criticised but must be accepted until it is reversed by the Appellate Division.[15]

Fortunately the law is more lenient in respect of an undue payment made in mistake of fact[16] – which is the case in the three situations that I have mentioned. The payer may recover the payment, provided the mistake was reasonable; where the error is inexcusable, he has no right of recovery. An exception to this rule is that where a person who has received another's money or goods and parts with them in bad faith, he will be liable for repayment. A person who appropriates money and uses it to pay his debts in the knowledge that it is not due to him, in any event makes himself guilty of theft.[17] For that reason alone, it would ordinarily be advisable for the recipient to repay money paid to him in error, without delay.

14 1962 (1) SA 598 (A).

15 Wille & Millin *op cit* 155 *et seq*; compare Carmen Nathan "Check before you write that cheque" *SA Practical Management* 1982 (1) 9.

16 *Ibid.*

17 *S v Graham* 1975 (3) SA 569 (A).

Assuming that a medical scheme has mistakenly paid money in respect of a member, or in respect of someone who is not yet a member or whose membership has terminated, and experiences problems in recovering from the practitioner the amount paid: may the scheme set its claim off against indebtedness that arises at a future date towards the same practitioner in respect of, (a) the same patient, or (b) another patient of that doctor?

As I see it, the possibility of set-off can occur only where the indebtedness of the medical scheme has arisen because of the statutory duty created by section 32(3) to pay the supplier of service direct.

As we have seen a right to recover a payment which was not due but was made in error, can arise only where the mistake of fact was a reasonable or excusable one. If the medical scheme's mistake was unreasonable, e g where it negligently failed to establish whether the patient was still a member before paying the doctor, no indebtedness (to repay) would arise on the part of the latter, so that the legal possibility of set-off against a future indebtedness would not occur at all – be it in respect of the same patient or another.

But if the mistake of the scheme was excusable, e g where the patient concerned had perpetrated a clever fraud towards the scheme, leading its staff to believe that he was still a member whereas in actual fact he was not, a right to recovery would arise, which could undoubtedly be set off against a future indebtedness towards the same doctor, in any event where the same patient was involved.

Set-off ("skuldvergelyking") is a legal process whereby debts which are liquidated (i e having a clearly ascertained or readily or arithmetically ascertainable money value) mutually owed between the same parties, are extinguished.[18] There is a single rider to be added to this: where a protracted and intricate enquiry is necessary before it can be determined whether the debt does in fact exist, the courts will usually not allow set-off. Borderline cases involving a dispute as to whether or not the payer's mistake was reasonable may fall within this category.

Where the future indebtedness arises in respect of the same patient and the earlier mistaken payment was made in excusable error, set-off is undoubtedly permissible. After all, exactly the same (three) parties were involved.

The question whether set-off is permissible where the indebtedness sought to be set off has arisen in respect of another patient, is more problematic. On the face of it, the two parties directly involved are the same, namely the medical scheme and the doctor. The argument may be put forward that the scheme's indebtedness towards the doctor has arisen not *ex contractu* but by reason of a statutory obligation, and that it is therefore irrelevant who the patient is.

My difficulty with that argument is that it is "the truth but not the whole truth". The obligation was not created simply because of the incidental presence of a set of facts as envisaged by the Legislature. As I have said before, a precondition for the obligation to pay the doctor direct, is the existence of a contract between the member concerned and the scheme. It can also be said that a *stipulatio alteri* which is statutorily "co-determined" exists in these cases, and such a *stipulatio* invariably involves three parties.

The better view therefore seems to be that there is not true reciprocity of the parties for the purposes of set-off where the indebtedness arises in respect of another patient. This view is reinforced by consideration of the object of a medical scheme as defined in the Act, section 1 *s v* "medical scheme"; one of the two objects stated is "the granting of assistance to members ... in defraying expenditure incurred by them" in connection with the rendering of any "service" as defined. It can therefore be argued that the adoption of the statutory procedure whereby the practitioner has the right to direct the account to the medical scheme, should not be understood as

18 Wille & Millin *op cit* 165 *et seq*.

undermining the underlying contractual obligation, namely that it is the patient who is indebted to the practitioner, and that payment by the scheme is made *on behalf* of the member in discharge of the scheme's undertaking in favour of the member to defray the expenditure incurred by that member.[19]

It goes without saying that where a medical scheme has applied legally justified set-off in a case of an earlier undue payment to a doctor, the doctor would not be entitled to sue the patient for the amount thus set off. As far as the patient is concerned, the right of the doctor to claim his fee (which has been in accordance with the scale of benefits) has been extinguished by the act of set-off. To put it in simple terms, the debt has been settled, i e paid on behalf of the member, already at the stage when the earlier "excusable" overpayment took place.

What I have said regarding set-off of overpayments made to doctors would apply in an equal measure to undue payments made by a medical scheme to patients.

Non-payment of claims by a medical scheme

Not all medical schemes are equally expeditious when it comes to the payment of claims. The time within which benefits due to members should be paid is fixed in the rules of a medical scheme and thus forms part of the contract between the scheme and the member. In the event of a scheme failing to pay the benefit within the time stipulated, it will be guilty of breach of contract and may be sued by the member.

Where suppliers of a service are entitled to be paid direct, in terms of their statutory right, they are likewise entitled to sue. What is more, their rights are apparently reinforced by a criminal sanction. Because the duty to pay the doctor direct – to the extent that it exists – is imposed by the Act itself, failure by the medical scheme to pay within the statutorily fixed period of six weeks,[20] would seem to constitute a criminal offence.

The Medical Schemes Act is one of those statutory instruments which, in the words of Van den Heever J in *R v Bethlehem Municipality*[21] "bristles with commands and directions" which are then sought to be brought under a "blanket penalty clause" by the Legislature. As is demonstrated by that case, the decision whether or not an omission on the part of a public official would fall within the penalty clause, can depend on rather complex and subtle considerations.

Here, of course, we are not concerned with a public official but with a body that can be described as no more than a "semi-public" organisation. Nevertheless, bearing in mind the considerations stated in that case, it would seem as if a persuasive argument can be presented that failure by a medical scheme to comply with the duty embodied in section 32, read with regulation 11, would fall within the ambit of section 40, the penalty clause.

If that assumption is correct, the next question is: who must put the criminal process in action? The answer is quite simple: any interested party, either the member, the aggrieved doctor, or the registrar of medical schemes. One would assume, however, that resort will be had to the criminal sanction in extreme cases only.

A rather more interesting question is whether a doctor would have a right of recourse against the patient if he (the doctor) got no satisfaction of his claim directly against the medical scheme by virtue of section 32 because of the inability of the scheme to pay, e g on account of insolvency.

As we have seen, a medical scheme is, by definition, a scheme which provides *inter alia* for "the granting of assistance to members thereof in defraying expenditure in-

19 I have had the benefit of seeing a legal opinion given by a colleague, with whom I respectfully agree.
20 Section 32 of the Act read with regulation 11 (4) contained in Government Notice R2768 of 21.12.1984 (*Government Gazette* 9533).
21 1941 OPD 227.

curred by them in connection with the rendering of any service" (as defined). It may therefore be argued that the doctor, in rendering service to a patient, has entered into a contract with the patient and that he would be entitled to look to the patient where the scheme fails to make good the undertaking given on behalf of the patient, which undertaking is given statutory backing by section 32. This line of reasoning is based on the assumption – which I would submit is correct – that the medical scheme in essence acts as the guarantor of payment to the doctor of benefits that are in accordance with the scale of benefits. Any other point of view would lead to the conclusion that the supplier of the service must suffer the loss caused by inability of the scheme to meet its obligations, and that could hardly have been the intention of the Legislature.

It is true, as I have said, that the medical scheme's obligation to pay direct to the doctor flows from statute, but the statutory duty arises only after a contractual relationship has come into being between the scheme and its member.

The effect of non-payment of benefits to members of a medical scheme was considered in *Meaker N O v Roup, Wacks, Kaminez & Kriger and Another*[22], but it is not directly relevant to the point I have just canvassed. In this case it was held that failure of a medical aid society to pay the benefits due to members, entitled the latter to refuse paying their normal contributions to the scheme and also excused them from paying the special levy agreed upon in an endeavour to rescue the scheme from a financial catastrophe. (It was also held that an *employer* who collects and pays over on behalf of its employees to the medical scheme contributions due by the employees, could not set off the claims of the employees for benefits against the contributions due by them to the scheme, for the simple reason that there is no reciprocity of debts between the employer and the scheme.)

Cession of doctor's claim against a medical scheme

It has in the past been a moot point whether suppliers of services may cede their claims against medical schemes.

Cession of book debts by a medical practitioner was the subject of a recent decision by the Appellate Division in *Sasfin (Pty) Ltd v Beukes.*[23]

In that case the doctor, an anaesthetist, entered into a discounting agreement with a finance company in terms of which he ceded, by way of continuing covering security, all "claims, rights of actions and receivables which are now due and which may at any time hereafter become due". The effect of the agreement was that the company was given immediate and effective control of all the doctor's past, present and future professional earnings. The Appeal Court held that an agreement having that effect was "clearly unconscionable and incompatible with the public interest", contrary to public policy and therefore null and void. The court regarded it as "grossly exploitative" of the doctor.

The *Sasfin* case was extreme. It does not affect the validity of *ad hoc* cession of existing debts. But the SA Medical and Dental Council, for obvious reasons, frowns upon cession by a doctor of claims against patients, although pure factoring which does not entail cession, is in order.[24] The ethical considerations applying to claims against patients would seem not to apply to claims against medical schemes.

The draft bill of 1988 which envisaged certain amendments to the Medical Schemes Act also contains a clause which would render cession of claims against a scheme inoperative.

Paper read at the Centenary Conference of the Representative Association of Medical Schemes held in Kimberley in April 1989.

22 *Supra.*
23 1989 (1) SA 1 (A).
24 See below 57.

10 Discounting ("cession") of doctors' accounts and factoring

The following questions were put to me: "Can you explain the ethical and legal considerations involved in the discounting of a doctor's accounts? How does that differ from the financing of a practice's book debts?"

My answer is as follows:

Discounting in the strict sense of the word, in this context, refers to the cession of a claim which a creditor has against a debtor, to a third party, for valuable consideration. The third party "buys" the claim from the creditor for cash at a discount, i e at an amount which is less than the book value of the claim.

The advantage to the creditor (the cedent) is that he gets an immediate cash amount in respect of a claim which may only be paid by the debtor at a future date after considerable pressure on the part of the creditor.

The advantage to the third party (the cessionary), again, is that he may "buy" a perfectly enforceable claim at an amount which is considerably less than the book value thereof, and in this way will make money by collecting the full amount of the claim.

In practical terms it means this: A owes B R100, B cedes his claim to X for a cash amount of R75. B has no further claim against A. X, who has legally stepped into B's shoes, may now claim the full amount from A.

Naturally, X, the cessionary, takes a certain risk. If it appears that A cannot pay the amount and does not have assets against which a judgment for the debt may be executed, he (X) loses on the deal. But where discounting is done on a large scale, X will be able to calculate his risk on the basis of average return and will ensure that the discounting takes place at a rate which is safe to him – safe in the sense that at the end of the day he will make a handsome profit on his gross turnover.

Legally there is nothing wrong with such a scheme,[1] but from the point of view of medical professional ethics extreme caution must be exercised. The SA Medical and Dental Council frowns upon discounting. The Council has resolved that it "was not in favour of the formation of a company to provide financial discounting facilities for ... practitioners ... and considered the formation of a company of this nature undesirable".[2]

The reason for the Council's disapproval is obvious: The company steps into the shoes of the doctor and what has been a doctor-patient relationship becomes a purely financial one. To the company the patient-debtor is a complete stranger and the company knows nothing about the former's personal circumstances. Whereas the doctor in enforcing the patient's debts by legal process may be swayed by considerations of compassion – knowing, for instance, that the patient is in financial straits because of the very illness for which the doctor has treated him – the company may take a rather mercenary, sanguine view of the debtor.

Discounting of accounts must of course be distinguished from the useful schemes of credit management, collection and financing of a practice's book debts, offered by

1 See *Sasfin (Pty) Ltd v Beukes* 1989 (1) SA 1 (A) which is discussed above 56. As was held in that case, cession of debts would be legally null and void only if it is so extreme as to give the cessionary control over all the doctor's past, present and future professional earnings.

2 See 1979 *S Afr Med J* 1011.

certain financial firms (and some chartered accountants) for their professional clients. Discounting of accounts is not at all involved in these schemes.

Firms offering this factoring service have sophisticated computer facilities at their disposal. The firm virtually takes over the practitioner's bookkeeping. Accounts are sent out on the doctor's behalf (but in his own name). A close check is kept on the payment of the accounts and the doctor is regularly furnished with computerised statements indicating in exact terms the financial state of his practice as far as income is concerned.

On the basis of the doctor's total book debts at the stage when he joins the scheme, the firm will make available to him a cash amount which will be in proportion to that total. Continuing financing will thereafter be available to the doctor; this is calculated on a basis whereby almost the entire future monthly turnover is available to him in ready cash. An assessment is made of the doctor's practice and professional status.

The doctor does not cede his accounts to the firm and the firm accordingly does not sue patients for overdue accounts. Where a particular patient's account is overdue, say for six months, the firm will bring it to the attention of the doctor, who will then decide whether or not he will take legal action.

As consideration for these services the firm will negotiate a fee with the doctor which is usually based upon a fixed percentage of his monthly turnover, e g 4 per cent.

It goes without saying that this type of scheme is perfectly legal and in fact provides a very useful service. The practitioner is largely relieved of the burden of financial administration. He saves time and may save on staff. The scheme enables him to concentrate more on his patients and his professional skill, and he may have more time to spend with his family or on recreational pursuits.

As far as the ethical side is concerned, I can see nothing wrong with this type of scheme and that seems to be the generally accepted view in the medical profession. Needless to say, however, the Medical Council is the final arbiter on ethical matters.

11 Collection of debts: the perennial headache

Irrespective of how good the quality of a doctor's services and his bedside manner may be, a certain percentage of medical fees end up as bad debts.

The medical profession, imbued with the spirit of Hippocrates – and used to waiting quite a while before the medical scheme's cheque arrives – is generally very lenient when it comes to the collection of overdue patient fees. There is no reason to suspect that people treat their medical bills with greater reverence than other bills.[1] In fact, some who have been cured of their ailments may tend to put the medical bills near the bottom of the pile, with the electricity and water bill on top – otherwise the municipality cuts off its services! Next comes the garage bill, because the garage man has a lien over his customer's car, unlike the doctor who ordinarily has no object belonging to or supplied to the patient over which he may exercise a legal right of retention – even if it were ethically permissible to retain that object until his bill had been paid.

Since 1988 medical practitioners have been permitted by the SA Medical and Dental Council[2] to charge interest on overdue accounts, subject to the following conditions:

- a doctor may, within reason, decide the duration of the period after which he will begin charging interest;[3]
- interest may be levied only if the doctor has an agreement to that effect with his patient;[4]
- the rate of interest may not exceed such rate as is determined by the Minister of Justice (the current[5] rate being 18 per cent);
- prior to the treatment, the patient must have been provided with an indication of the costs involved;
- in the event of a matter referred to the Council the charging of interest shall be suspended until the Council has finalised the matter.

Since a high percentage of medical practices operate on an overdraft facility, practitioners actually end up financing those patients who are overdue with the payment of their accounts.[6] It is only fair that doctors should be able to charge an interest on such accounts and to some extent the decision of the SAMDC to allow this, has eased the financial burden of practitioners.

The adding of interest to accounts will have the effect of encouraging at least a percentage of patients to be more expeditious in settling their accounts. But there will always be debtors who simply do not come up with the money. Some of them are

1 See article by P Edwards *S A Practice Management* vol 7 No 4 (1986) 15.
2 See *SAGTR/SAMDC Bulletin* No 4 (June 1988) 2.
3 The original policy of the SAMDC was that interest could be levied only after 90 days had elapsed from the date of the service. The ruling set out in the text was made in April 1991. See *MASA News* 79 *S Afr Med J* (1.6.1991) ix.
4 *Ibid.*
5 February 1991.
6 Edwards *op cit.*

genuinely hard up, some are merely negligent in attending to their financial affairs, some are chancers, and there may be a few who harbour a grudge against the doctor.

Not all debtors will be sensitive to red stickers on the third or consecutive accounts to the effect that "this account might have escaped your attention" or "this account is long overdue and settlement is urgently requested". An effective method to get some recalcitrant payers to settle their account, may be a personal letter or telephone call to the debtor by the doctor's receptionist, bookkeeper or wife, or even the doctor himself, requesting payment.

But when all this has been said and done, there will still be a hard core of non-payers. The doctor's state of mind will not be improved by the knowledge that where his fees exceed the scale of benefits, many of these patients would already have received their medical scheme benefits in hard cash a long time ago.

The time has now arrived for the doctor to consider taking legal action against his debtors by handing over the outstanding accounts to his attorney for collection. Unfortunately there is no guarantee that the attorney, taking all steps that the law permits, will succeed in collecting all outstanding debts. Some debtors will be in such dire financial straits that legal steps in the form of summons, the taking of a judgment by default and the issuing of a warrant of execution against their property, will be of no avail. "As with all remedies", Carmen Nathan[7] aptly states, "there can never be absolute certainty of a cure, and on occasion, the bitter pill of an attorney's statement of account instead of a cheque must be swallowed."[8]

Therefore, continues Nathan, be selective in the matters which you hand over for collection. Attorneys charge for professional services rendered irrespective of results. If you know for sure or have every reason to believe that there is little prospect of success, do not hand the matter over for collection. Your attorney may reach the same conclusion at your expense. Aim to keep costs at a minimum. Certain costs (attorneys' fees and expenses) can be recovered from debtors. These costs are listed in a schedule and are known as party and party costs. Examples of such costs currently allowed in undefended matters are:[9]

❑ registered letter of demand	R6
❑ summons for claims less than R1 500	R30
❑ judgment for claims less than R1 500	R30
❑ sheriff's fee for service within 6 km of court	R10
❑ issue of warrant of execution	R19,50
❑ arranging sale in execution	R45

In addition, the attorney charges a small instruction fee as well as a commission of 10 per cent on all amounts collected.[10] He will deduct this commission from any amount collected before he pays over the money to his client. Where an attorney has taken steps against a debtor and the debtor requests to settle the outstanding amount by way of instalments, the attorney may, on behalf of his client, agree to allow that, subject to an undertaking on the part of the debtor to pay the collection commission. The Medical Association of South Africa recommends that doctors – in an effort to

7 *S A Practice Management* vol 6 No 2 (1985) 24.

8 A classical example of what may go wrong in a collection case is to be found in *De la Rey's Transport (Edms) Bpk v Lewis* 1978 (1) SA 797 (A). An (apparently) simple claim instituted in the magistrate's court for R35 led to a counterclaim. The case ultimately landed in the Appeal Court. Before its determination, it was adjudicated by a magistrate and no fewer than twelve judges!

9 See tariff embodied in the Magistrates' Court Rules.

10 In the Transvaal, for example, the instruction fee ranges from R5 for claims up to R200 to R100 for claims above R5 000; R6 is charged for each necessary letter and attendance; R15 is charged per 10 minutes of each necessary consultation with a debtor. As far as the commission is concerned, the maximum is R50 per instalment collected. See Transvaal Law Society Rules as amended, and Randell & Bax, *SA Attorneys Handbook* (3rd ed, 1983).

avoid eventual attorney's costs or to at least minimise these – incorporate in forms completed by new patients, a clause in terms of which the patient undertakes to pay attorney's costs if legal steps become necessary. This is good advice.

As Nathan has pointed out, attorneys will ordinarily not charge more than the tariff in collection matters. "However, if the service rendered warrants a higher fee, they are fully entitled to charge accordingly. A fee over and above party and party costs is known as an attorney and client fee, i e it cannot be recovered from the other party. A great deal of an average attorney's time is spent on the telephone. This is part and parcel of his work and an attorney who finds it necessary to telephone an instructing doctor for particulars concerning a debtor (for example, full names and addresses), would be fully justified in marking a fee. There is nothing in the tariff which makes provision for such a fee in an undefended matter and it could therefore not be recovered from the debtor. To keep costs to a minimum, give your attorney written instructions and include all the particulars available about the debtor."

The system of small claims courts introduced into South Africa since 1985, which makes provision for "lawyerless" and therefore almost costless adjudication of civil cases, was not really designed to serve as a vehicle for debt collecting. The Small Claims Court Act[11] says a summons may not be delivered in respect of a claim arising from a business or profession until a previous case by the same plaintiff has resulted in judgment. Because it may take several weeks or even months from the date of the sending of a letter to a debtor until judgment is delivered, debt collecting *en masse* by means of suing in the small claims court is altogether impracticable.

An alternative to handing over a debt to an attorney for collection, is to hand it over to a collection agency. There are some very efficient agencies in the country, but be careful in deciding upon an agency to handle your collections. I do not wish to generalise, but practices applied by certain agencies are of doubtful legality. A collecting agency can agree with his client (the creditor) that the latter will pay it a specified commission on amounts collected by way of remuneration for its services. However, it may not – in the absence of an agreement with the debtor – simply add commissions and "collection costs" to the doctor's account and pressurise the debtor to pay these. I have seen threatening letters by a certain collection agency to a patient in which the total amount claimed was almost double what the doctor's fee amounted to after "collection costs" were added.

If a doctor knowingly allows such a collection practice to be conducted, he will incur the SAMDC's displeasure. The Council's attitude is that a doctor in principle assumes responsibility for the conduct of his collection agency. If the agency's conduct and procedures are reprehensible and can lead to exploitation of the debtor-patient, the doctor will be held ethically accountable. It is regarded as unethical for a doctor to cede ("sell") his book debts to a collection agency or any other person.[12]

In 1990 the MASA resolved that doctors are allowed to become involved in debt collecting enterprises themselves subject to certain conditions:

- the doctor must retain control over his accounts at all times;
- no collection fees may be added to a patient's account;
- a medical practitioner may not conduct a debt-collecting enterprise on the same premises as those of his consulting rooms;
- a medical practitioner may not enter into a partnership agreement with a debt-collecting agency irrespective of the premises from which the agency is conducted;
- a member of the staff of a medical practitioner may collect his debts on his behalf, provided he retains control over his accounts.

11 Act 61 of 1984, section 29(1)(*b*).

12 See above 57. As we have seen, however, factoring *per se*, which does not involve cession, is a permissible practice.

For the professional man, the collection of debts is an unpleasant and time-wasting exercise at the best of times. It is nevertheless an aspect of practice management that must be attended to. If a professional person is too "soft" on his debtors – apart from those cases in which he decides for humanitarian reasons rather to abandon claims – he will soon acquire a reputation that his accounts can be dodged with impunity. This will lead to exploitation of the doctor.

A final word: There will always be those debtors who apparently vanish from the face of the earth without settling their debts. If a substantial sum is outstanding in respect of a particular debtor, it may be worth the expense and effort to try and trace him with the help of tracing agents. Collection agencies may have their own tracing agents. But do enquire in advance precisely what the cost of tracing a debtor will be. Where a relatively small amount is the issue the game will usually not be worth the candle.[13]

13 77 *S Afr Med J* (17/3/1990) *SAMJ News* p xxiv.

12 Is "blacklisting" of patients who have a record of bad debts permissible?

The following question was put to me: A group of doctors in a particular city are investigating the possibility of setting up a "blacklist" of patients with a record of bad debts. The blacklist is envisaged for patients with accounts which after 5 to 6 months remain unpaid and who do not heed requests or threats. Among these are those patients who go from doctor to doctor without paying their accounts – the so-called "travellers".

The blacklist is not intended for those patients who for good reasons have accounts which remain unpaid for a long period. What the doctors have in mind is this:

- The patient receives a letter together with his account in which he is cautioned to pay his account within 30 days or to make arrangements for payment by means of instalments which must be mutually agreed upon.
- He is cautioned that unless he complies with this demand his name will be put on a blacklist which will be made available to all doctors. This will have the effect that medical services will be refused to him and his family – except in emergency situations – until such time as he has made arrangements to settle his account.
- He is cautioned to get in touch with the accounts office if he does not agree with the particulars on his account.
- If he does not make arrangements for payment, his name is sent to a central office and he is notified that his name was sent.
- These names are made available in pocket-book form to doctors who wish to subscribe to it. The names of present and new patients are compared with those on the list. If the patient's name appears on the list, he must make arrangements for payment of his account or settle it. If he does so he is issued with a ticket which he may show in order to obtain medical services. If he cannot show such a ticket, only emergency services are rendered.

What are the legal ramifications of the proposed scheme?

My answer is: The proposed scheme amounts to a boycott of patients with a bad record of paying their accounts. Unfortunately boycott as such has received scant attention only by South African courts.[1] Our courts will probably approach a scheme such as this from the angle of whether or not it amounts to an actionable "interference with trade, business or employment".

A leading South African case is *Tothill v Gordon*:[2] The plaintiff was a retail chemist and druggist carrying on business in Johannesburg. The defendants were members of the executive committee of the Transvaal Chemists' and Druggists' Association.

1 See H J O van Heerden & J Neethling *Die Reg aangaande Onregmatige Mededinging* (1983) 189 *et seq*. As the authors have indicated, *primary boycott*, i e refusal on the part of a person to enter into a contract with another, is usually not unlawful (compare *Times Media Ltd v South African Broadcasting Corporation* 1990 (4) SA 604 (W)). *Secondary boycott*, i e an organised effort to withdraw and induce others to withdraw from business relations with another, on the other hand will be unlawful unless the actor acts in the protection of a legitimate interest. On boycott in general, see also N E Wiehahn *Boikot as Onregmatige Daad* (LLD thesis, Univ of South Africa, 1974).

2 1930 WLD 99.

One of the objects of the Association was to regulate the prices at which goods should be sold by chemists and druggists in the Transvaal.

The plaintiff was not a member of the Association and he was therefore not bound by the scale of minimum prices and charges laid down by it. The court held that it was not illegal for the defendants to place the plaintiff's name on a "stop-list", that is, a list published to the members of the Association of persons to whom by the rules of the Association it was forbidden to supply goods; nor was it illegal for them *bona fide* to attempt to induce third persons not to supply goods to the plaintiff.

The court intimated that the defendants' conduct might have been unlawful if their intention was not to further any legitimate business interests of their own but solely to injure the plaintiff. The touchstone, therefore, seems to be malice.[3]

McKerron,[4] an authoritative South African author on delict, contended that interference with the trade or calling of another is not unlawful and therefore not actionable unless the defendant either uses illegal means or was actuated by malice. Examples of illegal means are injurious falsehood, inducement of breach of contract, or infringement of copyright.

In *Tothill's* case the court relied *inter alia* on the following statement from an English decision:[5] "If the real purpose of the combination is, not to injure another, but to forward or defend the trade of those who enter into it, then no wrong is committed and no action will lie, although damage to another ensues."

The "blacklisting" of patients is clearly not malicious in the sense that it is designed to make life difficult for defaulting patients without promoting any reasonable interest of the doctors. On the contrary, the doctors seek to protect their own financial interests and are at pains to ensure that defaulting patients will nonetheless receive emergency treatment. This seems to be a benevolent approach considering the fact that from a legal point of view a doctor, generally speaking, is a free agent who can ordinarily decide whether or not he wishes to treat any particular patient.[6]

For many years a publication in which the names of all persons against whom civil judgments have been given, has been published in South Africa and circularised among business and professional men. An association of advocates has also on occasion blacklisted attorneys who failed to pay their fees, the members undertaking to refuse briefs from such attorneys.

It is therefore submitted that the proposed scheme is not unlawful.[7]

A real danger in circularising names of defaulting patients would arise where a patient is erroneously described as a bad debtor. This could lead to an action for defamation.[8] The utmost care must therefore be taken that the information in the list is correct.

Concluding that the scheme is not *unlawful* in the sense that promoters thereof will not make themselves guilty of a criminal offence or expose themselves to a delictual action (which may lead to liability for damages for a civil wrong) is not the end of the matter though. Because the participants will be doctors, there may be *ethical* considerations involved, which should be carefully considered.

In the past, when the SA Medical and Dental Council was requested to pronounce on comparable schemes whereby doctors would collectively have informed defaulting patients that no further credit would be available, or whereby a commercial

3 *Tothill's* case was criticised by Van Heerden & Neethling *op cit* 194 *et seq*.
4 R G McKerron *The Law of Delict* (7th ed, 1971) 272.
5 *Sorrell v Smith* [1925] AC 700 at 712.
6 But see the qualifications to the general rule which I discuss above 23 *et seq*.
7 The scheme presently discussed is clearly distinguishable from the type of boycott that formed the subject of the decision in *Hawker v Life Offices Association of South Africa and Another* 1987 (3) SA 777 (C) and which was unacceptable in that it would have made it difficult for the individual affected by it to earn a living.
8 See J M Burchell *The Law of Defamation in South Africa* (1985) 123-5.

agency would have circularised among doctors the names of regular defaulters, the Council took no stand as concerned the scheme *per se*; the Council did emphasise, however, that although a practitioner was at liberty to decide whom he would treat and whom not, "the doctor could be called upon to justify his conduct, should unnecessary suffering or death flow from his refusal to attend to a patient". Moreover, the Council warned, "in cases of emergency a practitioner is in all circumstances obliged to render assistance".[9]

In 1990, however, the Council emphatically ruled[10] that a blacklisting scheme was ethically unacceptable because it "could be detrimental to the doctor-patient relationship". The ruling was in response to an enquiry by a medical practitioner. He had suggested that doctors who wanted to solve the problem of bad debtors would either have to practise on a "cash only" basis or do extensive credit reference checks on patients before taking them on to their books. Both methods, he said, could be effective but were potentially harmful to the doctor-patient relationship. Apart from that, reference checks were time-consuming, expensive and required more personnel. According to the proposed medical credit-control system, participating practices would report their bad debtors to a credit-control company, which would inform patients and urge them to settle the matter. Patients who failed to reply to notifications would be placed on the listing as bad credit risks and the list would thereafter be distributed to participating practices. It was this scheme that the Council disapproved of.

The conclusion: blacklisting of patients who have a record of bad debts is ethically impermissible.

9 See SAMDC ruling made in March 1964, reported in the Council's *Codification of Previous Rulings in Ethical Matters* vol 3, 203; a similar ruling was given by the Council's Executive Council in 1985.

10 The ruling was reported in *SAMDC/SAGTR Bulletin* No 7 (Feb 1990) 3.

13 Doctor requested by third party to attend patient: who must pay doctor's fees?

The question was put to me, who is legally responsible for payment of a doctor's fees in the following situations?

- An employer calls a doctor to his home for the treatment of a domestic servant. Who is responsible for payment of the doctor's account: the employer or the servant? It happens in practice that the servant maintains that the employer is responsible, but later, when the doctor submits his account, the employer's attitude is that the servant is responsible, refuses to settle the account, and it transpires that the servant has left him in the meantime.
- A grandmother calls her doctor to see her grandchild who is staying with her. The child's parents are alive and working. Is the grandmother responsible for the account?
- A father calls his doctor to attend his son. The son is an adult and is working. Is the father responsible for the account? In both the latter cases the doctor answered the calls only because he was called by his patients. He would have refused to go out had he been called by the grandchild's parents or by the son himself; the doctor would have insisted that they call their own doctor.
- A woman calls her doctor. In the very recent past, her husband (who now lives apart from her) paid her medical accounts. Now the husband, all of a sudden, informs the doctor that he is separated from his wife and refuses to pay. Must the wife pay her own account? (The husband left the matrimonial home and the spouses are not yet divorced.)

My answer is: Whether the person who calls in a doctor to attend another is responsible for the doctor's account, would depend on the parties' intention. In the absence of an express undertaking the intent must be inferred from the surrounding circumstances. One must therefore look at the facts of each individual case and on the basis of common sense try to come to a conclusion.

Generally speaking, a person who summons a doctor to attend a patient, does not thereby make himself liable to pay the fees. *Prima facie* the patient is always liable, but as Price[1] has pointed out, a third party may become liable in one of two ways (in the absence of an express undertaking to pay the doctor's account):

1. His conduct may be such as to suggest to a reasonable man that he is prepared to accept responsibility for the fees. "Such conduct must be very clear, for the presumption that a third party is accepting responsibility for medical attendance to another is one that will not easily arise. Thus, the mere fact that a master calls in a doctor to attend a servant does not in itself suggest that he is accepting responsibility for the doctor's fees. There must be some definite indication to that effect before he can be held liable."

   In the case of *Crook v Griqualand West DM Co*,[2] a servant of a mining company in Kimberley was injured in the course of his employment, by a fall of ground.

1 Gordon, Turner & Price *Medical Jurisprudence* (3rd ed, 1953) 76.
2 (1886) 4 HCG 16.

The managing director of the company called a doctor to attend him and was held to be liable for the latter's fees. It appeared that the company had been in the habit of sending for the same doctor in similar circumstances and had paid his fees for attendance.

In the case of *Argus P & P Co v Van Niekerk*,[3] an employee of a printing establishment was injured while at work in the printing room. A director of the company called the doctor in to render medical assistance. The court held that the company was liable for the doctor's account. The judge laid down as a general principle that "when a director of a company causes a doctor to be called in to render professional assistance to an employee of the company, who has been injured in its service, there are reasonable grounds for the doctor to suppose that the company makes itself responsible for his fees".[4]

2. The third party may be held liable by operation of law. This will occur where the third party is compelled by law to support the patient. In such a case he is liable to defray the cost of necessary medical attention, provided that the patient himself is not in a position to do so.[5] Thus a parent must support his child (who may even contract as "agent" of the father with the doctor)[6] and a husband his wife. In certain circumstances the duty arises for a child to support his parents or for a wife to support her husband. The duty to support may even extend to grandparents[7] who are unable to maintain themselves, although today that would be unusual, in view of the State's old age pension scheme.

Another example given by Price,[8] of liability for medical care arising by operation of law, is the Workmen's Compensation Act,[9] under which certain employers may be liable to defray the costs of medical care given to a workman injured in the course of his employment.

To come back to the individual situations mentioned above: Where the employer has not in any way intimated that he would accept liability for the doctor's fees in respect of the servant (whose illness is not related to his employment), the doctor must look to the servant for payment.

The same applies in my opinion to the grandmother. Unless she expressly undertook to pay the account, the doctor will have to seek payment from the child's father. It may be argued that the grandmother acted as implied agent for the father in seeking medical aid. Another legal ground on which the doctor may hold the father liable, is *negotiorum gestio* (unauthorised administration). This is the legal principle whereby a person may in the absence of another, take positive action in administering the former's affairs. It is a common-law duty for a parent to provide adequate maintenance for his child, and this includes reasonable medical aid. It may be argued that in the absence of the parent, the doctor acted as *gestor*, and is entitled to reasonable remuneration for his services.

Where a father calls a doctor to attend his major, working son, there is no question that the doctor must look to the son for payment. A request by a parent to attend an adult child certainly does not create an implied contract on the part of the parent to pay for the services rendered by the doctor. The parent can be held liable only where

3 (1895) 2 OR 40.
4 Compare *Fulls v Mollentz* (1896) 13 SC 369. This was a case where the servant called in the doctor. He had been injured in his work, which was to cork bottles for his employer, V & Co. A bottle broke in his hand. The court held that in the absence of a request on the part of the employer, there is no contract between the latter and the doctor. The servant was liable for payment.
5 Price *op cit* 76.
6 P Q R Boberg *The Law of Persons and the Family* (1977) 584 n 17. And see above 7.
7 Boberg 275 n 93.
8 *Op cit* 76, 848.
9 Act 30 of 1941.

the circumstances are such as to reasonably justify the doctor to believe that the parent intends to pay.[10]

As far as the estranged couple are concerned: a husband is ordinarily responsible by virtue of matrimonial law to maintain his wife and that includes the duty to provide necessary medical services. In the ordinary course of events the husband is responsible for services rendered to his wife and she can bind him as against a doctor treating her.

Where the parties become estranged, the situation becomes somewhat complicated. If the common household has broken up through no fault of the wife, the husband's duty of maintenance remains.[11] Thus where the husband has driven his wife away by assaulting her or constantly ill-treating or insulting her, she will still be entitled to bind him in respect of reasonable expenses incurred for her maintenance, such as the cost of necessary medical treatment. But where the wife through her conduct – e g by refusing her husband marital rights, by being unduly intimate with other men or by making life with her generally unbearable – has caused the husband to leave, his duty of maintenance is suspended. The doctor is in a rather unsatisfactory position here: how can he assess the merits of the matrimonial dispute?

From a practical point of view, if the woman gives him information to the effect that the husband would *prima facie* seem to be the guilty party, he (the doctor) would be entitled to try and obtain payment from the husband. Should the husband refuse to pay, however, the doctor will have to decide how far he is prepared to push the matter. An unsuccessful action for a small fee may be a costly exercise.

In such a situation, the doctor would be wise, before rendering services, to agree expressly with the woman that should the husband refuse payment, she will be responsible for his account.

10 *Broadway v Jeffers* 194 SE 642 (South Carolina, 1938), and see C J Stetler & A R Moritz *Doctor and Patient and the Law* (4th ed 1962) 59.

11 This principle of common law – see *Behr v Minister of Health* 1961 (1) SA 629 (SR) – has nothing to do with the old divorce regime which existed prior to the Divorce Act 70 of 1979 taking effect, whereby "malicious desertion" (which could also assume the form of "constructive desertion") constituted a ground for divorce. See also H R Hahlo *South African Law of Husband and Wife* (4th ed, 1975) 178-179. It is to be noted that under the Divorce Act the basic ground of divorce is irretrievable breakdown of the marital relationship and that guilt on the part of the defendant need no longer be proved. Guilt is nevertheless not irrelevant and may affect issues such as maintenance and the divorce court's order as to costs. The position stated in the text is, therefore, unaffected by the Divorce Act.

14 May a dentist claim a fee for a denture from a dissatisfied patient?

The following problem was put by a dentist: "My understanding is that a fee for dentures cannot be recovered from the patient unless he is satisfied with the denture. What is the position if the patient says he is dissatisfied, but expert evidence indicates that the denture is clinically satisfactory?

"Does the same principle apply to crowns and bridges?

"The fee for denture work has been divided into professional and laboratory fees. Under the Medical Schemes Act the fee for treatment involving dental technicians is separated. Can the professional fee, i e for the dentist's services as opposed to the cost of the denture itself, be claimed from the patient even if he is dissatisfied with the denture?"

My answer is as follows: Even where a dentist has not given the patient an express guarantee of absolute satisfaction with his work, the dentist will have difficulties in recovering his fee – or at least his full fee – from the patient in the event of unsatisfactory work.

It is a principle of our law that where a contractor, such as a builder, has largely completed the work in accordance with his contract, but in some respects it is defective or incomplete, he cannot recover the full contract price but only a reduced amount.[1]

Legally speaking, the contract entered into by doctor and patient, would seem to be of the same type as that between builder and house-owner, i e *locatio conductio operis* ("the letting and hiring of work").[2]

As far as the dentist is concerned, however, there is a somewhat complicating factor, because the Transvaal Supreme Court decided in 1910 (in the case of *Tulloch v Marsh*[3]) that where a dentist supplies a denture to a patient, the transaction legally amounts to a sale and not to a letting and hiring of services.

One of the interesting implications of this ruling is that the equitable relief of the dentist claiming a reduced amount for the work done by him, irrespective of its shortcomings, does not apply in respect of dentures. (It was held by the Supreme Court that this principle does not apply to a transaction of sale[4] – a decision which, incidentally, has been criticised.[5])

I do not intend going into all the technical ramifications of the latter decision. Suffice it to say that the patient (the purchaser) who complains of a patently defective denture would be entitled to reject it, cancel his contract and claim damages for the breach of contract on the part of the dentist (the seller). In practical terms this means that the dentist gets back the denture and the patient does not pay the dentist's fee

1 *Hauman v Nortje* 1914 AD 293; *B K Tooling (Edms) Bpk v Scope Precision Engineering (Edms) Bpk* 1979 (1) SA 391 (A). Compare Wille & Millin *Mercantile Law of South Africa* (18th ed, 1984) 124. (As is pointed out by Wille & Millin, this principle was known as *quantum meruit*, prior to the *B K Tooling* case.) The reduction in the price is by an amount equivalent to the sum which would enable the contracting party to complete the work in exact accordance with the contract.

2 See E Kahn *Contract and Mercantile Law through the Cases* (1971) 316; Gordon, Turner and Price *Medical Jurisprudence* (3rd ed, 1953) 75. Cf *S v Progress Dental Laboratory (Pty) Ltd and Another* 1965 (3) SA 192 (T) 195 E-F.

3 1910 TPD 453; cf *S v Progress Dental Laboratory (Pty) Ltd and Another supra, loc cit.*

4 See *SA Wood Turning Mills (Pty) Ltd v Price Bros (Pty) Ltd* 1962 (4) SA 263 (T).

5 See Kahn *op cit* 377.

for supplying and fitting (or rather misfitting!) the denture at all. In the case of a latent defect, again, the patient would be entitled to either claim rescission of the contract,[6] or retain the denture and claim a reduction on its price.[7] These legal remedies are available to the patient even if the dentist did not expressly guarantee the patient satisfaction.

However, a rider must be added: if the patient retains the denture he will not be able to resist a claim for the full fee of the dentist,[8] unless he has given the latter a reasonable opportunity of adjusting the denture. If he has not done this, he is liable for payment of the full amount. Only once the patient has done this and the denture is still defective, would he have the legal remedies I have mentioned.[9]

The *Tulloch* decision was interpreted by dentists as meaning that a fee cannot be recovered unless the patient is satisfied with the denture. It was further maintained that the patient need only pay if he is (subjectively) satisfied in spite of expert evidence to the effect that the denture is satisfactory from a clinical point of view.

The first of these two views may be conditionally supported. If the denture is materially defective, the patient need not pay, provided he refuses to accept the denture.[10]

Whether or not the denture is so defective, however, is a matter of evidence. The subjective satisfaction or dissatisfaction of the patient is a factor, but a factor only. Expert evidence that the denture is clinically satisfactory, might well convince a court that the dentist duly performed what he had undertaken to perform – to apply reasonable skill in providing a denture which "objectively" fits – and that his work is therefore not defective, despite the fact that the patient is not happy with the result.

Do the same principles apply to crowns and bridges? In my opinion it is difficult to conceive of a sale in these cases. In the case of a denture, a separate "movable" (or "removable") object is delivered to the patient. But in the case of a crown or a bridge, the object is firmly (and, hopefully, permanently!) attached to the patient's jaw. The contract seems to be essentially one of services being rendered and should legally be treated as such.

Does the fact that under the Medical Schemes Act[11] the fee for treatment involving dental mechanicians is separate, make any difference in regard to the practical effects of the *Tulloch* decision? In particular, does it mean that where the denture is not to the satisfaction of the patient, the dentist can at least claim the fee for his professional services in taking the patient's impression and fitting the denture, as opposed to what the dental mechanician must be paid?

In my opinion the answer is no. If the providing of a denture is legally seen as a sale, it would seem that whatever fee the dentist charges when he ultimately delivers the denture, must be seen as the purchase price.

I would, however, respectfully doubt the correctness of the *Tulloch* decision in categorising the transaction as a sale. In my opinion it is today essentially a transaction in the nature of "a letting and hiring of services". My guess is that the technique in preparing the patient and taking his impression in order to have a denture made to size, in the year 1991 is a job which is more sophisticated and involves a technique superior to the selection from stock, as it were, of "false teeth" in the year 1910. In the USA, incidentally, it was expressly held that the dentist is not in the category of "a salesman of false teeth".[12] However, until overruled by another court in future, the *Tulloch* rule will remain in South Africa.

6 See Wille & Millin *op cit* 242 *et seq.*
7 *Ibid* 199.
8 *Oats v Niland* 1914 CPD 976.
9 *Kruger v Boltman* 1933 PH A3 (E). Compare *Shiels v Minister of Health* 1974 (3) SA 276 (RAD) which concerned an artificial leg.
10 *Sutherland v White* 1911 EDL 407.
11 Act 72 of 1967.
12 *Cox v Cartwright* 121 NE 2d 673 (Ohio), quoted by L B Wood *A Handbook of Dental Malpractice* (1967) 65.

PART III

Contracts between doctors

15 Drawing up a partnership agreement: some points to bear in mind

The first thing a doctor should establish when he contemplates setting up or joining a partnership, is whether he really wishes to practise in partnership and whether a different form of association with the prospective partner would not be preferable.

Partnership has distinct advantages but it also has distinct disadvantages.[1] The essence of partnership is that the parties pool their capital resources and labour, and share in both the profits and losses of their enterprise. The advantage of such a set-up is continuous mutual consultation as between the partners, whereby the knowledge and experience of each may be fully utilised. There is also the possibility of continuation of professional services during the absence of a partner on account of ill-health or leave.

On the other hand partnership poses a certain risk: if any of the partners does not display the expected ardour or competency, the others will suffer on account of that, not only because they are unhappy that they must work harder, and earn relatively less than the incompetent partner, but because the ultimate profit to be shared will be smaller.

In the event of a partnership estate becoming insolvent, it may have drastic consequences for individual partners. If the court sequestrates the estate of a partnership, it must simultaneously sequestrate the estate of every member of the partnership (except where a partner has undertaken to pay the debts of the partnership).[2] L Hodes[3] advises practitioners who wish to enter into any economic activity outside the partnership – such as owning a farm or clinic – to do this through a separate close corporation or private company where liability can be limited to the amount of money the members or shareholders invest in or lend to the corporation or company.

An important legal aspect of partnership that must be borne in mind, is that one partner is vicariously liable for the wrongful act of another when such act falls within the scope of the partnership business.[4] This means that if a doctor who is a member of a partnership negligently harms a patient, the partnership as such will incur liability for damages. In the absence of any agreement to the contrary, partners share in the losses in their joint business in the same proportion as they do in the profits.[5]

For these reasons – and for others, such as the desire for a greater degree of independence – many doctors nowadays prefer to practise in a looser form of association. A favourite form of "associate practice" is room-sharing agreements, whereby facilities such as the suite of consulting rooms, office equipment, reception and accounting facilities and staff, and specialised medical equipment are shared, but there is no sharing of profit and loss.

1 See, generally, S A Strauss & M J Strydom *Die Suid-Afrikaanse Geneeskundige Reg* (1967) 123 *et seq*; L Hodes "Legal and tax advantages of a partnership" 1985 *SAPM* No 3, 4.
2 Insolvency Act 24 of 1936, s 13(1). It is to be noted, however, that the sequestration of an individual partner's own estate does not result in the sequestration of the *partnership* estate, although it must be liquidated. Sequestration of a partner's own estate also has the effect that the partnership is dissolved. See De Wet & Yeats *Kontraktereg en Handelsreg* (4th ed, 1978) 410, 527.
3 See article cited in note 1.
4 *Lindsay and Others v Stofberg NO* 1988 (2) SA 462 (C).
5 Wille and Millin's *Mercantile Law of South Africa* (18th ed, 1984, by Coaker and Zeffertt) 531.

As S W L de Villiers[6] has pointed out, such a room-sharing arrangement may nevertheless legally amount to a partnership in so far as their room-sharing activities are concerned.

In the majority of cases, the advantages inherent in partnership certainly outweigh the risk attached thereto. If a doctor, having weighed the pros and cons, opts for a partnership, there are, however, a number of points which he should bear in mind.

So often prospective partners join forces on the basis of a simple, verbal agreement of fifty-fifty pooling of assets and labour, and profit-sharing in the same ratio. Such a relationship may last happily for many years, perhaps forever, but should a serious dispute at any stage arise, it may be extremely difficult for the parties to resolve the dispute in an orderly fashion.

No doctor should enter into partnership without a properly drawn partnership contract. The partners should not attempt to draft the deed themselves, but should have it done by an experienced attorney. In practice one of the prospective partners would ordinarily ask his attorney to draft the contract, which is then submitted to the others for signature. This could have the effect that the contract is not representative of all parties' wishes; an attorney's job, after all, is to look primarily after the interests of his own client.

I would therefore unhesitatingly recommend to prospective partners – especially if they are relatively inexperienced – to have the draft deed vetted independently by their own attorneys, before signing it. Insistence upon this can by no means be said to be "unfriendly" or "tactless". The parties may incur a bit of extra expense in the form of attorneys' fees, but it is "preventive medicine" in the legal field, and may in the long run save the partners thousands of rands and a lot of mental anguish.

Bearing in mind what I have remarked on the vicarious liability of partners for civil wrongs, it would certainly be advisable for professional persons who enter into a partnership to insist that each of them take out insurance against professional liability (or, in the case of doctors, to take out membership of a medical protection society).

An aspect which must be thrashed out very carefully in the deed of partnership is the contribution of capital, property or assets by the respective partners. This can be a complex matter, particularly where a young practitioner joins an old, established partnership. In the latter case the capital contributed by the joining partner may be specified as payments made in fixed instalments over a period of years. If these payments are to be made to a partnership in which the partners equally share the profits, such an arrangement practically amounts to the more senior partners *pro rata* drawing a greater share of the profits than the new partner. The capital contribution made by a new partner may of course also be expressed in terms of a provision whereby his share in the net profit will be smaller, over a specified period of years, than that of senior partners.

As Hirsh[7] has pointed out, where assets belonging to an individual partner may be used by the partnership, it is neither necessary nor always desirable for such assets to be brought into the partnership as capital. Thus a radiologist may find it advisable to rent his own equipment to the partnership. There are also income tax implications which must be carefully considered.

It may be advisable to avoid fixed property, e g a medical building, being brought into a partnership as capital. Should the partnership possess its own building, problems may arise when a partner dies or leaves the partnership, or when a new partner joins. In the latter case, making a *pro rata* contribution to assets of considerable value may present the new partner with a serious obstacle. One solution in regard to fixed property is for the existing partners, or a group of them, to form a company ("pty ltd")

6 "Sharing of Consulting Rooms", paper read at the Fourth International Symposium on Forensic Medicine, Pretoria, May 1976. The paper is reproduced below 77–8.

7 B D Hirsh "The Medical Partnership" 13 *De Paul L Rev* 28 (1963) 32.

or close corporation ("cc") which purchases the property and rents it to the partnership.[8] The tax implications of such a step are likewise deserving of close attention.

The capital contribution of a joining partner may be calculated on the basis of the goodwill of the practice. There is no absolute formula by means of which the value of the goodwill can be established. That value is relative to factors such as the scope of the practice, the amount of competition, the question whether the practice is situated in a developing or stagnant community, the type of patient drawn by the "old" partner or partners. I would always recommend that a new partner investigate the goodwill and try and put some value on it, before joining the partnership. This would indicate to the joining partner what contribution he could reasonably be expected to make.

Price[9] suggested that the value of the goodwill can be calculated on the basis of the annual gross income of the practice for at least the three preceding years. This is a useful formula, provided the joining partner has a good idea of the expenses of the practice over that period as well. The joining partner should firmly but politely insist on being given reliable information on these points – and the most reliable information can of course be obtained from auditor's statements. Marais,[10] again, feels that an acceptable basis of negotiation would be the net profit of the practice over a period of 12 to 18 months.[11]

A bride and groom do not enter into a marriage with divorce uppermost in their minds. Yet a wise spouse, when entering into an antenuptial contract, will be forgiven if he is not so infatuated that this eventuality has not escaped his thoughts altogether.

Likewise, prospective partners should never lose sight of the mechanics of, and the problems connected with, eventual termination of a partnership. Dissolution problems have caused a good deal of expensive litigation between partners.[12]

De Villiers, a leading authority on partnership, included in his invaluable check-list[13] on partnership agreements a number of vital points to be considered in regard to termination. Samples: Can the partnership be terminated by notice? If so, how and when can notice be given? Must provision be made for the expulsion of a partner and how is the expulsion to be affected? What grounds will justify termination? Will liquidation of the partnership follow its termination or are the remaining partners to have the option to succeed to its business? If so – how is the interest of the departing or deceased partner to be valued, how is payment for that interest to be made and how is the interest to be divided among the remaining partners?

What is of extreme importance, is to agree which partner, upon dissolution of the partnership will have the right to practise from the partnership rooms and to retain the existing telephone number. The dissolution clause should also state which partner will be entitled to retain the original patient records (linked with a duty, obviously, to furnish the "parting" partner(s) with a complete set of photocopies thereof).

One final point: the more senior partner(s) might be justified in insisting upon a restraint to be included in the event of dissolution of the partnership, upon practice in the same area by a younger partner who may leave the partnership. Sometimes, in fact, it may be the younger practitioner who joins a partnership who will insist on being protected by means of a restraint clause should a senior partner leave. Formu-

8 Hirsh *op cit.*
9 T W Price in Gordon, Turner & Price *Medical Jurisprudence* (3rd ed, 1953) 85.
10 H B Marais "Mediese Vennootskappe" in *Geneeskunde* of 28 October 1967, 252.
11 Yet another method, the "super-profits" method, in relation to the purchase price of a practice is described in *Robson v Theron* 1978 (1) SA 841 (A) at 859.
12 For an example of such a case, see *Robson v Theron, supra*, discussed in the text.
13 S W L de Villiers "Partnership" in *South African Encyclopaedia of Forms and Precedents* vol 13 (1976) 190.

lating a fair restraint is an aspect which must be carefully thrashed out in consultation with an attorney. Too severe a restraint clause may cause problems of its own.[14]

The type of problem that may arise when a partnership is dissolved and important points have not been covered in the partnership agreement, was well illustrated in the 1978 case of *Robson v Theron*.[15] A dispute arose between partners upon dissolution of their partnership as to the value of the goodwill. When the partnership had been entered into – on the basis of a simple "fifty-fifty" verbal agreement – some nine years before, the partners had not agreed on the goodwill value of their former practices. Now, upon dissolution of the partnership, Dr T retired from it and Dr R *de facto* retained the practice with full use and benefit of the partnership practice including its goodwill as a continuing partner. Dr T sued Dr R for an order declaring that the goodwill of the partnership was R62 987 and payment of one-half thereof. Dr T did not succeed in convincing the court that there was an actual or implied agreement at dissolution concerning the goodwill, but the court held that he was nevertheless entitled to relief. In the circumstances of the case it was impossible, impracticable and inadequate for a court in exercising its discretion to divide the goodwill between the parties or cause it to be auctioned and to have the proceeds thereof divided between the parties. It was therefore no defence for Dr R to contend that he had at all times been agreeable to the goodwill being realised by sale. The practical and equitable solution is for the court to place a valuation on the goodwill with due regard to the particular circumstances concerning its value at the date of dissolution of the partnership and to order Dr R to pay Dr T one-half thereof. On the basis of uncontradicted expert evidence by an accountant of the "super-profit" method of calculation of goodwill, the court in the event held that the share to which Dr T was entitled, was R15 000.

The problems which may arise for a partnership if one of the partners is suspended by the SA Medical and Dental Council for unprofessional conduct are discussed below.[16]

14 On restraint clauses generally, see Strauss & Strydom 146 *et seq* and see below 82. On this point and partnership generally, see further report of Partnership Agreements Study Group in *SA Medical Journal* 31 January 1970, 115.

15 *Supra*.

16 Page 378.

16 Sharing of consulting rooms

By SWL de Villiers†

The sharing of consulting rooms in its simplest form implies that two or more medical practitioners, each of whom practises for his own account, agree to share the use and enjoyment of certain common facilities. The shared facilities may consist merely of the suite of consulting rooms, but more frequently also involve office equipment, reception and accounting facilities and staff, and specialised medical equipment.

Some of the practical reasons which lead to room-sharing arrangements are:

- the availability of suitable numbers of rooms in prime locations;
- the high rentals for rooms;
- the high cost of reception and administration staff;
- the fact that expensive staff and space are often under-utilised in a one-man practice;
- the ease with which arrangements can be made for at least an emergency service to be provided for the patients of a room-sharer, who is on leave, by those who remain.

Medical practitioners embarking upon room-sharing clearly do not want to enter into a partnership in so far as their respective practice incomes are concerned. Frequently, however, their room-sharing arrangement could amount legally to a partnership in so far as their room-sharing activities are concerned. The danger may also exist that outsiders, particularly trade creditors, may regard room-sharers as practising in partnership by virtue of their room-sharing and they may be held liable as such on the principles of estoppel if they culpably represent to such an outsider that they are partners and he acts on that representation to his prejudice.

In practice, room-sharing is not confined to the medical and dental professions, but is also found in other professions with increasing frequency. Room-sharing arrangements work quite well, though they seem to work best when the parties have taken the trouble to have the details of their arrangement properly recorded in a contract drawn by an attorney.

I propose to deal with a few of the matters that could be dealt with in a room-sharing contract.

It is usual to record that each of the parties is practising for his own account and that they intend to share certain facilities for the sake of convenience. The duration of the contract is usually specifically dealt with, if only to say that it will endure for an indefinite period subject to a specified period of notice which can be given by either party. The period need obviously not be indefinite and may in fact be limited by the duration of e g the lease of the rooms.

The facilities to be shared should be very clearly described, preferably with the aid of attached plans of the floor-space of the rooms and attached inventories of the furniture, equipment, etc. Care should be taken to record which of the parties own which of the assets, which are owned jointly and by whom the lease of the premises

† During his life, Professor de Villiers was professor of Mercantile Law in the University of South Africa, and a highly esteemed colleague and friend. This is the text of a paper read by him at the Fourth International Symposium on Forensic Medicine, Pretoria, 1976. Reproduction here is by kind courtesy of his widow, Mrs Maggie de Villiers.

and/or equipment was entered into. The rights of the parties to the use of the shared facilities should be recorded, e g the times of access to certain equipment, if that is necessary. At the same time it is usual to write in some limitations on the use of equipment or facilities, e g that they are only to be used for the purpose of and in the normal course of practice; that neither party may pledge any shared asset or cede his rights in it as security or otherwise; that neither party should do or permit any act to be done which would result in any such asset being attached in execution of legal process; and that neither party should permit the use of any of the equipment by anyone except the parties and their staff. The contract also usually records the basis on which the acquisition of further equipment or improvements of the shared facilities will be effected.

A room-sharing contract also frequently contains a mutual undertaking to provide emergency services and possibly even normal services for each other's patients during absence from the rooms on vacation or due to fortuitous reasons. This again entails recording a leave and sick-leave arrangement in the contract as well as making provision for the reimbursement of the active party for services rendered. The normal arrangement is that the absent party sends an account to such a patient in the name of his own practice and, irrespective of whether he receives payment, pays his colleague at the usual rate within, say 90 days of his performing the service.

It is advisable to record the items of fixed expenditure to be shared and set out how, by whom and by when payments have to be made. Provision for a bookkeeping system in respect of shared expenses is essential.

A room-sharing contract should also provide for its termination. It is usual to allow the injured party to terminate the contract on notice in the event of the other party having breached any material terms of the contract; being guilty of serious misconduct, unprofessional conduct, or having committed an act of insolvency. Other factors resulting in termination of the contract are expiry of the period for which it is to run, the death of a party or his retirement for whatever reason. Provision should be made here for the retention of the facilities or shared assets by one of the parties or the division thereof between them. The injured or remaining party is often given the right to purchase the defaulting, deceased or retiring party's interest in the shared facilities for a purchase price to be determined according to an agreed formula.

In conclusion, it can be expected that the incidence of room-sharing will increase as the cost of suitable accommodation, equipment and staff continues to rise.

17 Contracts of employment entered into by general practitioners

The law does not require a medical practitioner who appoints an employee such as a professional assistant, a *locum tenens*, a nurse or a receptionist, to enter into a written agreement with the employee. Nevertheless, writing is always advisable. If the agreement is verbal, disputes may subsequently arise in connection with the exact terms of appointment which may cause ill-feeling and result in unnecessary – and expensive – litigation. Writing promotes certainty of terms, and at the very least there should be a letter of appointment, setting forth the essential conditions of employment.

In the case of a permanent appointment, however, I would always recommend a formal contract of employment to be entered into, and this should be drafted by an attorney. Apart from other considerations, a contract in writing compels the parties – and in particular the employer – to consider carefully all the terms and conditions which will govern the proposed relationship between employer and employee. This is of particular significance in view of the fact that the employer-employee relationship in the private sector (outside of domestic and agricultural employees and certain other categories) is affected by important labour legislation. The most important of these laws are the Basic Conditions of Employment Act[1] and the Labour Relations Act.[2] The former Act governs matters such as maximum working hours, overtime, leave and the termination of contracts of employment. The latter Act is the cornerstone of South African industrial legislation, regulating matters such as trade union recognition, collective bargaining, the industrial court and unfair labour practices.

It is to be noted that a *locum tenens* will not necessarily be an *employee* of the doctor going on leave. He may be appointed in that capacity, but the agreement may also be on the basis that the *locum* practises independently for his own account during the doctor's absence. The distinction is important. In the latter case, the *locum* is in the legal position of an independent "contractor" who would not in any way by his actions render the absent doctor liable in contract or in respect of civil wrongs.

Where the *locum* practises independently, the contract between the parties may be relatively simple. There are, nevertheless, several important points to be considered, e g the remuneration (if any) to be paid by the *locum* for the right to use the absent doctor's consulting rooms and other facilities, and a limitation (if any) on the *locum's* right to practise in the same area after termination of his contract – the so-called "bar clause" or "restraint clause" which may be of vital importance to the absent doctor in protecting his own practice.[3]

For present purposes, however, our attention is confined to employer-employee contracts, or, as they are sometimes referred to in legal parlance, "master and servant" contracts.

In drafting a contract, the following aspects, *inter alia*, must be considered:[4]

1 Act 3 of 1983.
2 Act 28 of 1956.
3 On restraint clauses generally, see Strauss and Strydom *Die Suid-Afrikaanse Geneeskundige Reg* (1967) 146 *et seq*, and see below 82 *et seq*.
4 See generally, Strauss & Strydom *op cit*, 137 *et seq*; W S McEwan on "Master and Servant" in *The South African Encyclopaedia of Forms and Precedents* vol 11 (1974), 429 *et seq*, in particular 478.

- The period of employment must be determined, unless the intention is that the relationship should last indefinitely. The hours of service should be specified in the case of an employee such as a receptionist.
- The employee's salary and how it will be payable, e g the last day of each month and additional remuneration for special services, must be mentioned specifically. The salary is usually specified as a fixed amount, but sometimes, in the case of a professional assistant, provision is made for additional remuneration in the form of a percentage (e g one-fourth) of all fees received by the employer in respect of certain services which will be rendered by the assistant (e g all confinements attended by him).[5]
- The nature of the services to be rendered by the employee. In the case of a professional assistant, this will usually be indicated in broad terms only, e g that he will be assisting full-time in a general practice. Where specific services are expected it may be advisable to indicate these expressly. An example is where a professional assistant is required to attend at consulting rooms elsewhere on, say Fridays between 09:00 and 13:00.
- The leave to which the employee will be entitled, e g 30 days per annum with full salary, and how the leave may be taken, e g 15 consecutive days in January and 15 consecutive days in the following December. If the employer specifies that additional leave will not be granted in respect of public holidays falling within the period of vacation, future arguments will be avoided. It is also advisable to specify how leave will be earned *pro rata* during the first year of service.
- Limitation of "outside" activities. If an employee is appointed full-time, this would of course imply that during working hours he may not undertake professional duties unrelated to the job for which he is hired. Many employers, anxious to discourage divided loyalties, would also place an absolute prohibition upon employees to engage upon remunerative work outside "office" hours, or at least to accept any remunerative appointment of a continuous nature. Since the appointment of a professional assistant will ordinarily not be on the basis of fixed consulting hours – general practice demanding the willingness to attend patients round the clock – the employer may deem it necessary to stipulate that the employee may not have an active interest in a business, such as a director of companies, or in a farming enterprise, or any other "outside" activity of a professional nature. Suitable exceptions may be made, such as limited teaching duties in a medical school. I would recommend a simple clause to the effect that no remunerative work outside the practice may be undertaken except with the employer's written consent.
- A prohibition upon the employee from disclosing to any other person information or particulars concerning the employer's practice. In the case of a professional assistant such a clause goes beyond his ethical duty of professional secrecy and embraces the "business" side of the practice as well. In the case of other employees, the clause serves as an injunction to maintain confidentiality, a breach of which may entitle the employer to dismiss the employee.
- A provision imposing upon the employee the duty to insure himself against professional liability by becoming a member of a medical protection society or otherwise. This is of special importance in the case of a professional assistant. Of course, by compelling an employee to insure himself, the employer does not rid himself of vicarious liability *vis-à-vis* patients injured by negligent actions of the

5 McEwan *op cit*, 480 n 36, recommends the draftsman to check whether such an arrangement (e g a percentage of the takings as stated) is permitted by the Medical Council. I am not aware of anything in the ethical rules preventing such an arrangement. The sharing of fees is prohibited in rule 8(4) only where it is an arrangement with a person who has not taken a commensurate part in the services.

employee performed within the scope of his employment. But it is undoubtedly to the advantage of the professional assistant and patients for the employer to make sure that a professional assistant has taken out insurance; a patient may have an enforceable claim against the employee, but may have difficulties in proving "scope of employment" so as to entitle him to sue the employer successfully.

- ❑ The mode of termination of the employment should be specified, e g a month's notice (or three months' notice), given at any time (or at the end of any calendar year).
- ❑ A restriction on medical practice by the employee within the employer's general area of practice, after termination of their relationship. Very careful consideration should be given to the scope of the restriction, because in our free-enterprise system the law has traditionally frowned upon such restrictive convenants. If it is too wide it may prove to be unenforceable as such and may lead to unnecessary and costly litigation. An example of too wide a clause would be to restrict a former *locum* from "practising as a general practitioner or in any speciality in Pretoria, Johannesburg or on the Witwatersrand for a period of 10 years". In deciding upon a reasonable restraint, expert legal advice should be sought.[6]

Medical practitioners should be aware of their legal responsibilities relating to compulsory registration for the purposes of, and payment of contributions for, workmen's compensation (if the earnings of the employee do not exceed R46 332 a year), and contributions for unemployment insurance (if the earnings of the employee do not exceed R18 000 a year). The figures quoted are those applying in February 1991. Full details may be obtained from the Department of Manpower.

Note that in terms of the ethical rules of the Medical Council, a *locum* may not be appointed for a period exceeding six months unless the notice requirements set forth in Rule 19 have been complied with.[7]

The Medical Association has drafted standardised employment contracts which are available to its members.

6 See also the discussion below 82.
7 See SAMDC rule 19, note (1).

18 Covenant restraining ex-partner or ex-employee from practising in same neighbourhood

Content

When a medical practitioner employs a professional assistant, it often happens that the former insists on including a condition that upon termination of the agreement, the assistant will not be entitled to practise within the general area in which the medical practitioner practises until a certain period has transpired. Similar conditions regarding junior partners are sometimes found in partnership agreements in favour of senior partners (or, on occasion, a restraint clause regarding the senior partner in favour of the remaining partners). Also when a medical practitioner sells a practice, the purchaser frequently insists on a similar condition in his favour.

Such restrictive clauses – popularly known as "bar clauses" or "restraint clauses" and in the law reports as "agreements" or "covenants" "in restraint of trade" – obviously do not only feature in agreements between doctors, but also in a variety of other contracts, such as between attorneys, accountants, architects, dealers, and consulting engineers.

Object of clause

The object of a restraint clause is self-evident: a senior practitioner has through his skill and ardour established a practice with such success that he needs assistance. With a view to this, he obtains the services of a young practitioner. Through being employed in this way the latter is introduced to a large number of patients gained by the senior over a number of years. In time, the junior can also win the confidence of patients.

This exposes the senior to the danger that the junior, on leaving, will take along a part of the practice. In order to diminish this risk, the senior endeavours to prevent the junior from practising in the same neighbourhood. The restraint clause simultaneously serves to prevent future competition including the drawing of new patients. Identical considerations apply in the case where a partner or seller of a practice is restrained by such a clause.

Validity

The justifiability of safeguarding yourself against future competition is recognised in principle by our courts. In *Weinberg v Mervis*,[1] which dealt with the validity of a restraint clause in a contract in which one practitioner sold his practice to another, the judge remarked as follows:[2] "I have never understood the law to be that the purchaser of goodwill can protect himself from competition by the seller in respect only of the existing clientele at the time of the contract of sale. What the purchaser is entitled to do is to protect himself against the seller's future competition in regard to activities normally falling within the confines of the type of business bought by the purchaser." Continued the judge:[3] "In the present type of case where the avowed object of the

1 1953 (3) SA 863 (C).
2 At 868.
3 At 870.

purchaser of the goodwill is to protect himself against the future competition of the vendor, one is not concerned only with the persons who are the patients of the practice at the time of the sale, but with potential patients."[4]

This type of clause has often been a subject of dispute resulting in litigation. In the past, the courts approached these clauses with considerable aversion because they could harm free trade (or professional activity). In fact, the point of departure of our courts was that such clauses were in principle null and void, and that the onus was on the person who wanted to enforce the clause – i e the ex-employer, senior partner or seller of a business or practice – to persuade the court that the restraint was reasonable and, therefore, enforceable. Since 1977, however, starting with the decision of the Natal full bench in *Roffey v Catterall, Edwards & Goudré (Pty) Ltd*,[5] a more favourable attitude on the part of our courts began to manifest itself. In 1984, in the important decision of *Magna Alloys and Research (SA) (Pty) Ltd v Ellis*,[6] the Appellate Division put its seal of approval on the new approach.

Summary of principles

The legal position may now be summarised as follows:

In principle, a clause in a contract which restricts a party's freedom to trade is not invalid and unenforceable. It is a principle of our law, however, that covenants which are not in the public interest cannot be enforced.

A covenant which restricts someone's freedom to trade is against public policy (and therefore unenforceable) if the circumstances of the case are such that the court is of the opinion that enforcement thereof would harm the public interest.

It may be assumed that a limitation of someone's freedom to trade which is unreasonable (i e unreasonable to him) would probably be harmful to the public interest as well. This would be the case where the person protected by the restraint (e g senior partner) has no practical interest in enforcing the restraint (e g where he stopped practising after dissolution of the partnership).

The person who alleges that he is not bound by a restraint clause – usually the former assistant or partner – bears the onus of proving that enforcement thereof would be against the public interest. He must therefore allege facts and adduce evidence on which he bases his attack on the validity of the restraint.

The court must have regard to the circumstances existing at the time it is requested to enforce the restraint. (This represents an important new point of view because the courts, in earlier cases, held the view that the reasonableness or otherwise of the restraint was to be assessed in the light of circumstances existing at the time the agreement was entered into. Changed circumstances may accordingly be of importance henceforth.)

The court is not limited to a finding that a restraint is enforceable (or unenforceable) in its entirety, but is entitled to decide that only a part of such clause is enforceable (or unenforceable). This, too, represents an important new point of view considering the fact that, in earlier decisions, the courts were not prepared to endeavour to "carve" from a void restraint the maximum upon which the protected party could have insisted – the entire clause was simply held to be null and void. This latter rule, known as "the blue-pencil rule", was cast aside in *Magna Alloys*, and the new principle is much more equitable.

Note that the *Magna Alloys* decision is of retroactive effect, in the sense that it affects all existing contracts containing restraint clauses.

In order to decide whether or not a restraint agreed upon is reasonable, the courts

4 See also *Forman v Barnett* 1941 WLD 54, at 63.
5 1977 (4) SA 494 (N).
6 1984 (4) SA 874 (A).

will, no doubt – as in the past – have regard particularly to circumstances such as: whether the area in respect of which the restraint operates is unreasonably wide, the period is unreasonably long and the scope of the activities from which the aggrieved party is excluded is unreasonably wide. A restraint clause is not open to attack, however, purely on the ground that it is of unlimited duration.

Every case is dealt with on its own merits. In considering the public interest, the court will have regard to *inter alia*, the availability of similar, alternative services. In order to avail himself of the restraint clause, the protected party must fulfil his obligations in terms of the agreement (e g as purchaser of a practice, by paying the purchase price).

In the past the courts, in requiring the protected party (e g former employer) to prove that the public interest would not be harmed by the restraint, attached considerable importance to the question of whether the contracting parties were more or less on an equal footing, e g as practitioners of more or less equal, independent status.[7] If they were, this fact afforded strong evidence that the restraint was reasonable. It is doubtful whether this factor will henceforth be of any particular significance. In *Roffey* the Natal court pointed out that with the advent of trade unions, economic progress and other modern phenomena (such as protective labour legislation) the employee may be in a more powerful negotiating position than the employer, nowadays.

It is doubtful whether the inclusion of an acknowledgement of the reasonableness of a restraint of trade in a service contract will *per se* be of much significance in future.[8]

Examples

Here are some examples, from our case law, of decisions on restraint clauses involving medical practitioners:

- ❑ Retiring partner in general medical practice with five partners restrained from practising for five years within an area of 50 miles from Riversdale. Upheld as reasonable restraint.[9]
- ❑ *Locum tenens* restrained from practising as a general practitioner in Boksburg North or within five miles thereof for five years. Upheld.[10]
- ❑ Seller of general practice restrained from practising within a radius of 10 miles from City Hall, Cape Town, except as a specialist or employee of health-care authority; no period stipulated – period therefore indefinite. Upheld.[11]
- ❑ Professional assistant restrained from practising for two years within a radius of 4 miles from employer's consulting rooms in Durban. Upheld.[12]
- ❑ Partner leaving specialist ear, nose and throat practice restrained from practising in this specialised field for three years, within a radius of 60 miles from Durban. Upheld.[13]
- ❑ Partner leaving general practice in Johannesburg restrained from carrying on general practice (but not specialist practice or as a health-care authority employee) in Johannesburg, for five years. Upheld.[14,15]

From the decisions quoted above – and many others in which persons other than doc-

7 See e g *Malan en Andere v Van Jaarsveld en 'n Ander* 1972 (2) SA 243 (C).
8 *David Wuhl (Pty) Ltd and Others v Badler and Another* 1984 (3) SA 427 (W).
9 *Malan's* case, *supra* note 7.
10 *Estate Mathews v Redelinghuis* 1927 WLD 307.
11 *Weinberg v Mervis* 1953 (2) SA 683 (C).
12 *Rogaly v Weingartz* 1954 (2) SA 791 (D).
13 *Savage and Pugh v Knox* 1955 (3) SA 149 (C).
14 *Hermer v Fisher and Others* 1960 (2) SA 650 (T).
15 For a survey of earlier decisions of our courts in cases other than those involving medical practitioners, see S A Strauss & M J Strydom *Suid-Afrikaanse Geneeskundige Reg* (1967) 153 *et seq*.

tors were involved – it is clear that an endeavour on the part of a doctor to protect himself with regard to an exceptionally large area and for an indefinite period, may lead to the court finding the restraint invalid, or limiting it to a reasonable extent. If the restraint concerns a rare kind of speciality practised by only a few doctors in the country, however, a large area would not readily be held to be unreasonable. A case in point would be *Pest Control (Central Africa) Ltd v Martin*[16] where a restraint clause for the entire areas of Zimbabwe, Zambia and Malawi for a period of two years in respect of a specialised commercial activity, where the potential number of clients was small, was upheld.

Penalty clause

Before concluding our discussion on covenants in restraint of trade, it must be pointed out that a penalty clause is sometimes attached to such a covenant.

A penalty clause is a provision in terms of which a party who acts in contravention of a contractual obligation, is liable to pay a sum of money to the innocent party (the creditor), whether by way of penalty or as liquidated damages: Conventional Penalties Act of 1962.[17] Such a penalty clause is enforceable.

However, the creditor is not entitled to claim damages in addition to the penalty sum; he may also not claim damages in lieu of the penalty sum, unless the particular contract expressly so provides. If, upon the hearing of a claim of a penalty sum, it appears to the court that the penalty sum is out of proportion to the loss suffered by the creditor as a result of the breach of contract, the court may reduce the penalty to the extent it may consider equitable in the circumstances.

An example of a penalty clause attached to a restraint clause is found in *Weinberg v Mervis*.[18] There the purchaser of a practice protected himself by stipulating that if the vendor contravened the restraint clause, he would have been liable to payment of three guineas (R6,30) to the purchaser in respect of each breach.

It is to be noted that the penalty clause should be as specific as possible – as in the case referred to. (The penalty clause in that case was formulated "as fixed liquidated and genuinely pre-estimated damages *and not by way of a penalty*" (my emphasis). The latter qualification has become superfluous since the enactment of the Conventional Penalties Act. Before the Act, "pure" penalty clauses *eo nomine* were not enforceable; what was enforceable was a genuine stipulation of pre-estimated damages. The 1962 Act rendered this distinction obsolete.)[19]

16 1955 (3) SA 609 (SR).
17 Act 15 of 1962.
18 *Supra*.
19 De Wet & Yeats *Kontraktereg en Handelsreg* (4th ed, 1978) 217.

PART IV

Emergency treatment

19 Rescue, emergency medical treatment and the law

Introduction

Although there are occasional references to emergency medical care in medical legislation,[1] the subject of emergency treatment is essentially governed by common law.

In considering the legal implications of emergency medical treatment, there are four aspects which come to the fore:

- the duty to rescue;
- the potential liability of the rescuer (or rescuing agency) to the patient in respect of unskilful medical treatment administered in an emergency;
- the right of the rescuer to be compensated by the patient for emergency medical treatment;
- the right of the rescuer to claim compensation from the author of the emergency, in respect of harm the former suffered as a result of measures taken to rescue the disaster victim.

A study of reported legal cases flowing from disasters reveals that persons injured in a disaster are inclined to sue the party who caused the disaster rather than doctors, nurses, paramedics or other providers of emergency services. The prime targets for legal actions are organisations such as railway administrations or companies, airline companies and insurance companies.

In disasters which flow from *vis major* – or, as it is sometimes translated, "God's Act" – it is of course more difficult to get at the defendant by means of legal proceedings! There is at least one recorded case,[2] however, of an American farmer who sued a church for the loss of his barn in a storm. The barn was struck by lightning and burned down during a storm following a prayer-day organised by the minister of the church, for deliverance from a severe drought. The judge threw out the case at the point when the lawyer representing the church argued there was no evidence that the church had prayed for anything but rain – and that the lightning was an entirely gratuitous gift from the Author of All Weather!

In regard to disasters flowing from God's Act, there will usually be no defendant. I advisedly say "usually" and not "invariably". As science advances, so does the predictability of some natural catastrophes. Where a human being is in charge of a technical "early warning" system – e g a radar station for predicting the movement of hurricanes – there is always the possibility of human error. And where there is human error, there is the possibility of a court finding that the error was the result of actionable negligence.

1 See e g the Nursing Act 50 of 1978, section 27, which in penalising unregistered practice as a nurse, exempts from liability – *ex abundanti cautela*, it is submitted – a person rendering assistance in a case of emergency. Compare the Medicines and Related Substances Control Act 101 of 1965, section 22A(15), which enables a pharmacist to supply a patient in an emergency with certain scheduled substances merely on the verbal instructions of a doctor or dentist. See also SAMDC rule 25. There is also a general provision in the Health Act 63 of 1977 (section 58) which exempts public-sector health personnel from liability for anything done in good faith under the Act.

2 The case is described by Bellamy Partridge *Country Lawyer* (1939) chapter 7.

To return to the rescuer himself: I know of no reported case in South Africa where action was brought by the victim of a mass disaster against a doctor or other person who rendered emergency treatment. Apart from an almost instinctive attitude of gratitude towards the doctor, the principles of our law are such that the likelihood of a successful action being brought in respect of emergency treatment administered in good faith, is minimal.

It is a well-known fact that in the USA, with its extremely high incidence of malpractice litigation, claims have often been brought against doctors who administered emergency treatment to accident victims – to such an extent that doctors have become reluctant to render aid to unknown persons. In a number of American states, legislatures have enacted so-called "Good Samaritan laws" to exonerate doctors from liability when they rendered assistance in good faith. There is no indication of a similar trend in South Africa and because of a number of points of difference in regard to the respective legal systems, such a development is highly unlikely to occur here. Legally there is no reason why doctors practising in South Africa should be reluctant to come to the aid of unknown accident victims.

The only reported case in South Africa involving emergency medical treatment administered is that of a surgeon who was unsuccessfully prosecuted following an anaesthetic mishap during which he came to the patient's rescue. The case is discussed below.[3]

The duty to rescue[4]

In principle there is no legal duty upon a person to rescue another, even if it could be expected of him, on purely moral grounds, to act positively to prevent the damage.[5] A duty to come to the rescue of another may arise from contract (e g in the case of the man who joins a municipal fire department as fireman, or the man who joins a hospital as ambulance driver or paramedic) or from statute (e g the duty imposed upon doctors, dentists and nurses who attend a child who has apparently been ill-treated or abused, to notify the Regional Director of Health and Welfare).[6] The scope of the duty to rescue in these cases will be determined largely by the terms of the contract or the provisions of the statute.

Quite apart from these situations, however, a duty to rescue may by common law arise from the circumstances in which the parties, i e the person in distress and the would-be rescuer, find themselves. In the landmark case of *Minister van Polisie v Ewels*[7] our Appellate Division gave express recognition to this duty in the context of defining the limits of delictual liability for a non-feasance: an omission, in essence, is wrongful where the circumstances are such that the omission would not only evoke moral indignation, but also that the juristic convictions of society would require that the omission be regarded as wrongful.[8] Applied to the medical situation, it is not difficult to conceive of circumstances in which there would clearly be a legal duty on the part of doctors,[9] nurses and other medically qualified persons to come to the rescue of accident victims by means of medical aid.

3 Pages 96, 276.
4 On the duty to rescue, generally, see also: K J Kemp "The Rescuer and the Law" 1980 *Obiter* 1; A K Blommaert "Negotiorum Gestio and the Life Rescuer" 1981 (2) *TSAR* 123; P Q R Boberg "Liability for Omissions: The Duty to Rescue" 1982 (11) *BML* 194-197, 230-232; D Giesen *International Medical Malpractice Law* (1988) 361 *et seq*. On American law generally, see J E George *Law and Emergency Medical Care* (1980).
5 See *Minister van Polisie v Ewels* 1975 (3) SA 590 (A) 596 H. See also F P van den Heever *Aquilian Damages in South African Law* (1944) 37.
6 Child Care Act 74 of 1983, section 42, discussed below 419.
7 1975 (3) SA 590 (A).
8 The case is discussed in detail above 24.
9 See above 25.

It is submitted that a duty to rescue someone by means of medical treatment will not arise where there is danger for the would-be rescuer. A situation that comes to mind is that of a doctor (or paramedic) who may save the life of someone who has apparently had a heart attack, by way of mouth-to-mouth resuscitation; the doctor has reason to believe that the patient is an AIDS carrier. Slight as the risk of contracting HIV infection may be in performing this procedure, it is nevertheless inconceivable that the juristic convictions of society would require the doctor to knowingly expose himself to that risk.

Consent required where possible

In modern Western societies personal inviolability and freedom of will – with patient autonomy[10] as one of its concomitants – are values that are highly rated. Legally speaking, the basic ground of justification for medical treatment is consent.

Even in an emergency situation, the will of a patient who is still capable of expressing it rationally, must be respected.

Medical treatment against the will of the patient is legally permissible within very narrow limitations only. The legal ground of justification upon which the doctor or other person may rely in these cases, is necessity (*noodtoestand*). A feature of the typical situation to which the doctrine of necessity generally applies, is that the interest of a person (the so-called "innocent third person") is sacrificed to protect or rescue the lawful interest of another who is endangered, either by a natural force ("inevitable evil") or by human agency. Therefore, where a doctor – in order to protect the social interest – administers medical treatment to a person against the latter's will, he (the doctor) may raise the defence of necessity against a charge of assault. Thus a doctor may treat a patient suffering from a dangerous infectious disease, against the patients's will, to prevent the disease from spreading. So too, a doctor may vaccinate healthy persons to prevent the outbreak of a dangerous disease in the community. In these cases, the doctor may act without the consent of the patient or even against his will.[11]

Although the defence of necessity may be relied upon even where the act intended to ward off the danger is directed not against the interest of an innocent third person, but against other interests of the person threatened by the danger,[12] such action, if undertaken against the will of the latter, can in my opinion only in exceptional circumstances be justified on the basis of the doctrine of necessity. The law will not protect the health fanatic who forcibly attempts to prevent me from using a lot of sugar in my coffee, because he maintains – quite correctly so – that in the long run it will harm my health and may even shorten my life. On the other hand, the doctrine of necessity will clearly avail the policeman who forcibly restrains me from committing suicide by jumping off a window-ledge in a high building.[13] A doctor would also clearly have the right to save the life of a would-be suicide who has taken an overdose of pills, by pumping out the content of the stomach or by administering a neutralising agent. Likewise, it is submitted, medical treatment can be administered to a prisoner who, in consequence of a hunger-strike, is at death's door.[14]

There must be a state of dire emergency which necessitates immediate action to save the life of the person who is endangered. It is submitted, however, that in regard

10 See above 8, 31.
11 A doctor may rely on the common-law defence of necessity, but compulsory immunisation is also provided for statutorily. In South Africa it is governed by the Health Act 63 of 1977, section 33, and the regulations thereunder.
12 See J V van der Westhuizen *Noodtoestand as Regverdigingsgrond in die Strafreg* (LLD thesis, Univ of Pretoria, 1979) 585, 609.
13 Van der Westhuizen 609.
14 See below 411 *et seq.*

to medical treatment of a person whose life or health is in serious danger as a result of injury, disease or ill-health, such treatment against his express will is in principle not justifiable on the basis of necessity, unless the act is directed solely to protection of the community interest[15] (to which I have referred above).

The reason for this is that in our society, the mentally competent individual's right to control his own destiny in accordance with his own value system, his *selfbeskikkingsreg*, must be rated even higher than his health and life[16] (unless it would clearly offend against the community interest).[17] It was an English judge, I think,[18] who gave expression to the notion of individualism in the legal system in words to the following effect: "It is the right of every man to go to hell in his own way."

There is one situation, however, in which in my opinion a doctor may, by virtue of the doctrine of necessity, treat a patient capable of expressing his will, without having first obtained the latter's informed consent. That is the situation where the doctor – after careful consideration and in good faith – deliberately refrains from informing a patient (who is anxious to be cured) of the nature of the (serious) disease diagnosed, because such information may have the effect that the patient would become depressed and desperate to such an extent that he refuses further medical treatment. The cancer patient comes to mind in this context.[19]

Where a mentally competent patient has not expressed unwillingness to undergo treatment, but is merely unable to give consent, on account of shock or unconsciousness, emergency medical treatment presents few legal problems. In these cases the doctor, nurse, paramedic or layman may rely on the common-law doctrine of *negotiorum gestio* (unauthorised administration)[20] to justify his actions.

Unauthorised administration

The essence of unauthorised administration is that a person is entitled – not obliged – to take steps to protect the interests of another person who is absent, where such interests are imperilled. The textbook example: My neighbour is away on leave; I notice that his horse is starving in his stable; I break open the stable door to feed the horse. In criminal law and the law of delict, the doctrine operates as a defence to protect the rescuer (*gestor*) against liability which he would otherwise have incurred. To put it in simple terms: If my object were not to feed my neighbour's horse, I would have been guilty of malicious injury to the property of my neighbour in breaking open the stable door.

This principle is extended to situations in which the person whose interests (life, health) are imperilled, is not physically absent but psychologically "absent". A man who is unconscious is as unable to take care of his own interests as a man who is a thousand kilometres away. Moreover, the doctrine of unauthorised administration is capable of application not only to proprietary interests but also to personality interests. In my opinion this doctrine can also be invoked in the following situation: A non-emergency operation is performed upon a consenting patient. After surgery has commenced and the patient is still under a general anaesthetic, a serious condition is discovered which would medically warrant an immediate extension of the operation in an endeavour to remedy the condition discovered, although such an extension was not contemplated by the parties.[21]

15 Cf Van der Westhuizen *loc cit*.
16 *Ibid*. See also the (German?) blood transfusion case and the views of Ebert cited by Van der Westhuizen 529.
17 See also my comments above 31.
18 Notwithstanding diligent search I was unable to trace the source and exact wording of this *dictum*.
19 The expression "therapeutic privilege" is used to indicate this type of situation. See above 18.
20 For a full discussion of this doctrine in relation to emergency medical treatment, see S A Strauss & M J Strydom *Suid-Afrikaanse Geneeskundige Reg* (1967) 238 *et seq*.
21 On extension of operations generally, see Strauss & Strydom 223 *et seq*.

The essentials of the doctrine in relation to medical treatment may be summarised as follows:

- ❑ There must be a real state of emergency.
- ❑ The patient must be unaware of the fact that he is medically treated, or must at least be incapable of properly appreciating the situation.
- ❑ The treatment must not be against the will of the patient.
- ❑ The treatment must be intended to be in the best interests of the patient.

The last of these requirements is self-evident, so that only the other three merit further discussion.

There must be a real state of emergency. By this is meant that in consequence of some event – natural disaster, an accident or disease – the patient must be confronted with the real possibility of death or serious bodily harm or a deterioration of his health. The danger must be such that immediate action is necessary to save the life or health of the patient. If a delay would not aggravate the patient's condition, his consent must first be obtained, at any rate where drastic surgery is envisaged.

In *Esterhuizen v Administrator, Transvaal* [22] a patient was subjected to deep X-ray therapy, without the necessary consent having been obtained. The defendant contended, *inter alia*, that because the patient's life expectancy had been one year only, it was a matter of "life and death". The court held, however, that there had been enough time to obtain the consent of the patient's guardian.

In the American case of *Jackovach v Yocom*[23] a 17-year-old was injured when he jumped from a moving train. He sustained a serious laceration on the head, a crushed elbow and other wounds and contusions. Dr Y tried in vain to get in touch with his parents and the patient requested the doctor "to fix him up". Two other doctors were called in to assist, and after consultation it was decided that the periosteum was damaged to such an extent that it was necessary to amputate the patient's arm. Afterwards the patient contended that the operation was performed without his consent. However, the court decided in favour of the doctor: "[I]f a surgeon is confronted with an emergency which endangers the life and health of the patient, it is his duty to do what the occasion demands within the usual and customary practice among physicians and surgeons ... without the consent of the patient."

The patient must be unaware of the treatment. This will usually be the case where the patient is unconscious, delirious or comatose. It is submitted, however, that total unconsciousness is not necessary. The patient's condition may be such, on account of injury or shock, that although he may have a certain awareness of the disaster and the fact that he was injured, he is incapable of properly appreciating the situation and of rationally considering the treatment proposed and giving meaningful consent. A severely injured person in great pain who implores medical personnel to leave him alone and let him die, may be in such a bad state of shock that his protestations are not of a rational nature. I have no doubt that the law will protect medical personnel who ignore such a person's resistance and come to his rescue.

However, if the patient is not in such a condition as to preclude him from making rational decisions, particularly where he is confronted with possible alternative forms of treatment, his wishes should be respected. Failure to do so, may result in legal action against the doctor.

A typical example of emergency treatment held to be lawful, is the American case of *Luka v Lowrie*[24]: A youth, 15 years of age, was hit by a locomotive when he was crossing a railway, and landed under the wheels of a railway coach. His left foot was severely injured. There was an open dislocation of the bones of the foot, and one of

22 1957 (3) SA 710 (T).
23 212 Iowa 914 (1931).
24 136 NW 1106 (1912).

the main bones of the arch, the scaphoid, was completely torn away, the flesh was crushed and torn on the upper side of the foot, so that muscles, tendons and bones were exposed. Shortly after the injury, he was taken to a hospital. He was partly conscious and was able to furnish the doctors in attendance with his name and the name of the street where he lived. Within 10 to 15 minutes after his arrival, he became comatose and later became completely unconscious. Unsuccessful efforts were made to revive him. Dr L was called in. He found the patient in a state of unconsciousness, with a weak pulse and dilated pupils. The foot was cold and dead because of interruption of blood supply. Dr L made enquiries whether there were any relatives present, but was told that there were none. After consultation with the four interns, it was decided mutually that an immediate amputation was necessary to save the patient's life. This was done and the patient recuperated. The court held that even if the doctor had made an error of judgment in deciding upon amputation of the foot, on account of the emergency he was entitled to operate; it would have been impracticable first to have sought consent. Evidence was led that death frequently ensued as a result of shock caused by serious traumatic injury. The patient's claim based upon the alleged unnecessary amputation of his foot without the necessary consent, was accordingly refused.

It is to be noted that it would be a wise precaution against possible subsequent legal action by a dissatisfied patient, for a doctor or hospital to document the medical need for proceeding with treatment without the patient's consent[25] (in so far as such documentation is practicable in the circumstances of the case), in particular where the treatment is of a drastic nature.

The treatment must not be against the will of the patient. According to our common law, unauthorised administration is considered a so-called quasi-contract and is based upon the presumption that the person whose interests are protected, would have given consent to the rescue action because it is in his interest. But an adult person of sane mind is considered to be the best judge of his own interests. Where, therefore, the person concerned has imposed a prohibition upon the rescue action, the rescuer cannot rely on unauthorised administration as a defence.

The fact that the patient's condition is critical, in itself will not justify medical treatment against his will where he expressly and while in full possession of his faculties of mind, forbade treatment or a specific form of treatment. A case in point is the Canadian judgment in *Mulloy v Hop Sang*.[26] The patient's hand was seriously injured in a car accident. The patient twice told the doctor who attended him not to amputate the hand, because he wanted his own doctor in a neighbouring town to treat him. The doctor told him, however, that he would be guided by the conditions established after anaesthesia had been administered. While the patient was under the anaesthetic, the doctor amputated the hand. In a civil action subsequently brought by the patient, the doctor was held liable.

A South African court has recognised the right of a person who was severely injured in a road accident to refuse a blood transfusion on religious grounds.[27]

May relatives issue a "veto"?

It is to be noted that relatives of an injured person, who himself would have been able to give consent had he been conscious, will not be entitled to place a prohibition on medical treatment. In the case of a mentally ill person[28] or juvenile below the age of 18,[29] a prohibition imposed by a person lawfully entitled to give consent to medical

25 See Health Law Centre *Problems in Hospital Law* (1968) 39.
26 1 Western Weekly Reports 714 (1935).
27 *Phillips v De Klerk* (1983, unreported) discussed in detail above 29.
28 See above 38.
29 See above 7. A minor who is 18 years or older, may independently consent; it is submitted that in the absence of a parent, such a minor may also independently veto an operation.

treatment, must be respected, provided – so it is submitted – the prohibition does not go against what objectively is in the interest of the patient. It is difficult to conceive on what legal ground the curator of a mental patient, or the guardian of a minor, may in an emergency situation dictate to a qualified medical practitioner, nurse, etc, to refrain from treatment which would manifestly be in the interest of the patient.

It is to be noted that in South Africa there are statutory provisions which expressly authorise certain officials to consent to emergency treatment of minors in the absence of parental consent,[30] or even in opposition to an unreasonable refusal on the part of a parent or guardian.[31]

Finally it must be mentioned that from a practical point of view, if a doctor were to disregard an injured person's prohibition, and treat him and save his life or his health, it is almost unthinkable that a patient will in South Africa be able to successfully sue the doctor for anything else than nominal damages for a technical assault (acting in violation of his will) which has injured his personality.[32] After all, where a man's life was saved or his health was preserved by the action of another, he can hardly claim that he suffered consequential damage calculable in pecuniary terms.

If all the requirements for successful reliance on the defence of unauthorised administration are met, the rescuer will be entitled to claim remuneration for his services from the injured person. However, our law allows recovery only where the rescuer at the time of the rescue action acted with the intent to claim remuneration. Where he has acted in the performance of duty, or purely as a Good Samaritan, or in accordance with moral duties arising from a family relationship, he will not be entitled to remuneration. The intent to claim remuneration may be inferred from the circumstances, such as the fact that the rescuer left a record of his expenditures. It is to be noted that remuneration is limited to recovery of expenses incurred or a loss sustained by the rescuer as a result of the services he rendered.[33]

There are two further aspects of the doctrine of unauthorised administration which in the context of emergency medical treatment deserve attention. The first is that there is a duty upon the rescuer to complete what he has commenced. Once he has taken it upon himself to look after the interests of the person concerned, he may not simply abandon his self-imposed task. Failure to complete what he commenced may lead to liability, should the person concerned suffer damage.

The duty of reasonable care

The other duty is for the rescuer to exercise reasonable care when embarking upon the act of rescue. Our law postulates that the rescuer must generally exercise the ordinary prudence which he would have displayed in taking care of his own affairs. Applied to medical treatment, this naturally does not mean the amount of care which the patient would have exercised had he himself undertaken the treatment. Particularly in cases of serious injury, the reasonable man will in the ordinary course of events not administer treatment upon himself (although such cases are of course not unknown: Paul Kruger amputated his own thumb with a hunting-knife following serious injury sustained to his hand when his gun exploded)[34] but entrust his body to experts, if possible.

Where a doctor administers treatment, he must apply the degree of care and skill which the average, reasonable doctor would display in the same circumstances. Likewise the action of a nurse or a paramedic will be judged in the light of the degree of

30 See above 6.
31 See above 6, 33.
32 Compare Neethling , Potgieter & Visser *Law of Delict* (1990) 195.
33 L Rubin *Unauthorised Administration in South Africa* (1958) 68-69.
34 J F van Oordt describes the incident in his book *Paul Kruger en der Opkomst der Zuid-Afrikaansche Republiek* (1898) 810-811.

care and skill which may reasonably be expected from the average professional person in this field. Depending upon the severity of the injury and the availability of better qualified professionals, a doctor, nurse, or paramedic may in a case of dire emergency – where the patient is at death's door – attempt measures which go far beyond his or her training, competency or experience.

In *S v Kramer and Another*[35] a relatively inexperienced anaesthetist, working with a surgeon in a tonsillectomy and adenoidectomy on a 10-year-old girl, failed to insert an endotracheal tube correctly. The patient became cyanosed and the surgeon noticed this. He then, with the aid of a laryngoscope, came to the conclusion that the tube was not in the trachea. At that stage the anaesthetist "froze". The surgeon immediately ordered further doses of fabantol and scolene (drugs used in connection with anaesthesia), removed the tube and re-intubated the patient with another tube. The patient was ventilated and her colour improved. She suddenly became cyanosed again and as no pulse was palpable, cardiac massage was started. Attempts were made to stimulate the deceased's heart with a defibrillator (an apparatus that delivers an electric shock) but to no avail. The patient died in the theatre. The court of appeal held that the surgeon had acted swiftly and reasonably in the emergency, in trying to create an airway, and that he had taken all reasonable measures to resuscitate the patient under the prevailing circumstances. The court held that the anaesthetist had been negligent in failing to insert the tube correctly and in failing to monitor the patient properly, by which the misplacement of the tube could have been discovered. It was further held that the surgeon could not be held liable for the negligence of the anaesthetist. Moreover, there was no legal duty on the surgeon to have looked down the trachea of the patient to check the position of the tube before commencing the operation.

Modern technology has provided the rescuer with a vast array of technical aids, in particular medical equipment, to use in the treatment of casualty victims. Failure to use these aids may in circumstances be judged to constitute negligence. It may be stated as a principle that the more sophisticated and available these aids are in a given situation, the more likely it is that failure to use them, or to utilise them fully, may be ruled legally blameworthy in the absence of an explanation for such non-use.

In cases of extreme emergency even unqualified laymen may render aid to the injured. It goes without saying that the actions of the layman will not be judged by applying standards pertaining to any branch of the medical profession. If a man has been critically injured and lies bleeding to death next to the roadside, the lay Samaritan who attends the victim, may render such assistance as is reasonable in the circumstances, even if it is of no avail. The court will not adopt the attitude of an armchair critic who is wise after the event, but will apply the standard of the reasonable man. In this regard, it must be observed that it would certainly be held unreasonable for a layman to treat a critically injured person if expert medical aid is immediately available. In practical terms, this means that when someone happens to arrive on the scene of a disaster where people are critically injured, it would be unwise for him to administer well-intended but unskilful first-aid unless he has first ascertained whether a doctor, or another professional with expert medical knowledge is available on the spot or within easy reach.

The administering of "scheduled" substances[36] in emergency treatment by persons who are not registered medical practitioners or nurses may be problematic. The possession and administration of scheduled substances are strictly controlled by the Medicines and Related Substances Control Act.[37] Generally speaking only pharmacists, doctors and nurses may possess and supply scheduled substances, subject to the conditions set out in the Act. Ambulance drivers, first-aiders and paramedics do

35 1987 (1) SA 887 (W).
36 I e substances listed in the schedules to the Medicines etc Control Act 101 of 1965.
37 Act 101 of 1965.

not have this right; however, in terms of section 22A(12) of the Act, the Director General of National Health and Population Development may issue special permits to persons or organisations to acquire, possess, use or supply any specified substance mentioned in the first four schedules to the Act. It is conceivable that paramedics, etc, may in a case of extreme emergency be justified to possess and administer scheduled substances: *nood breek wet*. Each case will have to be considered on its own merits. But *prima facie* the mere possession of certain scheduled substances by unauthorised persons may constitute a criminal offence.

Priority treatment

Can a rescuer be held liable for giving priority treatment to certain casualty victims? The dilemma of the rescuer who arrives on the scene of a disaster is nothing new in our age of mass casualties caused by crashes of jumbo jets, trains colliding or buses overturning. Through the ages, rescuers attending to casualties on battlefields or in cities struck by earthquake were called upon to make immediate life-and-death decisions in selecting those patients to be treated first.

I am not aware of a single reported court judgment in which a doctor or other rescuer was blamed for having erred in selecting the wrong patients in administering emergency medical treatment to casualty victims. If such a case were to come before a court, the judge would undoubtedly uphold the right of virtual freedom of selection on the part of the rescuer, as long as he has acted in good faith and reasonably in the light of the known circumstances. A rescuer is clearly entitled to make a selection of those cases which will probably still benefit from medical treatment, in preference to others. Depending on the magnitude of the disaster, the degree of injuries suffered by individual victims and the availability of other skilled assistance, immediate "on-the-spot" decisions must often be made. Giving due consideration to these different factors, a court would not judge an error of judgment made in the process of selection of victims too severely. Philosophers, theologians and jurists[38] have through the ages debated issues such as the following: when two persons are in equal danger, must the aged, full of knowledge, experience and wisdom, be rescued in preference to the young and inexperienced, but with the promise of life ahead of him? No court will expect a rescuer who, in an emergency situation involving a multiplicity of victims, was called upon to make an immediate decision to give preferential treatment to certain victims, to have given thought to these philosophical considerations.

In concluding this part of our discussion it is to be stressed that in an emergency situation, statutory provisions may become inoperative. In our own legal system, there are a host of statutory provisions relating to matters such as: the right to practise the healing profession or a particular branch thereof, or a particular type of expertise; certification of death; post mortem examinations and burial. In a grave emergency situation, statutory duties or prohibitions will temporarily become suspended by virtue of the common-law principle of *nood breek wet*. The interest of disaster victims and the social interest will override provisions enacted by the Legislature for everyday-life conditions. Thus nurses and paramedics would lawfully be entitled to undertake medical procedures ordinarily reserved for doctors, and general practitioners would be entitled to perform operations ordinarily reserved for specialists. As I have said, even complete laymen in a situation of dire emergency may administer such medical treatment as they deem necessary.[39] In a major catastrophe resulting

38 See for example the discussion by Antonius Matthaeus, the famous Roman-Dutch criminalist, in his treatise *De Criminibus* (1644) *ad* D 47.5.1.5, in connection with the justifiability of abortion, in which he quoted Plato and Calistratus.

39 This right is also expressly recognised in the Nursing Act. See note 1 above. This type of provision is not really necessary, because of the common-law doctrine of necessity which would protect a non-registered "practitioner" in regard to emergency treatment.

from an earthquake where there are tens of thousands of dead, it would become ridiculous – and dangerous to public health – if bureaucrats were to insist on compliance with the ordinary rules and regulations pertaining to matters such as death certification and burial.

May the rescuer sue others?

I want to turn now to the legal rights of the rescuer *vis-à-vis* others. In my introductory remarks I raised the question whether the rescuer is entitled to sue the author of the disaster for harm suffered by the rescuer in the course of the rescue operation.

In general there is no duty on the part of any person to expose himself to almost certain death or bodily mutilation in an endeavour to rescue another. The only absolute exception to this rule is a soldier in a military encounter, acting under lawful orders of a superior. Policemen and firemen must naturally in the course of carrying out the occupational duties which they have assumed by contract,[40] expose themselves to a greater or lesser extent to serious dangers, but a court of law would undoubtedly not find that their duties go so far as to expose themselves unreasonably to a risk which entails the certainty of death or, at the least, serious bodily harm. The law does not expect from mortals more than what is reasonable in the circumstances.[41]

But there are always heroic persons, in or out of uniform, who would selflessly rush into mortal danger in order to save others, thereby knowingly courting death or serious injury.

Ordinarily a doctor will not be injured himself in administering emergency medical treatment, but there is at least one reported case, *Barker v T E Hopkins Ltd*,[42] where a doctor was killed in attempting to rescue accident victims. The doctor had descended a well to rescue workmen overcome by fumes and was himself overcome. The defendant company, being found responsible for the accident to the workmen, was held liable in damages to the doctor's widow.

Can the party who negligently brought about the danger, escape delictual liability on the ground that the rescuer voluntarily assumed the risk of injury (*volenti non fit iniuria*), thereby waiving, as it were, his own right of recovery for injury, or that of his dependants, in the case of his death? Can the defendant alternatively disclaim liability on the ground that the rescuer was contributorily negligent in regard to the misfortune he (or his dependants) suffered?

The general trend of court judgments – in particular in cases where a rescuer attempts to save a life, as opposed to mere protection of property – is to the effect that where a man acts in the performance of a duty, it cannot be said that his exposure to the risk created by the negligence of another is voluntary. This duty need not be a legal duty; it may be a mere moral or social duty. The defendant can accordingly not deny liability by raising the defence of voluntary assumption of risk. Nor can it be said that the rescuer was guilty of contributory negligence, unless his act of rescue was unreasonable in that the risk incurred was out of proportion to the right asserted or the duty performed.[43]

A Pennsylvania judge in *Corbin v Philadelphia*[44] gave eloquent expression to this view: "A rescuer, one who, from the most unselfish motives, prompted by the noblest

40 Policemen also fall under the provisions of the Police Act 7 of 1958, but in *Ewels* at 596C Chief Justice Rumpff *obiter* intimated that a general duty to rescue could not be implied from section 5 of the Act although the general statutory duty was nevertheless a "factor" in the case.

41 *S v Goliath* 1972 (3) SA 1 (A) 25 B-D.

42 [1959] 1 WLR 966. The case is cited by S R Speller *Law of Doctor and Patient* (1973) 64.

43 S A Strauss *Toestemming tot Benadeling as Verweer in die Strafreg en die Deliktereg* (LLD thesis, Univ of S Africa, 1962) 73, 178 *et seq*, 323, 356, 398; McKerron, *op cit* 68-69.

44 195 Pa 461 (1900).

impulses that can impel a man to deeds of heroism, faces deadly peril, ought not to hear from the law words of condemnation of his bravery, because he rushed into danger, to snatch from it the life of a fellow creature, imperilled by the negligence of another, but he should rather listen to words of approval, unless regretfully withheld on account of the unmistakable evidence of his rashness and imprudence. The conscience and reason approve, and the best judgment of thoughtful and intelligent judges has declared it to be law of the land ..."

As the famous American judge, Cardozo,[45] put it: "Danger invites rescue. The cry of distress is the summons to relief. The law does not ignore these reactions of the mind in tracing conduct to its consequences. It recognizes them as normal. It places their effects within the range of the natural and probable. The wrong that imperils life is a wrong also to his rescuer. The risk of rescue, if only it be not wanton, is born of the occasion. The emergency begets the man. The wrongdoer may not have foreseen the coming of a deliverer. He is accountable as if he had."

Generally speaking, therefore, the rescuer (or his dependants in the event of his death) will be entitled to recover damages in respect of his injury, from the author of the catastrophe, provided that fault on the part of the defendant can be proved. A man who with humanitarian valour rushed into a danger can hardly be said to have willingly exposed himself to the risk of harm. Apart from that, the party whose negligence has caused the disaster, ought reasonably to have foreseen the possibility of heroic rescue attempts resulting in the loss of limb or life to the rescuer, and will for that reason be held accountable.

Even if a court were to find contributory negligence on the part of the rescuer, only a minor percentage of negligence would probably be apportioned to him in terms of the Apportionment of Damages Act.[46]

Based upon a paper read at the International Conference on Disaster Medicine held in Cape Town, August 1979.

45 *Wagner v International Railway Co* 232 NY 176, 133 NE 437 (1921) 437.
46 Act 34 of 1956.

PART V

Professional secrecy, patient records and medical certificates

20 Professional secrecy in relation to spouses

The doctor's position regarding professional secrecy[1] is particularly unenviable when he becomes involved in a legal confrontation between a husband and a wife, both of whom are his patients.

For many years he has been consulted by both spouses. He is fully familiar with their respective medical histories. His records contain details which may be highly relevant to the forensic duel between the spouses.

He has, for instance, treated the wife for a serious neurosis bordering on the psychotic, and he knows that she is not a good mother: the children would be better off in the husband's care. Or he has treated the husband for venereal disease which was contracted in an adulterous affair. Or he knows that the wife who claims to be medically unfit for sexual relations, is in good health and refuses to have relations with the husband simply because her feelings for him have cooled down.[2]

Now one of the spouses or the attorney handling the case, requires the doctor to supply medical information concerning the other spouse and to testify in court. How does the doctor handle such a request?

The very first consideration by which the doctor should be guided, is that the fact that he has been treating both spouses does not mean the medical details he has recorded on them form a "pool" to which both have access.

The medical relationship is a highly individual one and professional secrecy should be strictly observed towards each marriage partner individually. Outside the courtroom, that secrecy can ordinarily only be breached by the consent of the spouse concerned.

The personal "guardianship" of a husband over a wife, whatever it may have meant in days gone by, certainly does not give the husband the right to know what has transpired between her and her doctor – even where the latter is the husband's doctor as well.

The fact that the husband has for years paid the doctor's account, does not make any difference. It is part of his common-law duty to maintain his wife and it does not mean that the wife's confidential medical facts become his "property".

A party to a lawsuit or his attorney cannot compel a doctor to disclose confidential information before the trial. All that the party can do is to subpoena the doctor as a witness. The doctor must then attend court and may be asked questions relevant to the particular matter in issue. Strictly speaking, the doctor's duty to testify only arises when he is ordered by the court to reply to the questions put to him.

Medical practitioners who in accordance with their ethical duty protest to the presiding judge for having to testify in breach of their professional secrecy, are ac-

1 On professional medical secrecy in general, see Oosthuizen, Shapiro & Strauss (eds) *Professional Secrecy in South Africa* (1983) 3 *et seq.*

2 It is to be noted that although adultery is no longer *per se* a ground for divorce in South Africa, the adultery of a spouse may still be relevant to divorce proceedings. First, adultery may serve as proof (in terms of section 4(2)(*b*) of the Divorce Act 70 of 1979) of irretrievable breakdown of the marriage, which constitutes a ground for divorce; secondly, it may be relevant to the issue of maintenance of the innocent spouse (section 7(2) of the Act).

corded sympathetic treatment by judges. But, of course, they are ordered to testify if their testimony is relevant to the case.

A case in point is *Parkes v Parkes.*[3] A wife brought action against her husband for divorce on the ground of his adultery. The woman alleged that her husband was suffering from venereal disease which he had not contracted from her. A doctor who had refused to give any information concerning the husband to the wife's attorney prior to the trial, was subpoenaed as a witness by the wife.

Having been administered the oath, the doctor was asked in court whether he had treated the husband for venereal disease. The doctor claimed professional privilege and refused to reply to the question. The judge ruled, however, that he had to answer the question. He then told the court that he had treated the husband for such disease.

In his judgment, the judge made the following remarks: "I regret very much that the law compels me to elicit these facts from a medical man when in the witness-box relative to his patients, and the doctor has done all he possibly could to observe the professional confidence reposed in him, and I may say that I do not think that any other man could have done more to avoid a breach of professional confidence. He has taken every step to avoid the question put to him, and it is only the order of this Court that has compelled him to give the evidence relating to his patient."

It is to be noted that *Parkes's* case was a trial action. The Rhodesian court in *Ex parte James*[4] held that in motion proceedings – i e where oral evidence is not adduced but the matter is tried on the basis of affidavits – the court has no power to authorise and direct a doctor, or any member of the public, to make an affidavit.

The doctor's right to remain silent in court is recognised to a varying degree by virtue of express legislation in a number of states of the USA. But South African law, following English precedent, recognises professional privilege only in the case of legal practitioners.[5] (In the USA the doctor-patient privilege has been subjected to frequent criticism by legal writers.)

In the case of *Smit v Van Niekerk*[6] the South African Appellate Division was urged to rule that a clergyman has the right to remain silent on matters confessed to him, but the Court held that there was no such right. From remarks made in the course of the judgment, it is clear that there is no possibility at present of convincing the Court that a medical privilege should be recognised. The Natal case of *Botha v Botha*[7] also bears this out.

Since we are on the subject of the doctor's right or duty to testify concerning his patient's medical condition, mention may be made in passing of the fact that a statement made to a psychiatrist[8] by an accused whose criminal responsibility or fitness to stand trial is in doubt, and who was referred by a criminal court to a mental institution for observation, is protected against disclosure by virtue of the Criminal Procedure Act.[9] Section 79(7) of that Act provides that a statement made by such an accused at the relevant enquiry shall not be admissible in evidence against the accused at criminal proceedings, except to the extent to which it may be relevant to the determination of the mental condition of the accused.

A discussion of professional secrecy in relation to spouses would not be complete without making reference to the doctor's rights and obligations where he has diagnosed HIV positivity in a spouse. AIDS is different from other sexually transmissible

3 1916 CPD 702.
4 1954 (3) SA 270 (SR).
5 See Oosthuizen, Shapiro & Strauss *op cit* 25.
6 1976 (4) SA 293 (A).
7 1972 (2) SA 559 (N).
8 On professional secrecy and the psychiatrist in general, see: Oosthuizen, Shapiro & Strauss *op cit* 14; G Venniker "Confidentiality and the Psychotherapist-Patient Relationship" 1979 *NLR* 298.
9 Act 51 of 1977.

diseases in that it is an incurable and lethal condition. Because of that, the doctor is decidedly entitled to disclose the diagnosis of AIDS to his patient's spouse – in fact, there may be a duty, both ethically and legally, to inform the spouse. This aspect of professional secrecy is discussed in detail above.[10]

10 See above 16 *et seq.*

21 Medical certificates and professional secrecy: some legal issues

There are a number of legal problems relating to the issuing of medical certificates by private medical practitioners to employees for purposes of sick leave, and the doctor's duty of professional secrecy.

What particulars should the certificate contain? Must the certifying doctor tell the "full story" of the illness, including the diagnosis, or may he simply certify that the patient is ill and would be unfit to work for a specified period?

A statement of the diagnosis may sometimes have the effect that the employer becomes unwilling to employ the patient any longer on account of the nature of his disease – e g venereal disease – and may try to summarily terminate the employment, which may cause hardship to the employee.[1]

What is the doctor's position if an employer telephones him to seek more information regarding the patient's condition, where the patient has been given a "simple" certificate in the terms referred to above? May or must the doctor provide information to the employer? Is a doctor under any obligation to fill in lengthy forms supplied to him by the employer?

May a doctor in issuing a medical certificate to the effect that the patient has been ill for a certain period rely exclusively on what the patient tells him?

From the point of view of common law – i e apart from special duties that may be imposed upon a doctor by statute, in particular by industrial legislation – the position is quite simple and may be stated in the form of three propositions:

- By virtue of the professional relationship, a doctor who examines his own patient must basically maintain confidentiality in regard to everything pertaining to the patient. A breach of this duty will expose the doctor to a civil action for infringement of the patient's right to privacy.
- The very purpose of a medical certificate, however, is to give medical information to an "outsider", in the interest of the patient. The doctor must therefore inevitably disclose certain facts to the employer. What may and may not be disclosed is a matter for doctor and patient to agree upon.
- Both the law and medical ethics require that whatever information is given, the medical certificate must be truthful.

The patient's legal right to privacy is reinforced by medical ethics. Rule 16 of the SA Medical and Dental Council's code of conduct imposes a general duty upon a doctor to refrain from divulging in any form information which ought not to be divulged "regarding the ailments of a patient", except by consent or under judicial order. The duty of confidentiality is not absolute. Confidentiality must sometimes yield to the public interest. As we have seen, the SAMDC guidelines on the management of patients with AIDS make provision for a *duty* to divulge a diagnosis to sexual partners in certain circumstances.[2] The doctor would, on the other hand, ordinarily not be entitled to divulge such diagnosis to a patient's employer: the risk of transmitting HIV in the

1 Needless to say, such a summary dismissal will amount to breach of contract under common law and/or an unfair labour practice under the Labour Relations Act 28 of 1956.

2 See above 17.

normal work situation is very slight indeed so that the public interest cannot justify a disclosure not consented to.[3]

As far as the agreement between doctor and patient is concerned, and in so far as it relates to the contents of a medical certificate, it usually takes the form of a tacit agreement. The patient consults the doctor and asks him for a medical certificate for the purposes of sick leave. In the ordinary course of events the patient does not lay down any conditions regarding the contents of the certificate, e g by requesting the doctor specifically not to disclose the diagnosis.

In the absence of such a prohibition being imposed by the patient, the doctor would clearly be entitled to exercise his own discretion as to what he discloses and what he does not; there would certainly be no objection to a statement of the diagnosis. In fact, in most cases it would probably be advisable, in the occupational interests of the patient, to mention the diagnosis. The employer will then have little reason to suspect the authenticity of the certificate.

Without an indication of the diagnosis, the certificate may not be of much value to the employer in deciding whether or not the employee was entitled to sick leave in terms of the contract of employment.

There may be cases, however, where the doctor feels that it would be against the interests of the patient to mention the disease by name, and for that reason he may decide to omit such a reference; there is nothing to prevent a doctor from so doing. Where revealing the diagnosis to the employer could cause complications for the patient, the doctor would obviously be wise to bring this to the patient's attention.[4]

If the employer is in any way dissatisfied with the lack of detailed information supplied in the certificate, it is his problem. There is no way in which the employer can compel the doctor to supply more detailed information by telephone or otherwise; in particular the doctor is under no obligation to complete a lengthy questionnaire. In fact, the doctor is under an obligation *not* to provide further information unless the patient has consented thereto. It may of course frequently be in the interest of the patient to comply with a request reasonably made by the employer for further information, and if the doctor feels this may be the case, he should ask the patient's consent to make further information available to the employer.

Should the patient have expressly insisted on the diagnosis not being mentioned in the certificate and the employer is dissatisfied because of the lack of information and dismisses the employee – in so far as he would legally be entitled to do so – that is the employee's problem. The doctor is in no way concerned with the contractual relationship between employer and employee. If the patient loses his job, he can in no way hold the doctor liable.

The Medical Association has advised doctors that medical certificates should only be handed to patients and not direct to employers. The Association has pointed out, quite correctly, that it is the prerogative of the patient whether or not the diagnosis should be disclosed on the certificate.[5]

So far we have only dealt with the situation where a patient consults his own doctor. The position is of course different where the doctor is also employed by the employer, and where he is under a duty to the employer to examine employees and to record, and report to the employer, medical facts pertaining to employees. Part of the employee's conditions of employment may be to submit to such medical examinations and/or treatment by a "company" doctor as are reasonably necessary in the interests of employer and employee. It is clear that in these cases there can be no limitation

3 See my article "Employees with AIDS: Some legal issues" in *Huldigingsbundel vir W A Joubert* (1988) 140 at 142.

4 I respectfully associate myself with the views to this effect, expressed by a spokesman of the Medical Association of South Africa, reported in the *Medical Chronicle*, August 1980.

5 See *Medical Chronicle*, August 1980.

whatsoever on the nature of the information disclosed by the doctor to the employer; the patient has by contract agreed to this when he entered the employment and the doctor is in turn contractually obliged to supply to the employer such information as was stipulated by the latter.

We must now turn to statutory law. There are a number of enactments, particularly in the field of industrial legislation, where references are found to medical certificates.

Thus, for example, the Basic Conditions of Employment Act[6] (applying to workers in industries, shops, and offices of private concerns) provides that an employer may, as a condition precedent to paid sick leave for a period of more than two consecutive days, require the employee to produce a medical certificate "stating the nature and duration of the employee's incapacity". This provision clearly implies that the employer may insist on an express indication of the diagnosis, and doctors ought to bear this in mind when issuing medical certificates.

Under the Manpower Training Act[7] a prospective apprentice, in order to legally bind himself as such, must have obtained a certificate of physical fitness. Such a certificate must be issued free of charge to the prospective apprentice by a district surgeon. However, a certificate on the same form by any other registered medical practitioner may be accepted.[8] The prescribed form makes provision for the precise details to be stated. It must be noted, however, that there is no statutory duty upon doctors who are not district surgeons to issue such certificates.

There are a number of provisions in the Workmen's Compensation Act[9] relating to medical examinations. The amount of compensation payable to workmen for disablement caused by accidents or industrial diseases is in accordance with a sliding scale based upon the degree of disablement. For this a thorough examination or examinations are of course necessary, but these will ordinarily be conducted by doctors appointed by either the Workmen's Compensation Commissioner or the employer.[10] It goes without saying that in these cases the doctor will furnish a complete report, indicating the exact nature of the injury or disease and describing in detail the resultant disablement. A workman has the right to nominate a doctor, at his own expense, to be present at such an examination. Apart from these provisions, the Commissioner has the right to make regulations for the submission, without additional charge, of reports to him by medical practitioners who have attended or been consulted in respect of injured workmen.[11]

Finally, mention may be made of the fact that statutory duties are imposed upon medical officers – and sometimes upon private practitioners – to report to official agencies specified conditions discovered in the course of a medical examination. It is not intended to describe these duties in detail here, however, because we are presently concerned with medical certificates only. By way of example, mention may be made of the following duties: the duty of a doctor in terms of the Mental Health Act[12] to report to a magistrate or to the Police a mentally ill patient who is dangerous to others; the duty of a doctor in terms of the Health Act[13] to report to a local authority deaths resulting from notifiable diseases; the duty of a doctor, dentist and nurse in terms of the Child Care Act[14] to report cases of child abuse to the Regional Director of Health and Welfare.

6 Act 3 of 1983, section 13.
7 Act 56 of 1981, section 17*(b)*.
8 Regulations in terms of the Act, contained in GN R2366 of 2/11/81, reg 8.
9 Act 30 of 1941.
10 Section 60. See also *NGPG Bulletin* vol 3 no 6 (1991) 12.
11 Section 78 (2).
12 Act 18 of 1973, section 13.
13 Act 63 of 1977, section 47.
14 Act 74 of 1983, section 42.

Note that a fraudulent medical certificate exposes the certifying doctor to a criminal charge of fraud – which, needless to say, is a serious matter – as well as to disciplinary action by the Medical Council, which may have equally serious repercussions. A doctor should at all times comply with ethical rule No 17 which proscribes the following conduct: "Granting a certificate in his professional capacity unless he is satisfied from personal observation that the facts are correctly stated therein, or has qualified the certificate by the words 'as I am informed by the patient'." This rule clearly renders it improper for a doctor to certify that a patient has been medically unfit for a certain period, unless it is on the basis of his own (i e the doctor's) examination or unless he has added the quoted words.

Attention should also be drawn to section 39 of the Mental Health Act[15] which provides that a medical practitioner giving a certificate or making a report under chapter 4 of the Act (State President's Decision Patients and mentally ill prisoners) must state therein that the opinion he expressed has been formed after personal examination or observation of the patient by the doctor himself.

15 Act 18 of 1973.

22 The keeping of medical records and the rights of doctor and patient to these

General principles

It goes without saying that it is of vital importance that every doctor keep proper records of each patient. These records should include details such as the dates on which he saw the patient, his diagnosis, what treatment or advice he gave the patient, medicines he prescribed, referral to specialists, etc. The same applies to hospitals and clinics.

Apart from the obvious necessity of this in enabling the doctor to gauge the progress of the patient, such records may be of the utmost importance in the unfortunate event of a malpractice case being brought against the doctor or a disciplinary inquiry being instituted.

Elementary as the professional duty of keeping records is, it has nevertheless been pointed out by lawyers from time to time what disastrous consequences the failure to keep adequate records has had to medical defendants. As Ficarra[1] says, the patient's medical record may be the first line of defence against malpractice litigation.

The ownership of records made by the doctor for his own purposes cannot be legally in doubt. He is the exclusive owner of these records and is presently under no legal duty to allow a patient to read his records. The doctor has a moral obligation to keep the patient informed on his health, but he does not have to let the patient read his medical record.

According to South African law the patient would only be able to have access to medical records if he had already formally instituted action in court by means of summons or otherwise.[2] The Supreme Court rules[3] provide for a party to a suit to require the other party to make discovery on oath of all documents relating to any matter in question which are in the control of the other party. Such notice may not, except with the leave of a judge, be given before the close of pleadings. Failure by a party to disclose a document may lead to dismissal of his defence.

Our courts will not be prepared to make an order upon the application of a prospective plaintiff whereby a search of the defendant's premises will be authorised to look for documents or other things that may afford evidence to support a possible cause of action. This would amount to a so-called "fishing expedition". However, where there is a strong *prima facie* case as far as the prospective plaintiff's main action is concerned, and there is reason to believe that the objects or the information may be removed, concealed or destroyed – which will have the effect of defeating the ends of justice – a court will be prepared to order the defendant to permit access to the plaintiff and a search.[4] It is clear that in respect of actions against doctors or

1 B J Ficarra *Surgical and Allied Malpractice* (1980) 610.

2 Herbstein and Van Winsen *The Civil Practice of the Superior Courts in South Africa* (3rd edition by L de V van Winsen, J P G Eksteen and A C Cilliers, 1979) 398-399. Compare *Economic Data Processing (Pty) Ltd and Others v Pentreath* 1984 (2) SA 605 (W).

3 Supreme Court rule 35.

4 *Ex parte Dyanti and Another* 1989 (4) SA 826 (CKGD) and authority cited therein. As was pointed out by Mr Justice Heath, the Transvaal court had ruled against this view. However, in *Universal City Studios Inc and Others v Network Video (Pty) Ltd* 1986 (2) SA 734 (A) the Appellate Division *obiter* ruled in favour of this relief.

hospital authorities this situation will arise in the rarest instances only, e g where a doctor has threatened to destroy a patient's records.

The rule that a patient will ordinarily have access to medical records only by way of discovery, presents a major obstacle to patients who are still contemplating legal action against a doctor. It is submitted that we should in fairness to patients follow the trend in other countries[5] – by means of statutory provision if necessary – whereby a patient is allowed access to his own medical records prior to the formal institution of action. At the very least the patient should be allowed to inspect his records and to have copies made at his own expense. A de Klerk[6] has argued convincingly in favour of such legislation.

Bromberg and Hirsch[7] have made the point that "[a]vailability of the record actually decreases, rather than increases, the incidence of filing malpractice suits". They warn that by refusing to release records to a patient, the doctor is only inviting the former to file an action and to obtain access by procedural means. "The refusal will only serve to arouse the suspicions of the patient to a state of paranoia. Therefore, the best advice for a physician is to always maintain accurate and complete records in such a manner that they can readily be duplicated and turned over to the patient upon payment of duplicating costs."

Where a doctor, who is not a party to the litigation (i e is neither plaintiff nor de-

5 In *England*, by virtue of the Administration of Justice Act 1970, section 32, a patient may apply for a court order, enabling him to get access to medical records. In *McIvor v Southern Health and Social Services Board (Northern Ireland)* [1978] 1 WLR 757 the House of Lords ruled that this right was not restricted to doctors nominated by the patient. Parliament then responded to objections raised by the medical profession, and in terms of the Supreme Court Act 1981, section 34, disclosure is now limited to the patient's medical and/or legal advisers. See: J L Taylor (ed) *Medical Malpractice* (1980) 80; I Kennedy in *Medical Responsibility in Western Europe* (eds E Deutsch and H-L Schreiber, 1985) 147-8.

In *Germany* the courts have ruled that there is a legal duty upon doctors and hospitals to allow a patient to inspect the records pertaining to him, and to furnish him with a photocopy or a computer print-out after termination of his treatment, if the patient has a justifiable interest therein. Ascertaining whether or not the patient has a claim in consequence of professional negligence is regarded as a justifiable interest. See E Deutsch *Arztrecht und Arzneimittelrecht* (1983) 134.

In the *Netherlands* the trend is also to allow the patient access to medical records. The *Medisch Tuchtkollege* of Amsterdam ruled that a patient was entitled – at his own expense – to receive a copy of an X-ray plate of himself in the possession of a hospital (unless there are reasonable grounds for fearing that the patient could be harmed by knowledge of the plates or interpretation thereof by incompetent persons, and the risk of such harm could not be removed by means of a written explanation or warning). See *TvGR (Tijdschrift voor Gezondheidsrecht)* 1979, 209. The *Rechtbank* of Amsterdam ordered a hospital to deliver copies of medical reports relating to treatment by a gynaecologist so as to enable the patient's father to assess whether or not there were grounds for the institution of a civil action for damages. See *TvGR* 1979, 210, and compare the ruling by the *Kantongerecht* of Tillburg, *TvGR* 1979, 254. But in another case, the *Gerechtshof* of The Hague ruled against a patient who demanded the original X-ray plates taken by a hospital, refusing to accept copies; the ruling was confirmed on appeal by the *Rechtbank*. See *TvGR* 1981, 112. In yet another case, a bank which had advanced monies to a client was in possession of medical reports concerning the client's occupational disablement. The court ordered the bank to make photocopies of the medical reports available to the patient. The only exception to the principle that a patient is entitled to a copy of medical reports, the courts held, is when the nature of the medical particulars is such that direct cognisance thereof would be harmful to the patient: unreported decision of *Arrondissementrechtbank*, Amsterdam, of 3 March 1983 (KG 83/213). (I am indebted to Professor H J J Leenen of Amsterdam for making this decision, as well as the others referred to, available to me.)

As to the legal position in the USA see note 15 below.

On foreign law generally, see also: A de Klerk's thesis cited in note 6 below; D Giesen *International Medical Malpractice Law* (1988) 424 *et seq*.

6 A de Klerk *Die Reg van die Pasiënt om Insae te Verkry in Geneeskundige Dokumentasie betreffende Homself* (LLM thesis, Univ of S Africa, 1987). See also articles by De Klerk in 1989 *TSAR* 14; 8 *Med Law* 475 (1989).

7 J Bromberg & H Hirsch "Medical Records and Hospital Reports" 1982 (1) *Medicine and Law* 253 at 255.

fendant), is required as a witness at a trial to produce a document relevant to the case, that may be achieved by means of a subpoena *duces tecum*.

It is not only unethical[8] for a doctor to disclose medical facts to a third party without authorisation, but it is illegal in that it amounts to an actionable violation of the patient's right to privacy.[9]

The following are exceptions to this rule:

- where a doctor is called as a witness in a court action between a patient and another party, and is ordered by the presiding officer to testify on such medical facts;
- where a patient sues a doctor for malpractice, the patient himself puts the medical facts in issue, and the doctor will of course be entitled to testify, in his own defence;
- where a patient lays a complaint with the SA Medical and Dental Council, the doctor in answering the charge or in defending himself, may have to disclose medical facts pertaining to the patient;
- where a doctor acts in terms of the statutory duty to report a notifiable disease,[10] "dangerous" mental illness in a patient treated or examined by him,[11] or to report a case of suspected child abuse;[12]
- where the public interest is manifestly at stake, e g where a doctor informs sexual partners of a patient who has been diagnosed as HIV positive.[13]

It is to be noted that a patient's medical record may not be sent to another doctor without the patient's permission, which ought to be taken in writing.

A doctor should not surrender the original copy of his records but should preserve them. They will constitute the best evidence in the event of a dispute concerning the entries made on such records.

Ficarra,[14] writing on American law, is of the opinion that a patient has a property right to the information contained in medical records and therefore is entitled to a copy thereof,[15] but in my opinion this cannot be said of South African law. Medical records are made exclusively for the doctor's purposes, and information which happened to be recorded by the doctor ought to be imparted only in so far as it is necessary for the doctor to obtain an informed consent. As I have indicated above, however, it is doubtful whether this situation is fair to patients.

What Ficarra[16] says of telephone requests for information on a patient's medical record certainly applies to South Africa as well: a telephone request for a patient's record should not be honoured by a doctor, even if the request comes from a colleague related to the patient.

No doctor has the right to give a patient's family or employer detailed information

8 Ethical rule 16.
9 J Neethling *Die Reg op Privaatheid* (1976) 203, 253, 321; cf D J McQuiod-Mason *The Law of Privacy in South Africa* (1978) 176, 193.
10 See e g the Health Act 63 of 1977, sections 45 and 47.
11 See the Mental Health Act 18 of 1973, section 13.
12 Child Care Act 74 of 1983, section 42.
13 See above 16.
14 *Op cit*, 616.
15 As is pointed out by H L Hirsh "Medicolegal Implications of Medical Records" 1975 *Legal Medicine Annual* 171 *et seq* at 172, the American courts have in more recent decisions departed from earlier decisions in which it was held that a health-care facility had an exclusive proprietary right to a patient's records. The recent decisions are to the effect that although the health-care provider has absolute ownership and a right to possession of the original record, the patient also has the right to information contained in the record and is absolutely entitled to a copy of his hospital record. See also Bromberg & Hirsh *op cit* 254. As the latter authors reported, by 1982 at least 18 American jurisdictions had statutes permitting direct access by a patient to either hospital or physician records for the purposes of inspection or copying.
16 *Op cit*, 616.

on his medical record, without the patient's consent. An exception to this rule would of course be the giving of information to parents (or guardians) concerning a minor who is treated upon the request of his parent. Another exception would be where, in terms of industrial legislation,[17] an employee must undergo a medical examination and the doctor must certify whether or not he is suffering from a particular disease.

It must be mentioned that it is wise not to destroy medical records too soon. A delictual claim becomes prescribed after three years,[18] but it only arises from the moment that the claimant acquires knowledge of the facts from which the claim arises, or could have acquired such knowledge by exercising reasonable care.[19] There is no period of prescription for allegations of unprofessional conduct that may lead to a disciplinary inquiry. I would therefore advise doctors to keep their records for as long as this is practicable. From a practical point of view I would recommend that records be kept for at least ten years.[20] If the patient is a minor, the records should be kept until he has achieved majority and for some period beyond that. The reason for this is that prescription does not run against a person as long as he is a minor, and for one year afterwards.[21]

X-ray plates

The legal position regarding X-ray plates does not seem to be quite as unequivocal as in the case of written medical records. In terms of the South African Copyright Act[22] the ownership of the copyright in an "artistic work" vests in the author thereof.[23] "Artistic work" does not, as the term would seem to indicate, necessarily mean a work of art in the generally accepted meaning of that expression. The Act stipulates that among other things it includes, "irrespective of the artistic quality" thereof, photographs. "Photograph" is defined in the Act as embracing "any product of photography" – which without a doubt, would include an X-ray plate. "Author" in relation to a photograph is defined in the Act as "the person responsible for the composition of the photograph".[24]

There can be no doubt that the person "responsible for the composition" of the X-ray plate is the radiologist who has taken the plate or under whose direct supervision the plate was taken by a radiographer. In accordance with the Copyright Act he would seem to hold the copyright.

However, copyright and ownership are not identical concepts. I may be the owner of a photograph which I have bought from a photographer who is the owner of, and has the copyright to, the negative.

In private medical practice the doctor who treats a patient sends him to a radiologist with the request that X-ray plates be taken. The patient ordinarily pays the radiologist direct for his services, but the latter supplies the negative with his report to the doctor for final diagnosis. Frequently the doctor, with the tacit consent of the patient, keeps the X-ray plates as part of his records. In such a case, the plates would in my opinion become the property of the doctor.

The question of the ownership of X-ray plates has as yet not been the subject of a

17 See e g the Workmen's Compensation Act 30 of 1941, section 60. Implicit in the latter section is a duty on the part of the doctor who examines a workman, to report to the Workmen's Compensation Commissioner fully on the workman's condition, to enable the Commissioner to properly assess the compensation for which the worker would qualify.

18 Prescription Act 68 of 1969, section 11(*d*).

19 *Ibid*, section 12(3).

20 The Medical Association of South Africa (MASA) recommends to doctors that medical records be kept for six to nine years (see *S Afr Med J* vol 73, 20 Feb 1988, p x).

21 Prescription Act, section 13(1).

22 Act 98 of 1978.

23 Section 3.

24 The definitions are contained in section 1 of the Act.

reported decision by a South African court, nor, as far as can be ascertained, by an English court. In Michigan, however, it was held in *McGarry's* case[25] (1935) that in the absence of any agreement to the contrary, X-ray negatives are the property of the doctor who has them made pursuant to his treatment of the patient, despite the fact that the patient may have paid for them. The court pointed out that retention by the doctor of the negatives constitutes an important part of his record in any particular case, and that in the aggregate these negatives may preserve much of value incident to a doctor's experience.

"They are as much part of the history of the case," the court said, "as any other record made by the physician, differing little, if at all, from microscopic slides of tissue made in the course of the diagnosis or treatment of the patient.

"In the event of a malpractice suit against a physician, the X-ray negatives which he has caused to be taken and preserved incident to treating the patient might constitute the unimpeachable evidence which would fully justify the treatment of which the patient was complaining."

Although I was unable to trace any later American decision specifically on X-ray plates, it must be pointed out that American legal authors for the past 40 years generally seem to have quoted the *McGarry* decision with approval; this is true of English writers as well, although Speller[26] (1973) has pointed out that there are also cogent arguments to support the view that the patient should be considered the owner of the X-ray print accompanying the radiologist's report.

Speller says it may justly be argued that an expert's report normally becomes the property of the person paying for it even though obtained through the intermediary of a third party. He gives the examples of an attorney obtaining counsel's opinion, or an architect the opinion of a consulting engineer. Such further opinion he says, is obtained partly, at all events, with the object of divesting the attorney or architect to some extent of personal responsibility in the matter. But to obtain such relief, the expert's opinion must be communicated to the client.

But, argues Speller, this argument is not necessarily applicable to medical practice, since it would not always be in the patient's interest to disclose to him all the facts with reference to the nature and treatment of the disease. Furthermore it is not always practicable to do so in a form understandable by the patient: a radiologist's film or print, even accompanied by a report would not necessarily be intelligible to him.

Still, it must be conceded, says Speller, that "merely because a report a man has paid for is unintelligible to him, is no ground for depriving him of any right he may have to possession of such report or a copy of it".

The most telling argument against the patient's right to claim the film or print, according to Speller – and I respectfully agree – is to be found in the general custom of the medical profession in the matter. He argues that what the patient pays for is not a photograph but the expert reading by the radiologist of the film and his opinion being communicated to the medical practitioner by whom the patient was referred for his guidance.[27]

Apart from the narrow issue of *ownership* of records, there is of course the issue of *access* to medical records in general. According to English law a patient may by order of court have access to medical records.[28]

In Holland it was held (1981)[29] that X-ray plates made by a hospital of a patient,

25 *McGarry v J A Mercier Co* 262 NW 296 (Mich 1935).
26 S R Speller *Law of Doctor and Patient* (1973) 157.
27 See also J Seear "Dental Malpractice" in *Medical Malpractice* (ed J Leahy Taylor) (1980) 295 at 301-302. Seear makes the qualification that the patient will be the owner where the taking of radiographs has been performed at the express request of the patient and is not involved with the provision of treatment by the practitioner.
28 See above n 4.
29 See the report published in *TvGR (Tijdschrift voor Gezondheidsrecht)* 1981, 112.

treated in the hospital, are the property of the hospital and in the absence of an agreement to the effect that the plates would be handed over to the patient he was not entitled to claim delivery thereof. In this case the patient refused to accept copies of the plates which the hospital was prepared to make available to him.[30] In a case[31] which served before the Amsterdam medical disciplinary body *(Medisch Tuchtkollege)* in 1978, it was decided that a patient is entitled – at his own expense – to receive a copy of an X-ray plate of himself which is in the possession of a hospital, unless there are reasonable grounds for fearing that the patient could be harmed by knowledge of the plates or interpretation thereof by incompetent persons, and the risk of harm could not be removed by means of a written explanation or warning.

In the USA the latest trend is to give the patient a statutory right to have access to medical records generally for the purposes of inspecting or copying.[32] By 1982 18 jurisdictions had such laws, differing in their coverage and impact.[33] The trend in German law is likewise to give the patient the right to obtain copies of hospital records at his own expense.[34]

Price[35] (1953) reasoned that where a practitioner sends a patient to the specialist, the specialist's reports, film, etc, are made and sent to the practitioner for his personal information, not for the patient's. Price thought that there was no reason why a South African court should not adopt the same attitude as that adopted in *McGarry's* case and I would respectfully support his view. As I have mentioned above, however, I support the view that a patient should be legally entitled, at the very least, to receive a *copy* of medical records pertaining to himself. It goes without saying that he should bear the cost of such copies. The qualification stated by the Amsterdam *Medisch Tuchtkollege*, to which I have made reference, seems to be eminently reasonable. But at present our law is silent on these issues.

It is to be noted that where a doctor hands the patient the X-ray plates after having made his diagnosis, the doctor clearly transfers ownership. Likewise, if the doctor when making the plates agrees to hand them to the patient, the latter will be entitled to claim delivery.

The keeping of stacks of bulky X-ray plates may pose a "logistical" problem to the doctor. For that reason some doctors simply hand the plates to their patients after they (the doctors) have no further use for the plates. The patient is regarded by some practitioners as the best custodian of X-ray plates because of his interest (*quaere*: obsession in some cases?) in his complaint. However, this is not necessarily so. A doctor should never lose sight of the fact that should an allegation of negligence be made against him (the doctor) at a later stage, he may be unable to rely on important evidence embodied in the X-ray plates. As I have mentioned, it is wise for doctors to keep patient records for a considerable period.

As a result of the high price of silver today, there are firms which are keen to buy old X-ray plates from doctors. A doctor who sells these, should be mindful of the medico-legal risk attached to disposal of the plates.

If a doctor decides to let the patient have the plates, the latter should be warned of the importance of keeping these with a view to future reference. The patient should be required to sign a document acknowledging receipt. It goes without saying that under no circumstances should the doctor part with the original radiological report based upon the plates.

30 In this case the hospital was actually prepared to put the X-ray plates in the hands of the patient's family doctor or another doctor attending him.
31 See the report published in *TvGR* 1979, 209. The case was decided in 1978.
32 See above n 15.
33 See Bromberg & Hirsh *op cit* 254.
34 Deutsch *op cit* 134.
35 I Gordon, R Turner & T W Price *Medical Jurisprudence* (3rd ed, 1953) 82.

Patient-retained record cards: advantages and disadvantages

Certain hospital authorities have recently considered the possibility of introducing a system of patient-retained record cards. The objective is to alleviate the burden of keeping and storing record files on the very large number of patients who come to these hospitals, either for treatment over a period, or on an out-patient basis. (The overwhelming majority are out-patients.) The keeping of many thousands of files presents a problem in two respects: a) space must be made available for storage purposes, and b) staff must be employed to keep the files properly organised, in particular to retrieve a file when a patient again presents for treatment.

The proposed scheme entails that each patient or his parents or guardians will become responsible for the safe-keeping of his own medical records, save for dispensary notes issued by members of the staff, pathology reports, and X-ray negatives and radiological reports.

The idea is that the patient will be issued with a booklet in which clinical data – other than the items specified – will be entered; such as the date when the patient presented, a note of his symptoms, the diagnosis made by the clinician, the treatment, instructions to the patient and any other relevant information such as allergies. When the patient returns at any future date for further attention, he will be required to produce the booklet so as to enable the clinician to check or acquaint himself *de novo* with the medical history of the patient.

An advantage of the proposed system is said to be the fact that a patient may consult other doctors or health personnel not connected with the hospital, who will then be in a position to acquaint themselves fully with the patient's medical history. This would enable the latter health-care professionals to give better medical care. They would also not have to waste time trying to find out who had previously treated the patient and to establish contact with such personnel, which may be logistically very difficult since many of the patients may be relatively unsophisticated, illiterate or semi-literate and may experience language problems.

In theory the proposed system certainly has considerable advantages. In practice, however, very serious problems may arise. First, there is the problem of loss of booklets. It may be safely assumed that a percentage of patients will lose their booklets or misplace them. Booklets may be stolen together with other personal belongings or may be destroyed by accident. Secondly, there is the possibility of damage to the booklets, or obliteration of details because of "wear-and-tear" or other factors. Many of the patients will be domestic, farm or industrial workers, and experience with identity books has taught that these documents, which are often carried on the individual's person, become very tattered and soiled in due course.

There can be no objection to a doctor or hospital giving a photocopy of patient records to the patient but, to part with the original and only documentation (save for the exceptions mentioned above), may give rise to serious problems. First, there is the danger that a doctor or other health-care worker who must continue a course of treatment or who needs background on the patient's medical history to confirm a diagnosis, or has to decide on a modality or course of treatment, may be unable to do the correct and proper thing because of loss of or damage to the booklet. He or she will be fumbling in the dark, in a manner of speaking. Secondly, in the event of an untoward result such as death, injury or ill-health, or an allegation of malpractice or unethical behaviour by the patient, the documentation of a patient becomes of vital importance to the hospital authority, doctor, nurse or other health-care personnel.

A lawyer who is called upon to defend a doctor, nurse or hospital authority in a lawsuit or ethical inquiry, will regard it as a nightmare to do so in the absence of documentary evidence of what treatment was given on a previous occasion or occasions. How do you contest an allegation of malpractice if your client has no remembrance of either the patient or the exact nature of the examination or treatment, and, even if he can remember some details, cannot back up his version of what happened with documentary evidence?

Where a witness in a court of law wants to make use of a document to refresh his memory, it is a requirement of the law of evidence that the document must have been made or written contemporaneously with the event or transaction in question, or so shortly afterwards that the facts were still fresh in his memory.[36] A document compiled long afterwards can, therefore, not be used for that purpose and will be valueless in proving the existence of a fact.

Many a defence in a lawsuit against a doctor or hospital has failed because of *defective* records, not even to mention non-existent records.

In my opinion the disadvantages of a system of patient-retained record cards outweigh its potential advantages. A hospital authority should rather consider alternative methods, such as a more streamlined filing system and/or photocopying of documents (for the patient's benefit), acquiring or leasing additional storage facilities or microfiche equipment. These methods may in the long run prove to be more cost-effective than to run the risk of landing in indefensible litigation.

Mention should also be made of the possibility of fraudulent entries into the booklet by the patient himself or by others at his request. This can be most embarrassing to health-care personnel. Although we are not proud of them, there are some highly skilled forgers of official documents in this part of the world!

36 C W H Schmidt *Bewysreg* (3rd ed, 1989) 298.

PART VI

Mental patients, psychiatry and the law

23 Criminal responsibility and mental abnormality

Fundamental views

The criminal responsibility of mentally abnormal persons who have committed a crime is one of the most difficult problems of criminal justice.[1] Trial of the mentally abnormal, and in particular the question of responsibility, poses several fundamental problems of a philosophical kind. First, there is the question: what is the purpose of criminal law? And then the directly related question: does man have a free will?

Freedom of will

There are two approaches regarding the freedom of the human will: determinism and indeterminism.

- *Determinism* is a doctrine according to which the fate of human beings is determined by factors beyond their control. The individual's destiny is, as it were, already decided for him; he cannot choose it himself. In a criminal-law context this means the individual's psychological constitution determines whether he will be a criminal or not;[2] and, as some authorities hold, one's psychological constitution is simply the inevitable product of the cells of one's body. What one is, or is going to be, is therefore already determined in the protoplasm.

  According to the most extreme deterministic point of view there is no sense in punishment. In the criminal we have a sick person, and sick people should be medically treated and not punished. Crime is simply symptomatic of an illness. All criminals are sick people, or, differently put,[3] only sick people commit crimes. We do not punish a man because he has measles or scarlet fever. How then can we dare to punish a man whose mind is sick or who is mentally abnormal? Criminal law therefore has no purpose. Some adherents of determinism even refuse to use the term "criminal law", replacing it with the expression "social defence". They would like to see prisons converted into hospitals for the mentally deranged.
- *Indeterminism* is the doctrine which proceeds from the premise that the human will is essentially free; it is not incontrovertibly predestined to any particular line of conduct. Therefore human beings are responsible for their actions and can be called to account in a criminal court. The traditional system of criminal justice is based on this premise.[4] The criminal law nevertheless acknowledges that a certain degree of mental abnormality may have the effect that the individual con-

1 The criminal responsibility of the mentally abnormal formed the subject of a formal inquiry following the assassination of Dr H F Verwoerd, then Prime Minister of South Africa, by Demetrio Tsafendas in 1966. The government appointed a commission known as the Commission of Inquiry into the Responsibility of Mentally Deranged Persons and Related Matters, under the chairmanship of Mr Justice F L H Rumpff, judge of the Appellate Division of the Supreme Court. Its report was published as RP 69/1967. The report is referred to here as the *Rumpff Report*. The recommendations of the Commission were implemented in chapter 13 of the Criminal Procedure Act 51 of 1977.

2 *Rumpff Report* par 5.28.

3 *Ibid* par 1.23.

4 *Ibid* par 2.4.

cerned will not be criminally responsible or – at the very least – will not be fully accountable for his deeds.[5]

Once indeterminism is accepted as a point of departure, it follows that criminal law does have a purpose and that punishment is justifiable. Criminal law is not only an instrument for social defence, it is above all an instrument for social retribution. This does not mean criminal law cannot have other objectives as well, such as deterrence and rehabilitation.[6]

Retribution should not be understood, in the narrow sense of the word, as revenge. Juridically it has a wider meaning.[7] Some authorities hold that the notion of retribution is not restricted to criminal law. It is a basic tenet of law in general; it can in fact be said to constitute a jurisprudential basis of law.[8]

Criminal capacity a legal concept

Retribution being recognised as proper in law, it follows that crime is a legal concept and not merely a term to diagnose socially abnormal behaviour. As a legal concept, crime includes the concept of criminal capacity (or criminal responsibility, accountability, *toerekeningsvatbaarheid*).

Some psychiatrists, although not disputing the role of criminal law, are of the opinion that assessing criminal responsibility is a medical matter. Whether or not a man should be punished is for psychiatrists to decide, not for lawyers.[9]

This is an oversimplification. True, mental illness and its causes, its classification and its cure are matters falling within the ambit of medical science. Psychiatry is essentially a therapeutic science.[10] But mental illness is also of direct relevance to the administration of law and in particular criminal law. As soon as we recognise the concept of individual accountability, we are in the realm of normative science, i e law. Law deals with what human conduct *ought* to be (the *sollen*) as opposed to a study of what *is* (the *sein*), which is the realm of natural science. It is the task of the law to define the social norms to which men are bound and it is the task of the courts to decide whether or not specific conduct conformed to these norms.[11] Criminal responsibility is therefore a legal concept and a question to be decided by a court of law.[12]

In doing so, the court must of course be guided by psychiatrists and psychologists. These are the experts in the field of the *sein* of human behaviour.

A practical problem confronting the courts in assessing criminal responsibility, is that judges are sometimes called upon to make a choice between opposing views held by experts.[13] This is not something unusual, however. In adjudicating upon both criminal and civil matters, courts are often faced with conflicting expert views on questions such as the cause of death, whether or not an accused was intoxicated, paternity, whether or not a machine was defective. In a situation like this, a court must make a rational choice as best it can. In doing so it is aided by the rules defining *onus*. A difficult dilemma in choosing between opposing expert views is sometimes avoided, because the factual basis upon which a particular opinion rests is unacceptable to the court.[14]

5 *Ibid* par 9.51.
6 *Ibid* par 1.22.
7 *Ibid* pars 9.55, 9.57, 9.58.
8 This view is attributed to the Dutch legal philosopher, Herman Dooyeweerd. See *Rumpff Report* pars 9.62, 9.63.
9 *Rumpff Report* pars 5.10, 5.20.
10 *Ibid* par 9.39.
11 *Ibid* pars 9.48, 1.30.
12 *Ibid* pars 4.40, 4.43, 5.28.
13 *Ibid* par 4.67, 4.73.
14 See below 131.

The insanity defence: a juristic criterion

Formulating a juristic criterion for the assessment of criminal capacity (or its opposite, criminal incapacity – "insanity" was the term favoured by generations of lawyers) has proved to be a subject of considerable controversy. Generally speaking, lawyers and psychiatrists do not see eye to eye on this issue. The approach of psychiatry to criminal responsibility differs from that of the lawyer. Modern psychiatry, which is a therapeutic science, does not even use the term "insanity".[15] Psychiatrists use "mental abnormality" as a general term to cover all forms of mental disease, mental deficiency and disorders of personality. "Mental disease" or "disease of mind" is used in a narrower sense.[16] Various types of mental disease are identified by special names, but some apparently defy classification, other than "indeterminate types".[17] There is still a good deal of controversy among psychiatrists on the classification of and terminology for mental diseases.

So far, lawyers have not succeeded in formulating a criterion for insanity which psychiatrists find fully acceptable. The endeavour should nevertheless be to seek a formula as compatible as possible with modern psychiatric views. The legal criterion must necessarily be of a general nature. It would be impossible and even dangerous for a court to endeavour to find a general symptom by which a mental disease can be recognised.[18]

It was perhaps inevitable for legal formulae relating to insanity to suffer from oversimplification. On this issue criticism stemming from psychiatrists was quite correct. An example of oversimplification can be found in the *M'Naghten* rules[19] which reduced the test for insanity essentially to the ability to distinguish between right and wrong.[20] The "irresistible impulse" doctrine by which the "right-and-wrong" test was amplified in South Africa and some American jurisdictions, is more sophisticated, but has also been rejected by psychiatrists as too narrow.[21] Perhaps the American *Durham* test[22] (1954) has come the closest to acceptance by psychiatrists but it can indeed be asked whether this is still a legal criterion at all.[23] (In essence *Durham* ruled that the accused was blameless if the crime was the product of mental disease or defect. Although initially hailed as a breakthrough, the test did not find much favour with the American courts in the long run. In later decisions the test for criminal nonresponsibility was narrowed. In a few states, the insanity defence was even abolished altogether, legislatively, which means that the accused could not be acquitted on the ground that he was suffering from mental illness. If proven guilty of the criminal act charged, he is convicted and is then treated as a mental patient.)[24]

Today it is recognised that a legal criterion should be based on modern psychology which views personality as an integrated concept. You cannot split personality up into different parts. The doctrine of "partial insanity" is today considered outmoded.[25] Various aspects of human personality may be distinguished, but they all relate to an integrated whole and cannot be divorced in reality from an individual case. These aspects are the cognitive (relating to perception and intellect),[26] the affective (relating to the emotions)[27] and the conative (relating to will).[28] Any legal criterion

15 *Rumpff Report* pars 9.73, 9.74.
16 *Ibid* par 7.2.
17 *Ibid* par 7.3
18 See *S v Mahlinza* 1967 (1) SA 408(A) 417.
19 Formulated in the well-known English case of *M'Naghten* (1843) Cl & Fin 200, 8 ER 718.
20 *Rumpff Report* par 7.17.
21 *Ibid* par 7.18.
22 Formulated in *Durham v United States* 214 F 2d 862 (1954).
23 *Rumpff Report* par 7.19.
24 R Slovenko "The Continuing Saga of the Insanity Defense" in *Essays in Honor of Dean Paul K Ryu* (1988) 46, at 60.
25 *Rumpff Report* par 5.16.
26 *Ibid* par 9.13.
27 *Ibid* par 5.16.
28 *Ibid* 9.20 *et seq.*

which does not provide for consideration of all three of these cannot properly be described as scientific.

Accused's fitness to stand trial

In our law every person is presumed to be sane until the contrary has been proved. However, if an accused is on account of mental illness or defect, unfit to appreciate the proceedings so as to conduct his defence properly, it is inconceivable that he can be tried before a criminal court. "I can try a man who does not at least have the basis of a rational mind just as little as I can try a dog or a lifeless instrument," said Mr Justice Beyers in the case of *S v Tsafendas*.[29] If it is established that such an accused cannot be tried, he will – in terms of the provisions of chapter 13 of the Criminal Procedure Act – be dealt with under the administrative machinery contained in the Act. The investigation into the capacity of an accused to be tried precedes, and has no connection with, the inquiry into his responsibility.

Inquiry and report

Section 77 of the Act provides that if it appears, at any stage of criminal proceedings, that the accused is by reason of mental illness or defect not capable of understanding the proceedings so as to make a proper defence, the court must direct that the matter be inquired into and reported on in accordance with section 79. With a view to the inquiry the court may commit the accused to a mental hospital or other place designated by the court, for such periods as the court may determine from time to time, not exceeding 30 days at a time.[30] If the accused is charged with an offence for which the sentence of death may not be imposed, the inquiry must be conducted and reported on by the medical superintendent of the hospital, or by a psychiatrist appointed by the superintendent at the request of the court.[31] In the case of a capital offence (or if the court in any particular case so directs) the inquiry must be conducted by a panel of psychiatrists constituted in terms of section 79.[32] The section prescribes what matters are to be included in the psychiatric report.[33]

If the finding in the psychiatric report is unanimous and is not disputed by the prosecutor or the accused, the court may determine the matter on the report without hearing further evidence.[34] If it is not unanimous or is disputed, a proper hearing must take place in court.[35] If the court finds that the accused is capable of understanding the proceedings, the case continues in the ordinary way. If the court's finding is that the accused is not thus capable, the court must direct that he be detained – in a mental hospital or prison – pending the decision of the State President.[36] The accused then becomes what is known as a "State President's patient". This means that his detention will be indefinite and his eventual discharge subject to special procedures.[37]

29 1966 CPD, unreported. The full text of the judgment (in an Afrikaans version) is to be found in G C Steyl's book *Regters aan die Woord* (1971) 7.
30 Section 79(2).
31 Section 79(1) (*a*).
32 Section 79(1) (*b*). The panel consists of: (1) the medical superintendent (or other psychiatrist appointed by him); (2) a court-appointed psychiatrist who is not in the full-time service of the State, and (3) a psychiatrist appointed by the accused if he so wishes.
33 Section 79 (4). The report must include a description of the nature of the inquiry, a diagnosis of the accused's mental condition, and whether the accused is capable of understanding the proceedings. If the panel is not unanimous, that fact must be mentioned and each of the panel members must give his own finding.
34 Section 77 (2).
35 Section 77 (3). Note that the party disputing the finding may subpoena and cross-examine any person who under section 79 has inquired into the mental condition of the accused.
36 Section 77 (6).
37 See J Snyman "The Declaration of a Person as a State President's Patient" in *Law and Medicine* (eds Bennett *et al*, 1988) 128.

Mental illness or defect

The procedure prescribed by section 77 relates only to incapacity to appreciate proceedings as the result of mental illness or mental defect and not to other factors such as intoxication or temporary mental aberration due to the use of habit-forming drugs. The mental illness or defect need not be permanent, however. "Mental illness" and "mental defect" are not defined in the Act and an eventual finding on whether the accused is mentally ill or defective will be made on the basis of expert psychiatric evidence. But to make an order for committal of the accused for the purposes of an inquiry into his condition, it is not necessary for the court to first hear expert evidence. It will suffice if the court forms an impression on the basis of its own observation.[38] The court may act *suo motu* (on its own initiative) or upon application made by either the prosecution or the defence.[39] At this stage, in practice, the court will frequently be guided by the evidence of a district surgeon in forming an impression.

The fact that there is no more than a reasonable suspicion in the mind of the court that the accused is incapable of understanding the proceedings so as to make a proper defence, is sufficient for the making of such an order. A bare allegation by the defence of such inability is, however, not enough; it must be an allegation "of substance". In *S v Majola and Others*[40] committal was ordered despite the fact that the district surgeon had informed the court that, in his opinion, there was nothing wrong with the accused. Factors taken into account were, *inter alia*, that there was evidence that in the past the accused had received blows on his head with a hammer, and that defence counsel could get no coherent version out of the accused.

Other procedural aspects

The fundamental principle that judicial proceedings must take place in the presence of the accused, was underlined in *S v Eyden*.[41] In this case, when the accused was brought before the court, there was reason to believe that he was mentally ill or defective. The magistrate accordingly ordered that he be committed to a mental hospital for observation. Some weeks later the case was called again and the prosecutor handed in a psychiatric report to the effect that the accused was in fact mentally ill. The accused was not present in court as he was, at that stage, still in the mental hospital. The magistrate made an order that the accused be detained in a mental institution as a President's patient. Upon review, the court found that the proceedings at which the order had been made were irregular because the accused had not been present. Deranged as the accused might have been, the Criminal Procedure Act gave him the right to a trial.

There is no *onus* on the accused at this stage to prove either that he is incapable of understanding the proceedings or that he was in fact not criminally responsible for the offences.[42]

The question of the fitness of the accused to stand trial can be raised at any stage of the proceedings, even after his conviction and before sentence is passed.[43]

The provisions of section 77(6) are peremptory. Once the court has found that the accused is incapable of understanding the proceedings, the court is obliged to direct that he be detained in a mental hospital or prison, pending the signification of the decision of the State President.[44]

38 Cf *S v Majola and Others* 1980 (3) SA 705 (W).
39 *S v Ebrahim* 1973 (1) SA 868 (A).
40 *Supra*.
41 1982 (4) SA 141 (T); see also *S v Kahita* 1983 (4) SA 618 (C).
42 *S v Mogorosi* 1979 (2) SA 938 (A) 942.
43 *S v Leeuw* 1980 (3) SA 815 (A). Compare *S v Ebrahim, supra*.
44 *S v Skeyi* 1981 (4) SA 191 (N).

Certifiability

Incapacity to be tried in terms of the Criminal Procedure Act and certification of a person as mentally ill in terms of the Mental Health Act are two completely separate matters. The fact that a person has been certified in terms of the latter Act and admitted to a mental hospital does not mean that he will necessarily be found by a court to be incapable of being tried.[45] It is possible that e g a psychopath or a person with epilepsy who has been institutionalised in terms of the Mental Health Act can be found by a criminal court to be fit to stand trial. "Mental illness" is defined by the Mental Health Act, but this definition applies only for the purposes of that Act; the Criminal Procedure Act does not refer to that definition for its own purposes.

Deaf mute

The trial of a deaf-mute person may confront a court with special problems. Deaf-muteness is not necessarily the result of mental illness or mental defect.[46] If it is possible to communicate with such a person through another person, he will be tried in the ordinary way.[47] If there is reason to believe that a deaf-mute is mentally ill, the court may order an inquiry in terms of section 77 of the Criminal Procedure Act. But it would be irregular for a court to commit such a person to a mental institution pending the State President's decision merely on the ground that he is deaf and mute.[48]

Appeal

An accused against whom a finding is made that he is fit to stand trial and who is eventually convicted, may appeal against the finding. Likewise the accused may appeal against a finding that he is not fit to stand trial, unless he himself at the trial alleged that he was incapable, by reason of mental illness or defect, of understanding the proceedings.[49]

Criminal incapacity or non-responsibility

Legal criterion for non-responsibility

Criminal responsibility is a legal concept and not a medical or psychiatric concept.[50] In South Africa the criterion for criminal responsibility is contained in section 78 of the Criminal Procedure Act, which provides as follows:

"A person who commits an act which constitutes an offence, and who at the time of such commission suffers from a mental illness or mental defect which makes him incapable –
(a) of appreciating the wrongfulness of his act; or
(b) of acting in accordance with an appreciation of the wrongfulness of his act,
shall not be criminally responsible for such act."

45 *S v Mnyanda* 1976 (2) SA 751 (A) 764 F.
46 *R v Mamyila* 1913 TPD 464; *In re Pupu* 1959 (3) SA 480 (SR).
47 *In re Pupu, supra.*
48 *S v Matjhesa* 1981 (3) SA 854 (O). If it is impossible to communicate with a deaf-mute who is mentally normal, it would be impossible to try him. As proof of *mens rea* is legally impossible in such a case, such a deaf-mute accused should be acquitted. Cf *Pupu's* case *supra*. As noted in the Rumpff Commission's report (par 10.45) the acquittal of such a deaf-mute is inconceivable, however, where *prima facie* evidence points to the fact that he has committed a serious offence. The Rumpff Commission raised the possibility of detaining such a person in a suitable prison after an administrative inquiry. There is no legislation, however, to cover such a case and it is a *lacuna* in our law.
49 Section 77(8).
50 J C de Wet & H L Swanepoel *Strafreg* (4th ed, 1985) 113.

Responsibility a prerequisite for criminal liability

Criminal responsibility is an indispensable prerequisite for criminal liability in regard to any offence,[51] whether *mens rea* be required in the form of intent or negligence, or whether no *mens rea* be required for the crime in question.[52] Before the question can be asked whether the accused had a specific form of fault – where fault is in fact required – it must be established that he was responsible at the time of the act.[53] The criterion of non-responsibility embodied in section 78(1), in particular the use of the word "incapable" in the context of the subsection, confirms this view. It would be juridically untenable to assess the responsibility of the wrongdoer by asking whether he had the intent to commit the deed with which he is charged.[54]

Mental illness or defect

In order not to be found criminally responsible for his conduct, it must first be established that the accused was suffering from a mental illness or defect at the time of the act.

As I have mentioned, "mental illness" and "mental defect" are not defined in the Act. Whether mental illness or defect was present or not is therefore a question of psychiatric evidence, as indicated expressly in section 78.[55] It is impossible, and dangerous too, for a court to try and seek a general symptom by which a mental disorder can be recognised.[56] As we have seen, "mental illness" has been defined in the Mental Health Act, but certifiability under that Act does not per se lead to the conclusion that an accused is not criminally responsible or that his responsibility will be diminished.

"Mental illness" or "mental defect" refers to a pathological disturbance of the mental faculties of the accused[57] and not simply to a temporary mental aberration in a normal individual, which is not attributable to mental abnormality or is due exclusively to external stimuli such as brain concussion, the use of alcohol,[58] drugs or medicines, or is the result of provocation.

It must therefore be shown that the condition of the accused constitutes a recognised pathological deviation.[59]

The fact that the mental condition of the accused could have deviated to a certain degree from what is normal is not proof of a state of illness.[60] "Intelligent people also sometimes think and do stupid things, more particularly when emotions are ar-

51 *S v Mahlinza, supra,* at 414-5.

52 By virtue of express statutory exclusion, so that liability will be "strict" or "absolute".

53 De Wet & Swanepoel *op cit* 117; *S v Mahlinza, supra*; *Rumpff Report* par 12.26.

54 *S v Adams* 1986 (4) SA 482 (A) 901 C-E.

55 If the issue of non-responsibility on account of mental illness is raised at criminal proceedings, the court must in terms of section 78(2) direct an inquiry in accordance with section 79 – as to which, see above.

56 *S v Mahlinza, supra,* 417.

57 *Ibid* 418; *Rumpff Report* par 9.4.

58 See e g *S v Stellmacher* 1983 (2) SA 181 (SWA): A farmer who was on a strict diet, after a day of hard work in the sun, went to a bar and drank brandy on an empty stomach. He had a pistol with him. He fired several wild shots in the bar, killing another customer without any apparent motive. He claimed in court that he had gone "blank". According to medical evidence, excessive consumption of alcohol could cause temporary brain dysfunction in a healthy individual, as a result of hypoglycaemia. The court held that this does not constitute mental illness. However, it caused the accused to act automatically, in a state of amnesia, and he was accordingly found not guilty. Note that if the Criminal Law Amendment Act 1 of 1988 had been in force at the time (and of application to South West Africa/Namibia) the accused could have been convicted in terms of section 1 of that Act (see text and see below 353).

59 The formal report of the psychiatric examination of the accused in terms of section 79 of the Criminal Procedure Act must contain, *inter alia*, a diagnosis of his mental condition (section 79(4)(*b*)).

60 *S v Harris* 1965 (2) SA 340 (A) 360.

oused."[61] It would likewise be wrong to interpret an inclination to violence in the accused as being in itself an indication of mental illness.[62]

It is not necessary, however, to prove that the origin of the accused's mental illness or defect lies in his mind. It could just as well be organic in origin, e g arteriosclerosis (hardening of the arteries).[63] So too, functional (as distinguished from mere temporary, alcohol-induced) hypoglycaemia (shortage of blood-sugar) can occasion mental illness[64] as can a traumatic head-injury.

On the other hand, however, mere concussion, which causes a temporary interruption in the flow of blood to the brain and loss of consciousness, does not constitute mental illness;[65] such a condition could in fact cause automatism, which means that legally the accused is regarded as not having acted at all.[66]

Moreover, it need not be proved that the mental illness was of a permanent nature[67] or that it is incurable.[68] The doctrine of partial or limited mental illness – according to which one part of a person's mind is normal and the remaining part abnormal[69] – no longer has any support.[70]

The illness of the accused must have existed at the time of the conduct. A person who suffers from mental illness and commits an unlawful act during a *lucidum intervallum* can in fact be found to have been responsible at the time of the act. This would be so even where a court had previously held that the person was mentally deranged.[71]

Although, as we have seen, mere occasional mental aberration as a result of the use of alcohol does not constitute mental illness, the consumption of alcohol, especially if it is chronic, can result in a condition which can be clearly diagnosed as mental illness, e g *delirium tremens*.[72] The same would apply to the long-term use of drugs or medicines which results in serious brain dysfunction.

Psychopathy

The definition of "mental illness" contained in the Mental Health Act includes a psychopathic disorder. But in criminal law, psychopathy as such does not amount to mental illness that may result in criminal non-responsibility.[73] A psychopathic personality can be defined as the type of person in whom an emotional immaturity and instability exist, a condition which manifests itself in an inability to adapt to accepted moral and social norms from an early age.[74]

The typical characteristics of psychopathy are said[75] to include the following: superficial charm, and good or apparently good intelligence; untruthfulness and insincerity; lack of remorse or shame; inadequately motivated antisocial behaviour; failure to learn by experience; pathological egocentricity; general poverty in major

61 Chief Justice Steyn, in the *Harris* case at 358.
62 *Cf* C J R Dugard 1967 *SALJ* 134.
63 *Cf* the English case of *R v Kemp* [1957] 1 QBD 399; [1956] 3 All ER 249, cited with approval in *Mahlinza, supra*, 417.
64 Cf *S v Bezuidenhout* 1964 (2) SA 651 (A).
65 Cf the submission in *Kemp, supra*, 253F.
66 See below 129.
67 *Mahlinza, supra*, 417.
68 *Kemp, supra*, 253.
69 Cf *R v Kruger* 1958 (2) SA 320 (T).
70 Cf *Rumpff Report* par 5.15; E M Burchell & P M A Hunt *South African Criminal Law and Procedure* (2nd ed, 1983) 265.
71 *S v Steyn* 1963 (1) SA 797 (W).
72 *Cf R v Bourke* 1916 TPD 303, 307; *R v Holliday* 1924 AD 250.
73 *R v Kennedy* 1951 (4) SA 431 (A); *R v Von Zell* 1953 (3) SA 303 (A); *R v Roberts* 1957 (4) SA 265 (A); *S v Mnyanda, supra*.
74 *Kennedy, supra*, 434; *S v Nell* 1968 (2) SA 576 (O); *Rumpff Report* pars 8.18 *et seq*: J P Roux *Die Psigopaat* (1975) 14 *et seq*.
75 In *S v Kosztur* 1988 (3) SA 926 (A) the court referred to the 16 characteristics of psychopathy listed by H Cleckley in his book *The Mask of Insanity* (1982).

affective reactions; specific loss of insight; unresponsiveness in general interpersonal relations; and failure to follow any life plan.

In the Mental Health Act (section 1) "psychopathic disorder" is defined as "a persistent disorder or disability of the mind (whether or not sub-normality of intelligence is present) which has existed in the patient from an age prior to that of eighteen years and which results in abnormally aggressive or seriously irresponsible conduct on the part of the patient".

In *Mnyanda's* case[76] attention was drawn to certain problems arising from that definition. The court held that in the absence of any exceptional symptom, a "full-fledged" (*volwaardige*) psychopath is criminally responsible. "He is responsible because he realises what is wrong, and mentally he has the ability to act in accordance with that realisation."[77] The mere fact that an accused is considered to be a psychopath does not even mean that his responsibility is diminished.[78]

Automatism and amnesia

As already noted, there are mental conditions which would not amount to mental illness or defect, yet constitute a complete defence. Such a state is the so-called "sane" automatism or involuntary conduct. Sometimes mention is also made in this context of "blackout" or amnesia (loss of memory).[79] It must be noted however that mere inability to remember what took place does not constitute a defence.[80] A non-pathological condition such as shock, concussion, hypoglycaemia or the consumption of a sedative unknowingly can indeed occasion involuntary conduct with an accompanying loss of memory.[81]

In such a case the conduct of the accused is not regarded as an act in criminal law and he will ordinarily be acquitted.[82] There are two exceptions to this rule, though. First, if the impairment of the accused's faculties was the result of the voluntary consumption of liquor or any other substance, such as drugs, he can be convicted of a statutory offence.[83] Secondly, where negligence is an element of the offence in question, the accused can be convicted thereof if the circumstances were such that, at a stage when he was still in full control over his faculties, he ought reasonably to have foreseen that automatism could set in. An example of such a situation would be where a person who suffers from epilepsy fails to take medication that would prevent a seizure; he drives a vehicle in the knowledge that a seizure may occur which will disable him. If that in fact happens and he is involved in an accident, he can be convicted of negligent driving,[84] and, if someone has died, of culpable homicide.[85] In this type of case, the accused is blamed for his negligent omission at a stage preceding the catastrophe, when his conduct was still voluntary.

A person who is acquitted because of involuntary conduct that is not the result of

76 *Supra*, 762-3.
77 My translation of the words of Chief Justice Rumpff.
78 See below 133.
79 *R v Du Plessis* 1950 (1) SA 297 (O). On amnesia in general, see P H J J van Rensburg & T Verschoor 14(2) *TRW* 1 (1989).
80 *S v Piccione* 1967 (2) SA 334 (N); *R v Johnson* 1970 (2) SA 405 (R).
81 *S v Trickett* 1973 (3) SA 526 (T); *S v Van Rensburg* 1987 (3) SA 35 (T).
82 *R v Schoonwinkel* 1953 (3) SA 136 (C); *R v Dhlamini* 1955 (1) SA 120 (T); *R v Botha* 1959 (1) SA 574 (O); *R v Ahmed* 1959 (3) SA 776 (W); *S v Trickett, supra*; *S v Van Rensburg, supra*.
83 Section 1, Criminal Law Amendment Act 1 of 1988.
84 Compare *S v Trickett, supra. Trickett's* case, however, did not involve epilepsy. The accused fell into a state of (foreseeable) automatism when she was driving her car when probably in a state of drowsiness or extreme exhaustion of which she was aware before commencing the trip (see pp 531, 537-8). On epilepsy, see also below 136.
85 *S v Johnson* 1969 (1) SA 201 (A). On this point, namely liability for a *gevolgsmisdaad*, *Johnson* was not overruled in *S v Chretien* 1981 (1) SA 1097 (A). See also below 352.

mental illness, may not be declared a State President's patient. It should also be noted that there is no burden of proof on him.

The courts approach defences such as automatism and amnesia with caution. Even if such a defence is supported by medical evidence it is suspect, as such evidence is frequently based on the assumption that the accused's account is the truth.[86] To raise a defence of sane automatism there must be evidence strong enough to create doubt as to the voluntary nature of the alleged *actus reus* (unlawful act). It must be supported by medical or other expert evidence indicating that the voluntary act was quite possibly due to causes other than mental illness or disorder. If at the end of the trial doubt exists as to whether the act was voluntary or not, the accused must enjoy the benefit of the doubt.[87] A verdict of automatism cannot be based on a mere presumption that the accused acted involuntarily.[88] The accused must, as it were, lay the foundations of his defence.[89]

It should be carefully considered whether the case is one of sane automatism or a manifestation of mental disease. If the automatism is due to mental illness – so-called "insane" automatism – section 78(1) will apply and a special finding of not guilty owing to mental illness (or defect) will have to be returned.[90]

The effect of mental illness on the accused

In addition to proof of mental illness or defect in the accused, it must be proved that the condition from which he was suffering at the time of the act had a specific effect on him. The result must have been that he was incapable of:

(a) appreciating the wrongfulness of his act; or
(b) acting in accordance with an appreciation of the wrongfulness of his act.

Criterion (b) is an alternative to criterion (a). This means that even where it is found that the accused, in spite of his mental illness, appreciated the wrongfulness of his act he will be acquitted if it is proved that on account of his illness he was incapable of acting in accordance with that appreciation.

In criterion (a) the basic element of the old *M'Naghten* rules[91] was retained, i e the ability to distinguish between right and wrong. It is submitted that the word "wrongfulness" used in section 78(1) does not refer to *unlawfulness* in the strict sense that it is used in criminal law, viz an element of a crime.[92] The assessment of criminal responsibility, in my view, turns on the accused's general ethical sense of responsibility and not so much on the projection of this mental attitude towards the *unlawfulness* of his act.

If "wrongfulness" were to be understood as referring to unlawfulness in its restricted sense, the defence of mental illness would not succeed if an accused, despite his illness, was aware that his conduct was unlawful (i e contrary to the law) but was under the delusion – precisely because of his illness – that it was not wrong because a moral or God-given duty rested on him to commit the act. That result would be unacceptable.[93] It is submitted, therefore, that "wrongfulness" should be interpreted as "legally and morally wrong".[94] It is further submitted that in this context, "morally

86 L Blackwell 1962 *SALJ* 16.
87 *Trickett's* case, *supra*, 537.
88 *S v Ramagaga* 1965 (4) SA 524 (O).
89 *Trickett, supra* 534; C W H Schmidt 1973 *SALJ* 329.
90 Under section 78(6). Compare *R v Mokwanazi* 1959 (3) SA 782 (W) and see below 132.
91 See above 123.
92 M C J Olmesdahl 1968 *SALJ* 276 distinguishes between "moral wrongfulness" and "unlawfulness". Significantly, in the Afrikaans text of the Act, the Legislature used the word "ongeoorloofdheid", which has a wider meaning than "wederregtelik". See further Burchell & Hunt *op cit* 269-272.
93 See the court's remark in the American case of *US v Freeman* 257 F 2d 606 (1966) cited in the *Rumpff Report,* par 7.20. Compare R Petersen and C Steytler 1972 *Responsa Meridiana* 175; C R Snyman *Strafreg* (2nd ed, 1986) 174.

wrong" means "in conflict with the usual moral attitudes of reasonable people".[95] The test, accordingly, is an objective one: in order to be judged criminally responsible it must be established that the accused's assessment of the wrongfulness of his act was in accordance with general moral attitudes prevailing in society at the time.

Criterion (b) goes further than the "irresistible impulse" of earlier times. Although irresistible impulse can still be a defence,[96] the accused now need not show that his deed was the result of a violent urge which was impulsive and flared up suddenly.[97] It will suffice if he proves that owing to mental illness or defect at the time of commission of the act, he was incapable of controlling his will, i e of acting in accordance with his appreciation of the wrongfulness of the act. Such a lack of self-control can be the result of a gradual process of personality disintegration.[98]

Evidence

A finding that the accused lacked criminal capacity can only be made on the basis of expert psychiatric evidence. The court cannot arrive at a verdict on the basis of its own observations.

Where expert witnesses give conflicting evidence, the court must to the best of its ability make a choice between the different points of view. Where the evidence submitted for the prosecution conflicts with that submitted for the defence, the court is of course entitled to consider that the burden of proving non-imputability rests on the accused.[99]

The court is not obliged to accept any psychiatric evidence as conclusive proof. If it is found that the evidence concerning facts upon which the psychiatric opinion is based is not credible, the court is entitled to refuse to accept a psychiatric diagnosis.[100] If the evidence shows conclusively that the accused apparently acted rationally this will be a strong indication that he knew what he was doing, and the court will be guided by this, despite alleged non-imputability at the time of the act.[101]

Psychiatric evidence is worthless unless it is related to the facts of a specific case. "Without connecting psychiatric and psychological opinion with the facts laid before the court, it is abstract theory."[102]

The provisions of section 78 regarding the psychiatric examination of the accused are mandatory; this means that where an allegation of non-responsibility is made, or if it appears to the court that the accused was not responsible, it must direct that an inquiry take place.[103]

As we have seen, there are two types of inquiries: (a) an inquiry in terms of section 77(1) whether the accused is fit to stand trial, and (b) an inquiry in terms of section 78(2) whether the accused was criminally responsible. The psychiatric panel will, strictly speaking, be bound by the terms of the order committing the accused. In prac-

94 Burchell & Hunt *op cit* 271-2 are of the opinion that our courts will probably hold that "wrongfulness" means either unlawful *or* morally wrong. But that, in my opinion, would be too wide a meaning.

95 See the Australian case *R v Stapleton* (1952) 86 CLR 358 and see Burchell & Hunt *op cit* 272. *Contra*: Petersen and Steytler 182 *et seq*.

96 Decisions such as *R v Smit* 1906 TS 783, *R v Westrich* 1927 CPD 455 and *R v Koortz* 1953 (1) SA 371 (A) are, therefore, still valid precedents. But it does not mean that a psychopath who commits a criminal act in a fit of rage will necessarily be found not responsible. See *Rumpff Report* par 9.90. Compare *R v Kennedy* 1951 (4) SA 431 (A) on the responsibility of a psychopath who experienced an "emotional storm".

97 See *Rumpff Report* pars 9.90 *et seq*.

98 The broader scope of the new test is well illustrated by *S v Kavin* 1978 (2) SA 731 (W).

99 *Cf S v Harris* 1965 (2) SA 340 (A) 356.

100 *R v Kennedy, supra*; *R v Von Zell* 1953 (3) SA 303 (A) 311; *S v Harris, supra*, 365; *Rumpff Report* 4.40.

101 *Harris, supra*, 360.

102 Chief Justice Rumpff in *S v Mngomezulu* 1972 (1) SA 797 (A) 799 A; compare *S v Du Preez* 1972 (2) SA 519 (SWA).

103 Section 78(2).

tice, however, it often happens that the accused is committed under the wrong subsection. Accordingly the usage has come about that the inquiry is undertaken either under both subsections or the other subsection. This usage, although not strictly in accordance with the statutory provisions, has been accepted by the courts. With a view to greater legal certainty, however, a court should order committal under both subsections. This would enable the psychiatric panel to go into all aspects pertaining to the accused's mental state.[104]

Burden of proof

In law there is a presumption that every person is sane. The burden of proving a defence of criminal non-responsibility on account of mental illness or defect therefore rests on the accused. Proof beyond a reasonable doubt is not required; it is sufficient if the defence is proved on a preponderance of probabilities.[105] Even where a person has previously been declared by a court to be *non compos mentis*, the *onus* to prove non-responsibility in subsequent criminal proceedings will rest on him.[106]

The same applies to so-called "insane" automatism, i e automatism brought about by mental illness or defect.[107] Where, however, "sane automatism" is raised as a defence, it is for the State to prove beyond a reasonable doubt that the accused knew what he was doing and acted with the necessary *mens rea*.[108]

Special verdict

If the court finds that the accused committed the act in question but that he was not criminally responsible at the time, because of mental illness, the court must find the accused "not guilty by reason of mental illness". If the finding of non-responsibility is made only after the accused has been convicted of the offence but before sentence has been imposed, the court must set aside the conviction and likewise find the accused "not guilty by reason of mental illness".[109]

Such a finding does not mean that the accused is free to go home. The finding must be followed invariably by the order that the accused be detained in a mental hospital pending the decision of the State President.[110] This order must be made even if the accused's mental disorder was only temporary or where the accused has recovered from his illness; at best the court can make a recommendation that the accused be discharged from prison or mental hospital as soon as possible.[111] It goes without saying that where there was no evidence that the accused was mentally ill at the time he committed the deed, he may not be declared a State President's patient.[112]

A finding of not guilty because the accused did not legally act on account of automatism can, of course, not lead to the special verdict, unless the automatism was "insane", i e caused by mental illness.[113]

104 *S v V* 1984 (1) SA 44 (T).
105 *R v Kaukakani* 1947 (2) SA 807 (A); *Kennedy's* case, *supra*; *Mahlinza's* case, *supra*.
106 *S v Steyn* 1963 (1) SA 797 (W).
107 The references to *onus* to prove automatism, in the cases of *S v Van Zyl* 1964 (2) SA 113 (A) and *S v Bezuidenhout* 1964 (2) SA 651 (A), are apparently to automatism arising from mental disorder.
108 *R v Ahmed* 1959 (3) SA 776 (W); *R v Botha* 1959 (1) SA 547 (O); *S v Trickett* 1973 (3) SA 526 (T) 530.
109 Section 78(6).
110 *Ibid.*
111 *S v McBride* 1979 (4) SA 313 (W).
112 *S v Matolla* 1976 (1) SA 268 (C).
113 *R v Kumalo* 1956 (3) SA 328 (N); *R v Mokwanazi* 1959 (3) SA 782 (W); *R v Ngema*; *R v Cele* 1960 (1) SA 137 (A).

Appeal

An accused in respect of whom the special verdict is made and who is consequently declared a State President's patient, may appeal against it in the same manner as in the case of conviction by the court for an offence – unless he himself raised the defence of mental illness.[114] Leave to appeal must first be sought from the trial court.[115] Should the appeal against the special verdict succeed the court of appeal must remit the case to the trial court and the proceedings will then be continued in the ordinary course.[116]

Diminished responsibility by reason of mental illness

If a criminal court finds that, at the time of the act, the accused was criminally responsible but that his capacity to appreciate the wrongfulness of the act or to act in accordance with such appreciation was diminished by reason of mental illness or mental defect, it may in terms of section 78(7) take the fact of diminished responsibility into account when sentencing.

This provision of the Act is of special significance where the accused is proved to have been suffering from a lesser degree of mental illness or defect at the time of the act. The issue of diminished responsibility will be particularly relevant to cases of brain damage, mental retardation, epilepsy and – possibly – psychopathy.[117]

A court is likely to find extenuating circumstances only where the accused's mental defect appears to be substantial and related to the commission of the crime in question. It is apparently not necessary that a specific form of mental illness or defect be mentioned in the psychiatric reports. In *S v Sibiya*[118] extenuating circumstances were found to be present where a psychiatrist had testified that the accused (who was convicted of murder) was "a person who suffered from a persistent disorder or disability of mind which induced in him abnormally aggressive or seriously irresponsible conduct".

In *S v Smith*[119] the fact that a woman who had murdered her husband had an immature personality and was suffering from focal epilepsy was taken into consideration in extenuation of sentence together with factors such as coercion by members of her family and sustained provocation by the deceased. A specialist neurologist testified that the accused's immature personality, coupled with the effects of focal epilepsy, could have made her more susceptible to influence by others.

Whether or not psychopathy can lead to diminished responsibility is a controversial and oft-debated question.[120] Generally speaking, our courts are not prepared to find that psychopathy as such has diminished the criminal responsibility of the accused.[121] In *S v Lehnberg*[122] Chief Justice Rumpff declared that psychopathy as an extenuating circumstance should be treated with great circumspection "since it would otherwise be easy thereby to slip the doctrine of determinism into our criminal law through the backdoor".[123]

On the other hand, the Appellate Division held that it is possible that in certain cases a psychopath would not be able to offer the same resistance as an absolutely normal person would, and in such cases the accused's weakness may properly be

114 Section 78(8).
115 Section 316.
116 Section 78(9).
117 Compare *Rumpff Report* pars 8.13 *et seq.*
118 1984 (1) SA 91 (A).
119 1984 (1) SA 583 (A).
120 See e g : S A Strauss 1971 *THRHR* 11; A Kruger *Kante van Imputasie in die Nederlandse en Suid-Afrikaanse Strafreg* (1972) 281, 289; J P Roux *Die Psigopaat* (1975) 194-5.
121 *Mnyanda, supra,* 764 F, 766 G.
122 1975 (4) SA 553 (A).
123 At 559 (my translation).

taken into consideration as an extenuating circumstance.[124] Only when – in respect of a specific crime – it is found the psychopathic disorder is of such a degree that the person's power of controlling his will was weakened to such an extent that, in terms of a moral assessment, he was less blameworthy than he would have been had he not had such a weakened power of control, a finding of diminished responsibility can be made.[125]

Each case must therefore be judged on its own merits on the basis of all circumstances. In most reported cases where psychopaths were found guilty of murder, the courts refused to find that there were extenuating circumstances.[126]

In other cases, psychopathy together with other factors led to a finding of extenuating circumstances. Thus, psychopathy together with drug addiction and the fact that the accused was subject to a severe emotional conflict at the time of the act, were taken into account in mitigation of sentence.[127] So, too, the fact that the accused was a juvenile, together with his psychopathic tendencies, led to a finding of extenuating circumstances.[128]

It is to be noted that section 78(7) deals specifically with diminished responsibility by reason of mental illness or defect. It goes without saying that a finding of extenuating circumstances may be made by a court of law even where it has not been established that the accused was mentally ill or defective.

Thus it was held that when an accused is not able to resist his urges to the same extent as a normal person – owing to a mental condition which is *not* a mental illness or defect (e g an inadequate personality) – it is also relevant when, for example, the discretionary death sentence for rape is considered.[129]

Non-responsibility on grounds other than mental illness or defect

Mental illness or mental defect is, of course, not the only ground on which an accused may be found to be criminally non-responsible. Youth has since time immemorial been a ground which could result in a finding that the accused is not responsible at all for his deed.[130]

A serious degree of (voluntary) alcoholic intoxication was also at one stage recognised in our law as a circumstance that could lead to a finding of complete non-responsibility.[131] However, the position was legislatively changed in 1988.[132] Intoxication will now provide a complete defence in highly exceptional cases only.[133]

A trend currently manifesting itself in our criminal courts is that severe emotional distress or personality disintegration, unrelated to mental illness or defect, may result in a finding of criminal non-responsibility. This can occur where it is established that the accused's emotional distress was of such a serious degree so as to render him (a) incapable of appreciating the wrongfulness of his act, or (b) if thus capable, incapable of acting in accordance with such appreciation. What is especially interesting about this development is that the courts avail themselves of the terminology of the criteria embodied in section 78(1) of the Criminal Procedure Act, though without coupling the test with mental illness.

124 *Ibid.*
125 *Mnyanda's* case at 766. Compare *S v Pieterse* 1982 (3) SA 678 (A).
126 See e g *R v Von Zell* (2) 1953 (4) SA 522 (A); *R v Roberts* 1957 (4) SA 265 (A); *S v Nell* 1968 (2) SA 576 (A) 579; *S v De Bruyn* 1976 (1) SA 496 (A); *S v Mnyanda, supra*; *S v Pieterse, supra*; *S v Kosztur* 1988 (3) SA 926 (A).
127 *S v Webb* (2) 1971 (2) SA 343 (T).
128 *S v J* 1975 (3) SA 146 (O); *S v Lehnberg, supra.*
129 *S v M* 1985 (1) SA 1 (A).
130 C R Snyman *Strafreg* (2nd ed, 1986) 181.
131 *S v Chretien* 1981 (1) SA 1097 (A).
132 Criminal Law Amendment Act 1 of 1988, discussed below 353.
133 See below 353.

The courts have recognised this defence in cases such as the following: where a man killed his young wife in a fit of extreme jealousy following sexual taunting on the part of the woman;[134] where a woman killed her husband who had subjected her to continuous and extreme humiliation.[135] In *S v Wiid* [136] the Appeal Court upheld a defence of non-pathological incapacity, resulting in an acquittal, where a woman had shot and killed her husband shortly after he had seriously assaulted her. The court held that where the defence is raised, the *onus* rests on the prosecution to *rebut* it; however, it is for the defence to lay this foundation in its evidence. Whether this foundation has necessarily to be laid by way of expert psychiatric evidence, was not considered by the court.[137]

134 *S v Arnold* 1985 (3) SA 256 (C).

135 See *S v Campher* 1987 (1) SA 940 (A). Two of the three judges (Mr Acting Justice Boshoff and Mr Justice Viljoen) were of the opinion that the defence of criminal non-responsibility need not be limited to cases of mental illness or defect. (Compare the views of Mr Justice Viljoen in *S v Adams* 1986 (4) SA 882 (A) and of Mr Justice Joubert in *S v Laubscher* 1988 (1) SA 157 (A).) Mrs Campher was nevertheless convicted of murder with extenuating circumstances; Mr Justice Boshoff held that the defence of non-responsibility can only be decided with the aid of expert psychiatric evidence, which had not been adduced in this case.

136 1990 (1) SACR 561 (A).

137 On the defence generally, see also C R Snyman 14 (1) *TRW* 1 (1989).

24 Epilepsy and the law

The Mental Health Act

In the old Mental Disorders Act of 1916[1] a mentally disordered or defective person was defined essentially as a person who in consequence of mental disorder or disease, or permanent defect of mind, was incapable of managing himself, or constituted a danger to himself or to others.[2] The Act contained a fairly comprehensive classification of mentally disordered or defective persons. There were six "classes" ranging from mentally disordered persons through epileptics.[3] An epileptic was defined as "a person suffering from epilepsy who is a danger to himself or others or incapable of managing his own affairs".[4] It is to be noted that by virtue of this definition only those epileptics who were dangerous or incapable of managing their own affairs, were regarded as mentally disordered or defective for the purposes of the Act. One of the purposes of the Act was to make provision for compulsory hospitalisation of mental patients.

The classification in the Act of mentally disordered and defective persons, and in particular the definition of an epileptic, were subject to severe criticism through the years.[5] In 1970 Bird[6] pointed out that the legislation had been enacted in 1916 when very little was known about epilepsy. Then it was still regarded as being a mental illness, which in most cases had to be treated in mental hospitals because of a lack of any effective drug therapy. Modern neurologists regard epilepsy as an organic and not a mental illness.[7] Because everyone subject to fits without warning is in danger of injuring himself or others, Bird was of the opinion that a case could be made out that virtually every epileptic could be regarded as insane and incapable of standing trial on a criminal charge.

That was not the view of the criminal courts, however. The courts held the view that an epileptic was criminally accountable for his conduct unless there was positive proof that he did not know or could not reasonably have foreseen that it would be dangerous for him to embark upon a certain course of conduct. A case in point is *R v Schoonwinkel*:[8] The accused was charged with culpable homicide, after a road accident when the car he had driven, collided with another. According to the evidence the mind of the accused immediately before the collision became blank because of an epileptic fit, described as psychomotor epilepsy, a minor form of epilepsy. It appeared that he had had only two minor attacks before, one or both of which had been in bed. There was no evidence that the accused knew that, subject as he was to these fits, it would be dangerous for him to drive a vehicle. The court was not satisfied that

1 Act 38 of 1916.
2 Section 2.
3 Section 3.
4 Class VII (class VI, "social defectives", was repealed by Act 37 of 1957, section 1).
5 The Van Wyk Commission of Inquiry into the Mental Disorders Act (see its *Report* RP 80/1972, par 3.3.2) described the classification as "out of date" and held the view that greater flexibility was desirable in the certification and classification of mentally ill persons.
6 A V Bird "Epilepsy and the Law in South Africa" 1970 *S Afr Med J* 1093.
7 Bird *op cit.* According to the British Royal Commission on Capital Punishment, mental disease may also arise in cases of epilepsy and cerebral tumors.
8 1953 (3) SA 136 (C).

he could or should reasonably have foreseen the danger of driving on a public road, and accordingly found him not guilty. The court also held that the accused did not fall within the ambit of the epilepsy classification in the Mental Disorders Act because he was not a danger to himself and others.

The Mental Disorders Act was repealed by the Mental Health Act of 1974[9] which came into operation in 1975. The new Act scrapped the 1916 classification altogether and contains a very brief and general definition of mental illness as "any disorder or disability of the mind" which includes "any mental disease, any arrested or incomplete development of the mind and any psychopathic disorder".[10] The term "patient" – which has important implications for the purposes of application of the Mental Health Act – is defined as "a person mentally ill to such a degree that it is necessary that he be detained, supervised, controlled and treated" and it includes a person suspected of being ill to such an extent.[11]

It is not for a lawyer to say whether or not epilepsy can be said to constitute a "disorder or disability of the mind" so as to bring it within the ambit of the Mental Health Act. That is a question which must be answered by medical experts. Suffice it to say that some persons with epilepsy are still being received and treated in mental hospitals in terms of the Act. It is quite clear, however, that epilepsy *per se* would not justify an order of involuntary hospitalisation.

It is also clear that although the 1973 Act does not refer to the factor of a mentally ill person constituting a danger to himself or others as a general criterion justifying a reception order, this may be considered by a magistrate in deciding whether the person is mentally ill "to such an extent" that he should be detained as a patient.

There are references elsewhere in the Act to the factor of dangerousness. Thus a duty is imposed upon a doctor to report to a magistrate or the police the fact that a patient he examined or treated, is – in his opinion – mentally ill to such a degree that he is a danger to others.[12] Police officers are also charged with the duty to apprehend and detain persons whom they believe to be mentally ill and constituting a danger to themselves or others.[13]

As Perper[14] has observed with reference to the "dangerousness" criterion, it is difficult to perceive how the presence of epilepsy *per se* can justify compulsory hospitalisation, with the exception of cases of psychomotor epilepsy.

Criminal liability: a voluntary act?

To be found guilty of a criminal offence, it must be proved that the accused who was mentally competent at the time of the offence charged, committed an act *(actus)* as defined by the law; the act must be unlawful *(reus)* and must be accompanied by a blameworthy state of mind *(mens rea)*.

Not all human conduct is regarded as an act for the purposes of the criminal law. The act must be voluntary conduct, not in the sense that the actor in actual fact willed or intended the act, but in the sense – at the very least – that at the time of the act he was capable of exercising his powers of volition over his conduct. A man who walks or performs other actions in his sleep, [15] experiences a mental blackout,[16] acts purely reflexively,[17] or is in a state of automatism, on account of excessive consumption of

9 Act 18 of 1973.
10 Section 1.
11 *Ibid.*
12 Section 13.
13 Section 14.
14 J A Perper "Medicolegal Implications of Epilepsy 27 *Medical Trial Technique Quarterly* 9 (1980).
15 *R v Dhlamini* 1955 (1) SA 120 (T); *S v Ngang* 1960 (3) SA 363(A); *S v Naidoo* 1971 (3) SA 605 (N); *S v Ncube* 1978 (1) SA 1178 (R).
16 *R v Du Plessis* 1950(1) SA 297 (O).
17 *Cf S v Ngang (supra).*

alcohol[18] or otherwise, is not considered by the criminal law to have committed any act during that period. The same applies to any activities or movements performed by a person while experiencing an epileptic fit.

Several cases of the latter type were tried by our courts. An example of such a case is *R v Mkize*.[19] The accused, his three sisters, his brother and the latter's wife, were having a meal of roast meat. The accused had a pocket-knife in his hand which he used to cut the meat. One of the accused's sisters remonstrated with him when he threw down a wooden platter they had been using. In the course of the ensuing altercation, a sister of the accused was stabbed. Another sister, M, intervened and was fatally stabbed. The accused was charged with murder. It appeared that he was an epileptic. The court found that the accused was probably suffering an attack of epileptic equivalent when he stabbed M. "It follows that he was in an unconscious state, having neither judgment, will, purpose or reasoning, that the act ... of stabbing was a result of blind reflex activity", the judge found. The judge further held "that muscular activity during unconsciousness (whatever the cause of the unconsciousness) cannot be said to be a voluntary act". The accused was accordingly found not guilty.[20]

It must not be thought that a person with epilepsy will invariably be found not guilty if it is proved that at the time of the commission of the act in question (the stabbing, the driving of a car, etc) he was subject to an attack. In establishing criminal liability, a criminal court does not look at the final occurrence in the causal chain of events only. Liability may have been incurred at an earlier stage, i e before the onset of the epileptic seizure. The same principle is applied in regard to alcohol-induced automatism.[21] This is the so-called antecedent or anterior liability which applies particulary in regard to offences where the emphasis is on the causation of an unlawful result, such as murder or culpable homicide. In these cases, the accused is blamed not for what occurred at the moment when the fatal blow was struck, when he was unconscious of what he was doing, but for the fact that at an earlier point in time, when he was still in possession of all his faculties of mind, he actually foresaw or ought to have reasonably foreseen the possibility of finding himself in a position where harm might be caused to other persons, and for failing to take steps to avoid such an eventuality.

A good example would be the person with epilepsy who, well-knowing that he is subject to periodic seizures leading to total unconsciousness, hides this fact and allows himself to be employed as a bus-driver. The principle of antecedent liability would likewise apply to an epileptic driver who fails to take medication which would enable him to avoid potentially dangerous seizures while driving. The theory of the law is that in these cases the decisive act for which the accused is ultimately held criminally liable was his omission to avoid putting himself in a potentially dangerous position; that act was the first in the causal chain of events culminating in the catastrophic event. This was the basis on which the accused in *R v Victor*[22] was convicted of reckless driving. The accused was subject to epileptic fits and the court found him guilty on the ground that the negligence the accused committed was not so much in the driving of the vehicle, but in his driving at all, knowing of his physical disability. The accused was 28 years of age and had been driving a car for eight years. His health was normal, except that occasionally he suffered from epilepsy. He had had attacks since the age of 14 or 15 and generally had a "warning feeling" five or ten minutes

18 *S v Johnson* 1969 (1) SA 201 (A); *S v Piccione* 1967(2) SA 334 (N).
19 1959 (2) SA 260 (N).
20 *R v Victor* 1943 TPD 77; *R v Schoonwinkel supra; R v Kumalo* 1956 (3) SA 238 (N); *R v Mokwanazi* 1959 (3) SA 782 (W); *R v Ngema, R v Cele* 1960 (1) SA 137 (A).
21 *S v Johnson, supra,* and see above 129.
22 1943 TPD 77.

before an attack. There were times when he had a giddy feeling which was part of the warning; at other times he had this feeling without any attack.[23]

When a person has been injured in a traffic accident and has sustained a closed head injury, a neurologist who examines the patient may, in his report compiled with a view to "third party" litigation, mention that the patient (who has no previous history of epilepsy) might, in future, suffer from epilepsy. It is a well-known fact that purely on the basis of statistical experience, epilepsy may occur as a *sequela* of such an injury in a small percentage of cases. Will such a statement in a medical report have the effect of *per se* rendering the patient guilty of antecedent liability, if he does in fact, without any prior warning, experience an epileptic seizure at a later stage when engaged in a potentially hazardous activity, such as driving a car, thereby causing injury to another? It is submitted that the mere statement contained in a report, will not have this effect. Because the overwhelming majority of patients do not in fact subsequently suffer from epilepsy, a patient would, in my opinion, incur liability only if, after his head injury, he had already had a warning of a seizure and nevertheless embarked upon the potentially hazardous activity.

Criminal responsibility: the Criminal Procedure Act

The next question to be considered in regard to the criminal responsibility of the epileptic, is whether he may be dealt with under chapter 13 of the Criminal Procedure Act.[24]

The criterion for lack of criminal capacity (*ontoerekeningsvatbaarheid*) is whether the accused, at the time of the commission of the act, on account of mental illness or defect, was incapable of appreciating the wrongfulness of his act and if not incapable thereof, whether he was incapable of acting in accordance with an appreciation of the wrongfulness of his act.[25]

It is to be noted that "mental illness or defect" is not defined in the Criminal Procedure Act. What amounts to these conditions is for a court to decide on the basis of expert medical evidence. A court is not bound by the definition of that concept in other statutes, such as the Mental Health Act. If epilepsy is considered as a form of mental illness or defect, the accused may be dealt with under these provisions. This will have the effect that declaration as a State President's patient becomes mandatory.[26] A President's patient is detained indefinitely in a mental hospital or prison pending the signification of the State President's decision.

In some cases before our courts, the accused was dealt with on the basis of lacking criminal capacity on account of suffering from a "mental disorder or defect".[27] In other cases, however – as I have pointed out – the acquittal was justified on the basis of absence of the first and foremost requirement of criminal liability, viz a voluntary act.

What is significant is that prior to the Criminal Procedure Act of 1977 coming into operation, when the courts found an epileptic accused not guilty of murder on the latter ground (i e "non-act" by virtue of an epileptic seizure) the courts nevertheless held that by virtue of section 29 of the Mental Disorders Act of 1916 (relating to the procedure to be followed when it appeared that the accused at the time of the act "was mentally disordered or defective so as not to be responsible according to the law for the act ... charged") the accused had to be declared a State President's patient.[28] In

23 *S v Trickett* 1973(3) SA 526 (T) affords a good example of antecedent liability where a night driver fell asleep as a result of exhaustion and was involved in a collision. The court held that the driver's lapse of consciousness was such as she could and ought to have foreseen before it occurred. "The negligent act complained of is the fact that she drove the car when she did drive it, not the way in which she drove it at the time of the collision." See below 352.

24 Act 51 of 1977. See also above 126 *et seq*.

25 Criminal Procedure Act, section 78(1).

26 *Ibid*, section 78(6).

27 See e g *R v Smit* 1906 TS 783.

28 See e g *R v Kumalo, supra,* and *R v Mokwanazi, supra.*

a 1959 case, that of *Mkize* (to which I have referred above) the Natal Court (Mr Justice Jansen) held the opposite view, arguing rather technically that because the acquittal of the accused rested on the basis only of finding that the accused had committed no act in the criminal sense of the word and not on the basis of a finding of criminal incapacity, section 29 was inapplicable. However, soon afterwards, in the case of *Ngema* and *Cele*,[29] the Appellate Division reaffirmed the earlier view.

There is nothing in the wording of the 1977 Criminal Procedure Act suggesting that the Legislature intended to change the position. The conclusion is that it is compulsory for a court which acquits an epileptic patient on the ground that he suffered from a seizure at the time of the act, to declare him a President's patient.

It may well be asked whether this result is still acceptable in view of the fact that the modern neurological view of epilepsy is that it is an organic and not a mental illness. From a practical point of view it may be asked whether an order of indefinite detention in a mental hospital or prison is the ideal result in the case of an epileptic who has caused the death of another, but who is found not guilty on the ground that he experienced an epileptic seizure at the time when the act was committed. The attitude of the courts so far has been – rightly or wrongly – that it is not necessary to prove that the origin of the accused's mental illness or defect lies in the mind; from the legal point of view it could just as well be organic in origin,[30] e g traumatic injury to the brain or hypoglycaemia.

Also in England, a finding that an accused is not guilty of criminal conduct induced by epilepsy will result in the court making a confinement order. In *Sullivan's* case[31] the House of Lords justified this rule as follows: "To some this may seem a harsh decision; but it should be remembered that persons who, through disease, cause injury to others and may do so again, are a potential danger to all who may come into contact with them. It is in the public interest that they should be put under medical care for as long as is reasonably necessary for the protection of others, but no longer. The modern order for confinement following a special verdict gives the Secretary of State a wide discretion as to the kind of hospital to which a defendant should be sent and how long he should stay there." The prospect of confinement has induced persons with epilepsy on occasion to plead guilty to the charge rather than to rely on the defence of automatism. In the words of Brahams,[32] commenting on the *Sullivan* case, "confinement in an unknown place for an unknown time is not appealing".

Epilepsy associated with the commission of a crime may be a factor in the assessment of diminished criminal responsibility or extenuating circumstances.[33]

Fitness to stand trial

Before concluding this discussion on the position of the person with epilepsy in criminal law, reference should be made to the decisions handed down by courts in respect of the triability of such persons. The Criminal Procedure Act[34] makes provision for an inquiry into the capacity of an accused to understand the proceedings, to be ordered in a case where doubt exists. For the purposes of such an inquiry, the court may commit the accused to a mental hospital (or other place designated by the court) for periods of not more than 30 days at a time.[35] The accused is then subjected to psychiatric examination, the results of which are subsequently reported to the court. If

29 *Supra*.
30 See *S v Mahlinza* 1967 (1) SA 408 (A) 418; *S v Ncube* 1978 (1) SA 1178 (R) 1183.
31 *R v Sullivan* [1983] 2 All ER 673 (HL). The decision of the Court of Appeal is discussed critically by D Brahams 51(2) *Medico-legal Journal* (1983).
32 See preceding note.
33 See *e g S v Smith* 1984 (1) SA 583 (A) discussed above 133.
34 Section 77.
35 Section 79. See also above 133.

the court finds that "the accused is not capable of understanding the proceedings so as to make a proper defence" he must be declared a State President's patient. Such declaration has the effect that the accused may be neither acquitted, nor convicted at that stage. Should the accused's condition improve at a later stage to such an extent that he would understand the proceedings, he may be tried.

The case of *Pratt*,[36] who in 1960 shot at and wounded the then Prime Minister, Dr H F Verwoerd, was dealt with by the court under section 28 of the Mental Disorders Act of 1916. That section made provision for an inquiry to be conducted where, in the course of criminal proceedings, it appeared to the court that the accused was "mentally disordered or defective". At Pratt's trial application was made for such an inquiry. Mr Justice Rumpff (then judge-president of the Transvaal) who tried the case, observed that the court, for the purpose of section 28, was not really concerned with the crime charged, "but simply with the question of the present mental state of the man in the dock". The judge drew attention to the fact that one of the expressly stated classes of mental disorder in terms of the Act was epilepsy, as defined, and then observed: "It is clear that whatever anomalies may flow from the law as it stands, the legislature has decided that epilepsy is a disease of the mind and that if an epileptic is a danger to himself or others or incapable of managing himself or his affairs, he should not be tried. He must be regarded as mentally disordered or defective in terms of the Act." On the evidence before the court there was no question that Pratt was an epileptic and a danger to himself and others. Two years before the attack on Dr Verwoerd, a psychiatrist had already found that Pratt had suicidal tendencies and was a danger to himself and others. The court accordingly declared him mentally disordered and declared him a "Governor-General's patient" (the term then used).

It is to be noted that under the legislation then in existence (the Mental Disorders Act and the old Criminal Procedure Act) there was a certain amount of confusion in that the impression was created that where application was made under section 28 of the former Act, all that was at issue was whether the accused was certifiable in terms of that Act.[37] In accordance with the recommendation of the Rumpff Commission, that confusion was removed altogether by the new legislation, i e the Mental Health Act of 1973 and the Criminal Procedure Act of 1977. Fitness to stand trial and "certifiability" are today completely unrelated.[38]

The present position is therefore quite flexible and not as rigid as under the old legislation. A criminal court will be guided solely by the psychiatric reports submitted after observation of the accused. It is quite possible that on the psychiatric evidence a court will find that an accused is triable, although he has been diagnosed as an epileptic. On the other hand, another epileptic may not be triable on account of his general mental condition. It is clear that quite apart from the issue of certifiability, on the psychiatric evidence led in Pratt's case – and also on the basis of his demeanour in court – he was incapable of being tried.[39]

Other legal aspects involving epileptics

There are a number of other legal issues concerning epileptics that should be mentioned.

First, there is the question of civil delictual liability, i e liability for harm caused by one person to another through a civil wrong committed by the former. Suffice it to say that as far as the epileptic is concerned, the principles I have outlined when discussing criminal responsibility, will in equal measure apply to delictual liability.[40]

36 *R v Pratt* 1960 (4) SA 743 (T).
37 See *Report* of the Rumpff Commission, pars 10.26, 10.27. See also the *Richards* case (involving a person with epilepsy) referred to in the *Report*, par 10.30.
38 See *S v Mnyanda* 1976 (2) SA 751 (A) 764 F.
39 See the remarks of Mr Justice Rumpff, at 1960 (4) SA 747H.
40 Compare Perper, *supra*.

The capacity of a person to enter into a contract is, of course, not affected by the mere fact that he has epilepsy. Whether or not a person has the capacity to contract will depend on whether he is *compos mentis* at the time he enters into the contract. When a person's understanding is affected by liquor, drugs, extreme physical debility or mental illness to the point at which he is incapable of appreciating that he is entering into a contract, or of grasping its terms, he lacks the capacity to contract. Any agreement he would enter into while in that condition, is void.[41]

If a person with epilepsy does not inform the party with whom he enters into a contract of his disability, it may affect the validity of the contract when such disability is material to the contract. This is of particular importance to insurance policies where the person who wants to take out insurance is pertinently required to furnish certain details concerning his state of health and life style.

This principle was well illustrated by the judgment in *Pickering v Standard General Insurance Co Ltd*:[42] P applied for comprehensive motor vehicle insurance. On the form he had to fill in, the question was asked whether he was suffering from any physical or mental infirmity. He answered "No". Later he became involved in a car accident and was sued by a person injured in the accident, for a substantial amount of damages. It then came to light that P had had a history of severe migraine attacks, associated with visual disturbance, nausea and paresthesia. These attacks decreased as he passed beyond adolescence. But in 1974 he experienced a fit as a result of strenuous exercise while on military training. It was suspected by a military doctor that P had suffered an epileptic *grand mal* seizure. In 1977 he was called up for military service and when asked whether he had ever suffered from fits and convulsions, answered in the affirmative. After the accident P was examined very thoroughly by a neurosurgeon, who came to the conclusion that he had never really been a victim of epilepsy. The neurosurgeon was of the opinion therefore that the answer given by P when he applied for the insurance was, objectively speaking, true. The court nevertheless held that the insurer was entitled to avoid liability under the policy by reason of the fact that P had not disclosed the fact that epilepsy was suspected at the stage when he applied for insurance.

Under older legislation, a person applying for compulsory motor vehicle insurance to cover "third party" liability, had to fill in a lengthy form requiring information to be supplied on a number of points, *inter alia* whether he had ever "had a fit" or had any physical infirmity.[43] The effect of a fraudulent non-disclosure on any material issue could have been that, even though the motorist was covered by the insurance in the sense that the insurer would pay compensation to the injured party, the insurer had a right of recourse against the motorist[44] – which, naturally, might have had catastrophic financial implications for the latter.

Today there is a totally different system of "third party" compensation under the Multilateral Motor Vehicle Accidents Fund Act.[45] A car owner no longer takes out insurance but is automatically covered by the provisions of the Act in the sense that he or the driver of the car can ordinarily not be sued by someone who is bodily injured (or the dependants of someone killed) in consequence of his (the motorist's) negligence. An injured party must claim from the MM Fund or an insurance company appointed as its agent. The Fund is funded by the State.

Failure by a person with epilepsy to disclose facts pertaining to his condition, in particular where his epilepsy is not adequately controlled by the use of drugs, may also have effects in regard to other contracts he enters into. Legally such failure may

41 Wille and Millin's *Mercantile Law of South Africa* (18th ed, 1984, by J F Coaker and D T Zeffertt) 72.
42 1980 (4) SA 326 (ZAD).
43 Suzman & Gordon *The Law of Compulsory Motor Vehicle Insurance* (2nd ed, 1970) 70.
44 *Ibid*, 225.
45 Act 93 of 1989.

amount to a misrepresentation. This may constitute a ground on which an employer, who employed a person with epilepsy to undertake tasks which may be affected by the employee's disability, may be entitled to avoid the contract. It is clear that the person with epilepsy here finds himself in a most unenviable dilemma. If he makes a full disclosure, the potential employer may become unwilling to employ him, irrespective of his other qualities of excellence. We are all too aware of the amount of ignorance and prejudice still prevailing in regard to epilepsy. There may still be regulations pertaining to occupations closed to those suffering from seizures. Bird[46] has convincingly argued that these regulations should avoid the use of the words "epileptic" and "epilepsy" and should refer in general terms to "any disease or physical disability which is or will be likely seriously to interfere with the ability to carry out duties of the post for which application is being made". Each case can then be considered on its own merits – in regard to official appointments, hopefully by an unprejudiced body.

Protection to employees with some disability is afforded by the Labour Relations Act.[47] An employer who unilaterally changes the conditions of employment in a manner which will affect an employee's job security or limit his career opportunities, may make himself guilty of an unfair labour practice. Likewise termination of employment in an unreasonable manner may amount to unfair dismissal. An employee's employment may be terminated if he is no longer capable of carrying out the functions for which he was employed, but a fair hearing must first be conducted.[48] There are a number of factors to be considered. One of these is whether the employee's handicap could create a situation of danger for his co-employees.[49] Where appropriate, it is required that a competent authority should conduct a test to ascertain whether the employee is indeed incapable.[50] The underlying idea is that the assessment of incapacity should be an objective and verifiable one. The industrial court does not tolerate arbitrary and capricious action by the employer. An important aspect is that, according to decisions of the court, where the employee's incapability has indeed been proved (or admitted by him), alternative employment – and not in the first place dismissal – should be considered; the employer should consult with the employee in this regard.[51] It is manifestly clear, therefore, that the mere fact that epilepsy has been diagnosed will not enable an employer to dismiss the employee.

Counteracting an unwillingness on the part of employers in recruiting prospective employees to employ persons with a history of epilepsy, is a more difficult problem. In South Africa we do not as yet have legislation forbidding employment discrimination against persons with handicaps.[52] A heartening development elsewhere in the world – particularly in the USA – is modern legislation appearing on statute books, positively encouraging the employment of persons with epilepsy.[53]

As a matter of policy the attitude of the South African Public Service towards the employability of persons with epilepsy is a positive and sympathetic one.[54]

Some of the earlier – and most unreasonable – limitations to the civil rights of persons with epilepsy relate to compulsory eugenic marriage laws and eugenic sterili-

46 *Op cit.*
47 Act 28 of 1956.
48 M S M Brassey, E Cameron, M H Cheadle and M P Olivier *The New Labour Law* (1987) 445-6.
49 *Ibid* 445.
50 *Ibid* 446.
51 *Ibid.*
52 Nearly all the states of the USA have some type of law forbidding this form of discrimination. The federal Rehabilitation Act of 1973 applies to employers which are federal agencies. See pamphlet "Epilepsy – Legal Rights – Legal Issues", published by the Epilepsy Foundation of America (1987). See also R T Fraser *et al* in *Advances in Epileptology* (Manelis *et al*, eds, 1989) 474.
53 See Perper *op cit.*
54 Paper "The Attitude of Public Service to Employability" by H P Schoeman (Government Medical Officer, Department of National Health and Population Development) at Symposium on Epilepsy, Employment and Industry, Faculty of Medicine, University of Pretoria, 1 October 1988.

sation. As Perper[55] has observed "[t]he great variation in the etiology of seizure disorders implicitly denies the rationale of such legislation". South Africa does not have eugenic marriage legislation. The Abortion and Sterilisation Act[56] makes provision, *inter alia*, for voluntary eugenic sterilisation of mentally defective persons, but it does not refer to epilepsy as such.[57]

Reference should further be made to legal disabilities in regard to driver's licences. In terms of the Road Traffic Act[58] a person is disqualified from obtaining or holding a driver's licence if he is suffering from one of the following diseases or disabilities, *inter alia*:

- uncontrolled epilepsy;
- sudden attacks of disabling giddiness or fainting due to hypertension or any other cause;
- any form of mental illness to such an extent that it is necessary that he be detained, supervised, controlled and treated as a patient in terms of the Mental Health Act.

A provincial administrator may cancel or suspend a driver's licence if he is of the opinion that the holder is disqualified by virtue of any of the conditions described (or other specified conditions). For this purpose the administrator may request the holder to submit to an examination by a medical practitioner to determine his physical and mental fitness to drive a motor vehicle.[59]

The courts are empowered by the Act[60] to order endorsement, suspension or cancellation of a driver's licence when a person is convicted of an offence relating to the driving of a motor vehicle or failure to stop after or report an accident.

In older texts of provincial ordinances, reference was simply made to "epilepsy" as a disqualifying condition.[61] The objections which could be brought against the latter disqualification have been largely removed by later statutory texts referring to *uncontrolled* epilepsy. As far as the third of the above disabilities is concerned, it must be noted that in terms of the Mental Health Act epilepsy is no longer an express class of mental illness. Even if epilepsy were still to be regarded *per se* as a form of mental illness or defect, the explicit references in the Road Traffic Act to "uncontrolled epilepsy" give expression to the Legislature's intent to confine the disqualification to an uncontrolled condition only.

However, the new wording has not given effect to Bird's suggestion that the legal prohibition to drive a car should be couched in general terms as referring to any disease or disability which would or might interfere with driving ability, without any particular disease or disorder being specified.

Finally, mention should be made of the duty resting upon a medical practitioner in terms of the Mental Health Act[62] to report a mentally ill person he has examined and whom he regards as dangerous to others, to a magistrate or the Police. In so far as epilepsy is regarded as "mental illness" in terms of the Act, a patient may fall within the ambit of this duty.

Based on a paper read at the Third South African Conference on Epilepsy, held in Cape Town, September 1979.

55 *Op cit.*
56 Act 2 of 1975.
57 On the Act in general, see also below 214.
58 Act 29 of 1989, section 18.
59 *Ibid*, section 30.
60 Section 55.
61 Cooper & Bamford *SA Motor Law* (1965) 154.
62 Section 13.

PART VII

Organ and tissue transplantation; rights to tissue

25 The law relating to organ and tissue transplantation

Introduction

The comprehensive legislation in South Africa on human organ and tissue transplantation – the Human Tissue Act of 1983[1] – has its origin in the first successful heart transplant operation performed by Professor Christiaan Barnard and his team in December 1967.[2] But seminal legislation already existed at the time in the form of the Post Mortem Examinations and Removal of Tissues Act of 1952.[3]

Anatomical donations by living persons

In the first place, the Human Tissue Act governs the removal of tissue, blood or gametes from the bodies of living persons for therapeutic and other uses. The Act defines "tissue" as "any human tissue, including any flesh, bone, organ, gland or body fluid, but excluding any blood or gamete", and "any device or object implanted, before the death of any person, by a medical practitioner or dentist into the body of such person".[4] In the Act, "gamete" is defined as "either of the two generative cells essential for human reproduction", i e the male sperm and the female ovum.[5] It is submitted that for the purpose of the Act, a foetus is tissue of the woman in whose womb it is.[6]

The Act provides for the use of tissue, blood and gametes removed or withdrawn from the body of a living person for medical and dental purposes. These purposes include the transplanting of tissue, the production of a therapeutic, diagnostic or prophylactic substance, the transfusing of blood, the production of a blood product and, in the case of a gamete, artificial insemination.[7] (It is to be noted that the Act makes no reference to purely scientific research and experimentation, and it is doubtful whether such activities could be described as "medical".)[8]

Tissue, blood or a gamete obtained from mentally ill persons may not be used for any of the said purposes,[9] nor may tissue of a minor which is not replaceable by natural processes, or the gamete of a minor, be used.[10] (A minor may therefore donate blood,[11] skin and the like.) Similarly, a gamete obtained from a habitual criminal may not be used.[12]

1 Act 65 of 1983.
2 For the history of the Act, see the second edition (1984) of this book, pages 147-8.
3 Act 30 of 1952.
4 Section 1.
5 *Ibid.*
6 This, of course, does not mean that the woman is entitled to freely dispose of the foetus. Intentional termination of pregnancy is governed by the strict provisions of the Abortion and Sterilisation Act 2 of 1975.
7 Section 19.
8 Compare J M Burchell "Experimentation on Children" in *Attitudes to Clinical Experimentation in South Africa* (eds G C Oosthuizen, H A Shapiro and S A Strauss, 1985) 94 at 99.
9 Section 19, proviso (i).
10 *Ibid*, proviso (ii).
11 Apart from the fact that blood is replaceable by natural processes, "tissue" is defined by the Act in terms specifically excluding blood. The prohibition in section 19 relating to minors does not exclude blood.
12 Section 19, proviso (iii).

Placenta, foetal tissue and umbilical cord may not be used, except with ministerial consent.[13]

Tissue destined for transplantation may be removed only in a hospital or other authorised institution (i e authorised by the Minister of National Health and Population Development). The medical superintendent of the hospital or institution must provide a written authorisation and may not carry out the transplant himself.[14] Note that these provisions do not apply to blood or gametes.

The removal of tissue, blood and gametes for any of the above-mentioned purposes may be effected only with the consent of the donor – in the case of a minor, the consent of his parents or guardians.[15] This consent must be given in writing,[16] except in the case of blood or tissue replaceable by natural processes, where consent may be given orally.[17] Moreover, in the case of donors of 14 years or older who are mentally competent, no parental consent (or consent of a guardian) is required before replaceable tissue and blood may be removed.[18] The Act also provides that tissue removed (with the necessary consent) for the sake of the health of the person concerned (e g bone from a leg amputated after a road accident) may be used for any of the above-mentioned purposes.[19]

The use of a gonad for transplantation [20]– if the result thereof could be procreation – is illegal, unless the Minister's written consent thereto has been obtained in advance.[21] The Act defines "gonad" as "the human organ which produces gametes",[22] i e a testicle in the case of a male and an ovary in the case of a female. Artificial insemination – the Act uses the term "artificial fertilisation" – is governed by regulations promulgated under the Act. This subject is discussed in detail below.[23] It may be noted here that artificial fertilisation is defined in such wide terms as to include *in vitro* fertilisation (IVF).[24]

Only medical practitioners, dentists or persons acting under their supervision may remove and transplant tissue, withdraw blood, and administer blood or a blood product for any of the above-mentioned purposes.[25]

It must be noted that the Act does not provide any guidance as to how drastic the operation to remove the tissue may be. The 1952 Act did contain such a provision, viz that, in the opinion of at least two medical practitioners, the removal of specified

13 *Ibid*, proviso (iv).
14 Section 20.
15 Section 18.
16 *Ibid.*
17 *Ibid*, proviso (*aa*).
18 *Ibid*, read with section 1 (*v*). The question arises whether section 39(4) of the Child Care Act 74 of 1983, which enables a minor over the age of 18 years to consent independently to medical operations, makes it possible for such a minor to consent to the removal of non-replaceable tissue or gametes for purposes of transplantation. This question must clearly be answered in the negative. Section 19, proviso (ii), of the Human Tissue Act prohibits in absolute terms the use of non-replaceable tissue and gametes of minors, for any of the purposes mentioned in the section. That constitutes a special law – and *generalia specialibus non derogant.*
19 Section 18, proviso (*bb*).
20 "Transplantation" in this context refers to use of the gonad "in the body of *another* living person" (see section 21 – the italics are mine) and the prohibition accordingly does not affect *in vitro* fertilisation of an ovum obtained from Mrs X and subsequent replacement thereof into her uterus. As is observed in the text, it is to be doubted whether the provisions of the Act relating to artificial insemination affect the latter type of procedure. (The terms "embryo transfer" is often used to refer to this type of procedure, but as Dr Patrick Steptoe has pointed out in a letter to *The Listener*, 3 November 1983, page 23, the term should be limited strictly to cases where the embryo is transferred from one woman to another.)
21 Section 21.
22 Section 1.
23 See 181 *et seq.*
24 Section 1.
25 Section 23.

tissue would in no way prejudice the donor.[26] It was generally conceded that this test was far too stringent, and that no doctor could certify to this effect where major surgery (e g the removal of a kidney) was involved. Quite apart from the usual risks inherent in any such operation, the removal of a healthy kidney from a donor would diminish the donor's chances of survival by 50% in the event of his remaining kidney failing. Subsequent legislation therefore eliminated the prejudice test altogether.

The Human Tissue Act purports to legalise tissue transplantation in absolute terms (subject only to the statutory conditions relating to consent, official authorisation, etc). However, it is to be doubted whether a court of law will be prepared to interpret the provisions of the Act as conferring an absolute discretion concerning the removal of tissue upon either the authorising doctor, the surgeon undertaking the removal or the donor. Should such a case come before our courts, section 19*(a)* will probably be interpreted against the background of the common-law principle of *volenti non fit iniuria* (to him who consents, no wrong is done). This will mean that an operation for the removal of tissue will be ruled as unlawful if it is of such a nature that it is considered to be contrary to public policy. A court will have to decide this by carefully weighing the donor's interests against those of the recipient. An obvious condition is that the operation should not substantially imperil the life and health of the donor. Naturally, the removal must be performed in accordance with scientifically-approved methods as in the case of therapeutic operations. The advantage for the patient should be commensurate with the disadvantage suffered by the donor.[27] It would in my opinion have been preferable if a more concrete test had been inserted into the Act, such as was proposed in the first draft of the 1969 Bill which later became Act 24 of 1970, viz (a) that the risk involved in the removal of the tissue would be justified in terms of the purpose sought to be achieved, and (b) that the removal would not constitute an immediate or substantial threat to the life of the donor.

The removal of tissue from dead bodies

The removal of tissue and organs from dead bodies for the purpose of transplantation into a living person is a controversial subject. Societal views are highly divergent[28] and the Legislature, in the Human Tissue Act and its predecessors, endeavoured to harmonise conflicting views in a manner which was, hopefully, acceptable to the majority. In their most vivid relief, these conflicting interests may be stated as follows: On the one hand, there are medical men who feel that each human being should automatically be considered a donor of tissue unless he has indicated a contrary intention while alive. This would mean that, in the absence of such an indication, a doctor may remove tissue from a corpse without the consent of the deceased's next of kin.[29] On the other hand there are people who, on religious or other grounds, maintain that the removal and transplanting of tissue from human beings can never be justified.

The Human Tissue Act deals primarily with the removal of human tissue from

26 Act 30 of 1952, section 3.

27 P Noll *Uebergesetzliche Rechtfertigungsgründe, im besondern die Einwilligung des Verletzten* (1955) 91.

28 For a collection of South African views prevailing in the early seventies, see G C Oosthuizen (ed), *The Ethics of Tissue Transplantation* (1972).

29 Professor Rudolf Pichlmayer of Germany, a pioneer in the field of kidney and liver transplantation, made the point that the term "donation" of organs gives the impression that it is something exceptional or extraordinary. Part of our culture is that people upon their deaths "pass on" their earthly goods. This is a normal thing, and the same attitude should be adopted in future to bodily parts. "Handing on" ("Weitergeben") of an organ is a more acceptable term, says Pichlmayer. See *Frankfurter Allgemeine Zeitung*, 6 April 1983, p 8. Several European countries have already legislatively opted for the system that removal of tissue from the body of a deceased for transplantation purposes is legal, unless the deceased has vetoed it during his life. See D Giesen *International Malpractice Law* (1988) 620.

dead bodies which is, juridically speaking, more problematic than tissue donation by live donors. The reason for this lies in the fact that, in society, there is a deep-seated respect for the dead and compassion for the bereaved. According to Roman-Dutch law the violation of a corpse is a punishable offence, and may constitute an *iniuria* to the next of kin.[30] The Act also deals with diagnostic *post mortem* examinations.[31]

The donation of human bodies or of tissue from dead bodies is governed by chapter 1 of the Act. The provisions of this chapter are very extensive. It must be noted that the donation of eye tissue is particularly "favoured" by the Act, as was also the case under the 1970 legislation. It was testified before the Parliamentary Select Committee of 1969[32] that, in practice, the strict provisions of the 1952 Act had rendered the acquisition of eye tissue, which today is widely used, extremely difficult.

GENERAL CONDITIONS FOR LEGALITY

The "donor" must be deceased

Self-evident as this requirement appears to be, no other aspect of anatomical donation has been more intensively debated. Before the days of organ transplants, there was little controversy on the certification of death for the purpose of tissue removal or for other purposes. An organ, it must be noted, differs from other tissue in that it is "a somewhat independent part of the body that performs a special function",[33] such as the heart, lungs, liver, kidneys and testicles. Whereas tissue such as the corneae or skin need not be removed or transplanted to the recipient immediately, but may be stored for an indefinite period, removal of an organ must take place almost immediately after death and must be transplanted without any delay.

Until fairly recently, the test for death has primarily been the absence of heart activity. In the first heart transplant operations, Professor Barnard and his team applied the following test: the absence of cardiac activity for five minutes as measured by the electro-cardiograph, the absence of spontaneous respiratory movements and the absence of reflexes.[34]

However, the traditional test is no longer universally accepted in the medical world. Increased medical knowledge, modern methods of resuscitation and the demands of successful organ transplantation have led to an entirely new approach. Today, medical science does not accept that there is any one moment at which a human being dies. It rather sees death as a process which may sometimes be extended over a period of time.

It is generally accepted that, for the continuance of life in the human organism, the combined activity of the brain, heart and lungs is essential. Grave harm to or interference with the function of one of these organs has an almost immediate effect on the others. The most vulnerable of these organs is the brain. When the flow of blood to the brain is interrupted, unconsciousness follows within ten seconds and regular respiratory movements cease within a minute. According to doctors, irreparable damage to the brain occurs after five minutes.

Before the advent of antibiotics which prevent infection of the respiratory organs, and of technical devices controlling blood circulation, cases like this were hopeless. Today, however, there is a variety of drugs and machines (e g the heart-lung machine) which have greatly dimished the absolute interdependence of the three organic systems. The mere fact that a heart stops beating does not mean, nowadays,

30 W A Joubert *Grondslae van die Persoonlikheidsreg* (1953) 87; *cf* C F Klopper 1970 *THRHR* 38.

31 The Act further governs a variety of matters such as the disposal of bodies of deceased destitutes, inspectors of anatomy and the import and export of human tissue.

32 See *Report of the Select Committee on the Anatomical Donations and Post Mortem Examinations Bill* SC 11 – '69.

33 *Dorland's Medical Dictionary sv* "organ".

34 See C N Barnard 1967 *S Afr Med* J 1271.

that its "owner" is dead. In certain circumstances, the activity of the heart can be restored by means of massage or electrical shock.

As we know, resuscitation of the heart does not necessarily mean that the patient has been placed on the road to recovery. Although the circulation of blood has been restored, damage to the brain might already be such that the patient has reached – or will soon reach – the stage that may be described as "brain death" or "cerebral death". When this stage is reached, there is one of two possibilities: either treatment ceases and "heart death" follows within minutes, or treatment is continued and the heart may still function for some time and then cease beating. The occurrence of brain death may be determined by means of the electro-encephalograph, an instrument used to measure electrical impulses caused by brain activity. The experience of doctors is that, as soon as a reading on this instrument, taken at body temperature, shows "nil" (i e "still" or "iso-electric"), it can mean only one thing in a given clinical context, and that is irreparable brain damage which, in the absence of further measures, will swiftly be followed by the cessation of other bodily functions.

At this stage, the question is: must death be described as the cessation of both heart and brain activity, or is brain death sufficient? If one accepts the latter, it simply means that the physicians may disconnect their apparatus. It also means that an organ intended for use in a transplant may be removed from a body in which the heart is still beating. Certain physicians emphasise that the removal of an organ before the circulation of blood has ceased involves a considerable advantage. This advantage is that the duration of ischemia (degeneration of the organ by reason of insufficient "feeding" by the blood), where minutes are important, is curtailed. With little hesitation, therefore, prominent medical men suggest that brain death should legally be accepted as death. In fact, the contention is that after brain death the patient leads merely a vegetative existence, the only measurable spontaneous reactions being a heart-beat and a measure of blood circulation, which is totally dependent on the artificial lung and increasing doses of drugs. It has been suggested that, in these cases, we are dealing with nothing more than a living corpse.

While many might still recoil from the suggestion of removing organs from a body of which the heart is still beating, it is clear that there is now substantial support – also among doctors – for the view that cerebral death is an acceptable criterion.[35] However, a difficulty is that absolute unanimity as to the symptoms or indications of irreversible cerebral damage has not been achieved so far.[36] For this reason, our Legislature refrained from including a definition of "death" or "corpse" in the Human Tissue Act. Whether or not death has ensued is therefore a question of fact, the decision of which will, in the event of a dispute, be influenced to a large extent by expert medical evidence.

The Act[37] simply provides that, for the purpose of removing tissue, the death of the person concerned must be established by two doctors, one of whom must have been practising for at least five years. These two doctors may not be members of the transplantation team. Eye tissue is specifically excluded from the aforegoing provisions. In respect of eye tissue, an ordinary death certificate will suffice. It would appear that the certification rule embodied in the Act does not apply to the removal of tissue in the course of a medico-legal *post mortem* examination (which is discussed below).

In *S v Williams*,[38] a murder case, the accused raised the defence that the revolver shot he had fired had not been the cause of the deceased's death, but disconnection

35 Giesen *op cit* 616; E Deutsch *Arztrecht und Arzneimittelrecht* (1983) 153 *et seq*.
36 Giesen *op cit* 612 *et seq*; Deutsch 153 *et seq*. As Giesen 613 has pointed out, several jurisdictions now have statutory criteria for determining death.
37 Section 7(2).
38 1986 (4) SA 1188 (A).

of the respirator, which – it was contended – constituted an *actus novus interveniens*. The trial court found that, according to traditional medical standards, the moment of death is when brainstem death sets in. The accused was accordingly convicted of murder and sentenced to death. The Appellate Division confirmed that verdict and sentence. Chief Justice Rabie, however, did not consider that it was necessary to decide whether the medical standpoint of brainstem death was also to be accepted in law. He observed that the issue is one of great interest not only to criminal law, but also as it concerns other areas of the law, e g the law of succession – where the precise moment of a person's death can be of cardinal importance. "Medical science," the Chief Justice remarked, " understandably perhaps, approaches the problem from a purely mechanical or physical point of view, but in my view moral or even religious considerations, as well as societal attitudes, may become relevant."[39] The moment of death, therefore, remains an open question in South African law.

To whom donations may be made

A donation of the whole body, or of specific parts thereof, may be made to a hospital, a university or technikon and any other institution authorised thereto by the Minister. A specific doctor or dentist may also be indicated as a donee, or, naturally, in the case of tissue, any person requiring therapy in which the tissue can be used.[40] If no donee is nominated, or an institution or person other than those mentioned is nominated, the donation is of no force or effect.[41]

However, where the donor makes a donation to an institution it is not necessary for him to mention a specific institution by name. Thus, if he simply donates his body to "a hospital", the nearest hospital is deemed to be the donee.[42] If the donation has been made to a specific institution which is not within easy reach at the time of the donor's death, the nearest institution in the appropriate category is regarded as the donee. If a doctor, dentist or patient has been nominated, however, and such person is not within easy reach, the donation likewise falls away.[43]

If the donor has made conflicting donations, effect is given to the donation made last. However, if the donor had first donated his whole body to one donee and thereafter donated specific tissue to another, the first donation becomes effective.[44]

Purpose of donation

A dead human body or specific tissue may be donated to an institution, doctor or dentist for the purposes of medical or dental training, research, the advancement of medicine, dentistry or therapy (this includes the use of tissue in living persons), or for the production of a therapeutic, diagnostic or prophylactic substance. If the donee is a private individual, it may be donated for therapy. The tissue donated may be used only for these purposes. The purpose of a donation need not be expressly stated, but a donation is of no force or effect when made for any other purpose than those stated.[45] Thus, if A donates his skull to his friend to be kept as a grisly *memento mori*, the donation will be void!

Consent

Consent to the removal of tissue from a dead body is a prerequisite except in those

39 My translation.
40 Section 3(1).
41 Section 3(2).
42 Section 3(3).
43 Section 3(4).
44 Section 3(5).
45 Section 4.

cases (discussed below) where removal of tissue may take place in the course of medico-legal autopsies. Consent may be given in one of the following ways:

1. By the deceased prior to his death. Such consent may be given in a will or in any document attested to by two competent witnesses, who must be 14 years of age or older. It may also be given by means of a statement made orally in the presence of at least two such witnesses.[46] Thirdly, a prospective donor may wear a prescribed identity tag issued by an authorised institution, by which he identifies himself as an anatomical donor.[47] The donor may revoke any donation prior to his death.[48] However, a relative of the donor can obviously not revoke or veto a donation by the deceased.
2. By the spouse, a major child, a parent, guardian or a major brother or sister of the deceased, after his death. Such consent can be given only if the deceased has not (prior to his death) forbidden it.[49] The Act does not provide for revocation of such a donation, and it is submitted that such a donation is incapable of being revoked. Nor, it is submitted, can one relative veto a donation made by another.
3. If none of the persons mentioned in the preceding paragraph (i e the spouse, etc) can be traced, the Director-General, National Health and Population Development (or person delegated by him) may, instead of such persons, donate specific tissue for transplantation purposes.[50] There are two conditions for the validity of such a donation: the deceased must not – prior to his death – have given a contrary instruction; and the Director-General (or person authorised by him) must be satisfied that all reasonable steps have been taken to trace the person referred to in the preceding paragraph.[51] The question arises whether the official concerned may make such a donation if the identity of the deceased is unknown. In my opinion, this question must be answered in the negative. It is difficult to see how the official can be satisfied that all reasonable steps have been taken to trace a relative if the deceased is unidentified. Further, it is to be noted that the Act clearly does not visualise revocation of a donation by the official.

Official authorisation

For lawful removal of tissue from a dead body, an act of official authorisation is necessary. This must be obtained upon request, by a medical practitioner or dentist, from any one of the following officials:

- the magistrate in whose district the deceased has died or where the body of the deceased is (or another magistrate authorised by him);
- the medical practitioner in charge of a hospital or authorised institution in which the deceased has died, or of a mortuary where his body is;
- any other medical practitioner employed at such hospital, institution or mortuary and who has been so authorised by the medical practitioner in charge.

The authorising official must be satisfied that the body or tissue was in fact donated, and that the body is no longer required for an official *post mortem* examination. He must also be satisfied that the removal of tissue is necessary for any of the purposes mentioned above.[52]

The authorisation must be in writing, in the prescribed form.

46 Section 2.
47 *Ibid.*
48 Section 5.
49 Section 2(2).
50 *Ibid.*
51 *Ibid.*
52 Section 14(2).

No official authorisation is necessary in the case of the removal of eye tissue.[53] The authorising official must forthwith forward a written report with regard thereto to the inspector of anatomy in whose care the body is. Persons to whom and institutions to which bodies are donated, must keep registers in the prescribed fashion.[54]

Removal of tissue under medical supervision only

The removal of tissue from a dead body for the purposes of the Act (i e for medical training, research, the advancement of science, therapy, etc) may be done only by or under the supervision of a medical practitioner or dentist. Obviously, the tissue must be removed before the body is buried.[55]

Gonads excluded

The transplanting of a gonad removed from the body of a deceased person which may result in procreation is prohibited in absolute terms.[56]

Body not required for post mortem examination

Official authorisation may not be given unless the magistrate or medical practitioner is satisfied that the body is no longer required for the purposes of an examination in terms of specified statutes. These are: section 3 of the Inquests Act 1959[57] (*post mortem* examinations where the deceased apparently died from other than natural causes); section 46 of the Health Act 1977[58] (*post mortem* examinations to establish the possible presence of an infectious disease); section 25 of the Births, Marriages and Deaths Registration Act 1963[59] (*post mortem* examination where the deceased is a still-born child, or where the deceased was not treated by a medical practitioner during his last illness, or where the deceased was so treated but a medical practitioner was unable to issue a death certificate); section 34 of the Occupational Diseases in Mines and Works Act 1973[60] (*post mortem* examination of former mine and industrial workers).

It is to be noted that, in regard to examinations in terms of the Inquests Act, an exception is made: where the district surgeon or pathologist of the area concerned certifies that, in his opinion, the removal of any specified tissue will in no way affect the outcome of the examination, he may consent to such removal.[61] The rationale of this exception is that the bodies of healthy young persons who have died as a result of a criminal attack or from accidental causes are an excellent potential source of tissue for transplantation. Moreover, it will frequently happen that where the victim of an assault or accident is brought to a hospital in a dying condition, it is already unmistakably clear what the cause of death will be.

If an organ or tissue were to be removed immediately after the death of such a victim, this would not affect the outcome of the *post mortem* examination, which may take place only days afterwards. Take the example of a patient being brought to a casualty ward with a fatal stab wound in the aorta. There would be no objection to the removal of his corneae after his death but before the *post mortem* examination takes place.

Special provision is therefore made for the granting of official authorisation for the

53 Section 7(3).
54 Section 17.
55 Section 14(1)(a).
56 Section 16.
57 Act 58 of 1959.
58 Act 63 of 1977.
59 Act 81 of 1963.
60 Act 78 of 1973.
61 Section 14(3).

removal of any specific tissue in medico-legal *post mortem* cases, if the doctor who is to conduct the examination (or cause the examination to be conducted) certifies that –

- he is satisfied that the removal of the tissue will in no way affect the outcome of the examination, and
- he has no objection to the removal of such tissue.[62]

It should be noted that these provisions do not dispose of the consent requirements. Accordingly, the body or tissue must have been duly donated for transplantation purposes, either by the deceased, a relative, or, in the circumstances described above, by the Director-General (or person delegated by him). However, the Act contains special provisions relating to the removal of tissue or organs during *post mortem* examinations without prior consent or official authorisation, which will now be discussed.

REMOVAL OF TISSUE DURING POST MORTEMS

Dead bodies which form the subject of medico-legal *post mortem* examinations or "hospital" *post mortems* are an important potential source of human tissue.

Because such a body will be dissected in any event, in order to establish the cause of death, the provisions of the Act are less stringent.

The Act[63] empowers a medical practitioner who conducts a *post mortem* examination under either the Inquests Act[64] or under section 8(*b*) of the Human Tissue Act – i e the "hospital" *post mortem* examination conducted to determine "more precisely the cause of death or for a specific scientific purpose" – to remove tissue.

A ministerial authorisation is necessary. The Minister may authorise a person or institution to obtain tissue. Authority may be granted for the non-recurrent acquisition of tissue, or for acquisition for a stated or unspecified period. Tissue thus removed by a medical practitioner must be handed over to the holder of the authority.

It is of importance to note that no formal donation of a body – either by the deceased prior to death, or by his next of kin after his death – is required in these cases. (If the body has in fact been thus donated, it is dealt with under other provisions of the Act.)[65]

The medical practitioner who performs the *post mortem* must, however, be satisfied that –

- the removal of tissue will in no way affect the outcome of the examination;
- the deceased has not before his death given a direction forbidding removal of tissue.

In the past authorisations were issued for removal of the following types of tissue or organs, *inter alia*: pituitary, kidney, bone tissue, tendon, cartilage, skin, heart valve, eye, bone, dura mater, liver, aorta, heart, auricle.

REMOVAL OF TISSUE FROM BODIES OF DECEASED DESTITUTES

A body handed over to an institution such as a hospital, university or technikon,[66] by virtue of a formal order by the inspector of anatomy in terms of section 12[67] (relating to the bodies of destitute persons or the inmates of public institutions)[68] of the Act,

62 *Ibid.*
63 Section 9.
64 For the background to the introduction of this provision into our legislation on anatomical donations, see the 3rd edition of this book (1984), page 156.
65 Section 9(2) (*b*) forbids a removal of tissue under this section if the doctor concerned has reason to believe that the body or tissue has been donated.
66 Or other institution authorised in terms of section 3(1).
67 "Public institution" is defined in section 1 as an institution supported wholly or in part by State or provincial funds.
68 Read with sections 10 and 11.

may be used by such institution in accordance with the regulations for any of the statutory purposes such as medical training, research and transplantation.[69] It would appear that the provisions of the Act relating to consent and official authorisation do not apply to such use.[70] However, if a body of a pauper or institutional inmate was duly donated by the deceased prior to his death, or thereafter by another person legally entitled to make a donation, it must clearly be dealt with in terms of the donation.[71]

PROVISIONS DESIGNED TO FACILITATE TISSUE ACQUISITION

The Act contains a number of provisions designed to facilitate the donation and acquisition of human tissue. Thus the authorising official is empowered to act upon a will if, on the face of it, it appears to be legally valid, irrespective of the fact that the will has not yet been lodged with or accepted by the Master of the Supreme Court.[72] As was mentioned above, it is not a requirement for the lawfulness of an anatomical donation that the person making the donation must expressly specify the purpose of the donation. The Act further contains directions regarding conflicting donations. Provision is also made for the nearest hospital to become the donee if the hospital mentioned by the donor is not within easy reach.

TIME LIMIT FOR REMOVAL OF TISSUE

Except in the case of the entire body being donated, the donee of tissue has 24 hours following the death of the donor within which he may remove the tissue donated. After 24 hours have elapsed, whether or not the tissue has been removed, the body may be claimed by the relatives of the deceased, or by the person or persons otherwise entitled thereto, with a view to burial or cremation of the remains.[73] Proper registers must be kept in respect of anatomical donations.[74]

General considerations relating to both deceased and living donors

RIGHTS CONCERNING DONATED TISSUE

The person who acquires tissue (including blood or a gamete) in terms of the Act, upon delivery of the body or tissue to him by means of use or otherwise, is vested with exclusive rights over it, subject to the prohibition of the sale of tissue.[75] The provision was especially designed to eliminate the possibility of the relative of a deceased donor and the relatives of a deceased recipient becoming involved in a distasteful conflict over the remains of the latter.

SALE OF TISSUE PROHIBITED

No person or body – except an authorised institution, or, in the case of tissue or gametes being imported, the importer – may receive payment in respect of the import, acquisition or supply of tissues or gametes for any of the purposes sanctioned by the Act. The same prohibition applies to blood or blood products, in respect of which only prescribed institutions and persons are exempted.[76] The rationale for these prohibitions is that most people find commerce in "human flesh and blood" ab-

69 See section 12. For criticism of the use of bodies of institutional inmates, see article by A J van der Walt 1984 *TSAR* 154.
70 This is indicated in my opinion by the imperative "shall" used in section 10.
71 This is the meaning which in my opinion must be given to the words "subject to the provisions of sections 2 and 8" used in section 10.
72 Section 14(4).
73 Section 7 (1).
74 See the regulations contained in GN R287 of 29 December 1989 *GG* 12234.
75 Section 36.
76 Section 28(1).

horrent.[77] Authorised or prescribed institutions are specifically excluded from the prohibition to enable institutions such as tissue banks (which must incur costs in acquiring and preserving tissue) to be remunerated.[78]

The prohibition on the sale of tissue does, of course, not prevent a medical practitioner from receiving remuneration for any professional services rendered by him to any person.[79]

The unlawful sale of human tissue is a criminal offence.[80] If payment has been made for tissue, gametes or blood in contravention of the Act, the person who made such payment is entitled to a refund.[81]

GENETIC MANIPULATION PROHIBITED

Genetic manipulation of gametes or zygotes outside the human body, is absolutely prohibited by the Act.[82] (A zygote is the cell resulting from the fusion of two gametes, i e the fertilised ovum.)[83]

SECRECY

At the time of the first heart transplants, a highly controversial issue with regard to tissue donation and transplantation was whether the donor and/or recipient should be protected against publicity. It was argued that if the identity of a recipient were known, there would be the possibility of "blackmail" on the part of the donor or his next of kin. It was also contended that the fear of publicity could deter potential donors. On the other hand, it was felt that the personal freedom of an individual was of too great importance to be fettered by a prohibition against the disclosure of the fact that he was a donor or recipient of human tissue. The Legislature ultimately followed a middle course by making lawful disclosure of the identity of the parties dependent upon their consent.

The Act contains a prohibition against the publication to any other person of any fact whereby the identity of the donor of the body of a deceased person or of any tissue thereof, or the donor of tissue removed from the body of a living person, may be established, unless consent thereto in writing has been given by the deceased prior to his death or by the living donor, or after the death of the person whose body tissue has been donated by one of the specified relatives who may consent, or by the district surgeon who donated the tissue. The Act contains a similar prohibition regarding the recipient. Such disclosure is unlawful, unless the recipient has consented thereto in writing. If the recipient has died without giving consent or without having indicated that he would not be prepared to give such consent, consent may be given by one of the following persons: a spouse or a major child or a parent or a major brother or a major sister of the recipient.[84]

77 According to a report in the *Rand Daily Mail* of 7 October 1982 (with a New York date-line), a surge in successful heart and other organ transplants has drastically outstripped the donor supply and raised fears that "a grisly, lucrative black market may develop". Giesen (*Arzthaftungsrecht – Medical Malpractice Law* (1981) 370) reports that "there are already cases of wealthy Asians travelling to Australia with paid donors in their entourage to have kidney transplant operations"! A report in *Die Vaderland* of 25 April 1984 referred to a "diabolical plan" of a Durban man to recruit persons in Transkei to sell their kidneys for transplantation purposes. The scheme was brought to the attention of the SA Medical and Dental Council. According to a report in *The Citizen* of 20 June 1989 a Turkish peasant claimed that he had been "robbed" of one of his kidneys. The report contains details of the international "trade in human organs".

78 Section 28(1).

79 *Ibid.*

80 Section 34(*j*).

81 Section 28(2).

82 Section 39A.

83 *Dorland's Illustrated Medical Dictionary* s v "zygote".

84 Section 33.

It must be noted that the unlawful disclosure of identity constitutes a punishable offence.[85]

Exclusion of civil and criminal liability

The Act exempts from civil and criminal liability a doctor who, for any of the purposes stated in the Act has, in good faith, removed any tissue from a dead body or from a living donor, in the event of any donation subsequently being found to be legally invalid. The same protection is afforded to a magistrate or medical practitioner who has authorised the removal of tissue.[86]

IMPORTING AND EXPORTING OF TISSUE

The Act strictly controls the importing and exporting of tissue, dead human bodies, blood and gametes. For this a permit signed by the Director-General of National Health and Population Development is required.[87] If tissue is imported contrary to the provisions of the Act, it must either be destroyed or removed from the Republic at the expense of the importer, or it is forfeited to the State (in which event it may be destroyed or be dealt with otherwise in such a manner as the Director-General may deem fit).[88] The illegal importation or exportation of tissue constitutes a criminal offence.[89]

OFFENCES

The Act creates a number of criminal offences which are punishable by a fine of R2 000 or imprisonment for a period not exceeding one year (or both).

Among the offences are the following:

- ❑ acquiring, using or supplying the body of a deceased person, or tissue, blood or a gamete from a living person, in any manner or for any purpose other than is permitted by the Act;
- ❑ using a gonad in the body of a living person contrary to the provisions of the Act;
- ❑ removing tissue from the body of a living person, or using or transplanting tissue thus removed, by a person who is not a medical practitioner or a dentist;
- ❑ disclosing the identity of a donor or recipient of tissue, otherwise than in accordance with the Act;
- ❑ contravening a provision or condition relating to the importing or exporting of tissue, blood, a blood product or a gamete.[90]

Diagnostic ("hospital") post mortem examinations

A *post mortem* examination of the body of a deceased person may be conducted before burial, if the deceased gave consent thereto prior to his death, or if the autopsy is necessary to determine more precisely the cause of death, or for a specific scientific purpose.[91] The provisions of the Act make it clear that consent by the deceased before his death is not an absolute requirement. All that must be established is that the autopsy is, in fact, necessary for the purpose stated. The Act contains no indication that the deceased's relatives have to be consulted or that they have any right to veto an autopsy.

The provisions of the Act[92] relating to official authorisation for the removal of

85 Section 34(*k*).
86 Section 35.
87 Section 25.
88 Section 26.
89 Section 34(*i*).
90 Section 34.
91 Section 8.
92 Contained in section 14.

tissue from a dead body for purposes of donation (discussed above) also apply to *post mortem* examinations, except that the authorising official need not, of course, be satisfied that the deceased's body was donated for scientific or therapeutic purposes.[93]

Where a person consents to a *post mortem* examination of his body, such consent must be obtained in the same manner as if he were donating his body for scientific or therapeutic purposes.[94]

Note that a *post mortem* examination may be performed only by a medical practitioner personally.[95]

93 Section 14(2)(*a*) expressly excepts the magistrate or medical practitioner from being satisfied, in the case of a *post mortem* examination conducted under section 8(*b*) for the purpose of determining more precisely the cause of death or for a specific scientific purpose, that the body had been donated.

94 Section 8(*a*) read with section 2(1).

95 Section 8 read with section 14(1)(*b*).

26 The patient's rights to tissue removed during an operation

The following questions were put to me:

"A patient consents to an operation which involves the removal of a diseased tissue (or organ) from his or her body, e g an appendix, gall-bladder or uterus.

"In our hospital the procedure is that after the tissue has been removed in the theatre, it is kept there. The patient is taken back to the ward and the tissue is sent to the incinerator for destruction.

"If the patient were to request that tissue removed from his body be handed to him and it transpires that the hospital staff has already destroyed the tissue, without having sought the patient's consent, will the hospital in any way incur legal liability?

"The same situation arises where an arm or a leg has been amputated. Sometimes it happens that after the patient has been brought back to the ward he requests the member removed so as to have it buried or embalmed. Is the hospital entitled to destroy the member without the patient's consent? And what is the position where a foetus is removed in a lawful abortion? Can the woman demand to be given possession of it?"

My answer is as follows:

On a number of occasions I have seen ex-patients proudly displaying to their friends or relatives gall-stones removed from their bodies, or an appendix carefully preserved in a little bottle – not to mention children boasting of a tooth pulled out by a dentist. Possession of these bodily parts by patients is certainly harmless enough.

One does feel a certain amount of aversion, however, to possession of an amputated leg or arm, the preservation of which may present the possessor with a difficult practical problem. The keeping of a well-developed foetus in a bottle by a woman from whose body it was removed in the course of a legal abortion, likewise would not appeal to many people: it may be felt that in a way the foetus has a kind of "personality" of its own, and once removed from the uterus, it can hardly be considered as part of the mother's body.

Yet the law must be consistent and in principle there seems to be nothing in our law against possession by a person of parts severed from his own body.

It is true that a corpse has traditionally been viewed as an unownable thing – the possession of an Egyptian mummy by a museum would clearly constitute an exception to this rule – and this principle may also be considered as applying to the possession of parts of a corpse (although a clear exception of lawful ownership of such parts would be the possession of anatomical specimens for scientific purposes by a recognised medical school or scientific institution).[1]

But if the possession of parts of a corpse is seen as socially undesirable and there-

1 This is clearly envisaged by the proviso to section 13(1) of the Human Tissue Act 65 of 1983, which authorises institutions such as universities to remove "and preserve separately" any tissue of cadavers. Such bodies or tissue may be used *inter alia* for training and research (section 4(1) read with sections 12 and 13). C F Klopper "Diefstal van 'n Lyk" 1970 *THRHR* 38 at 42 is correct when he states that theft of a corpse is legally impossible, but I am unable to agree with his suggestion that the same is invariably true of parts of a corpse. Anatomical specimens lawfully (and carefully) collected by a medical school in the course of years, constitute a valuable asset of the school. They are *res in commercio*, i e capable of being owned, are in fact owned, and, *ergo*, are capable of being stolen.

fore forbidden by the law, the same considerations do not necessarily apply to possession by a living person of parts removed from his own body (or from the body of another living person, if the patient has consented to such possession).

It is also true that Roman-Dutch jurists propounded the view that no one is *dominus membrorum suorum* (master of his own bodily members).[2] But by that they signified nothing more than that a man cannot consent to arbitrary removal of parts of his body – e g by allowing his hand or leg to be chopped off for no medical reason.

Price[3] (in 1953) stated categorically that a portion removed from a patient's anatomy in the course of an operation is the patient's property and if he demands it, it must be surrendered to him. There does not seem to be anything in our law to contradict this. The Human Tissue Act[4] in fact allows a patient from whose body tissue – and this concept includes flesh, bones, organs and glands – has been removed in the interest of his health, to consent to the use thereof for transplantation purposes. If a person has the right to donate such tissue, surely he has the right to decide not to donate it and keep it for himself.

If the patient does not make any claim to the part removed from his body, which certainly occurs in the vast majority of cases, the part would become *res nullius*, i e a thing belonging to no one – and any person can lay claim to it by *occupatio*, either with intent to possess it as owner or to destroy it. Should it be felt that the possession of fairly substantial parts of a body, such as an amputated leg, genitals or a foetus, either by the patient or by another, offends against public policy or morality, it is for Parliament to legislate against such possession. However, the problem hardly seems to be of such magnitude as to warrant legislative regulation. Surely society can afford to allow one out of ten or twenty thousand patients to "hang on" to severed bodily parts.

In the absence of such legislation, the only question of importance appears to be: from what moment does the part removed become *res nullius*? The patient may of course declare in advance that he does not want the part and that the hospital may do with it as it pleases. He may also after the operation make such a statement. In both cases there would be no problem at all.

Problems may arise, however, where the patient has not entered into any express arrangement regarding the disposal of parts of his body which will be or have been removed – which undoubtedly is the position in the vast majority of cases. Here the time factor and the physical condition of the patient are circumstances which may play a role.

If the patient's condition is such that he is mentally capable of enforcing his rights, and he does not claim the part removed within a reasonable time, it may be assumed that he has abandoned it.

What should be considered a reasonable time? In the unlikely event of litigation being brought by a patient in such a case, a court would probably be guided by what is considered reasonable by medical practitioners and hospital staff, in the light of practical realities. In the case of drastic surgery under a general anaesthetic, it would seem to be unlikely for a patient to be able to meaningfully exercise any right of this nature within 24 hours; in less drastic surgery the period may be substantially shorter.

It would seem, in any event, that the part removed cannot be considered as *res nullius* immediately after the operation, that is before the patient could reasonably have been expected to apply his mind to whether or not he would lay claim to the

2 See S A Strauss *Toestemming tot Benadeling as Verweer in die Strafreg en die Deliktereg* (LLD thesis, Univ of S Africa, 1961) 369 *et seq*.
3 I Gordon, R Turner & T W Price *Medical Jurisprudence* (3rd ed, 1953) 82-83.
4 Act 65 of 1983, section 18, read with section 19.

part removed. Should the hospital therefore destroy the part immediately, it may technically lay itself open to a claim by the patient.

A hospital can decidedly not be expected to confront every patient upon admission or afterwards, with the question whether or not he wishes to lay claim to parts which will be or have been removed from his body.

The matter can best be resolved by making waiver by the patient of his rights to bodily parts so removed, a condition of admission to the hospital. This can be accomplished by inserting a clause into the hospital admission or consent form (routinely signed by the patient or his guardian upon admission to the hospital), to the following effect: "It is agreed that it is a condition of my admission to the hospital that I waive all rights that I may have in regard to any tissue or bodily part removed from my body during any operation performed upon me in the hospital. I accordingly hereby waive such rights and I authorise the superintendent of the hospital or any employee of the hospital to dispose of such tissue or part in any such manner as they may see fit."

Should a patient upon admission to the hospital refuse to agree to this clause it is for the superintendent to decide whether he would refuse admission to the patient – in so far as this may legally be done[5] – or whether he would be prepared to delete the clause, in which event the patient should be given the part(s) removed from his body if he so insists.

Tissue, organs, etc removed from a patient's body would ordinarily have no economic value, so that a claim by the patient for actual damage suffered by him would seem to be out of the question.[6] The question may be asked whether intentional destruction of a bodily part after removal of it, before the patient has effectively abandoned it, could be considered as constituting an infringement of a right of personality of the patient, for which a court may award sentimental damages to him. Professor Boberg[7] is of the opinion that it would be difficult to construe such an act as an *iniuria* to the patient. He argues that such destruction is not an invasion of the patient's dignity or his reputation. Nor can it be regarded as an invasion of his person, for having been removed, the part no longer forms part of his person. Boberg sees the part merely as a piece of the body of the patient which, though it may belong to the patient in a technical sense, is no longer a portion of his body in the sense required for protection under the *actio iniuriarum*. Says Boberg: It would of course be a totally different matter if the bodily part were destroyed in circumstances contumelious to the patient – e g the defendant held the patient up to ridicule by publicly burning his genitals!

5 As far as State or provincial hospitals are concerned, patients may have a qualified right of admission (see e g the Transvaal Hospitals Ordinance 14 of 1958, section 33(1)) and an unreasonable refusal to admit a patient might lend itself to an attack in court on the ground that the superintendent has not properly applied his mind to the matter. It would seem grossly unreasonable for a patient suffering from a serious condition to be refused admission simply because he is not prepared to agree to a waiver clause of this kind.

6 A tooth with a gold-filling is clearly an exception.

7 Professor P Q R Boberg of the Faculty of Law of the University of the Witwatersrand expressed this opinion in a letter to me. Publication of his opinion here is with his kind permission.

27 May a hospital destroy the remains of a still-born foetus?

The following questions were put to me:

"A premature child is still-born in a hospital and the foetus is destroyed in the incinerator by the hospital staff. Must the hospital first obtain the parents' consent in writing to have the foetus destroyed, or may it be assumed that such a child is premature and not viable according to the law, that is, if it was born before 28 weeks?

"If the child was born before 28 weeks and it breathed – a live birth, in other words – but expired shortly afterwards, say within half an hour, may the hospital likewise destroy it in the incinerator, or must it be buried?"

My answer is as follows:

As far as could be ascertained, statutory law does not provide an answer to these questions.

The Registration of Births, Marriages and Deaths Act[1] does in fact define "viable", in relation to a child, as meaning "that it has had at least six months of intra-uterine existence". "Still-born", in relation to a child, is defined as meaning "that it was viable but showed no sign of life after complete birth". "Birth" means "the birth of any viable child whether such child is living or dead at the time of birth". "Body" means "any human dead body, including the body of any still-born child".[2]

The Act deals primarily with the registration of births, marriages and deaths, and the definitions were of course designed with that purpose foremost in the Legislature's mind. However, the Act also contains important provisions relating to death certificates and burial orders. Thus a duty is imposed upon doctors and midwives who were in attendance at a birth, to issue to an undertaker a certificate stating that the child was still-born.[3] Other provisions of the Act govern the issuing of a burial order by a registrar of births.[4] These provisions do of course not apply to a foetus ("child") which has had less than six months' intra-uterine existence.

The Act further ordains that save in exceptional circumstances, e g where the deceased has died from an infectious disease, no burial may take place in an urban area unless a burial order has been issued.[5] This provision applies to "bodies", and the definition of a "body" referred to above, clearly excludes the "child" or foetus with an intra-uterine life-span of less than six months.

The Act, however, does not stipulate what must be buried and how burials must take place, and what need not be buried. Funerals and cremations are essentially governed by provincial ordinances and municipal regulations.[6] In the Transvaal, for in-

1 Act 81 of 1963, section 1.

2 J Taitz and S Clow 73 *S Afr Med J* 240 (1988) state that a medical calculation in "weeks and days" is more accurate that a "month" and that the provisions of the Act should be reviewed. In my view the existing provisions are quite satisfactory. A doctor is not required to determine the exact age of the foetus; all that he is required to do is to determine that the foetus had an existence of "at least" six months. To the best of my knowledge the practical application of that criterion causes no problems.

3 Section 20.

4 Section 21.

5 Section 28.

6 On funerals in general see F F W van Oosten in *The Law of South Africa* (eds W A Joubert and T J Scott) vol 21 (1984) 27 *et seq*; C Nathan 8 *Med Law* 445 (1989).

stance, there are the Cemetery Ordinance[7] and the Crematorium Ordinance.[8] Local authorities are vested with powers regarding the establishment and control of cemeteries and crematoria. In the Transvaal, this is provided for in the Local Government Ordinance.[9] In terms of the latter Ordinance,[10] a municipal council is empowered, *inter alia* "to compel the burial of dead bodies in a proper burial ground or cemetery". The Ordinance does not indicate whether a non-viable foetus should be regarded as a "dead body".

The Cemetery and Crematorium By-Laws for the Municipality of Pretoria[11] are probably typical of municipal regulations concerning burial and cremation. These by-laws provide that burials must take place in municipal cemeteries[12] and cremations in municipal crematoria.[13] ("Cremation" is defined[14] as "disposal of a body by means of incineration" – destruction of a body in a hospital incinerator will accordingly fall within that definition.)

The municipal regulations to which I have referred, apply to "bodies", and a "body" is defined[15] as "any human dead body including the body of any still-born child". It can be assumed that "human dead body" would not include a non-viable foetus, and "still-born child" would undoubtedly be interpreted by reference to the definition of that concept in the Registration of Births, Marriages and Deaths Act, quoted above. There is no reference in the by-laws to a non-viable foetus, so that the by-laws may not provide an answer to our problem either.

The issue can only be resolved by referring to the general principles of common law. A point of departure would be the view that a dead body is *res extra commercium*[16] and as such is not capable of being owned by anyone, and should be buried. The detailed statutory regulation of burials and cremation can lead to no other conclusion. In an old Transvaal case, *Klingenberg's Exor v Lademan*[17] (1898), it was held that a dead body does not form part of the deceased's estate and that the executor has no right to possession of the body. The famous 17th century Roman-Dutch jurist, Voet,[18] stated that even a complete stranger may carry out a funeral so that dead bodies shall not lie unburied. Dead bodies or parts thereof may clearly remain unburied only by specific statutory provisions regarding schools of anatomy,[19] *post mortem* examinations, etc. (The keeping of an Egyptian mummy by a museum clearly constitutes a "common-sense" exception to the rule that a dead body is incapable of ownership!)

However, the fact that dead bodies should be buried (or cremated) does not mean that the same rule applies to foetuses. As was pointed out, the statutory provisions relating to burial and cremation apply only to dead bodies, including *viable* foetuses. Judged in the light of general principles, it would seem as though non-viable foetal remains would definitely not qualify as human bodies and should therefore simply be dealt with on the basis of being a tissue removed from the mother's body. It is therefore submitted that a foetus may lawfully be destroyed in a hospital incinerator, unless the woman has before removal or shortly afterwards laid claim to it.[20]

7 Ordinance 8 of 1932.
8 Ordinance 18 of 1965.
9 Ordinance 17 of 1939.
10 Section 93(3)(*a*).
11 Introduced in terms of section 101 of Ordinance 17 of 1939, by Administrator's Notice 82 of 30 January 1957 (see the Transvaal *Provincial Gazette* of the same date) and subsequently amended.
12 Section 4.
13 Section 61.
14 Section 1.
15 *Ibid.*
16 Literally, "a thing outside commerce", i e incapable of being owned.
17 (1898) 5 OR 105.
18 *Commentarius ad Pandectas* 11.7.7.
19 Section 13(1) of the Human Tissue Act 65 of 1983, read with section 4(1) of the same Act.
20 See further my remarks above 160 *et seq.*

The question remains whether a foetus with a life-span of less that six months which was born *alive* and then expired, must be dealt with on a different basis than in the case of a still-born foetus. In my opinion there would be no reason for such a distinction. Despite live birth, such a foetus is not a "viable child" or "still-born child" in terms of the Registration of Births, Marriages and Deaths Act.[21] Nor would its remains in my opinion qualify as a "human dead body" or "still-born child" in terms of the municipal by-law quoted.

It is to be noted that a foetus ("child") which has breathed, is regarded as a human being for the purposes of murder and culpable homicide (in terms of the Criminal Procedure Act)[22] and a foetus ("child") which "has completely proceeded in a living state from the body of its mother, whether ... it has breathed or not, and whether it has an independent circulation or not, and whether the navel string is severed or not", is regarded as "human being" for the purposes of the Transkeian Penal Code.[23] It might perhaps be argued that in view of these provisions such a foetus should be regarded as a human being and should be given to its parents for burial if they so desire.

However, as Hunt[24] has pointed out, the "breathing test" was introduced into our law to bridge any possible gap ("absurd and undesirable") between the crimes of abortion and murder. It is one thing for the law to say that a person who kills a foetus which has proceeded from the body of the mother and has breathed, is guilty of infanticide. It would be a completely different matter to say that a doctor who destroys such a foetus which has died, is guilty of a criminal offence. There is no authority in our law for the latter proposition.

Likewise, the fact that such a foetus is for the purpose of the law of infanticide regarded as a human being, does not justify the conclusion that it is such for the purpose of cemetery by-laws. As I have mentioned, a doctor is not even required in the case of a foetus which is younger than six months to issue a death certificate in terms of the Registration of Births, Marriages and Deaths Act.

The position is somewhat more problematic when it concerns a foetus which has in fact had an intra-uterine existence of more than six months, but which dies *in utero*; it is removed medically from the womb in a macerated condition. It would be somewhat artificial to construe such a procedure as a "birth" in terms of the Registration of Births, Marriages and Deaths Act. It is submitted that such a foetus may also be incinerated.

For the sake of completeness it should be mentioned that incineration of a non-viable foetus can in no way be regarded as constituting the offence of concealment of the birth of a child. In *R v Matthews*[25] it was held that a foetus "is not a child for the purposes of the statutes unless it has reached a stage of development sufficient to have rendered its separate existence apart from its mother a reasonable probability". Accordingly the court held that where birth was given five months after conception, the foetus was not a child. In coming to this conclusion the court relied upon a similar provision of the 1923 Births, Marriages and Deaths Registration Act[26] which imposed an obligation to report the death of a still-born child which was likewise defined as a foetus of over six months' intra-uterine existence. From this the judge concluded: "I cannot think that there has been any concealment of birth of a *foetus* where the law imposes no necessity of reporting it."[27]

21 Section 1.
22 Act 51 of 1977, section 239.
23 Section 83 of the Penal Code of 1983. The provisions are identical to those of section 134 of the Code's predecessor, the Native Territories Penal Code 24 of 1886 (C). Although the latter Code applied only in Transkei it had a marked influence on South African criminal law in general.
24 P M A Hunt *South African Criminal Law and Procedure* vol II, *Common Law Offences* (2nd ed, 1982, by J R L Milton) 372-3.
25 1943 CPD 8.
26 Act 17 of 1923.
27 See also the comments on *Matthew's* case by J R L Milton and N M Fuller *South African Criminal Law and Procedure* vol III, *Statutory Offences* (1971) 271.

Note that in terms of the Abortion and Sterilisation Act[28] the fruit of coitus undoubtedly is a foetus for the purposes of that Act as long as it is *in utero*, i e before birth. In terms of the Human Tissue Act,[29] again, a foetus *in utero* clearly is "tissue" for the purposes of the latter Act. However, these two Acts do not in any way prevent a woman from consenting to the destruction of a still-born foetus. In particular such consent does not amount to an anatomical donation by virtue of the Human Tissue Act. On the other hand, there is nothing in the latter Act to prevent a woman from donating for medical or scientific purposes a foetus lawfully removed from her body in terms of the Abortion and Sterilisation Act.

28 Act 2 of 1975.
29 Act 65 of 1983.

PART VIII

Contraception, sterilisation, artificial insemination, surrogate motherhood, genetic manipulation

28 Legal problems connected with contraception and sterilisation

Contraception and the married woman

Does a doctor expose himself to liability when he inserts an intra-uterine device in a married woman or prescribes an oral contraceptive without her husband's consent? May a doctor do so in the case of an unmarried minor female without her parents' consent?

These questions have given rise to controversy in the past. There is no statutory law in South Africa, nor are there any court decisions, dealing directly with these questions. (A 1909 statutory provision[1] in the Transvaal prohibiting the advertising of contraceptive methods, instruments, etc was repealed in 1975 by the Abortion and Sterilisation Act.)[2] In venturing an opinion, the lawyer can only argue inferentially from broad juridical principles.

In assessing the legality or otherwise of contraception, and the doctor's liability in a hypothetical lawsuit, the court would in the final analysis be guided by "public policy" or the *boni mores.*

It can categorically be stated that for operations or treatment not involving a married woman's procreative functions, the husband's consent will not be required. In *Palmer v Palmer*[3] the judge ruled that "the personal guardianship of a husband over his wife ... does not today give the husband the right to interfere with the wife's personal freedom to the extent that he can force her to undergo a medical examination against her will ...". *E contrario* it can be argued that the wife does generally not need the husband's consent for medical treatment.

In the case of *W v H*,[4] again, it was held that where a husband without good cause refused to have intercourse with his wife without the use of contraceptives, such conduct constituted malicious desertion, entitling the wife to divorce. The judge stated that "to deny the wife, *stante matrimonio*, the right to motherhood without good cause is a wrongful refusal of marital rights". At the time (1965), malicious desertion was still a ground for divorce. The Divorce Act of 1979[5] brought about a new divorce regime and irretrievable breakdown of the marriage is now *per se* a ground for divorce; proof of malice in deserting a spouse or of marital infidelity is no longer required. The philosophy behind the decision in *W v H* might perhaps have provided substance for reasoning that a third party, a doctor, would have violated the husband's right to procreation by prescribing an oral contraceptive to his wife or inserting an IUD without his (the husband's) consent. In earlier times there was support for the view that spouses shared a mutual right to procreation; the husband's right could then conceivably be violated by a third party interfering with his *wife's* procreative capability, or *vice versa*.[6] There is little support for this view in modern times,

1 The Criminal Law Amendment Act 38 of 1909 (T) section 2(8).
2 Act 2 of 1975.
3 1955 (3) SA 56 (D).
4 1965 (3) SA 740 (O).
5 Act 70 of 1979.
6 See e g P Noll *Uebergesetzliche Rechtfertigungsgründe, im besondern die Einwilligung des Verletzten* (1955) 93 – 7. This view was also supported in the previous editions of this book.

though. The modern view of marriage is that each spouse is autonomous as far as his or her body is concerned.[7]

Each spouse may accordingly practise contraception without the consent of the other and there is no question of liability on the part of the doctor who provides contraceptive advice or means to a married person, without consulting or seeking the consent of his or her spouse. The conduct of a married person in applying contraceptive measures without his or her spouse's approval may strain the marriage relationship and may lead to irretrievable breakdown thereof, but that is not the concern of the doctor.

Although there are still certain churches and religions that disapprove of artificial methods of birth control, the legality of contraceptives is beyond question today.

Sterilisation of spouse

Our legislation on sterilisation – the Abortion and Sterilisation Act of 1975 – does not deal comprehensively with sterilisation. It is narrowly confined to sterilisation of persons who are mentally incapable of consenting and is applied particularly to mentally defective minors. (The provisions of the Act are discussed below.)[8]

An assessment of the lawfulness of sterilisation of mentally competent persons therefore depends on common-law considerations.[9] The Abortion and Sterilisation Act is significant in this context only in so far as it is indicative of the fact that the South African Legislature is not averse to sterilisation as such.

Whatever past attitudes to sterilisation have been, there can be no doubt that the procedure is not regarded as *contra bonos mores* today, provided that a socially approved objective is sought to be attained. The legality of therapeutic sterilisation is beyond question, e g where a hysterectomy is proposed because of a diagnosis of cancer. Where the patient is married, his or her spouse's consent is not necessary. Just as a husband is not entitled to dictate to his wife that she must be medically examined or treated,[10] so, it is submitted, he may not veto medically indicated treatment that will be highly beneficial to her. "The law does not authorize the husband to say to his wife, you shall die of cancer – you cannot be cured."[11]

Where a married couple already have a child or children and either of them desires to be sterilised, there can be no question that it will be lawful for a doctor to perform the operation. "Sterilisation has become an accepted form of contraception for married couples. The State is conducting a campaign of family planning, the aim of which is to curb the growth of the population. It is in the interests of society that the size of a family should not exceed the limit beyond which it would not be possible for it to maintain a reasonable standard of living."[12]

It is perhaps somewhat more problematic legally to justify in such absolute terms sterilisation, purely for convenience, of a married person who has not yet generated offspring. Sterilisation, whether of a male or of a female, must generally be regarded as an irreversible operation. There are a number of ethical issues relating to this situ-

7 See J C Sonnekus "Sterilisasie – Toestemming deur Nie-pasiënt-gade" 1986 *De Rebus* 369.
8 Page 214.
9 See S A Strauss & M J Strydom *Die Suid-Afrikaanse Geneeskundige Reg* (1967) 250 *et seq*. Compare F Bosman (ed) *Social Welfare Law* (1982) 529.
10 See *Palmer v Palmer, supra*.
11 Statement quoted with approval in the American case of *Pratt v Davis* 118 Ill App 166 (1907) 167; compare the English case of *Bravery v Bravery* [1954] 3 All ER 59.
12 Mr Justice Thirion in *Edouard v Administrator Natal* 1989 (2) SA 368 (D) at 376 A. The *Edouard* decision was confirmed by the Appellate Division in *Administrator, Natal v Edouard* 1990 (3) SA 581 (A). Such operations have become quite common in South Africa. In 1983 it was reported that during the 4-year period 1979 to 1982 (inclusive) 9 175 laparoscopic sterilisations had been performed in certain rural regions of the Cape Province. See article by A J Nieuwoudt *et al* 1983 *S Afr Med J* 1972.

ation which would not apply to a couple who have already satisfied their procreative desires. However, considering the great emphasis modern legal systems place on the personal autonomy of the individual, it is doubtful whether a South African court of law would rule that a sterilisation performed by a doctor in these circumstances constitutes an (illegal) assault on a person who has given his or her informed consent.

In 1976 the South African Medical Council ruled as follows on the ethical permissibility of sterilisation: "Except where it is done on purely medical grounds, a sterilisation operation may not be performed unless: (a) the full implications are explained to the patient; (b) the patient is married or over the age of 18; (c) written consent has been obtained from the patient." Although this is a purely professional-ethical ruling and the Medical Council cannot create law, it is a good indication of the contemporary attitude to the justification of sterilisation.

Is the consent of the other spouse, i e the husband or wife of the person who is to be sterilised, a legal requirement? The older view was that such consent was required, because of "a mutual right to procreation" to which I have made reference above.[13] This view is no longer held. J C Sonnekus[14] has argued persuasively that each spouse is autonomous as far as his or her body is concerned.

Many doctors regard it as professionally correct that the spouse of a patient who has requested a sterilisation should not be kept in the dark. But a doctor who is of this view need not go further than recommending to the patient that his or her spouse be informed.

Although the consent of a spouse is not a legal requirement, it is to be noted that in view of the possibility of a doctor being held liable at a later stage in respect of a "pregnancy claim" – which is discussed in detail below[15] – it may be wise for the doctor to take a proper written consent-*cum*-waiver signed by *both* spouses.

The lawfulness of a sterilisation performed on a young, unmarried (consenting) person, is not beyond doubt. This matter is discussed in the next section.

The minor female

May a doctor prescribe an oral contraceptive to a minor (unmarried) female or fit her with an intra-uterine device? May he advise her in general on sexual matters and contraception? Must he consult with the girl's parents and obtain their consent?

In terms of section 39(4) of the Child Care Act[16] a minor over the age of 18 years may independently consent to medical treatment. This provision was introduced into our law in 1976.

What is also certain is that any person under the age of 21 years who is married, in the eyes of the law is a major and can independently give consent to medical treatment or an operation.

Prior to 1976 there was some doubt on the question whether or not a minor could independently consent. The view was put forward that any minor could indeed so consent, provided that his intellectual maturity was such as to enable him to know what the treatment or operation entailed and to satisfactorily express his will.[17]

Assuming this view to have correctly reflected the position in common law, the question arises: Did the 1976 legislation supplement common law? Or did it substitute the common law altogether?

13 See e g C J Stetler & A R Moritz *Doctor and Patient and the Law* (4th ed, 1962) III; see also p 91 of the booklet *Sterilization: The World's Laws on Voluntary Sterilization for Family Planning Purposes* (Apr 1973) published by the Dept of Medical and Public Affairs (George Washington Univ Medical Centre).

14 See note 7, above.

15 Page 175.

16 Act 74 of 1983.

17 See Strauss & Strydom *op cit* 189 *et seq.*

It is submitted that the 1976 provision which was incorporated into the Children's Act,[18] the predecessor of the Child Care Act, was merely declaratory and did not substitute common law.[19] What the Legislature wanted to do, in other words, was to declare beyond any doubt that a patient who is 18 years or older can consent independently. It has thus made 18 years the general age of medical consent, thereby making it unnecessary for a doctor or anyone else to inquire into the individual's intellectual maturity – much in the same way that 21 years is by common law the general age of majority.

The age of sexual consent in respect of females is 16 years. A man who has sexual intercourse with a girl under that age, or who attempts to have such intercourse, is guilty of a criminal offence in terms of the Sexual Offences Act,[20] even if such conduct has taken place with the consent of the girl. If the girl is under the age of 12, the man will be guilty of the common-law offence of rape (or attempted rape, as the case may be). (*It is to be noted that a Bill was published early in 1991 which envisages an amendment to section 39(4) whereby the age of consent to medical* treatment– *as opposed to a medical operation – will be lowered to 14 years.*)

If section 39(4) of the Child Care Act as it reads at present were to be interpreted as denying a minor under the age of 18 the right to consent to medical treatment, it would lead to the anomalous result that although a girl of 17 can lawfully have a sexual relationship with a man, she would be unable to consult a doctor on her own with a view to obtaining contraceptive measures. There can be no doubt that the prescribing of an oral contraceptive or the insertion of an IUD amounts to medical treatment. Even if that interpretation of the subsection were the correct one, it must be pointed out that a doctor who prescribes "the Pill" to a minor under 18, does not contravene the Child Care Act.[21] However, this is not the end of the matter for the doctor. The question may be asked: can it not perhaps be argued that by prescribing to a minor (of whatever age) he is interfering with the parental authority?

In *Gordon v Barnard*[22] a father successfully applied to court for an interdict restraining a married man from meeting or communicating with his unmarried daughter aged 18. The judge held that the respondent's conduct in building up a surreptitious intimate relationship with the girl, which included having sexual intercourse with her, was a direct and unlawful challenge to the father's parental authority.

Assuming that a doctor who was familiar with the situation had put the girl on "the Pill", would the father be able to obtain a court order against the doctor as well? I do not think a case can be made out for that. For a man to have a sexual relationship with a minor female is one thing; it is ethically a completely different thing for a doctor to come to the aid of a girl who is legally regarded as capable of consenting to medical treatment, and to supply the means for contraception. By so doing, he is not aiding and abetting her immoral or illicit affair; he is merely aiding her in preventing the birth of an illegitimate child. The argument that the doctor is facilitating adulterous intercourse would not be very convincing. The sexual urge is not made more powerful by the availability of contraception!

The same may in my opinion be said of the argument that a doctor who provides contraception to a girl under the age of 16 is criminally guilty of aiding and abetting a contravention of the Sexual Offences Act (which penalises intercourse with a girl

18 Act 33 of 1960, section 20(8A).

19 In the previous editions of this book I argued in favour of the opposite view – but that was before the House of Lords decided *Gillick's* case!

20 Act 23 of 1957, section 14(1)(*a*).

21 Section 39(4) simply declares a person over 18 years of age capable of consenting. The subsection is not couched in such terms as to suggest that a doctor medically treating a "consenting" child under that age is guilty of an offence.

22 1977 (1) SA 887 (C).

under the age of 16, except where the accused can raise any of three expressly specified defences).

To be punished as an aider and abettor an accused must at least be found to have impliedly encouraged the commission of the offence. This does not seem to be the case here.

The question whether a doctor may furnish contraceptive advice and treatment to a minor girl without her parents' consent was the subject of an important case that came before the English courts in the 1980s, *Gillick v West Norfolk and Wisbeck Area Health Authority and Another.*[23]

At the outset it must be pointed out that the English legislation under which *Gillick* was decided is not quite identical to ours. Our section 39(4) says that a person who is 18 years or older may consent independently to medical treatment (the English age of medical consent is 16), but does not contain a provision similar to that of the English Act which declares that the section in question is not to be construed "as making ineffective any consent which would have been effective if this section had not been enacted".

Mrs Gillick, the mother of five daughters all under the age of 16, in 1983 sought a court order against the health authority, restraining its family-planning clinics from providing contraceptive advice and treatment to her daughters, unless it was with her consent. She complained that in so doing the authority was condoning and conniving at unlawful conduct on the part of males against females below the age of 16, namely the committing of offences of unlawful sex with an infant.

The judge who heard the case refused the application and Mrs Gillick appealed to the Court of Appeal. The appeal was allowed by the court on the ground, essentially, that a child under 16 could not validly consent to contraceptive treatment. This judgment was taken on appeal to the highest court of appeal in England, the House of Lords, which at the end of 1985 decided the case against Mrs Gillick.

In a majority ruling it was held that having regard to the reality that a child became increasingly independent as it grew older and that the parental authority dwindled correspondingly, the law did not recognise any rule of absolute parental authority until a fixed age. Instead, parental rights were recognised by the law only as long as they were needed for the protection of the child and such rights yielded to the child's right to make his own decisions when he reached a sufficient understanding and intelligence to be capable of making up his own mind.

Accordingly, the Law Lords held, a girl under 16 did not, merely by reason of her age, lack legal capacity to consent to contraceptive advice and treatment by a doctor.

The House of Lords also had to decide whether or not there was a possible contravention of the provisions of the Sexual Offences Act 1956 which penalise sexual intercourse with young girls. It was held that it was unlikely that a doctor, who in the exercise of his clinical judgment gave contraceptive advice and treatment to a girl under 16, could be said to have been aiding and abetting the commission of unlawful intercourse. The reason for this was that the *bona fide* exercise by the doctor of his clinical judgment negated the *mens rea* (guilty mind) which was an essential ingredient of those offences.

It followed that a doctor had a discretion to give contraceptive advice to a girl under 16 without her parents' knowledge or consent, provided the girl had reached an age where she had a sufficient understanding and intelligence to enable her to understand fully what was proposed. Such an act would therefore not amount to an infringement of parental rights.

Lord Fraser of Tullybelton, in his judgment, pointed out that notions of parental authority over a child had changed considerably since Victorian times. "In practice most wise parents relax their control gradually as the child develops and encourage

23 [1985] 2 All ER 402 (HL).

him or her to become increasingly independent ... Social customs change, and the law ought to, and does in fact, have regard to such changes when they are of major importance." Once the rule of the parents' absolute authority over minor children is abandoned, "the solution depends on a judgment of what is best for the welfare of the particular child," the Lord said. Nobody doubts that in the overwhelming majority of cases the best judges of a child's welfare are his or her parents. "That is why it would and should be 'most unusual' for a doctor to advise a child without the knowledge and consent of the parents on contraceptive matters." But, the Law Lord added, "there may be circumstances in which a doctor is a better judge of the medical advice and treatment which will conduce a child's welfare than her parents". The doctor is entrusted with a discretion, but should nevertheless "always seek to persuade her to tell her parents that she is seeking contraceptive advice". Earlier in his judgment, Lord Fraser was at pains to point out that although contraceptive advice and treatment are essentially medical matters, they may also raise moral and social questions on which many people feel deeply, and in that respect they differ from ordinary medical procedures.

Can the *Gillick* decision be of any value to us in South Africa in interpreting section 39(4) of the Child Care Act? Our courts are of course not bound by foreign judgments, but the views of the Law Lords have in the past commanded, and still do, great respect here and have considerable persuasive value in our courts.

As I have mentioned, our statutory provision, although similar to that of England, is not identical in all respects.

Lord Fraser regarded it as "verging on the absurd" to suggest that a girl or boy aged 15 could not effectively consent to ordinary medical procedures. If that is true of a 15-year-old, I would suggest that it is true, *a fortiori*, of 16 and 17-year-old juveniles.

Perhaps the correct approach for us would be to regard section 39(4) of our Child Care Act as merely declaratory – and not prohibitory, as I have argued above – and to treat of the effectiveness of juvenile consent to medical treatment in all its forms, including contraceptive advice and treatment, as a factual issue which does not depend on any specific age.

At the same time it must be said that some of the views set forth in the minority opinions in *Gillick* unquestionably still find wide support in this country (as also in England, no doubt). To mention only two: Providing contraceptive advice and treatment to a girl under 16 would make it more likely that she and her lover would have illegitimate sex, by removal of the risk of unwanted pregnancy (Lord Brandon). Before a girl under 16 is supplied with contraceptive facilities, the parent who knows most about the girl and ought to have the most influence with her, is entitled to exercise parental rights of control, supervision, guidance and advice (Lord Templeman).

However, if the 1991 South African Bill – to which I have made reference above – were to become law and the age of consent to medical *treatment* lowered to 14 years, these issues may become largely academic.

The subject of sterilisation of mentally defective persons – minors or otherwise – is covered by the provisions of the Abortion and Sterilisation Act and is discussed below.[24]

A word or two must be said about sterilisation of mentally competent minors. If such an operation were to be performed purely for the sake of convenience and without any medical indication, there can be little doubt that even if consent was given, the operation would be regarded as *contra bonos mores* and therefore unlawful. It is submitted that the juristic notions of South African society at this juncture do not approve of minors, or parents on their behalf, agreeing to be deprived of the ability to procreate. In fact, a question mark hangs over the lawfulness of voluntary sterilisation for purposes of convenience, exclusively, of childless young majors, whether married or unmarried.

24 Page 214 *et seq.*

29 Failed sterilisation: liability for "wrongful conception"

A discussion of sterilisation would be incomplete without some reference to liability for "wrongful conception". Over the past two decades or so, a number of cases have come before the courts – particularly in the USA – involving allegations of medical negligence in respect of contraception, sterilisation, genetic screening and abortion which resulted in the birth of an unwanted child – a child who, in addition to being unwanted, in some cases was also seriously handicapped. The general label "wrongful life" (or "wrongful birth") was attached to this type of case.

In the USA courts initially held that a doctor would not be held liable for negligence in the performance of sterilisation operations which resulted in the birth of an unwanted, normal child, on the ground – as it was put in a 1957 case – that "to allow damages for the normal birth of a normal child is foreign to the universal public sentiment of the people".[1]

Later the judicial outlook changed, and doctors were held liable in some cases of this nature. Generally speaking, courts were prepared, in cases of proved negligence on the part of the doctor (e g in performing a sterilisation, or in failing to advise genetic screening of a pregnant woman, or in failing to advise her to have the pregnancy terminated) to order the doctor to pay damages in the form of medical expenses in connection with the birth of the child. In exceptional cases the doctor was held liable for maintenance of the child, but usually the courts were not prepared to go to such an extreme.

There have been several such cases in England since 1980. In some of these the plaintiffs have succeeded in recovering damages and in other cases their claims have failed. It is difficult at this stage to extract hard and fast rules from the English cases. Four of the reported cases concerning failed sterilisation are discussed briefly.

In *Udale's* case[2] a sterilisation was performed negligently on a woman. She fell pregnant and a normal child was born. Her claim for the cost of enlarging the family home to accommodate the new baby and for the cost of the child's upbringing until the age of 16 was refused on the ground that it would be "contrary to public policy". The court held, however, that public policy did not preclude an award of damages for lost income and also for pain, suffering, inconvenience and the disruption of the family's finances caused by the unexpected pregnancy.

In *Emeh's* case[3] an abnormal child was born following a negligently performed female sterilisation. The Court of Appeal held that the woman's refusal to undergo an abortion did not constitute a *novus actus interveniens* (new intervening act breaking the causal sequence) or a failure to mitigate her damages. Irrespective of whether the child was normal or abnormal, she was entitled to damages under the following heads: future loss of earnings, the cost of maintaining the child from birth to trial and future maintenance, for the layette and for pain, suffering, and loss of amenities due to the need to care for the handicapped child. One of the judges was of the opinion that "where the arrival of the child has mitigating features" in the form of the value

1 *Shaheen v Knight* 11 D & C 2d 41 (1957).
2 *Udale v Bloomsbury Area Health Authority* [1983] 2 All ER 522 (QBD).
3 *Emeh v Kensington, Chelsea and Fulham Area Health Authority and Others* [1984] 3 All ER 1044 (CA).

of the child's aid, comfort and society during the parents' life expectancy, these could lead to an appropriate diminution in the damages awarded.

In *Thake's* case[4] a married man underwent an unsuccessful vasectomy and a sixth child was born to his wife and himself. The couple instituted an action for damages against the medical practitioner who had performed the vasectomy. The Queen's Bench held that the medical practitioner had committed breach of contract. On appeal, the Court of Appeal held that there had been no implicit guarantee that the husband would be sterile. In the absence of an express guarantee of the success of any operation or treatment performed by a medical practitioner, he does not give the patient such a guarantee; medical science is too unpredictable for this. All that a medical practitioner implicitly undertakes is to take reasonable care in effecting treatment. The plaintiffs therefore did not have an action for breach of contract against the medical practitioner. The plaintiffs' action (which was successful) was based on negligence on the ground of the practitioner's failure to comply with a contractual agreement, and to exercise a delictual duty to take care, in that the medical practitioner failed to warn them that the husband could again become fertile. The court held that the plaintiffs were entitled to damages for prenatal stress, pain and suffering as well as the reasonable cost of rearing the unplanned child.

In *Eyre's* case[5] a woman who had undergone a sterilisation operation nevertheless gave birth to a child. She could not prove that the operation had been performed negligently, nor did she allege that the doctor ought to have warned her that the operation may have been unsuccessful. Accordingly her claim was rejected.

The first decision on "wrongful conception" in South Africa was handed down in *Behrmann and Another v Klugman.*[6] In that case Mr and Mrs B sued Dr K, a specialist surgeon, for R299 609 in damages after the birth of a normal child which had been conceived following a vasectomy the doctor had performed on Mr B. The plaintiffs' action was based upon alleged breach of contract on the part of the doctor, and alternatively, negligence. The plaintiffs alleged *inter alia* that there had been an express or implied agreement that the doctor would properly and skilfully carry out the vasectomy, taking all necessary precautions to ensure that the vasectomy rendered Mr B permanently sterile and to prevent recanalisation of the *vas deferens* (sperm duct). The plaintiffs contended that the doctor had failed to advise Mr B to have a sperm count, before intercourse without contraception was resumed. The doctor denied that he had breached the agreement or had been negligent.

The decision in the *Behrmann* case essentially turned on whether the plaintiffs had been adequately warned about the necessary sperm counts to establish infertility. The plaintiffs testified that statements by the doctor caused them to believe that the operation was irreversible and would render Mr B sterile after ten weeks. Dr K testified, however, that it was his practice to tell patients that it could take up to nine months to achieve two negative sperm counts and that he would first have to declare the husband sterile. Mr Justice Melamet found in favour of the doctor. The judge found on the evidence of the plaintiffs that they had in fact waited 16 to 20 weeks after the operation before commencing intercourse without contraceptives; accordingly the judge had grave reservations whether Mr and Mrs B had in fact believed that Mr B would be sterile after 10 weeks.

The court agreed with the view expressed by the English Court of Appeal in *Eyre* that in the absence of an express warranty, the court should be slow to imply that a medical man gives an unqualified warranty as to the results of an intended operation. Mr Justice Melamet concluded that Mr and Mrs B, on a balance of probabilities, had

4 *Thake and Another v Maurice* [1986] 1 All ER 497 (CA).
5 *Eyre v Measday* [1986] 1 All ER 488 (CA).
6 1988 WLD, unreported. The case is discussed in 1988(4) *SA Practice Management* 6.

failed to establish that the contract between them and Dr K contained an express or implied term of warranty as to the permanent success of the operation.

The following remarks by the judge are also of interest: "At the outset I raised a query as to whether an action for damages of this nature was not *contra bonos mores* particularly in the light of the fact that the boy was born in wedlock and was apparently a healthy child. Defendant accepted that such action was permissible and did not wish to raise any objections in this regard. The trial proceeded without any decision in this regard – it apparently being the first trial of this kind in South Africa – although the matter has been considered in England where it has been decided that such an action would not be contrary to public policy despite doubts previously expressed in this regard."

In the light of the grounds on which the plaintiffs' action was dismissed, the decision left open the question whether such an action is not *contra bonos mores*. On the other hand, the decision does not afford authority for the proposition that an action for damages might not have succeeded if the facts as alleged by the plaintiffs had formed the basis of the court's decision.

In a comparable case, *Edouard v Administrator of Natal*,[7] the verdict went in favour of the parents of a child. In that case, the parents had agreed with a provincial hospital that a tubular ligation was to have been performed on the woman, at the time of her giving birth by Caesarean section to her third child. The hospital staff failed, however, "to cause the said surgery to effect the tubular ligation of the [woman's] fallopian tubes, to be performed at all".

The woman and her husband believed that the sterilisation procedure had been performed and accordingly took no precautions to prevent pregnancy. Approximately four months after the birth of her third child the woman fell pregnant again. She gave birth by Caesarean section to a normal child and a tubular ligation was then performed on her by Dr F.

The child's father brought action against the Provincial Administrator in his capacity as the executive of the provincial administration, for damages allegedly suffered in consequence of breach of contract. The defendant conceded that the administration was liable for damages for breach of contract as a result of its failure to effect the tubular ligation that had been agreed upon and contended that payment of the cost of the surgery (R622,79) subsequently performed by Dr F would discharge its liability. (A factor in this case, it is to be noted, was that the defendant had also conceded that the woman had requested the procedure because she and her husband could not afford to support any more children.)

The plaintiff, however, averred that he was entitled to receive further compensation, namely –

- general damages for the discomfort, pain and suffering, and loss of amenities suffered by his wife (with whom he was married in community of property and on whose behalf he sued);
- the cost of maintaining the child until she reached the age of 18 years.

The defendant denied liability for such further compensation on the ground that although the contract for the woman's sterilisation was valid and enforceable, it would be contrary to public policy to allow the parents of a healthy and normal but unplanned child to recover the cost of bringing up the child where the parents refuse to give the child out for adoption.

Counsel for the defendant argued that it was the notion that the court – in assessing "damages" of this nature – was called upon to decide whether a value in monetary terms had to be given to a healthy life, which was offensive, in the light of the South African view of the sanctity of life "in the context of our anti-abortion laws". The cost

7 1989 (2) SA 368 (D).

of maintaining a child, it was submitted, is "but one of those incidents of parenthood – that Pandora's box of joy, expectation, disillusionment, worry, expense and resignation and hopefully in old age, reward".

The trial court held, however, that damages in the form of maintenance for the child were recoverable. Sterilisation, the judge said, had become an accepted form of contraception for married couples. "It is in the interest of society that the size of a family should not exceed the limit beyond which it would not be possible to maintain a reasonable standard of living."

There would be nothing inconsistent in the attitude of parents if they were to say that they had not wanted another child but now that the child has been born they love it and refuse to part with it. The acceptance of the responsibilities of parenthood, however, would still leave the parents in the dilemma which they had wanted to avoid with the sterilisation, i e that they have a child whom they are unable to support.

The loss which the parents complain of is an economic loss which cannot and need not be weighed against the value of the life of the child. The emotional benefits which the birth of the child bestow on the parents do not increase their patrimony and are irrelevant in the determination of the *quantum* of damages.

"It would be fair and equitable," Mr Justice Thirion said, "that liability to provide for the maintenance of a child should fall on the doctor through whose neglect it was born, rather than it should fall on the parents, who because of their inability to provide adequately for the child had not wanted to have it. Fathers are regularly ordered by the courts to bear the cost of maintaining their illegitimate offspring. It would be a novel argument for the father of such a child to claim that by fathering a child he had conferred a benefit or a blessing on the mother which outweighs the cost of maintaining the child."

The court regarded the argument – that it is morally wrong that a normal healthy life should be the basis of a compensable wrong – as "squeamish and pedantic". Compensation would not be awarded for the fact that a child has been allowed to be born. It would be awarded for the loss which the parents suffer in having to support the child whose conception the doctor negligently failed to avoid and whom they cannot support.

No court would require parents to mitigate their loss by having the child adopted. An innocent party who has suffered loss as a consequence of breach of contract has to take only reasonable steps to mitigate his loss. To require that parents should give away their child would not be reasonable. That would run counter to our accepted community values.

The judge felt that although the assessment of damages in wrongful birth actions may raise difficulties, those difficulties are not by any means insurmountable.

Fears that imposition of liability would lead to awards of damages quite disproportionate to the moral culpability of the doctor or might tend to warp professional standards – in that doctors might be tempted to improperly advise patients to have abortions or make practitioners unwilling to undertake sterilisation operations – were exaggerated.

He added that the operation was a fairly simple procedure and it would be a simple matter for the doctor to explain to the patient that there is, despite the operation, a possibility that she might still fall pregnant. It would be easy for the doctor to contract out of liability.

In the event, the court came to the conclusion that it would not be contrary to public policy to recover damages in respect of the child's maintenance. The defendant was accordingly ordered to pay the plaintiff R22 500, the amount on which the parties had agreed.

The court was not prepared, however, to award general damages for the woman's pain and suffering, etc. "The question whether liability on contract for damages should be extended so as to cover damages for non-pecuniary loss flowing from a breach of the contract, involves considerations of legal policy," the judge said. Considering the ease with which a delictual claim – i e an action based on a civil wrong, for which general damages may be claimed – can be conjoined with a contractual claim, the judge saw no real need for extending liability in contract to that kind of loss. (In this case a delictual claim was not so conjoined because the plaintiff had failed to give timeous notice of his intention to bring such an action, as is statutorily required.)

It is to be noted that the judge for the sake of convenience used the terms "wrongful birth" to describe this type of case. Legal terminology is not quite settled as yet, however.

The following terms seem to have gained fairly general acceptance in American legal literature now:

- "wrongful pregnancy" or "wrongful conception" for cases of healthy but unwanted children where a claim is brought by the parents;
- "wrongful birth" where a claim is brought by the parents of an abnormal or disabled child;
- "wrongful life" where a claim is brought by the abnormal or disabled child itself.[8]

Edouard's case was taken on appeal and the judgment of the trial court was confirmed unanimously by a five-judge bench of the Appellate Division.[9]

The court of appeal held that in principle the precise nature of the breach of contract or neglect giving rise to the birth of an unwanted child, is immaterial in relation to the question whether a claim for child-raising expenditure was sustainable. As far as terminology was concerned, Mr Justice van Heerden preferred the simpler designation of a "pregnancy claim" for this type of case.

The court rejected the argument that the birth of a normal child is a blessing which in law cannot constitute a wrong: "Parents who cannot afford a further child may well be overjoyed by the birth of another, but unwanted sibling, but will naturally be dismayed by the additional financial burden cast upon them. It is, after all, that burden and not the child as such which is unwanted." In any event, the birth of a normal child does not invariably constitute a blessing: the child may "turn out to be a drug addict or a violent psychopath".

The Appeal Court rejected the argument that it was against public policy – and an interference with the sanctity accorded by law to the parent-child relationship – that the basic legal duty of parental support be transferred to the hospital authority. The judgment in favour of the child's father, in respect of child-raising expenditure, in no way relieved him or his wife from the obligation to support the child. There was, accordingly no *transfer* of that obligation. Should the money be lost for some reason, the father would remain obliged to support the child from their available sources.

An important qualification was added by the court to its finding that a claim for maintenance was good in law: this conclusion "is intended to pertain only to a case where, as here, a sterilization was performed for socio-economic reasons".

The *Edouard* decision leaves little doubt that in South Africa liability will arise (a) in the "classical" situation of "wrongful conception" (pregnancy resulting from medical negligence in respect of sterilisation and a normal child is born), as well as (b) for "wrongful birth", i e where it is alleged that the birth of a defective child should have been medically prevented by means of a lawful abortion.[9]

It is still an open question, however, whether our courts will uphold a claim for

8 See B Keplinger & J J Cramer "Wrongful Pregnancy: A House Divided" 23(2) *Tort & Insurance Law Journal* 496 (1988); J R Botkin "The Legal Concept of Wrongful Life" 259(10) *JAMA* 1541; D Giesen *International Medical Malpractice Law* (1988) 242-3. Compare S Brownlie "Wrongful Life: Is it a Viable Cause of Action in South Africa?" 5(1) *Responsa Meridiana* (Sept 1985) 18; P L Louw "Wrongful Life: 'n Aksie gebaseer op die Onregmatige Veroorsaking van Lewe" 1987 *TSAR* 199.

9 *Administrator, Natal v Edouard* 1990 (3) SA 581 (A).

"wrongful life" in the narrow sense, i e where a suit for damages is brought on behalf of the impaired infant rather than the parents. The infant does not claim that the doctor caused the impairment but that he (the doctor) was responsible for the infant's very existence.[10] Different policy considerations may apply in respect of such a claim.[11]

In view of the *Edouard* ruling a doctor who undertakes a sterilisation and wants to protect himself against liability should take a proper informed consent, in writing, by which the patient and his/her spouse also waives any eventual claim. A suggested consent form is published below. It must be noted, however, that such a consent will be of no avail if the doctor has forgotten to perform the sterilisation! The enforceability of a waiver in a case of negligence (in particular where the negligence was "gross") is also doubtful.[12]

CONSENT TO PRIMARY STERILISATION

I, the undersigned ______________________________ (name), a married person, hereby consent to undergo the operation of vasectomy/tubular ligation*, the nature of which has been explained to me. I have been told that the object of the operation is to render me sterile and incapable of parenthood. I have also been told, however, that no guarantee can be given that I will thus be rendered sterile. As concerns the proposed vasectomy, I have been advised that appropriate sperm tests must be performed so that it may be established whether sterility has in fact been achieved. Should it transpire that the operation has not been successful and a child be born to my wife/me*, I hereby waive any claim that I may have for any loss in the form of medical or hospital expenses, child-rearing expenses or otherwise suffered by me as a result of such a birth. I understand that if successful, the procedure may be irreversible.

I also consent to the administration of a local or other anaesthetic and any procedure incidental to the operation.

Date: ____________ Signature: ______________________

Place: ____________________ Witness: ______________

STATEMENT BY SPOUSE

I, the undersigned ______________________________ (spouse), married to the abovementioned, hereby state that I have read the above consent and that I agree to the said operation being performed on my spouse. I further agree to waive any claim that I may have for any loss suffered by me should a child nevertheless be born to me/my wife.*

Date: ____________ Signature: ______________________

Place: ____________________ Witness: ______________

* Delete that which is not applicable.

10 See Botkin *op cit* 1541.
11 See Brownlie *op cit*, Louw *op cit*, Botkin *op cit*.
12 See below 305. Strauss & Strydom *op cit* 324.

30 Artificial insemination

Introduction

There are two types of artificial insemination: artificial insemination where use is made of the husband's semen (AIH) and artificial insemination where use is made of semen obtained from another man, i e a donor (AID). The latter type, particularly, raises complex legal problems.

The main indication for AID is the husband's infertility. Infertility affects 10 to 15 per cent of married couples and in about 30 to 40 per cent of these cases the problem is one of the male infertility. As is the case in other countries, the procedure is extensively used in South Africa. According to an estimate made in 1980, about 1 500 children had already been born in South Africa following AID. Currently about 400 women are probably being artificially inseminated in Johannesburg a year.

In the past there were several legal uncertainties regarding artificial insemination, in particular where donor semen was used. The lawfulness of the procedure itself was open to doubt and the legal status of a child conceived by AID was uncertain. Legislation has removed these uncertainties.

Statutory regulation

Artificial insemination is a lawful procedure, provided it is performed by a medical practitioner (or a person acting under his supervision, such as a nurse) in accordance with the regulations promulgated by the Minister of National Health and Population Development in terms of the Human Tissue Act.[1] It is to be noted that the legislature in 1989 substituted the term "artificial insemination" in the Act with "artificial fertilisation".

The artificial insemination regulations generally are not applicable to AIH but apply only to AID. The only regulation applicable to AIH is regulation 11, which requires the doctor who performs the procedure to be registered with the Director-General, National Health and Population Development, and to work in approved premises.

Strict control is exercised over donation of gametes. "Gamete" is defined in the Human Tissue Act as either of the two generative cells essential for human reproduction. No person, except a medical practitioner or somebody acting under his supervision, may remove or withdraw a gamete from the body of a living person for the purpose of artificial insemination.

A doctor intending to obtain gametes for the purpose of artificial insemination, must open a personal donor's file. A comprehensive written consent must be obtained from the prospective donor.

The donor must consent to: a physical examination and interview by the doctor; the taking of samples of gametes for the purpose of testing, analysing or processing; certain personal details of himself (except his name, date of birth and ID number) being made available to the ultimate recipient; certain personal details, including his

1 Act 64 of 1983, section 22. The regulations were published in Government Notice R1182 of 20 June 1986 (*Government Gazette* 10283). The regulations are currently under review.

family history, being made available to the doctor who will perform the artificial insemination; and certain confidential details regarding himself being made available to the Director-General, National Health and Population Development.

If the doctor has reason to believe that at least five children have been artificially produced by means of gametes from the donor, the latter must be informed that no further donation may be made by him.

Before undertaking a removal of gametes, the doctor must establish that the donor has undergone, no more than one year earlier, medical tests for sexually transmitted diseases as well as a sperm analysis (in the case of male donors) or a gynaecological examination (in the case of female donors).

In the case of a married donor, the spouse's consent must be obtained in writing.

The donor file kept by the doctor who handles the donation must contain an entire range of very specific details provided for in the regulations. *Inter alia* there should be an evaluation of the psychological suitability of the donor for the purposes of artificial insemination.

The donor file must be kept in safe custody. Certain prescribed details must be made available to the recipient and her husband. Each January the doctor must confidentially transmit certain specified particulars to the Director-General. No other person may be furnished with any details on file, except where it is provided otherwise by law or if a court so orders.

The donor may be compensated for any reasonable expenses incurred by him to effect the donation. The Human Tissue Act, however, prohibits the sale of gametes. Artificial inseminations may only be effected on married women whose husbands must consent in writing. A case was reported in the South African press in 1989 of an unmarried woman who performed an artificial insemination of herself. Depending on the circumstances in which the donor's semen had been obtained, the woman may have been guilty of contravention of certain of the regulations.[2]

A gamete obtained from a specific donor may not be used for artificial insemination if the doctor involved knows or suspects that two or more pregnancies exist as a result of artificial insemination and that the possibility exists of two more simultaneous pregnancies as a result of that procedure, or that at least five artificially produced living children have been born as a result of the use of that donor's gametes.

A doctor who intends to effect artificial insemination of a recipient must open a personal recipient's file, in which a series of details prescribed in the regulations must be recorded. These include details of medical examinations and tests and a written consent.

Before an artificial insemination can take place, the doctor must ensure that the recipient and her husband be informed by appropriate experts of the possibilities of natural conception as well as of all the implications of artificial insemination, including: potential problems with the technique, the chances of success, the financial aspects, the consequences for the marriage, the ethical, psychosocial and educational implications, etc, and legal advice which may be obtained with regard to artificial insemination.

The doctor handling the recipient must make sure that the latter is physically, socially and mentally suited for artificial insemination. The wishes of both the donor and the recipient must be respected regarding the population and religious group of the child to be procreated.

Where the recipient or donor comes from a population group in which the individual runs a high risk of being a carrier of a specific genetic defect e g Tay-Sachs disease or thalassemia, they must be properly tested.

Likewise, where, on account of the family history, a possibility exists that the recipient or donor is the carrier of a defect which can be transmitted by genes or chro-

2 The regulations in question are regs 3 and 8(2).

mosomes, examinations and tests must be carried out. If the tests are positive, genetic counselling must be given to the recipient couple and the donor's semen may not be used.

A proper recipient file must be kept containing the prescribed information, and certain details must be transmitted to the Director-General in January of each year. Proper confidentiality must be maintained at all times.

Doctors who were involved in artificial insemination on 20 June 1986 were required to apply to the Director-General for special registration within 12 months from that date. Doctors who intend undertaking these procedures in future, must likewise apply for such registration. Doctors so registered may perform the procedures only in premises approved by the Director-General and subject to special or general conditions imposed by him.

A doctor who has effected an artificial insemination must report the birth within 30 days to the doctor who handled the donation. Should the child display a genetic defect, the former doctor must attempt to determine if the cause thereof can be traced back to the donor or the recipient. If the effect can be traced back to the donor, the doctor who handled the donation must be notified.

It is a criminal offence for a doctor to act otherwise than in accordance with the regulations.

The legal status of the AID child

The 1979 case of *V v R*[3] was the first decision of a South African court on important legal issues relating to artificial insemination. The judgment of Mr Justice Steyn of the Transvaal court primarily concerned the legal status of a child conceived by artificial insemination of a married woman with semen obtained from a donor who was not her husband (AID).

The case originated from a dispute between former spouses regarding the guardianship of a child conceived, with their mutual consent, by artificial insemination during their marriage. When the child was three years old, the spouses were divorced and custody was awarded to the woman, with the usual right of access given to the husband.

Subsequently the woman remarried. She then sought a court order to the effect that her ex-husband was not the natural and/or lawful father of the child, and that accordingly only her consent was necessary, in terms of the Children's Act,[4] for adoption of the child by her new husband.

The judge was of the opinion that the only ground on which such a child could be considered illegitimate, was if it could be said that the mother had committed adultery by receiving the semen of an unknown donor in "an unnatural" process of insemination. However, in artificial insemination there is neither satisfaction of the sexual urge nor does the woman surrender her reproductive power to the donor. Artificial insemination accordingly does not amount to adultery, the judge said.

The judge was also of the opinion that the correct social and legal assessment of a child so conceived within the marriage relationship ought to be that the child is not deemed to be illegitimate for the purposes of the provisions of section 71 of the Children's Act of 1960 relating to the adoption of illegitimate children.[5]

However, the judge said, contemporary juristic thought in South Africa still followed the basic tenets in regard to illegitimacy laid down by the old Roman-Dutch authorities and held that a child so conceived was illegitimate. Moreover, the main Judeo-Christian religious denominations of the country all held the view that artificial

3 1979 (3) SA 1006 (T).
4 Act 33 of 1960, later replaced by the Child Care Act 74 of 1983.
5 See now section 18 of the Child Care Act.

insemination with the semen of an unknown donor constituted a "sinful practice". The judge observed that it would be preposterous for a single judge to hand down a contrary decision and it was "with regret" that he felt constrained to declare the child in question illegitimate for the purposes of the Children's Act.

Nonetheless, the "putative father" of such a child, in the judge's opinion, stood in a special relationship to the child and, at least as long as the marriage existed, was legally obliged to maintain the child and had the right of guardianship in respect of the child.

The judgment in *V v R* gave rise to much discussion among the general public and in particular also in religious circles and in the legal and medical professions. Although some leading religious figures expressed opposition to heterologous artificial insemination (AID), strong pleas were made that the Legislature ought to intervene and declare children conceived in AID and born within wedlock as legitimate where the husband was a consenting party. A clause to this effect was inserted into the Child Care Bill of 1981 which was designed to replace the Children's Act, but the clause fell by the wayside and did not become part of the Child Care Act of 1983.

In a 1984 decision *Riback v Riback* [6] Mr Justice Kriegler regarded himself as fortunate "in not having to bastardise the parties' children" who had both been born by artificial insemination; the legal maxim *pater est quem nuptiae demonstrant* ("the marriage indicates the father") was held to apply.

The question whether the husband of a woman who gave birth to a child conceived by way of AID without the husband's consent, is legally bound to maintain the child was the subject of a 1985 decision of the Cape court, in *L v J*.[7] The court ruled that such a child was illegitimate. It is clear, Mr Justice Berman said, that no duty is imposed on a husband to provide maintenance for the child if he is not that child's natural father, the sole difference between the cases where the child is born by AID or out of an adulterous relationship being that in the former case no accusation of adultery can be levelled against the wife – "the child's legitimacy, or rather illegitimacy, remains unaffected by his or her mother having undergone medical treatment or having enjoyed the thrills of illicit passion". The court further held that there is no duty to continue – after divorce – to support such a child merely because the husband treated the child as his own as an inevitable concomitant of the maintenance of the household while he had the *consortium* of the child's mother.

In the meantime the Human Tissue Act of 1983 had been enacted and this Act, together with the artificial insemination regulations promulgated thereunder in 1986, created *in extenso* regulation of AID practised within a marriage, thereby giving the Legislature's blessing to the procedure as such. But a question mark continued to hang over the legal status of children thus conceived, in consequence of the two Supreme Court rulings.

In 1987 the Legislature finally removed all doubt by enacting the Children's Status Act.[8] In terms of section 5 of the Act, a child born to a woman in consequence of AID which has been practised with the consent of her husband, is deemed for all purposes to be the legitimate child of the woman and her husband. The section further provides that it is legally presumed until the contrary is proved that both spouses have given consent. A consenting husband is accordingly legally responsible for the maintenance of a child conceived by means of AID.

As we have seen above, the artificial insemination regulations require consent to AID to be in writing. It has, therefore, become of the utmost importance for medical practitioners to comply strictly with that requirement to obviate a subsequent dispute

6 The case is unreported but is referred to in *L v J*, *infra*, 377.
7 1985 (4) SA 371 (C).
8 Act 82 of 1987.

of the kind that arose in the two cases referred to. If the consent requirement is disregarded, the unfortunate result will be that the child will be regarded as illegitimate.

The Children's Status Act defines artificial insemination in such terms that it includes *in vitro fertilisation* (IVF).[9] It further provides that no right, duty or obligation shall arise between a child born as a result of artificial insemination and the donor of the gamete or gametes and his/her blood relations, unless, (a) the donor is the woman herself who gave birth to the child, and (b) the donor is the husband of the woman at the time of the artificial insemination.[10] Also in this respect, the new Act has brought complete legal certainty.

Registration of the birth of a child conceived by means of AID was problematic at the stage – prior to enactment of the Children's Status Act – when such a child was regarded as illegitimate; there was an inducement to make a false statement to the Registrar of Births, etc as to the paternity of the child. But these problems have now fallen away in consequence of the Act.

The potential liability of the doctor

A few aspects deserve consideration as far as the potential liability of the doctor who performs an artificial insemination is concerned.

It must be stressed that even apart from the requirements contained in the Artificial Insemination Regulations, the taking of a fully informed consent from all parties concerned is of vital importance. It is submitted that AID performed upon an unconsenting female will by common law constitute a gross *iniuria* towards her. (*Iniuria* is a common-law wrong which, generally speaking, means the violation of the rights of personality of a person, and which may have a criminal sequel (*crimen iniuria*) as well as delictual (i e civil liability for damages).[11]) Likewise a husband can complain of an *iniuria* being perpetrated towards him, if AID was performed on his wife at her request, without his (the husband's) consent. In these cases of lacking consent, the doctor performing the act may be held liable.

If artificial insemination were to be performed upon an unmarried female under the age of 16, with or without her consent, such an act might perhaps be regarded as constituting an "indecent act" in contravention of the Sexual Offences Act[12] and may lead to criminal prosecution of the doctor. (It is unthinkable that a responsible doctor would perpetrate such an act, but I am stating the hypothetical possibility.)

If a doctor were to be negligent in the selection of semen, e g by obtaining semen from a donor suffering from venereal disease or related too closely to the recipient, so that a defective child is born, the doctor might be held delictually liable on the basis of so-called "wrongful birth".[13]

It has been suggested that a doctor might be held contractually liable if he were to guarantee that semen used in AID came from a specific (identified) donor or that the donor belonged to a certain population group, and the doctor does not fulfil his guarantee. The proof of pecuniary loss caused by such a breach of contract – a requirement of our law – in these cases would afford a problem to the plaintiff, however.

By common law there is nothing against the keeping of a "semen bank" as such. However, donation of semen now qualifies as tissue[14] donation under the Human Tissue Act and must comply with the stringent provisions of the Act. As I have men-

9 Section 5.
10 *Ibid.*
11 What can be claimed is damages in the form of "satisfaction" (*genoegdoening*); damages in respect of patrimonial loss is recoverable by means of the Aquilian action. See Neethling, Potgieter and Visser *Law of Delict* (1990) 272.
12 Act 23 of 1957, section 14(1)(*b*).
13 See below 197.
14 See the definition of "tissue" in section 1.

tioned above, the regulations make provision for a gamete donor to be compensated for reasonable expenses incurred by him in order to effect the donation.[15] It is to be noted that if semen is sold to a recipient it will constitute a criminal offence, unless the sperm bank is an "authorised institution" in terms of the Human Tissue Act.[16] There is a total prohibition on the use of semen obtained from mentally ill persons, minors and habitual criminals.[17]

Inspectors of anatomy are vested with the power to enter, at any reasonable time for the performance of their duties and without prior notice, premises on which artificial insemination is effected or is reasonably suspected to be effected.[18]

15 Regulation 7.
16 Section 28.
17 Section 19.
18 Section 31(1)(*a*)(iii).

31 In vitro fertilisation and surrogate motherhood: some issues

A procedure first successfully applied to animals, is the transfer of a fertilised ovum from "mother" A to "hostess" B. In this manner a far larger number of children of A may be born than A would have been capable of bearing herself. A champion cow, for instance, will ordinarily produce an ovum every three weeks which may be fertilised. However, the period between conception and birth of the offspring is approximately nine months. Now science has developed a method whereby the cow's ovum may be fertilised within the cow itself and is then shortly afterwards removed and implanted into the uterus of the "hostess" cow. By means of hormonal stimulation, the cow may even be induced to hyper-ovulate and may produce up to 20 ova per ovulation. All these ova are then simultaneously fertilised in the normal manner and are shortly afterwards removed from the cow and individually implanted into other cows' uteri.

Such a mass production of human offspring is of course unthinkable and would grossly offend the *boni mores*.

However, a comparable procedure – which does not amount to an actual transfer – may be employed to aid a woman who is afflicted with a conception problem. This was in fact done for the first time with the so-called "test tube" baby which was conceived in England and born in 1978 (as a result of the work of Doctors Steptoe and Edwards). The woman, Mrs Lesley Brown, could not fall pregnant on account of an abnormal condition of her Fallopian tubes (the tubes through which the egg in the normal course descends into the uterus). By means of a needle, a ripe ovum was removed from the ovary. It was placed in a laboratory dish (the medical term is *in vitro*, i e "in glass") and sperm from her husband was added. The egg was fertilised and after a few days, the developing embryo was placed into the woman's uterus. There it attached to the wall of the uterus and developed in the normal manner until the child was born.

There can, of course, be no ethical objection to such a procedure – which serves a therapeutic purpose – and it is altogether lawful, as long as the practitioner complies with the provisions of the Human Tissue Act[1] and the regulations[2] thereunder.

Artificial insemination is defined in the Act[3] in such terms that includes *in vitro* fertilisation. "Artificial fertilisation" – the term used by the Legislature – means "the introduction by other than natural means of a male gamete or gametes into the internal reproductive organs of a female person for the purpose of human reproduction, including -

(a) the bringing together outside the human body of a male and a female gamete or gametes with a view to placing the product of a union of such gametes in the womb of a female person; or

(b) the placing of the product of a union of a male and a female gamete or gametes which have been brought together outside the human body, in the womb of a female person

1 Act 65 of 1983.
2 The regulations in question are those pertaining to artificial insemination. See above 181.
3 Section 1.

for such purpose".

Where the sperm of a woman's husband is used for *in vitro* fertilisation and eventual implantation of the ovum into her womb, the artificial insemination regulations under the Act are not applicable;[4] these regulations essentially regulate donor insemination.

But if donor semen is used for fertilisation or the ovum of another woman is used, the procedure is only lawful if it has taken place in accordance with the regulations.

The definition of "artificial fertilisation" in the Human Tissue Act is wide enough to embrace *in vitro* fertilisation with a view to the introduction of a fertilised ovum into the womb of a "hostess" or "surrogate" mother. The regulations also apply to *in vitro* fertilisation. *In vitro* fertilisation is defined in the regulations as "the bringing together outside the human body of a male and a female gamete and the placing of the zygote in the womb of a female person". A zygote is defined as "the product of the union of a male and a female gamete outside the human body".

Although the Human Tissue Act and the artificial insemination regulations were not designed to regulate surrogate motherhood, they nevertheless affect certain important aspects thereof. But the legal relationship between the genetic parents of the child and the surrogate is not addressed by the Act at all, nor is the legal validity of a surrogacy agreement.

A distinction is made between two types of surrogacy : full surrogacy and partial surrogacy. In full surrogacy the genetic material (sperm and ova) are provided by the commissioning couple and the surrogate merely acts as a hostess ("gestational" or "birth mother"). In partial surrogacy the surrogate is artificially inseminated with semen from the commissioning husband; she therefore contributes genetically to the child.[5]

The motivation for a married couple to avail themselves of surrogate motherhood to have a child may either be medical or social. A medical indication will be present where the woman is unable to produce oocytes or is physically unable to carry a baby to term. Surrogacy will be sought for social reasons where a normal, healthy woman is unwilling to put up with the inconvenience of a pregnancy or wishes to avoid temporary inability to be fully active occupationally. Ethical assessment of surrogacy will probably be less favourable where it is resorted to purely for social reasons.

As far as the hostess or surrogate mother is concerned, there may also be different motivations. Her willingness to act as surrogate may be actuated purely by a desire to be of assistance, gratuitously, to a friend or relative (altruistic surrogacy), or may have its origin in a desire to make money by being generously compensated for her "services" (commercial surrogacy).[6] Without a doubt current societal attitudes are more favourable towards the former.

A few cases on surrogate motherhood have come before the courts in the USA and England.[7] In England the Surrogacy Arrangement Act 1985 made the conducting of commercial surrogacy a punishable offence, but only where third parties are involved. Criminal sanctions are imposed on commercial brokers who make, negotiate and facilitate a surrogacy agreement for payment. The Act does not, however, apply to the commissioning couple and a surrogate who conclude an agreement; and it would seem that no prohibition is placed on the payment of a fee to the surrogate mother.[8]

In the absence of legislation in South Africa prohibiting surrogacy arrangements, there is nothing to prevent parties from entering into such an agreement. The en-

4 With the exception of regulation 11. See above 181.
5 Compare L Tager 103 *SALJ* 381 (1986) 383; R Pretorius 1987 *De Rebus* 270.
6 *Ibid.*
7 *Ibid.*
8 On the Act generally, see L Tager *op cit* and R Pretorius *op cit*.

forceability of such agreements is speculative, however. Some local surrogacy cases have received considerable attention on the part of the media. Because of possible legal complexities it is advisable for the parties to a surrogacy agreement to enter into a carefully prepared and detailed contract.[9] Doctors involved in a surrogacy arrangement should also ensure that their interests, rights and obligations be spelled out clearly and satisfactorily in a contract.

The consensus of legal opinion in South Africa at this time appears to be that surrogacy agreements are not *per se* unlawful. If, however, the arrangement assumes a commercial or profitable character in that a substantial amount of money[10] is paid to the surrogate mother, the agreement will be unenforceable as being *contra bonos mores*. It is further accepted that, quite apart from the latter aspect, a surrogacy agreement would be unenforceable in absolute terms by the commissioning couple against the surrogate mother. Should a legal dispute arise, the Supreme Court will clearly be guided by considerations of what would be in the best interest of the child. But if the commissioning couple have a stable marital relationship and will provide a good home for the child, it is unlikely – in the absence of special circumstances – that a court of law will not order the surrogate mother to hand over the child. As far as the legal procedure to achieve this result is concerned, the provisions of the Children's Status Act of 1987 [11] must now be taken into account.

The Children's Status Act was placed on the statute book with the object, *inter alia*, of bringing certainty regarding the legal status of children conceived by artificial insemination. The Act was not designed to regulate surrogate motherhood as such. The Act defines artificial insemination in such terms that it includes *in vitro* fertilisation.[12] In terms of section 5 of the Act, a child born to a woman after AID with the consent of her husband, is deemed for all purposes to be the legitimate child of the woman and her husband.

It is clear from the wording of section 5 that cases of surrogacy will also fall within the ambit of its provisions. A child born to a surrogate mother is, therefore, now legally deemed to be the child of her and her husband, and not that of the commissioning couple (who, in a case of full surrogacy, will be the genetic parents). This legal result confronts the commissioning couple with a real problem.

A thorny question is whether the genetic parents would be legally entitled to formally adopt a child born from a surrogacy arrangement. The Child Care Act of 1983,[13] section 17, provides that a child may be adopted by a husband and wife jointly, "if the child is not a child born to one of them". The interesting further question now arises whether the phrase quoted refers to the genetic origin of the child or to physical birth. If it refers to genetic origin (and that would seem to be the correct interpretation), the genetic parents will be unable to adopt the child – and this will confront the parties to a surrogacy arrangement with a legal dilemma. In such a case, the only way out for the genetic parents may be to apply to the Supreme Court for an order whereby the guardianship of the children would be awarded to them. The Supreme Court is the upper guardian of children and may make an order which in its judgment would be in the best interests of the child. (In February 1991 the genetic parents of twin children born after a "full surrogacy" arrangement in the Transvaal were allowed to adopt the children.)

It is clear that, sooner or later, the Legislature will have to attend to the legal issues

9 For a full discussion of the possible content of a surrogacy contract, see R Pretorius 1987 *CILSA* 293.
10 But compensation for necessary medical expenditure in connection with the surrogate's pregnancy and maternity dresses, etc, would be unobjectionable.
11 Act 82 of 1987.
12 Section 5.
13 Act 65 of 1983.

involved in surrogate motherhood. The South African Law Commission has already launched an investigation.

In 1987 history was made in regard to surrogate motherhood when a married grandmother, Mrs Anthony of Tzaneen, on 1 October of that year, gave birth in Johannesburg to triplets, the genetic parents of which were Mrs Ferreira-Jorges (Mrs Anthony's own daughter) and her (Mrs Ferreira-Jorges's) husband. As far as is known, this was the first case of its kind in the world.

Even before the birth of the Tzaneen triplets, the question arose as to who would be regarded as the legal parents of the children. The first practical issue was: in whose names were the children to be registered? The eventual settlement of this issue was not without a touch of drama, in view of the fact that as the expected delivery date of the triplets approached, the Children's Status Bill with the provisions outlined above, had already had its passage through Parliament, but had not yet been signed by the State President and published in the *Government Gazette*.

As it happened, the birth of the babies preceded the promulgation of the Children's Status Act by a mere thirteen days. But the sequence was of the utmost importance and the Registrar of Births, Marriages and Deaths decided that the triplets had to be registered, not as the children of their grandmother who had actually given them birth and of her husband, but as those of their genetic parents: the ideal state of affairs for all involved. Had the babies been born thirteen days later, the inevitable outcome would have been that they would have been registered as the children of their genetic grandparents; *ergo* their genetic grandmother and "birth-mother" would legally have been one and the same person![14]

14 On surrogate motherhood in general, see also D Pretorius *Surrogate Motherhood: Legal Issues* (LLD thesis, Univ of S Africa, 1991).

32 Genetic manipulation: the potential legal liability of the practitioner

Super-calves and supermen?

"Genetic manipulation", "genetic experimentation", "genetic engineering" – to the layman in the field of genetics these terms are rather nebulous and somewhat frightening. Whatever their exact contents may be, and wherever the boundaries between them must be scientifically drawn (in so far as clear demarcation is at all possible), the layman conjures up in his mind the vision of a scientist at work in his laboratory, trying to create life – perhaps even human life – from non-living matter; "playing God", in the popular terminology of our time. After all, he has read of the piecing together by Wisconsin scientists in 1970 of a molecule link by link, thereby achieving the first complete snythesis of a gene.[1] He has read of scientists claiming in the same year to have produced the first man-made part of a human cell, the lyosome, in a laboratory in New York.[2] He has read of scientists in Massachusetts claiming to have synthesised and deciphered the chemical structure governing the "turning-on" of heredity instructions in a gene in 1974.[3] He has read of scientists at the same institute having made and implanted a bacterial gene a year or two later.[4] He has read of the construction of the first artificial mammal gene, in the form of synthesis of rabbit haemoglobin, in 1975, by scientists working at Harvard University.[5]

Our layman, who is a reasonably well-educated fellow, knows that techniques of human abortion and sterilisation, contraception, artificial insemination and amniocentesis have been virtually perfected in our time. He has also taken notice of the reports on the miraculous achievements of agricultural scientists who have fertilised animal eggs *in vitro* – "test-tubes" in the terminology of the mass media – and have transferred the embryos to "hosts". He has been informed of the most spectacular feat of all: the "creation" of a human embryo in a "test-tube" by Doctors Steptoe and Edwards in 1978. In fact, he has seen the baby who was subsequently born, on television – he has even through the same medium heard her cry, loud and clear, alive and well, like a real, natural baby with a real name, Louise Brown. He has heard of something called "cloning" – the photocopying as it were, of human beings. He has read about experimentation being conducted on human embryos. He has read about a baby being "produced" by its parents with the expressed purpose of providing a source of bone marrow for transplantation in a defective older brother. And he has been told scientists believe they have found a genetic trigger that determines an embryo's sex, which might enable parents to decide what the sex of their child should be.

Our layman is told that it is now possible for scientists to induce a "super-cow" to hyper-ovulate, to fertilise her eggs from sperm obtained from a "super-bull", to transfer the embryos to a number of hose cows and thus to produce some 40 "super-calves"

1 L A Sobel (ed) *Medical Science & the Law: the Life and Death Controversy* (1977) 71.
2 *Ibid* 72.
3 *Ibid.*
4 *Ibid.*
5 *Ibid* 73.

from the same "super-parents" within a period of 18 months![6] And he has been made aware of the fact that what is possible for animals, is possible for human beings. The possibility now exists, so our layman believes, for a megalomaniac ruler, assisted by his super-scientists, to order the breeding of a race of supermen who will ultimately conquer the world.

And he asks himself, where does all this lead to? From his minister of religion he wants to know: is this in accordance with the Law of God? And from his lawyer he enquires: is this in accordance with the law of the land? What is the legal liability of the doctor or scientist *vis-a-vis* society or towards the individual if anything goes wrong in the process?

Few crystallised rules

As far as the potential legal liability of the doctor or the scientist is concerned, it must at the outset be stated that this aspect cannot be divorced from the overall assessment of the lawfulness or otherwise of a particular procedure which may fall within the general meaning of the concept of genetic manipulation.

We have as yet precious few "crystallised" legal rules in our society in regard to the questions which have arisen in this field. There are, therefore, very few ready-made answers. But fortunately our legal system, which in essence is uncodified, is a dynamic system based on a rich structure of principles from which specific answers may evolve with the passage of time, even in the absence of statutory law being laid down by the legislature. Parliament is the surgeon of the juridical world. With one stroke of the legislative knife it can excise an existing rule or principle; it can quickly and effectively restructure the body of the law almost at will.

But because the law is essentially a conservative discipline, and because of conservative societal attitudes when it comes to matters such as human fertility, procreation, life and death, Parliament has traditionally been very slow in legislating on these matters. In respect of pressing political and economic issued on the other hand, our legislature has a record of speedy and effective action. However, it took many years of urging on the part of doctors and lawyers before the Abortion and Sterilisation Act[7] was put on the statute book in 1975. Despite the name of that Act, we have as yet no comprehensive statutory regulation of sterilisation. It took many years before we saw detailed statutory regulation of human artificial insemination (in 1986); as yet surrogate motherhood remains almost altogether unregulated. In 1989 the Legislature, in an amendment to the Human Tissue Act,[8] prohibited in absolute terms genetic manipulation of gametes[9] or zygotes[10] outside the human body; it did not attempt, however, to define "genetic manipulation" so that the precise effect of this prohibition is uncertain.

In so far as the lawyer ventures to answer some specific questions, these are largely speculative. The process of judicial "lawmaking",[11] although it may be quite effective in laying down concrete rules, is a slow and laborious one. Our courts do not hand down rulings *in abstracto*. A decision will only be given in a specific case brought before the court, and judges are ordinarily at pains not to travel beyond the narrow issued raised by the parties in their pleadings. Thus, after many years of

6 In 1983 it was reported in the press that 1 000 embryos of dairy cows had been flown from Britain to Egypt in a container the size of a suitcase. If the calves themselves had to be flown, so the report said, it would have cost R340 000! (In 1991 rands the cost would be about a million rands.)
7 Act 2 of 1975.
8 Act 65 of 1983, section 39A.
9 A gamete is a generative cell essential for reproduction, i e the male sperm or the female ovum.
10 A zygote is the cell resulting from the fusion of two gametes, i e the fertilised ovum.
11 In theory, of course, the courts do not make law; they only state what the law is – *iudicis est ius dicere sed non dare*. But in actual effect, this declaration of the law often breaks new ground and the precedents so created, are themselves considered law for all practical purposes.

speculation on the lawfulness of, and other issued relating to, artificial insemination where use is made of donor semen, it was only in 1979 that the first court judgment in South Africa, *V v R*,[12] was handed down, in which some issues relating to AID were canvassed. If anything, this case illustrated the pressing need for legislative regulation of AID. In venturing to give you a few thoughts on professional liability in the field of genetic manipulation, my approach will therefore be largely speculative.

Professional liability

At this stage I must define what is meant by "professional liability". By that is understood individual accountability before a court of law of a person – *in casu* the scientist or medical practitioner – which may take the form either of a civil judgment for delictual damages to compensate for harm wrongfully caused by him, or of a civil judgment compelling him to refrain from continuing with an unlawful course of action on which he has embarked, or of a criminal conviction for an offence which he was found to have committed. (As far as civil actions are concerned, the wrongful conduct may also take the form of a breach of contract,[13] but this form of liability will be excluded from the present discussion.)

Delictual liability may lie either for intentional wrongdoing, or for negligent conduct, which has resulted in damage being suffered by another person. Damage need not only take the form of actual pecuniary loss, but also infringement of the rights of personality of another. For this damages may be awarded in the form of satisfaction (sometimes called sentimental damages). In all these cases, the plaintiff must prove a causal connection between the conduct of the wrongdoer and the harm he had suffered. The harm must of course have been caused wrongfully. Conduct which otherwise would have been wrongful may be justified on specific grounds, such as self-defence and consent. The latter is particularly relevant to medical treatment and experimentation on human beings, and I shall return to this in a while.

As far as the element of wrongfulness in causation of loss to others is concerned, our law has through the centuries evolved principles which have become well-established, and which are capable of practical application in most situations in everyday life. When it comes to highly unusual or altogether new situations, however, it is not always possible for the lawyer to come up with a ready answer. In these situations the *boni mores* – understood by the lawyer as referring to the legal convictions (the *regsoortuiginge*) prevailing in contemporary society – will serve as touchstone to assess whether a particular form of human conduct will be held to be unlawful and to found an action for the harm caused. Sometimes the term "public policy" is used to denote the same notion.

In criminal law, however, the position is somewhat different. By virtue of the principle of legality accorded recognition in our law, it is forbidden for a court to rule that a particular act is criminal, unless that act falls within the wording of a statute by which it was expressly declared criminal or is at least covered by the definition of a common-law crime, i e has been considered criminal for centuries or millennia. However, in establishing the extent to which an alleged wrongdoer can rely on the defence of consent to avoid criminal liability, a court would be entitled in a previously "untested" situation to have recourse to the *boni mores or* "public policy".[14]

In the grey areas of law, the *boni mores* will therefore be taken into account in establishing whether a specific act will be ruled unlawful, and in particular whether the defence of consent will apply.

12 1979 (3) SA 1006 (T).
13 See e g *Administrator of Natal v Edouard* 1990 (3) SA 581 (A).
14 S A Strauss & M J Strydom *Die Suid-Afrikaanse Geneeskundige Reg* (1967) 182 *et seq*.

Ideological considerations

To bring the discussion back from the abstract *beginselstruktuur* to the form of conduct which forms the subject of the present discussion, viz genetic manipulation, it must immediately be stated that it would be impossible for the jurist to make an *ex ante* pronouncement covering all conceivable procedures undertaken by the men of science. Each procedure will have to be judged on its own merits. A problem for the lawyer is that as a layman in the field of natural science, he is not in a position to envisage the exact nature, scope and effects of a particular scientific procedure. It is for the scientist to describe and explain what the procedure entails, why it is undertaken, and what its ultimate implications are for a specific person or for mankind. The lawyer can then take over and make a concrete assessment. In this assessment, factors such as the following will play a role:[15] Is there a therapeutic objective as concerns the individual affected by the procedure? If not, can other human beings benefit from the procedure? Or is it a matter of "pure" scientific research, i e of research into physical possibilities or impossibilities, unrelated to the needs of mankind? Has the individual who is the subject of the procedure or who is directly affected by it, been apprised of all, and in particular of potentially harmful, consequences?

In making his assessment, the lawyer will not withdraw into his own particular ivory tower and emerge after a while with an answer he has "conjured up" on the basis of "pure" juridical thought, but will have recourse to, and try to seek evidence of, societal evaluation in the broadest sense of the procedure. The lawyer will particularly take note of the views of recognised religious denominations and theologians, and will also be guided by general ethical considerations, including medical professional ethics. Values protected by other laws will likewise be taken into consideration. The reasoning of Mr Justice F S Steyn in an "AID case", *V v R,*[16] affords an excellent example of how a jurist in a given "untested" situation proceeds to arrive at a "yes-no" type of answer. The judge was limited to a very narrow issue, viz whether or not for the purposes of section 71 of the Children's Act,[17] the child so conceived was illegitimate. It was not necessary for him to decide whether the doctor who had carried out the procedure was guilty of an unlawful act, although in no uncertain terms he intimated that the procedure as such could not be regarded as socially undesirable. In his judgment he was guided by traditional jurisprudential views, societal attitudes, and the consensus of religious opinion and of modern jurists.

From the abstract to the concrete

Let us relate the juridical testing method that I have described to other concrete examples.

Amniocentesis is a procedure used to detect serious or fatal genetic defects in the foetus. The procedure has been well-established in modern gynaecology and the risk to the mother and the foetus is very slight. Provided that the procedure is carried out with proper care and skill, there is no question of liability on the part of the doctor even if it transpires – for the sake of argument – that the foetus was damaged in the course of the procedure and the child born is now defective. The reason is simply that the objective sought to have been achieved by the procedure is scientifically, medically and socially recognised as not only fully justifiable, but indeed commendable. Moreover, there is no other known alternative to enable the doctor to make the same, accurate diagnosis. In so far as there may be a slight risk to the mother or to the child, the taking of that risk is therefore lawful.

15 *Ibid,* 246 *et seq.*
16 *Supra.*
17 See now the Child Care Act 74 of 1983, section 18(4) (*d*).

Let us contrast this situation now with a hypothetical one: Dr X is anxious to confirm the hypothesis that a human foetus can survive in an artificial environment, a man-made womb, as it were. A perfectly normal foetus in its third month is removed from its perfectly normal mother's womb and is transferred to a "tank" in which it is endeavoured to simulate all the conditions in the womb and to nourish the foetus artificially until it may be "delivered", i e be taken out of the tank, as a normal baby at the age of approximately 266 days. The mother has been fully apprised that this procedure may result in either the death of the foetus, or harm to it which will manifest itself in the form of a handicapped child once it is delivered, but has nevertheless given consent. There is not doubt that the *boni mores* prevailing in this country would thoroughly disapprove of such a procedure. The mere removal of the foetus from the mother's womb would therefore be ruled wrongful and the mother will be entitled to sue the doctor for damages for assault, notwithstanding the fact that she had given consent.

The doctor may also be criminally charged with assault. If the child were delivered alive and was physically or mentally defective, it would have an action for damages against the doctor, even if the latter had displayed superb skill and had exercised the utmost care at all times. But if the facts were different and, for the sake of argument, medical opinion were unanimous that the foetus would be doomed if it were to remain in the mother's womb, and unusual and desperate measures – even of an experimental nature – to endeavour to secure its survival were undertaken, the legal liability of the doctor would for obvious reasons be assessed in an altogether different light.

The hypothetical case I have just described, is perhaps a poor example, because we are talking about human genetic manipulation after all. I have used it because it is simple for the lawyer to envisage. If our geneticist friends can help us to introduce some hypothetical genetic objective into the removal of the foetus, the example might be a better one.[18]

As far as *in vitro* fertilisation of a human ovum and subsequent implantation into the mother's uterus is concerned, in the circumstances in which Doctors Steptoe and Edwards performed the procedure: this must in my opinion be regarded as altogether unobjectionable from the point of view of the *boni mores*. Nor can there be

18 Professor Trefor Jenkins, head of the Department of Human Genetics of the University of the Witwatersrand, responded to this suggestion in the following terms (and kindly gave me permission to publish his views, for which I record my sincerest appreciation):

"You raised the theoretical possibility of a couple being helped to have a normal baby by means of an artificial womb. I have now thought of an actual situation in which such a mechanical aid would be most desirable.

"It concerns the case of woman who has phenylketonuria (PKU), a recessively inherited inborn error of metabolism, and who, because she was diagnosed as having the disease soon after birth, and because she received the low phenylalanine diet, developed into a healthy woman of normal intelligence. Her husband does not carry the gene for PKU so their children cannot suffer from PKU – all will be carriers of the gene – but it has been observed that the developing foetus often suffers adverse effects because of the mother's elevated plasma phenylalanine levels. It is extremely difficult to maintain a satisfactory level during the period of gestation – too little phenylalanine can impair the brain development, as can too much.

"An artificial uterus would obviously be of great help in a situation like this; so would a surrogate mother into whom could be implanted the ovum of the PKU woman after *in vitro* fertilisation using her husband's sperm.

"The references I have concern the outcomes of pregnancies to women with PKU. The problem is generally well known so I think it would be unnecessary for you to quote them.

"Other situations come to mind in which a similar technological innovation might be helpful. Diabetic and epileptic mothers have a significantly greater risk of having babies with congenital abnormalities than do their normal fellows so, again, these women might opt for your artificial womb!"

In their section on ethics, *Time* of 11 June 1990 reported as follows: "In recent years .... scientists have learned how to build and maintain artificial wombs to give extremely premature infants a fighting chance."

any objection to the "deep-freezing" of a fertilised ovum for implantation in the woman at a later, more convenient or medically more suitable, stage – as long as the doctor acts in good faith.

Case law

In my introduction I have raised the issue of liability of the doctor if anything goes wrong in the process of what could in wide terms be described as genetic "engineering".

Over the past two decades or so, a number of cases have come before the courts – particularly in America – involving allegations of negligence in respect of contraception, sterilisation, genetic screening and abortion which resulted in the birth of an unwanted child – a child which in addition to being unwanted, in some cases was also seriously defective. The general label of "wrongful life" was attached to this type of case (a more unfortunate term would hardly have been invented!); as I point out below, the term "wrongful life" acquired a more restricted meaning in due course.

In the USA, courts initially held that a doctor would not be held liable for negligence in the performance of sterilisation operations which result in the birth of an unwanted, normal child, on the ground – as it was put in a 1957 case – that "to allow damages for the normal birth of a normal child is foreign to the universal public sentiment of the people" (*Shaheen v Knight*).[19] Later the judicial outlook changed and doctors were held liable in cases of this kind.[20]

In 1971 a Michigan court (in *Troppi v Scarf*)[21] held that a pharmacist who negligently filled a birth control prescription – he provided a tranquilliser instead – was liable to the parents although the child subsequently born was quite normal. The pharmacist was held liable for measurable damages, such as the mother's lost wages, medical and hospital expenses, and the economic costs of rearing the child. The court rejected the notion that the birth of a healthy child always confers an overriding benefit.

As Waltz[22] has pointed out, the reasoning of the latter decision has applicability to instances of negligence in genetic screening: if a mistaken diagnosis is caused by a screener's negligence and results in the birth of a defective child, the doctor would in his opinion be liable for "reasonably ascertainable" damages.

As long ago as 1967, the New Jersey Court (in *Gleitman v Cosgrove*)[23] denied both the infant and his parents recovery when the child was born deaf and blind as a result of the rubella from which his mother suffered during her pregnancy. The court arrived at this finding even though the doctor apparently knew of the possibility of this injury, and intentionally withheld this information. In 1975, however, the Texas court (in *Jacobs v Theimer*)[24] came to the opposite conclusion, and held that a claim brought by the parents for the amount of additional money necessary to spend solely because of the physical defects of the child, was good in law.

The principle that prenatal injury to a foetus which is subsequently born alive and as a child is defective on account of the injury, can lead to delictual liability on the

19 11 D & C 2d 41 (1957).

20 For a useful summary of American cases, see G M Lehr & H L Hirsh "Wrongful Conception, Birth and Life" 1983 *Medicine and Law* 199. See also D Giesen *International Medical Malpractice Law* (1988) 242 *et seq*, and see above 175.

21 31 Mich App 240, 187 NW 2d 511 (1971). The case is discussed by J R Waltz "The Liability of Physicians and Associated Personnel for Malpractice in Genetic Screening" in A Milunsky & G J Annas (eds) *Genetics and the Law* (1975) 139, at 144.

22 *Op cit*, 144.

23 49 NJ 22, 227 A 2d 689 (1967). The case is discussed by G J Annas & B Coyne "'Fitness' for Birth and Reproduction: Legal Implications of Genetic Screening" in 1976 *Legal Medicine Annual* 273, at 281.

24 519 SW 2d 846 (1975). The case is discussed by Annas & Coyne *op cit*, 281.

part of the person who negligently injured the foetus, has been recognised both in American decisions[25] and in South Africa.[26] That there is a sound jurisprudential basis for these decisions, cannot be denied. There is no reason why this principle should not be extended to injury *before* conception, provided that the requisite causal connection can be proved. Such injury was in fact held to be actionable if the injured party, the child, is born alive, in the American case of *Jorgensen v Meade-Johnson Laboratories Inc.*[27] The mother had taken contraceptive pills, but a child was nevertheless conceived and born. It turned out to be mongoloid.

American courts even went so far as to allow recovery of damages in the case of prenatal injury to a foetus where the foetus was not born alive, provided that it was viable at the time of the injury.[28]

Today three different categories of claims are distinguished and the following labels attached to each of these in American literature:

- "wrongful pregnancy" (or "wrongful conception") where a healthy but unwanted child is born, e g in consequence of medical negligence in performing a sterilisation, and a claim is brought by its parents for damages in respect of medical expenses involved in the pregnancy and confinement, maintenance of the child, etc;
- "wrongful birth" where a claim is brought by the parents of an abnormal or disabled child for the same kind of damages;
- "wrongful life" where a claim for damages is brought by or on behalf of the abnormal or disabled child itself; the essence of this type of claim is violation of an alleged right not to be born with defects, which in the circumstances amounts to a right not to be born at all.[29]

That the doctor may be held liable for damages in a suit brought by the parents of a child for "wrongful pregnancy" or for "wrongful birth" has now been established in a number of jurisdictions, *inter alia* America, Canada, England and Germany.[30] The landmark decision of the South African Appellate Division in *Administrator, Natal v Edouard*[31] – involving breach of contract in the form of a failure to perform a sterilisation agreed upon (resulting in the birth of an unwanted child) – has opened the door widely for recognition of these types of claims here. An issue on which there is a considerable divergence of opinion in the various jurisdictions, though, is what types of damages are recoverable. The courts of the majority of American jurisdictions refuse to award damages in the form of child-rearing expenses, but England does and so will the South African courts decidedly do in consequence of the *Edouard* ruling.

Liability for "wrongful life", on the other hand, is a completely different story. As Giesen[32] has pointed out, claims by the infants themselves have been regarded almost universally with disfavour: "The child is not claiming that the physician's negligence caused its defects, but that, had he informed its parents properly, it would never have seen the light of day at all. And the courts have refused, on policy grounds, to hold that life, even if experienced with severe handicaps, is or can be preferable to non-existence." Judging by the views expressed by South African jurists, it is highly unlikely that "wrongful life" will be upheld by our courts as a cause of action.

25 See M C Shaw & C Damme "Legal Status of the Fetus" in *Genetics and the Law* (*supra*) 1, at 5-6.
26 See below 199.
27 483 F 2d 237 (10th Cir, 1973). The case is discussed by Shaw & Damme, 6.
28 *Chrisafogeorgis v Brandenburg* 55 Ill 2d 368, 304 NE 2d 88 (1973). The case is discussed by L H Glantz "Legal Aspects of Fetal Liability" in *Genetics and the Law* (*supra*) 29, at 36.
29 See Giesen *op cit* 242 *et seq*, and see above 180.
30 Giesen *op cit* 242 *et seq*.
31 See note 13 above, and see above 177.
32 *Op cit* 250. But on the position in Israel, see A Carmi 9 *Med Law* 777 (1990)

In *McKay and Another v Essex Area Health Authority and Another*[33] the English court refused to allow a child plaintiff damages on the grounds that she had been born disabled because of the conduct of the doctor who had attended her mother in pregnancy. The child was disabled because the mother had contracted rubella in early pregnancy, and sued for damages *inter alia* for being allowed entry into a life in which her injuries are highly debilitating. The child contended the doctor should have advised the mother to have an abortion. The court dismissed the action, on the ground that to allow it would be against public policy, since it could never be said that being born was damage or harm, which the law should compensate.[34] A consideration by which the court was guided in coming to that conclusion was that if such a cause of action existed, an almost intolerable burden would be placed on medical advisers. The danger that doctors would be under subconscious pressures to advise abortions in doubtful cases through fear of an action, is a real one. It was also held that the duty owed to an unborn child was one not to injure it and, on the facts, the child had not been injured by either the doctor or the health authority but by the infection contracted by the mother without any fault on their part.

Possible future cases

Other possibilities of liability on the part of doctors raised by American jurists – and which in some cases already have led to litigation – are:

- ❑ negligent diagnosis with amniocentesis on account of which the mother agrees to the abortion of a perfectly healthy foetus;[35]
- ❑ failure of a doctor to refer his patient to a specialist for amniocentesis;[36]
- ❑ failure of a doctor to routinely perform amniocentesis on all pregnant women with potentially affected foetuses;[37]
- ❑ failure to obtain an informed consent in genetic screening;[38]
- ❑ unauthorised disclosure of confidential information obtained in genetic screening;[39]
- ❑ cloning which results in a defective child being brought to term;[40]
- ❑ the deliberate withholding of treatment in the case of a defective newborn infant.[41,42]

33 [1982]2 A11 ER 770 (CA).

34 The mother also brought action against the defendants on the ground, *inter alia*, that she had been deprived of the opportunity of choosing to abort the damaged child. The court made no adjudication on the mother's claim, except to allow it to proceed on trial. The outcome of the case is not known to me. In *Emeh v Kensington and Chelsea and Westminster Area Health Authority.* [1984] 3 All ER 1044 (CA) a mother successfully sued for damages for the birth of a defective child following sterilisation, but no suit was brought on behalf of the child itself.

35 Annas & Coyne, *op cit*, 292.

36 *Ibid.* In 1977 a New York court awarded damages to parents who alleged that their obstetricians had been negligent in not making use of amniocentesis, which could have prevented the birth of their mongoloid child. See H F Klodowski *Buffalo Law Rev*, vol 27 (1977-1978) 537, at 544.

37 Annas & Coyne *op cit* 282.

38 Waltz, *op cit*, 146 *et seq*.

39 Waltz, *op cit*, 150 *et seq*.

40 Sledenberg "Law and Cloning – the State as Regulator of Gene Function" in "*Genetics and the Law* (*supra*) 377 at 381.

41 R A Burt "Authorizing Death for Anomalous Newborns" in *Genetics and the Law* (*supra*) 435, at 436; J A Robertson "Discretionary Non-Treatment of Defective New-borns" in *Genetics and the Law* (*supra*) 451.

42 In an English case, *R v Arthur* (unreported, November 1981), a doctor, after consulting the parents of a new-born baby boy with Down's Syndrome, instructed that the baby be given "nursing care only". The baby died after 63 hours. The doctor was charged with murder, but the charge was subsequently reduced to attempted murder. The judge directed the jury that there were circumstances in which a doctor was legally entitled to "conduct a holding operation", to wait and see whether a severely disabled baby would rally and prosper, or whether it would die. He called this

In regard to potential liability in all these situations, the field is wide open for speculation, particularly if we restrict ourselves to considerations which might sway South African courts. What we can say with absolute certainty, is that a court here will allow a handicapped child who *in utero* suffered injury as a result of the negligence of any outsider (a motorist, an assailant of the mother, a doctor) to sue the guilty party for damages, if it can be proved that the injury was brought about by the negligence of the wrongdoer. This principle was expressly recognised by Mr Justice Hiemstra in the Transvaal case *Pinchin NO v Santam Insurance Co Ltd.*[43]

If a foetus injured prenatally were not born alive, the situation would be different. In my opinion there is no principle in South African law which would allow the parents to sue for damages for the loss of a potential child, except for harm which the mother herself might have suffered to her own body in consequence of the injury. We do not recognise in our law anything comparable to a right of "ownership" of children. A person can only bring an action for damages resulting from the wrongful death of another, if he can prove that the wrongdoer by his deed has caused him (the plaintiff) pecuniary loss.[44] Thus a child who is dependent can claim damages from the man who killed his father, but the father would only be entitled to claim in respect of the death of his child if he (the father) was financially dependent on the child. To put it in somewhat crude terms: I am entitled to claim damages from the man who wrongfully killed my dog, but I do not ordinarily have a claim for the killing of my child. The only conceivable damages I can claim, would be medical, death-bed and funeral expenses. (If a man were to deliberately kill a baby before the mother's eyes, she would undoubtedly have a claim against the wrongdoer for damages for her hurt feelings as well as for an impairment of her health as a result of nervous shock,[45] but that would be for the intentional wounding of her own feelings by the foul deed, and not because of the loss of her child.)

If according to our law a parent cannot sue for the unlawful killing of his child, a claim would *a fortiori* be denied him or her if no child was born, whatever the cause of that was – abortion of the foetus as a result of negligent diagnosis with amniocentesis, or otherwise.

Whether failure to refer a patient to a specialist, or to routinely perform amniocentesis on all pregnant women with potentially affected foetuses, will in our society be judicially considered as *per se* constituting negligence, seems extremely doubtful. As I understand the position, we do not as yet have adequate medical facilities to cater for even a substantial percentage of cases where this procedure would be advisable. Until that day arrives, I deem it unlikely that a court will come to such a conclusion as a general statement of the law. Failure to refer the patient for, or to perform amniocentesis might in a given situation be held to be negligent[46] – but that could only

second alternative, "letting nature take its course". The doctor was acquitted. (Particulars of the case supplied by I Kennedy in *Medical Responsibility in Western Europe* (eds E Deutsch and H L Schrieber, 1985) 131.) As Kennedy has pointed out, this case is difficult to reconcile with another English case, *Re B (a minor)* [1981] WLR 1421, decided seven months previously by the Court of Appeal, in which it was held that a baby born with Down's Syndrome and duodenal atresia ought to be operated upon to save her life, despite the fact that the parents and attending doctors were prepared to allow her to die. (These two cases are also discussed by Mason & McCall Smith *Law and Medical Ethics* (2nd ed, 1987) 106–7.

43 1963(2) SA 254 (W).

44 R G McKerron *The Law of Delict (7th ed, 1971) 148 et seq*; N J van der Merwe & P J J Olivier *Die Onregmatige Daad in die Suid-Afrikaanse Reg* (6th ed, 1989) 332 *et seq*.

45 See *Boswell v Minister of Police and Another* 1978(3) SA 268 (E). As far as damages for mental shock as a result of negligent killing of a child are concerned, see *Lutzkie v South African Railways & Harbours and Another* 1974(4) SA 396(W) and Van der Merwe & Olivier, *op cit*, 331 *et seq*. See also J C van der Walt "Skoktoediening: 'Wie sal die aftreksom maak?'" in *Huldigingsbundel vir W A Joubert (ed SA Strauss, 1988)* 247.

46 See note 36 above.

occur in the context of an action for damages for "wrongful birth", of which the eventual success is very doubtful at best.

As far as cloning resulting in a defective child is concerned, the principle of prenatal damage of a foetus is undoubtedly capable of application by analogy.

Deliberate non-treatment of a defective new-born child, is a more problematic issue. In the course of the celebrated *De Bellocq*[47] trial, in Pretoria in 1968, I heard an eminent paediatrician testifying that he would not have medically treated the infant – the grossly defective victim of the debilitating disease of toxoplasmosis – if it had been his own. Everyone in court sympathised with the doctor's view. The question of non-treatment, of course, puts us squarely into the troubled waters of euthanasia. I am not going to say anything here on that subject except for stating a personal opinion: if it amounts to euthanasia to withhold medical treatment of grossly defective newborns – who have no hope of being cured or of living for any length of time – and the withholding doesn't inflict starvation or any other form of cruelty and allows the baby to die a natural and hopefully early death, I for one, am in favour of that kind of euthanasia.[48]

Experimentation on embryos

Our discussion of embryo transfer would not be complete unless mention were made of experimentation on embryos.

Reports in the press in 1982 that Dr Edwards had experimented on human embryos fertilised *in vitro*, unleashed a torrent of criticism, but it was subsequently stated by the British Medical Association that he had not made himself guilty of any unethical conduct.

In terms of the Human Tissue Act, the Minister of National Health and Population Development is vested *inter alia* with the power of making regulations relating to research with regard to the product of the union of male and female gamete outside the human body.[49] Experimentation with gametes or zygotes, outside the human body, which amounts to genetic manipulation, would constitute a contravention of the Act.[50]

The South African Medical Research Council has laid down important ethical guidelines on research relating to *in vitro* fertilisation (IVF) and embryo biology: Research on IVF may only be conducted in approved institutions and in accordance with the provisions of the Human Tissue Act and the regulations contained in Government Notice R1182 of 26 June 1986 in so far as these are applicable. A research unit must maintain thorough documentation of all its activities. The unit will be subjected to regular inspections. The exclusive production of embryos for research is unacceptable. Embryo research cannot be conducted without the written permission of the donors of the gamete or the embryo. It is advisable to inform the donors of the gametes or embryo about the nature of the planned research. Without particularly

47 *S v De Bellocq* 1975 (3) SA 548 (T). The case was first reported and commented upon in 1969 *THRHR* 385. It is discussed below 339.

48 In 1982 a dispute arose in Cape Town involving a grossly defective 3-week-old. The child was born with Down's Syndrome and had no oesophagus. Surgery to construct an oesophagus would have been very complicated and expensive, and a successful outcome could not be guaranteed. The infant was put on a drip and fed intravenously. The parents in consultation with doctors decided against surgery, preferring the child to die a natural death in due course. Certain parties who knew about the case, threatened to seek a court order compelling reconstructive surgery. After taking legal advice the parents and doctors stuck to their guns. The threatened lawsuit did not materialise, nor were any criminal proceedings instituted. (I believe that it is the same case as the one referred to by Ellison Kahn in his paper "Murder as a Fine Art" in *The Sanctity of Human Life* (ed E Kahn) Senate special Lectures, Witwatersrand University (1984) 24 at 28.) See also the view of T Jenkins "Neonatal Euthanasia" in Oosthuizen *et al* (eds) *Euthanasia* (1978) 173 *et seq*; and see below 338.

49 Section 37 (1) (*e*) (vii).

50 See *supra* 157.

good reasons, the long-term freezing of gametes and embryo is not recommended (not longer than the expected reproductive life of the donors). Replacement of a manipulated (treated) embryo in the mother can only be done if prenatal tests, which can determine the success of the therapy, exist. No embryo will be allowed to develop for longer than 14 days.[51]

"Monsters" and a "super race"

Before concluding this discussion, I should like to return to some of the situations mentioned in my introduction. When the American experiments in genetics were disclosed, other scientists warned about the accidental creation of "dire diseases" or "human monsters". Thus a committee of scientists, endorsed by the American National Academy of Sciences, pleaded for a temporary ban throughout the world to halt certain types of experiments involving genetic manipulation of bacteria.[52] They argued that gene-transplantation experiments might accidentally increase the resistance of some micro-organisms to drugs or lead to the spread of some types of cancer-causing viruses.

It is decidedly not for the lawyer to express an opinion on the possibility of such a result. But if it were to happen, and if reputable scientists had timeously issued warnings, and if the consequence would be the spread of a disease affecting any number of individuals, the scientists who had initiated the experiments may in my opinion decidedly be held legally liable to the affected individuals for harm done to them. The lawyer will argue that the *boni mores* do not approve of purely experimental work, unrelated to any endeavour to bring about a cure for an existing disease, being allowed to cause harm to healthy people.[53] The scientists would be guilty of wrongful conduct and their liability would depend on the proof of fault.

As far as the accidental creation of "human monsters" is concerned, the case for legal liability is as strong, if not stronger. A defective human being is a financial burden on its parents or upon the State, and if the wrongful act of another person were responsible for his defectiveness, he or his parents would be entitled to hold the latter liable for his condition. As I have mentioned, this principle was expressly recognised by Mr Justice Hiemstra in the South African case of *Pinchin*.[54] The judgment in that case concerned the legal rights of a child damaged pre-natally by the negligence of a motorist who injured its mother, but the reasoning of the judge would also apply to damage brought about by a wrongful medical act or wrongful scientific experimentation. This is, of course, not "wrongful life" liability. The gravamen of the child's claim is the harm inflicted upon him *in utero*, and not the fact that he was allowed to be born.

As far as the creation of a "super race" by scientists is concerned, the question of liability is not so easy to answer. The point is that unlike handicapped human products of genetic manipulation, "super humans" whose existence is brought about by the same means, have no reason to complain. After all, they are presumable perfect human specimens with the perfect physique, perfect health and perfect brains! The law of delict is largely the law of damages and a person who has suffered no damage, either in the form of pecuniary loss or recognised injury to his *corpus, dignitas* or *fama*, has no claim against anyone. In the "AID case" Mr Justice Steyn held *obiter* that the husband of a woman who gave birth to a child conceived in AID, is legally obliged to maintain the child if he has agreed to his wife's insemination, and that ruling is perfectly acceptable – and laudable – on the basis of legal reasoning and "or-

51 South African Medical Research Council *Ethical Considerations in Medical Research* (revised edition, 1987) 27.
52 Sobel, *op cit*, 74.
53 Strauss & Strydom, *op cit* 247, 256.
54 *Supra*.

dinary justice between man and man". On the analogy of that ruling, a "super-race" scientist who has been causally responsible for the birth of a fatherless super-human baby, may at least be held liable for maintenance of the child as long as it is dependent! But that would be a "family-law" type of liability and not delictual.

However, what is conceivable from the point of view of delictual law, as concerns the "super-race" geneticist, would be a prohibitory court order (interdict) to restrain him from continuing with a patently wrongful course of conduct – unlawful because if offends against the current *boni mores*. But who would have the *locus standi* to bring the court application – a *curator ad litem* appointed by the court for the unborn, and as yet unconceived "super-human"?[55] Unlike the Romans we do not recognise the *actio popularis* and unlike the Americans we do not recognise "class actions"; it is a principle of our law that only a person with a special interest in the subject-matter of the case may institute action.[56] At any rate, long before anyone contemplates such an action, the legislature would in all probability have stepped in and by statute prohibited the geneticist from continuing with his project.

I hope I have not created the impression that I have been dealing facetiously with science-fiction possibilities. In this day of men walking on the moon, deep-space probes, heart transplants and test-tube babies, nothing seems to be impossible. I am reminded of the words of Arthur C Clarke, the well known space-fiction author: when an aging scientist says that something is scientifically possible, he is usually right; when he says that something is scientifically impossible, he is usually wrong. The lawyer is therefore in good scientific company when he speculates on the application of existing legal principle to legal issues that may present themselves tomorrow as a result of scientific advances.

Genetic screening: technological advances – and questions

As Baum[57] has pointed out, modern methods of genetic screening raise a number of difficult legal and ethical questions: "Use of the so-called DNA fingerprinting, for instance troubles some observers who question the reliability of such analyses carried out on a large scale and who worry about effects on civil liberties of widespread genetic testing for identification purposes."

Prenatal genetic screening has become much more sophisticated in recent years. Until recently, amniocentesis – invented in the 1960s – was not used to identify genetic diseases through direct analysis of DNA.[58] Rather, the technique has provided foetal cells that are grown in culture. A technique known as "restriction fragment length polymorphism" (RFLP) analysis, developed over the past decade, has widened the possibilities of identifying chromosomes carrying defective genes. Much research is being done which will result in other techniques of genetic screening for medical purposes. "Routine screening for genetic disorders," says Baum, "is a technology that is one the verge of being invented."

These are some of the questions[59] posed: can insurance companies require that genetic testing be done for a person to get coverage? Can they load their premiums for high risk individuals? Is legislation necessary to ensure that confidentiality be maintained? Will employers require testing of a condition of employment? Will society mandate premarital genetic testing? Would there be mandated genetic therapy for individuals who have correctable conditions? Will prenatal screening be made

55 In *Christian League of Southern Africa v Rall* 1981 (2) SA 821 (0) the court refused to appoint a *curator ad litem* to represent a foetus in connection with the termination of the mother's pregnancy.
56 *Bozzoli v Station Commander, John Vorster Square, Johannesburg* 1972 (3) SA 934 (T).
57 R M Baum *C & E N* (Aug 7, 1989) 10.
58 *Ibid.*
59 *Ibid.*

mandatory? Suppose foetal therapy or foetal surgery becomes possible:[60] What should be done in the case of a mother who does not want her foetus submitted to therapy or surgery? Will courts order therapy in a manner analogous to what already occurs with blood transfusions for children?

The ethicist and the lawyer of tomorrow will be faced with the task of providing answers to these questions.

Based on a paper read at a symposium on Genetics and Society *held at the University of Durban-Westville, July 1979.*

60 Foetal surgery has already arrived. See the report on "Major Surgery Before Birth" in *Time* of 11 June 1990 describing "the most impressive achievement yet in the field of fetal surgery" by Dr M Harrison and colleagues of California.

PART IX

Abortion

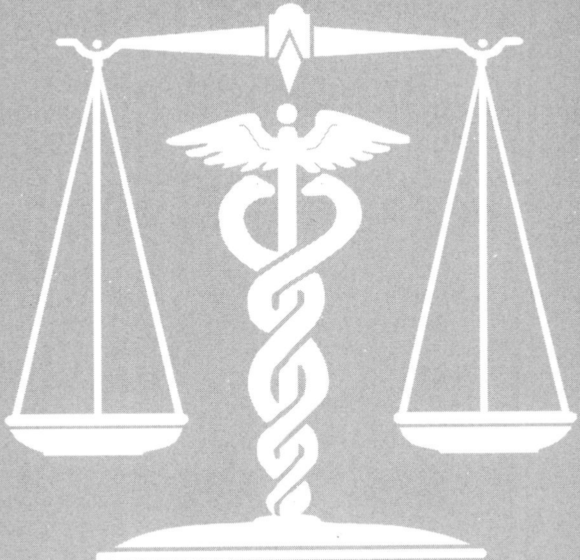

33 The Abortion and Sterilisation Act

Introduction

The Abortion and Sterilisation Act of 1975[1] regulates therapeutic abortion in detail, but it was not intended to pronounce conclusively on the lawfulness or otherwise of sterilisation. In so far as the Act deals with sterilisation, it only makes provision for consent to sterilisation of persons who are incapable of consenting thereto and certain incidental aspects. Sterilisation as such is therefore still essentially governed by the common law (i e non-statutory law). For the sake of convenience the provisions of the Act relating to sterilisation will also be discussed in this chapter.

The Act was, of course, not intended to bring about abortion on demand. It did not "legalise" abortion in that sense. It was intended to clear up legal uncertainties, and in a positive context, to give legal affirmation to a practice of therapeutic abortion which had for many years become settled in the medical profession. Prior to the Act the only legal certainty was that pregnancy could be medically terminated to save the life of the woman. The Act extended this common-law protection to several other indications.[2]

Abortion defined

"Abortion" is defined[3] in the Act as "the abortion of a live foetus of a woman with intent to kill such foetus". The Afrikaans text refers to "die afdrywing van 'n lewende vrug ..." As Hawthorne[4] has indicated, this means that there must be a killing as well as an expulsion.

In terms of this definition it would seem that even where a foetus is still alive after expulsion, but is medically a foetus, and is then killed, the act amounts to abortion, which would be lawful if the requirements of the Act are complied with. Conversely, in the case of an abortion not falling under the Act, the deed would in this case constitute criminal abortion and not infanticide (murder). If, however, the expulsion of an unborn child amounts to live birth (according to the respiration test), and the child is then killed, this would seem to constitute infanticide (murder) or at least culpable homicide.[5]

1 Act 2 of 1975.

2 The common law of abortion was discussed in detail in previous editions of this work. See the second edition of this book (1984) 207 *et seq.* Two 1971 court decisions on abortion accelerated the reform movement which resulted in Parliament passing Act 2 of 1975. The first of these cases was *S v King*, discussed in the second edition of this book on pages 217-9 (a résumé of the judgment is reported in 1971 (2) PH H103 (T)). The second was *S v Van Druten*, a regional court matter, also discussed in the second edition of this book on pages 219-224. On the Act in general, see also L Hawthorne *The Crime of Abortion : A Historical and Comparative Study* (LLD thesis, Univ of Pretoria, 1982) 248 *et seq.*

3 The statement referred to in the text is contained in section 1 of the Act, entitled "Definitions" but Hawthorne *op cit* 248 does not regard it as a definition. According to her this provision does no more than bring a certain type of abortion within the scope of the Act. On the deficiencies of the definition, see also P C Smit *Die Posisie van die Ongeborene in die Suid-Afrikaanse Reg met besondere aandag aan die Nasciturus-leerstuk* (LLD thesis, University of the OFS, 1976) 315 *et seq.*

4 *Op cit* 251.

5 Compare Smit *op cit* 316.

What is a foetus? This concept is not defined in the Act. Medical evidence is therefore necessary to establish whether a live foetus was aborted, and whether what was aborted is a foetus or a viable infant.

The effect of the decision in *Collop's* case[6] is that legally there is no distinction between a zygote, an embryo or a foetus. The moment the female ovum has been fertilised *in utero* a foetus comes into existence. It is submitted that fertilisation *in vitro* cannot be regarded as resulting in a foetus in terms of the Act, first because it is not capable of a natural existence, and secondly because the Act must be interpreted as requiring an expulsion. If an ovum is fertilised *in vitro* and is not implanted in the uterus but thrown away, no expulsion has taken place.

It would appear that it is not a requirement for a foetus to come into existence for the purposes of the Act that the fertilised ovum *in utero* must first have been imbedded in the wall of the uterus.

Legal indications for abortion

Abortion may be procured by a medical practitioner only. There are seven different indications:

1. Where the continued pregnancy endangers the life of the woman.
2. Where the continued pregnancy constitutes a serious threat to the woman's physical health.
3. Where the continued pregnancy constitutes a serious threat to the woman's mental health, and is of such a nature as to create the danger of permanent damage to her mental health, and the abortion is necessary to ensure her mental health.
4. Where there exists a serious risk that the child to be born will suffer from a physical or mental defect of such a nature that he will be irreparably seriously handicapped.
5. Where the foetus was conceived in consequence of rape.
6. Where the foetus was conceived in incest.
7. Where the foetus has been conceived as the result of illegitimate intercourse with a mentally defective woman who is unable to comprehend the consequential implications of, or bear the parental responsibility for, the fruit of coitus.[7]

An abortion not falling within these provisions, constitutes a criminal offence and is punishable by a fine not exceeding R5 000 and/or imprisonment not exceeding five years.

Intent an element of the crime

What is the legal position of a doctor who performs a hysterectomy on a pregnant woman and destroys the foetus in the process? If the doctor knew that the woman was pregnant and performed the operation in circumstances where there was no urgency, without complying with the provisions of the Act, the doctor may be found guilty under the Act. In performing the operation the doctor indirectly destroyed the foetus. Even if one of the seven legal indications were present, the pregnancy may not be terminated before the certification requirements[8] in terms of the Act have been met. If the doctor had no idea that the woman was pregnant and did not foresee that possibility, he cannot be found guilty of the crime. Intent to terminate a pregnancy by killing the foetus is an element of the crime.[9] A *bona fide* but mistaken belief

6 1981(1) SA 150 (A). This case is discussed in detail below 222. See also *S v Kruger* 1976(3) SA 290 (O).
7 Section 3(1) read with the definition of "unlawful carnal intercourse" in section 1.
8 See below.
9 P M A Hunt *South African Criminal Law and Procedure* (2nd ed, 1982) 325-6.

that the accused was lawfully entitled to procure an abortion would constitute a defence to the charge, whether the mistake was of fact or law.[10]

A difficult problem may arise where it is established that a woman is pregnant with twins and medical tests indicate that one of the foetuses is decidedly deformed or defective to the extent that it may lawfully be aborted by virtue of the fourth indication mentioned above. Its abortion will, however, expose the other foetus to the risk of also being killed. In my opinion a doctor would not incur liability for the death of the healthy foetus, provided he has complied with the certification requirements in respect of termination of the life of the defective foetus, and has exercised reasonable care in endeavouring not to harm the healthy foetus.

Common law substituted

One of the first reported cases decided under the Act was *S v Kruger*.[11] The accused, described as a "weed-exterminator in gardens" was convicted by a regional magistrate on a number of charges of abortion, attempted abortion, statutory "pimping" and rape. It appeared that the accused had recklessly used an enema apparatus, and in some cases a car wheelpump fitted with a home-made nozzle, to inject an irritating red fluid into the wombs of pregnant women. He charged fees of R150 or more per "case". Some of his "patients" addressed him as "Doctor".

On appeal, the question arose whether the common-law crime of abortion still existed or had been substituted by the Abortion Act. If the common-law offence still existed, the court could in the imposition of punishment merely be guided by the penalties prescribed in the Act; if the Act substituted the common-law offence, however, the court was bound to give effect to the prescribed penalties. Mr Justice Erasmus held that the Act had substituted the common-law offence. It was significant, the judge observed, that the penalty clause of the Act also referred to persons other than medical practitioners. He further ruled that for the purposes of a conviction in terms of the Act it was sufficient if there was evidence from which it could be inferred that the foetus was living, irrespective of how long the woman had been pregnant. Even where the product of conception is medically still known as an embryo, it constitutes a foetus for the purposes of the Act.

It does not mean that the common-law defence of necessity in life-and-death emergencies was abolished because the Act now states that abortion may be procured only in the circumstances described in section 3 – i e the seven indications outlined above. I am in respectful agreement with Hawthorne[12] when she says that where the circumstances are such that it is impossible to comply with the requirements of the Act, the common-law defence of necessity will still be available if the life of the woman is endangered.

Certification requirements and application for abortion

In all cases of proposed termination of pregnancy, certification by two other medical practitioners – i e other than the doctor performing the abortion – is required. At least one of them must have practised for four years. In the case of the psychiatric indication, one of the certifying doctors must be a psychiatrist employed by the State.

In the case of rape or incest, one of the doctors must be the district surgeon who examined the woman if a complaint has been lodged with the Police.[13] In these cases

10 *Ibid.*
11 1976 (3) SA 290 (O).
12 *Op cit* 269. As was correctly pointed out by Hawthorne 270, this defence only applies to the situation where the pregnancy constitutes a danger to the woman's life.
13 Section 3.

the Act requires a further certificate, to be issued by a magistrate,[14] to the effect – (i) that a complaint has been lodged with the Police (or that there is a good and acceptable reason why a complaint has not been lodged); (ii) after an examination of any relevant documents and such interrogation of the woman as he may consider necessary, that on a balance of probability, unlawful intercourse had taken place, and (iii) in the case of incest, that the woman is related within the prohibited degree to the man. The magistrate must further certify that the woman has stated under oath that the pregnancy is the result of rape or incest, as the case may be.[15]

The doctor who has issued a certificate may in no way participate in or assist with the abortion in question.

An abortion may not be procured unless authorisation in writing has been obtained from the medical superintendent of the hospital (or another doctor designated by him).[16] Application, fully substantiated and in the prescribed form, must therefore first be made to the superintendent. The superintendent may institute such investigation as he may deem necessary to satisfy himself that the application complies with the statutory requirements.[17]

If there is reason to believe that a woman will commit suicide, may this be considered a threat to her life in terms of section 3 (1) (*a*) (the psychiatric indication)? I do not think so. Section 3 (1) (*a*) specifies that "the continued pregnancy [must] endanger the life of the woman". If the woman threatens to commit suicide, it is her state of mind, or neurosis, so it would seem to me, that endangers her life, and not her pregnancy. Admittedly this is a fairly hard stance, but in my opinion, it is the only correct one.[18]

Is a psychiatrist in the employ of a provincial administration a "psychiatrist employed by the State" for the purposes of section 3 (3) (*b*)? I am inclined to think so. Section 1 (viii) is not exactly in point because it does not define "State" but only "State-controlled institution", and in the definition of the latter concept there is specific reference to the "the State (including a provincial administration)". However, where used generally in a statute, "State" will probably include a provincial administration as well.

Would a psychiatrist who is part-time in the employ of the State and who has a private practice, be entitled to charge private fees for patients in respect of whom he issues certificates in terms of section 3 (1) (*b*)? It would seem as though in principle he would be entitled to do so. All that the Act specifies is that the psychiatrist who certifies must be "employed by the State".[19] It does not say that in certifying he works *for* the State. However, he may of course be bound by his contract with the State not to charge private fees for any work done by him while doing work in an official capacity for the State.

14 "Magistrate" includes an additional and an assistant magistrate and must be a magistrate of the district in which the offence is alleged to have been committed. It need not be a regional magistrate, however. The effect of the decision in *Rall NO v Landdros vir die Distrik Heilbron* 1980 (3) SA 287 (O) was nullified by amendment of section 6(4) by Act 38 of 1980, section 2.

15 Section 6.

16 Section 6(1). In respect of State-controlled institutions, the Act refers to "the medical practitioner in charge of such institution". In the case of "designated" private institutions, the authorisation must be given by a doctor designated by "the person managing such institution".

17 Section 6(6).

18 In February 1980 Mr Justice De Wet of the Orange Free State court in an uncontested application brought by the father of a minor girl who had fallen pregnant and allegedly made several attempts on her life, ordered the superintendent of a provincial hospital to give an authorisation for an abortion to be performed on the girl under section 3 (1) (*a*) of the Act, i e the "life and health" indication. But according to my information, the hospital gynaecologists refused to perform the abortion. The judgment was not reported, but was referred to in *Christian League of Southern Africa v Rall* 1981 (2) SA 821 (O) at 825C. See also below 219.

19 Section 3 (3).

Some problems relating to consent to abortion

Next, I want to deal briefly with some problems relating to consent to an abortion. The Act is silent on the entire question of consent.

The consent problem arises in respect of married women and minors. In regard to a major woman herself, consent affords no real problem. The usual common-law principles will apply: she must be a consenting party, except where she is brought to hospital in an unconscious condition, and an emergency abortion is necessary to save her life, or possibly, where it is necessary to prevent a serious threat to her physical health. In these cases the *negotiorum gestio* principle will apply, in terms of which a doctor may, without consent, perform an emergency operation.[20]

Must a married woman's husband consent as well? The traditional view would seem to be that in principle his consent in necessary. Abortion without his consent would accordingly constitute an *iniuria* to him, exposing the doctor to an action for damages. This view is in line with the earlier standpoint that spouses share a mutual "right to procreation" which can be violated by a third party interfering with a spouse's procreative ability.[21] Today there seems to be little support for this standpoint, though, and the spouses' individual autonomy is stressed. Taken to its logical extreme, the idea of a mutual right to procreation would lead to the conclusion that a husband could force his wife to die in order to bear his child. [22] I entertain grave doubts as to whether modern public policy and enlightened sentiments would still support this extreme view. There are three potentially conflicting interests here; the right of the father to procreation; the right of the mother to her life and health; and the right of the foetus to be born alive (a qualified right in modern law). As Olmesdahl[23] has pointed out, for a court to decide which of these rights must take precedence, is an unenviable task.

I would submit that in view of the fact that the Act extended the legal possibility of abortion largely in recognition of the woman's interests,[24] the husband should have no veto right except in regard to the indication contained in section 3 (1) (*c*), i e the potentially handicapped child. (In England, incidentally, it has been held that a prospective father cannot by means of an injunction (interdict) restrain his wife from undergoing a lawful abortion.[25] It must be pointed out, however, that the English Abortion Act is a more liberal statute than ours.)

Must the consent of the man who made an unmarried female pregnant be obtained for an abortion in terms of the Act? Since the father of an illegitimate child is not the guardian of the child, it is submitted that he will have no say whatsoever in regard to an abortion and need not be consulted.

As far as a minor (unmarried) female is concerned: a minor of over 18 years can independently consent to a medical operation or treatment, in terms of the Child Care Act.[26] In the case of a child under the age of 18 years, parental consent is necessary, except in the emergency situations provided for in the Child Care Act. Here the question arises whether parents can force their minor child to undergo an abortion against her will. We may have the situation where the girl is pregnant by her lover, whom she wishes to marry and whose child she is anxious to bear. If she is over 18 years, she may consent independently. However, if she is under the age of 18 the legal position is more complex. I would submit that since parents may by virtue of the parental power force a child to undergo any operation or treatment in the interest of the

20 See *supra* 92.
21 See *supra* 171.
22 *Cf* M C J Olmesdahl 4 *Natal Univ LR* 213 (1975).
23 *Ibid.*
24 Compare the views of F van der Merwe in Aug 1979 *Responsa Meridiana* 50.
25 *Paton v Trustees of British Pregnancy Advisory Service* [1978] 2 All ER 987.
26 Act 74 of 1983, section 39 (4). See also above 7. (The Act may be amended in 1991.)

child, objectively viewed, they can enforce a (legal) abortion, provided that it is in her interest. However, in my opinion the court would be entitled to interfere with the exercise of parental authority and prevent the parents from forcing a minor to undergo an abortion, if the girl wanted the child and evidence showed that the shock of an abortion would seriously affect her mental or physical health.

In 1986 the Transvaal Supreme Court granted an interdict against the parents of an unmarried 17-year-old who had fallen pregnant in consequence of a relationship with her friend, preventing them from having her pregnancy terminated in an unlawful manner, which would have involved non-medical violent acts. The girl brought the application against her parents.[27] A similar interdict was granted in 1990 in a comparable case involving an 18-year-old unmarried girl, by the Witwatersrand Local Division of the Supreme Court.[28]

The converse situation was the subject of the decision of an English court in 1982.[29] A 15-year-old girl had become pregnant for the second time. She desired an abortion but the parents objected strongly on religious grounds. The court ordered that an abortion should take place against the parents' wishes, and ordered further that, with the approval and at the request of the mother, the girl be fitted thereafter with a suitable internal contraceptive device. (This was clearly a case in which the abortion would have been lawful in terms of the English Abortion Act.)

It is certainly desirable that the entire problem of consent to abortion should be statutorily regulated, by amendment of the Abortion Act.

A right to abortion?

Does the law give a woman the right to demand an abortion where her circumstances fall within the law? There are two aspects to this question. Firstly, can a woman say: "My situation conforms to all the essentials stated in section 3. Therefore the superintendent must authorise an abortion in my case, and if he refuses, I shall apply to the Supreme Court for a *mandamus* (mandatory order) to compel him to do so!" Secondly, assuming that the hospital superintendent has in fact given an authorisation, can a woman say: "Now there is a legal duty on the State in absolute terms to 'provide' me with the abortion, and should the institution for some reason refuse or fail to do so, and a child is born, I will hold it liable in law!"

I shall give my opinion on the first question and then return to the second.

Section 6 (6) of the Act provides that if an application complying with the requirements of this section is made to the medical practitioner referred to in this section, and after investigation by him he is satisfied that it so complies, "he *shall* grant the authority in question" (emphasis supplied). Now, although we have decisions of our Supreme Court holding that "shall" may in a specified context mean "may", I think this subsection is quite emphatic, namely that "shall" must be interpreted as having a peremptory meaning here: in other words, if an applicant to the satisfaction of the superintendent complies with the requirements set forth in section 6, the superintendent concerned has no further discretion, but *must* give the authorisation applied for. If, however, he has reason to believe that the case is not *bona fide* or is deficient in particularity, he may clearly refuse to give the authorisation.

It is to be noted that by virtue of the principles of administrative law there is a duty upon any official charged with a discretionary function of this kind to apply his mind properly to the matter before him. Failure to do so would entitle a party affected by his decision to approach the Supreme Court for review thereof.

The question arises whether – e g in regard to section 3 (1) (*a*), i e danger to the

27 The case was reported in *Die Beeld* (7 June 1986): "Swanger meisie vra bevel teen ouers."
28 "Granted interdict against parents : Girl goes home." Report in *The Citizen* of 2 May 1990.
29 *Re P (a minor)* (1982) 80 LGR 301 (discussed by I Kennedy & A Grubb *Medical Law: Text and Materials* (1990) 8.)

woman's life or physical health, or section 3 (1) (*b*), i e danger to her mental health – it would be sufficient for the certifying doctors simply to follow the wording of the Act. Or must they supply further detailed reasons or grounds for their opinion? I do not think one can be dogmatic here. If the superintendent has no reason to suspect the *bona fides* of the certifying doctors, a simple certificate may do. If, on the other hand, he has reason to doubt their *bona fides*, he may, of course, call for further substantiation.

It is clear that the *onus* to ensure that the application is *bona fide*, rests heavily on the gynaecologist. He is the applicant for an authorisation: "An application for authority ... shall be made ... by the medical practitioner who is to procure the abortion ..."[30] If he is in doubt on the *bona fides* of the psychiatrist's or other practitioner's reports, he would be entitled to refuse to apply – in fact, it may be argued that he ought to refuse to apply. *Mala fides* on his part may result in a possible charge of fraud.

I want to turn to the second question: assuming that authorisation was given by a hospital superintendent, does the woman now have an absolute and enforceable right to an abortion? The answer to this, I submit, can be neither an unqualified "yes", nor an unqualified "no".

To begin with: The fact that the Act makes provision for legal abortion, upon authorisation, in a State institution (or other approved institution) does not make the State (or other approved authority) a guarantor in absolute terms that an abortion will be performed. It is again to be noted that application for authorisation of an abortion is made "by the medical practitioner who is to procure the abortion" and *not* by the woman herself, and that the authorisation is given to that doctor.[31] The authorisation gives the doctor a right to procure abortion, and since he has ostensibly contracted with the woman to terminate her pregnancy subject to authorisation, she will have the right to *require him* to perform the operation (unless he exercises his statutory right to refuse).[32]

However, the mere fact that the superintendent has given authorisation does not mean that his institution is absolutely bound to make its facilities available to the doctor and the woman. It is quite possible that the hospital is full during the crucial time, or that the operating-theatre is fully booked. Must the superintendent, because of the fact that he gave an authorisation, now eject another patient to make room for the woman? In my opinion the rights of the doctor and the woman *vis-à-vis* the hospital are relative to what would be reasonable in the circumstances – what is *sosiaal adekwaat* in the juristic sense of that term. The superintendent would be entitled to exercise a choice, to elect priorities. (Hospital statutes sometimes expressly confer this right upon the superintendent. See e g the Transvaal Hospital Ordinance, [33] section 33 (1): "All persons shall be admitted into a provincial hospital in accordance with the urgency of their need for treatment, as determined by the superintendent ...") The purpose of the Act is without a doubt not to make State hospitals "abortion factories" to the detriment of other health services.

Supposing, however, that hospital facilities are in fact available and the superintendent in question wilfully and arbitrarily refuses access to the woman and her doctor, after he has already granted an authorisation. Can he then be compelled by means of a mandatory court order to allow the applying doctor to perform the abortion in his hospital? Reasoning on the basis of general principles of administrative law, there seems to be no reason why such action cannot be accomplished by means of a *mandamus*.

30 Section 6 (2).
31 Section 6(1) read with regulation 3 under the Act.
32 See below 215. It may be argued that where a doctor, after having seen the patient, submits an application to the superintendent he has waived his right of refusal.
33 Ordinance 14 of 1958.

Assuming that the superintendent wilfully or negligently delays making available his hospital facilities for the abortion and a child is subsequently born? Can he and his institution be held civilly liable? This raises the thorny issues of so-called wrongful life, and wrongful birth, which involve difficult questions of public policy that I have discussed elsewhere.[34]

May a hospital superintendent arbitarily refuse to allow certain forms of abortion in his hospital? In my opinion he may not.

While there is no obligation on the superintendent to guarantee that his hospital's facilities will be available, there is nothing in the Act to suggest that he is vested with arbitrary powers of selection, where these facilities are available. A selection seems to be proper only where there is a conflict of interest in cases of relative availability of hospital facilities. Thus he would obviously be entitled to refuse priority to a non-emergency abortion where his hospital's facilities are urgently required for emergency (life-saving) operations.

Is it lawful to refer patient to overseas abortion clinic?

Would it be lawful for a doctor in South Africa to refer a pregnant woman to an abortion clinic in England[35] or elsewhere for an abortion which may not be procured locally in terms of the Act?

It is submitted that such action on the part of a doctor will not be punishable. Generally speaking the jurisdiction of our courts is limited to criminal offences committed on South African territory. Our courts will not exercise jurisdiction in respect of an abortion procured in another country, even if it is illegal in that country.

In any event, if the abortion is lawful according to the law of England or any other country in which it is performed, there is no question of the South African doctor who made the referral being accused of complicity: by virtue of the "principle of accessoriness" he must be aiding and abetting the commission of an offence by another person.

As far as the ethical aspect is concerned: In 1973 the South African Medical and Dental Council was asked to rule on the question what a doctor should do if a patient requests assistance in obtaining an abortion overseas. The Council made the following ruling: "Any medical practitioner who contravenes any law of the country, including being an accessory to an illegal abortion, irrespective of where it is performed, exposes himself to disciplinary action ..."

On the face of it, it would seem as if the Council would regard such assistance as impermissible, but as I have said, a doctor who refers a patient to an overseas clinic for an abortion which would be lawful in that country, cannot be charged with being an accessory to an illegal act.

Sterilisation

"Sterilisation" is defined in the Act as "a surgical operation performed for the purpose of making the person upon whom it is performed, incapable of procreation, but does not include the removal of a gonad".[36] A gonad is a gamete-producing gland, i e an ovary or testis.[37]

34 See *supra* 195 *et seq.*

35 In 1981 128 555 legal abortions were procured in England and Wales. This figure includes 33 899 non-residents. Most of the non-residents came from Spain (20 454). 511 came from South Africa. Figures obtained from DPCSM Monitor *Legal Abortions* 1981, issued 7 September 1982, Tables 9 and 10 on page 8. This information was kindly supplied by Dr Barbara Huber of the Max Planck Institute for Foreign and International Criminal Law, Freiburg, Germany. In the *Weekend Post* of 27 August 1988 it was reported that R2,2 million had been spent in 1987 by South African women in England and Wales, procuring abortions. The number of women given was 477.

36 Section 1.

37 *Dorland's Illustrated Medical Dictionary* (24th ed, 1967) s v "gonad".

A sterilisation may not be performed on any person who for any reason is incapable of consenting or incompetent to consent thereto, unless the following three requirements are complied with:

1. Two medical practitioners, one of whom must be a psychiatrist, must certify in writing that the patient (a) is suffering from a hereditary condition of such a nature that if he or she were to procreate a child, the child would suffer from a physical or mental defect of such a nature that it would be seriously handicapped, or (b) due to a permanent mental handicap or defect is unable to comprehend the consequential implications of or bear the parental responsibility for the fruit of coitus.
2. The person who may in law consent to an operation beneficial to the patient must grant written consent to the sterilisation. If there is no such person or such person cannot after reasonable enquiry be found, a magistrate may – after such investigation as he may deem fit – grant written authority for the sterilisation.
3. The Minister of National Health and Population Development or a medical officer of his Department authorised by him, must grant written authority.[38]

Patients who could fall under these provisions would be minors under the age of 18 and mentally ill or defective persons. (It is to be noted that a minor over the age of 18 years may independently consent to any medical operation or treatment.[39]) A married woman may independently consent to surgery on herself, including a sterilisation for convenience only.[40] Note that a minor – i e a person under the age of 21 – becomes legally a major when he or she gets married.

"Conscience clause"

A medical practitioner (other than the medical practitioner in charge of a State-controlled or designated institution who is vested by the Act with the right and duty to grant an authorisation for abortion or sterilisation), a nurse or any person employed in any other capacity at such an institution, may refuse to participate in an abortion or sterilisation. The Act expressly provides that such doctors, nurses or other personnel are not obliged to participate, notwithstanding any contract (e g their contracts of employment) or any other law.[41]

It is to be noted that the right of refusal is not restricted to conscientious grounds. A doctor, etc may, therefore, refuse to participate without giving any reason for refusal, and cannot be compelled by a court order on the ground that he (or she) has not indicated that the refusal is on conscientious grounds.

Only in State hospital, or approved hospital

An abortion, or sterilisation of the type regulated by the Act, may be procured only at a State-controlled institution or an institution designated in writing for that purpose by the Minister of National Health and Population Development.[42] "State-controlled institution" includes a hospital conducted by a provincial administration.[43]

Prior to the abortion or sterilisation, a written authorisation must be obtained from the medical practitioner in charge of the hospital concerned. Application must be made by the medical practitioner who is to procure the abortion.[44]

The authorising doctor must make a written report to the Director-General, Na-

38 Section 4.
39 See note 19, *supra*.
40 See *supra* 18, 169.
41 Section 9.
42 Section 5.
43 Section 1.
44 Section 6.

tional Health and Population Development after the abortion or sterilisation, in the prescribed manner and within the prescribed period, containing the details required in section 7 (1) of the Act.[45] The person in charge of an institution where an operation connected with an abortion or the removal of the residue of a pregnancy is performed, must keep a record of the particulars.[46]

Formalities to be observed

The formalities to be complied with in regard to applications for abortions and sterilisations, authorisations, notes and records, etc, are set out in ministerial regulations made in terms of the Act.[47]

An application in terms of the Act to procure an abortion, or to perform a sterilisation on a person who cannot consent thereto himself (or herself) must be made on a form drawn up by the Department of National Health and Population Development.[48]

The doctor making application, and in the case of an abortion, the woman concerned, must declare that a similar application has not previously been submitted to the superintendent, or has been submitted and was refused by him (in which case the reason for refusal must be furnished).[49]

The person in change of an institution must, immediately after each operation connected with the removal of the residue of a pregnancy, complete the prescribed form on which the following details must be supplied:

- the name and address of the institution;
- the date of the operation;
- the full names and case number of the patient;
- the age of the patient;
- the marital status of the patient;
- the population group of the patient;
- the name of the person who referred the patient;
- the name of the doctor who performed the operation;
- which of the following gave rise to the operation –
  (i) an inevitable miscarriage, (ii) an incomplete miscarriage, (iii) a septic miscarriage;
- any noticeable signs of injuries, any foreign material, found in the internal genital tract of the patient during the operation.[50]

The doctor who has authorised an abortion or sterilisation must immediately after the operation see to it that the prescribed form is completed. On or before the 14th day following the last day of each month, all completed forms must be forwarded to the Director-General, National Health and Population Development.[51] These forms must be kept for one year. All other documentation relating to applications for abortion or sterilisation must be kept for five years after the operation. Documents must be kept in a safe or other safe place.[52]

45 Section 7. The details required are: the name, age, marital state, race and (in the case of sterilisation) the sex of the patient; the place where and date on which the operation was procured; in the case of an abortion, the reasons therefor; the names of the doctors involved (and the magistrate, where necessary); if the consent of any person other than the patient was required, the name of the person who consented, and his/her capacity.
46 Section 7(3).
47 See *Government Notice* R610 of 25/3/83 *GG* 8617, as corrected by R774 of 15/4/83 *GG* 8652.
48 Reg 2.
49 Reg 2(2).
50 Reg 4.
51 Reg 4(3).
52 Reg 5.

An assessment

Has the Act had any significant effect on illegal or backstreet abortion? As I have said at the beginning of this chapter, the Act was intended to regulate therapeutic abortion; it was certainly not designed to achieve total, or even substantial, eradication of illegal abortions. The same sordid cases keep coming before our criminal courts as in the past. Newspaper headlines tell the stories: "*Young girl dies in secret abortion bid*"; "*Wife tells of wire abortion*"; "*Vrugafdrywing in hotelkamer*"; "*Girl tells of her abortion agony*"; "*Former MOH Fined: Gave 5 women abortions*".

It is difficult to draw any firm conclusions from criminal statistics. Bearing in mind that the Act became operative on 12 March 1975, bearing in mind our constant population growth, and bearing in mind the fact that four national states achieved independence a decade or two ago, what does one make of the following figures? In the 12-month period 1 July to 30 June the number of convictions for abortions recorded in the Republic[53] were as follows for each of the periods indicated:

1968-69	43	1978-79	52
1969-70	39	1979-80	55
1970-71	34	1980-81	32
1971-72	31	1981-82	31
1972-73	23	1982-83	27
1973-74	27	1983-84	not available
1974-75	34	1984-85	31
1975-76	41	1985-86	23
1976-77	32	1986-87	1
1977-78	55	1987-88	25

On the basis of the experience of countries with very liberal abortion laws, we know that not even an "abortion on demand" law would completely eliminate backstreet abortion, although it would undoubtedly reduce the mortality figure very substantially. The continuation of backstreet abortion, even in societies where the law has been liberalised, seems to be attributable to several factors. Among these are an aversion to the "official" inquiry preceding legal abortion, and in the lower social strata, ignorance of the possibility of legal abortion, coupled with the knowledge that there is an "old woman" down the street who will do the job cheaply.

Nevertheless, as far as the South African Act is concerned, it will be a relatively safe guess that the Act must have had some effect on illegal abortion (if not on *backstreet* abortion – these are, of course, two different things).

The total number of abortions and sterilisations officially recorded in the annual reports of the Department of National Health and Population Development for the years[54] 1976 to 1990 is as follows:

Year	**Abortions**	**Sterilisations**
1976	625	(not mentioned)
1977	539	74
1978	541	70
1979	423	84
1980	347	113
1981	381	87
1982	464	74

53 I am indebted to Mr Willem Krugel, president of the regional court of Northern Transvaal and Miss Roelien Theron of the UCT Institute of Criminology, respectively, who kindly furnished me with these details obtained from official sources.

54 The "years" are not calendar years, but generally 12-month periods (although not invariably the same 12 months).

Year	Abortions	Sterilisations
1983	474	126
1984	566	173
1985	712	233
1986	770	200
1987	810	210
1988	1112	182
1989	963	153

Considering the population growth rate, these figures do not indicate more than a slightly rising trend in the incidence of legal abortion. Certain other trends have also manifested themselves. The most important single indication for legal abortions, statistically speaking, has been by far the psychiatric indication: in 1976 it was 52,3%, in 1977 51,2%, in 1978 48%, in 1979 46,3%, in 1980 44,9%, in 1981 48,5%, in 1982 52,8%, in 1983 47,6%, in 1984 45,7%, in 1985 51,6%, in 1986 54%, in 1987 55,9%, in 1988 56,1% and in 1989 62,4%. The demand for abortion in terms of the Act has essentially been a White demand, with the Coloured population in second place. Of the overall number of abortions in the years indicated, the percentage performed on White women and Coloured women, respectively, was as follows:

	Whites	Coloureds
1976	81,4%	12,3%
1977	74%	14,4%
1978	78,1%	14,4%
1979	70,9%	15,1%
1980	67,1%	18,1%
1981	69,2%	16,7%
1982	69,8%	15,3%
1983	75,1%	15,1%
1984	78,3%	12,4%
1985	78,4%	11,1%
1986	79,1%	14,8%
1987	78,5%	11,3%
1988	83,6%	9,8%
1989	76,3%	14%

Adapted from a paper read at the Fourth International Symposium on Forensic Medicine, held in Pretoria, May 1976 (first printed in (1977) 1 SACC *116).*

34 The Abortion and Sterilisation Act and the drama of Miss X

No other case of a woman desiring an abortion has been accorded greater publicity in South Africa than that of the girl who became known as Miss X,[1] early in 1980. The case triggered a nation-wide discussion of the merits and demerits of legal abortion and has highlighted several aspects of the application of the Abortion and Sterilisation Act.[2]

The dramatic events started when Miss X, a 19-year-old, accompanied a young man to a drive-in theatre and had intercourse with him in his car, as a result of which she fell pregnant. Later she told a magistrate she was raped after the man had threatened to mutilate her face with a broken bottle unless she allowed him to have his way with her. She explained that she did not lay a charge against the man because she feared her father would "chase her away" from home.

When it became known to her that she was pregnant, Miss X developed an acute state of anxiety and threatened to take her own life. She actually made several unsuccessful attempts to that end.

A psychiatrist in private practice who examined and treated her, came to the conclusion that a continuation of the pregnancy would endanger the life of the girl (as envisaged by section 3 (1) (*a*) of the Abortion and Sterilisation Act) and an abortion was indicated. The superintendent of the provincial hospital to whom application was made for the abortion to be performed, disagreed with this contention. He indicated that the provision of the Act that might be applicable to the situation was the psychiatric indication contained in section 3 (1) (*b*). But it appeared that no psychiatrist in the employ of the State in that area was prepared to issue the certificate required in terms of the latter clause. In view of that, the superintendent was not prepared to issue the necessary authorisation for the abortion.

The father of the girl accordingly brought an application to the Supreme Court for a *mandamus* ordering the superintendent to issue an authorisation for a gynaecologist to perform the abortion. The application was not defended and a judge in chambers granted the application.[3] Miss X was now approximately 18 weeks pregnant.

The application, although successful, brought no finality to the matter, however, because it soon transpired that no gynaecologist in the hospital concerned was prepared to perform the abortion, unless it could be done under the psychiatric clause – for which the required certification could not be obtained.

Miss X found herself on the horns of a medico-legal dilemma, and the press, ever alert to a human-interest story, got wind of the drama. Soon every major newspaper in the country splashed the story of Miss X. The father of the girl was quoted as saying that his daughter had in fact been raped, and it was suggested that an authorisation would be sought for the abortion to be performed under the "rape clause" of the Act.

Within a matter of days, the hapless girl's father was in court again, this time as

1 Miss X subsequently disclosed her identity to the press, which gave massive publicity to her case – colour photographs and all – but I prefer to use her fictitious name.

2 Act 2 of 1975.

3 The case was not reported, but a reference to the judge's decision is to be found in the *Christian League* case (see note following) at 825C.

the respondent in an urgent application brought by an organisation known as the Christian League of Southern Africa.[4] This organisation contended that because the prospective mother of the unborn child rejected the child, it had no guardian to protect its interest in relation to the contemplated abortion. They accordingly asked the court to appoint an advocate to act as curator of the unborn child.

The court issued an interim order to prevent the father from taking any further steps to obtain an abortion under the psychiatric or rape provisions of the Act, but three days later the application for appointment of a curator was refused. The court held that the Christian League had no *locus standi in iudicio* (legal standing) to bring the application and that there were no legal grounds for the appointment of a *curator ad litem* to represent an unborn child in regard to proposed termination of its mother's pregnancy.

In the meantime, the girl's pregnancy had advanced to almost 20 weeks. And still no gynaecologist would come to her aid notwithstanding the superintendent's authorisation issued in compliance with the court order. By virtue of section 9 of the Act no doctor or nurse can be compelled to give effect to an authorisation.

The family's attorney now put the case for abortion on the grounds of rape to a magistrate of the district in which the rape was alleged to have occurred. In the early hours of a Sunday morning the magistrate issued a certificate to the effect that after questioning Miss X, he was convinced on a balance of probability, that she had been raped. Soon afterwards, however, doubts arose in the magistrate's mind concerning his jurisdiction to issue such a certificate. (By law only regional magistrates could try rape cases.)

The next day the attorney approached the regional magistrate of the area for a certificate, but the latter was of the opinion that there were insufficient grounds for such a certificate to be issued. The district magistrate withdrew his certificate.

Time was marching on, and soon Miss X would reach the point where no doctor would be prepared to terminate her pregnancy, even if all the formalities were observed. Soon she would enter the 22nd week of pregnancy. In a last-ditch attempt, her father now approached the Supreme Court on an urgent basis for an order upholding the first magistrate's certificate. It was contended that although the Act provided that a magistrate "attached to the court having jurisdiction in respect of the alleged offence" was competent to certify, these words had to be read in conjunction with the definition of "magistrate" in the Act, as "including an additional or assistant magistrate", and that "jurisdiction" also included territorial jurisdiction.

However, the judge to whom the application was made – at his home at 21:00, one evening – declined to uphold these submissions and refused the application.[5]

Ironically, the House of Assembly at that stage had already passed a Bill designed to amend the Abortion and Sterilisation Act, which in express terms would have vested a district magistrate with the power of issuing a certificate, but the Bill had yet to come before the Senate and the State President.[6]

Miss X, having come to the end of the legal road, dramatically announced that she had now resigned herself to becoming a mother, and that she would have the baby "and give it the love it needs". Her parents told the press that they would give their daughter all the support she needed. A beautiful baby was born – and they all lived happily ever after, according to all accounts.

In the aftermath of the case, many questions were asked:

- is the procedure that must be complied with in order to obtain an abortion, not too cumbersome?

4 *Christian League of Southern Africa v Rall* 1981 (2) SA 821 (O).
5 *Rall NO v Landdros vir die Distrik van Heilbron* 1980 (3) SA 287 (O).
6 See now section 6(4) of the Act, and see above 209.

- when can it be said that a pregnant woman's threats or attempts to commit suicide are "endangering her life"?
- should the grounds for abortion not be extended?

The abortion debate continues ...

35 Can the use of an intra-uterine device amount to illegal abortion?

The Abortion and Sterilisation Act of 1975,[1] defines abortion as "the abortion of a live foetus of a woman with intent to kill such foetus".[2] "Foetus" is not defined in the Act and that has given rise to some discussion in medico-legal circles. In 1979 the issue of what a "foetus" is came up for decision in the Cape Provincial Division of the Supreme Court.

As is well known, a distinction is made medically between "embryo" which refers to the developing young in the human uterus up to the eighth week, and "foetus" which refers to the product of conception after that stage.[3]

In *S v Collop*[4] the accused was charged in the magistrate's court with several counts of criminal abortion. It appeared that she had treated her "patients" by injecting into their wombs a mixture of soap – the brand name of which ironically was Lifebuoy – glycerine and an antibiotic.

In respect of one of the charges the accused raised the defence that in view of the fact that the "patient" involved had conceded that she might have told the accused at the time of her "treatment" that she was between seven and eight weeks pregnant, the State had failed to prove that the accused had procured an abortion of a "live foetus".

At the trial medical witnesses testifying for the prosecution distinguished between a foetus and an embryo, although describing the term "abortion" as referring to the termination of pregnancy at any time after conception has resulted in a fertilised ovum in the uterus of the mother. One of the medical witnesses said that the term "foetus" covers the whole period from conception to childbirth, but that for a certain time during that period the fertilised ovum is also described as an embryo.

The accused was convicted and she appealed to the Supreme Court. In his judgment, Mr Justice van Winsen referred to the works of Roman-Dutch jurists and came to the conclusion that the state of the development reached by the fertilised ovum at the time of its expulsion from the uterus, was only of importance in regard to the penalty to be imposed for the crime of abortion, and that the offence itself was not limited to the expulsion of the fertilised ovum only after it has reached a more advanced state of development. Modern South African legal authorities support this view, the judge said.

Counsel for the appellant raised the interesting argument that in the light of modern law and social thinking in other parts of the world, the South African Legislature might well have intended to depart from the common law and to introduce a new concept of abortion which would have the effect of exempting from criminal liability all acts having the effect of terminating a pregnancy prior to some stage of the development of the fertilised ovum. In this context, reference was made to rulings of the United States Supreme Court to the effect that during the first trimester of pregnancy, termination thereof may lawfully take place at the request of the woman "if determined proper within the medical judgment of the attending physician".

1 Act 2 of 1975.
2 Section 1.
3 *Dorland's Illustrated Medical Dictionary s v* "fetus".
4 1979 (4) SA 381 (C).

The appellant's counsel further argued that if the Legislature had intended to proscribe all abortions done at any time after fertilisation, it would have the effect of prohibiting the use of a particular form of contraception, namely the insertion of an IUD (intra-uterine device) which does not prevent conception but prevents the fertilised ovum from establishing itself.

This contention, the judge observed, presents the problem of having to determine a period in the existence of the fertililsed ovum during which pregnancy could be regarded as legally terminable. Our common-law authorities, requiring to draw a distinction for the purpose of deciding on an appropriate punishment, described the dividing line as being reached when the child "quickened in the womb", but the differing points of view on when this occurred seem never to have been authoritatively settled, the judge said.

"Had our Legislature intended to perpetuate this division, it is more than probable that it would have grappled with the problem of defining from what point of time abortion became illegal. The failure to do so is a strong pointer to the fact that it never sought to draw such a distinction."

The judge concluded that the Act penalises the procuring of abortion of a live foetus, and that "foetus" refers to a fertilised ovum.

The effect of the ruling seems to be that the prescribing of the "morning after" pill and the insertion of an IUD (intra-uterine device) may technically amount to an unlawful abortion in terms of the Act.[5] If this were so, it seems most unlikely, however, that in practice such cases would ever be reported with a view to prosecution. Moreover, there would be the problem of proof: the prosecution would have to prove beyond a reasonable doubt that the foetus was alive at the time when it was interfered with.

Because of the requirement of *mens rea* (criminal intent) the prosecution must further prove that the accused at the time of his act must have known, or, at the very least must have foreseen, that the foetus was alive.

Note that it was expressly held by the Cape court in *Collop's* case that a mere admission by the defence that the accused interfered with the pregnancy so that it was terminated does not include an admission that the foetus aborted *was living at the time of abortion*.[6]

The appellant took the case on appeal to the Appellate Division.[7] Her counsel argued *inter alia* on the basis of medical evidence and dictionary meanings that the unborn offspring in the human uterus is an embryo, and not a foetus, before eight weeks of pregnancy. Mr Justice Diemont, however, found that there was no merit in that proposition: "Parliament would, I apprehend, be surprised to learn that in its wisdom, it had placed on the statute book a law which made legal an abortion procured by any unqualified person or quack carrying on business in a back-street, provided only that the operation was performed on the patient before the end of the second month of pregnancy. To place such an interpretation on the Act would ... cause public consternation and concern."

Counsel argued further that the use of the "popular post-conceptive device" of the IUD would be illegal and prohibited if the judgment were upheld. But Mr Justice Diemont said he was not persuaded that the manner in which a contraceptive device operates is calculated to shed any light on the interpretation of this statute. The judge accordingly did not rule on the legality or otherwise of the IUD.

5 Compare P M A Hunt *South African Criminal Law and Procedure* vol II (2nd ed, 1982, by J R L Milton) 325, n 167. On "interceptive" methods in general, in this context, see also Mason & McCall Smith *Law and Medical Ethics* (2nd ed, 1987) 68.

6 The State, in a cross-appeal to the Appellate Division, challenged the correctness of this finding, but in the circumstances of the case, the Appeal Court found it unnecessary to decide the issue. See report of the latter court's judgment (referred to in the footnote following) at 168 *et seq.*

7 *S v Collop* 1981 (1) SA 150 (A).

The judge drew attention to the dispute in the days of the Roman-Dutch jurists as to when the foetus began to quicken in the mother's womb. He felt that Parliament could not have intended to revive this age-old controversy.

The Appeal Court accordingly ruled that the appellant had been correctly convicted.

It is of interest to note the comments on the legality or otherwise of the use of an IUD, made by counsel for the State Mr J Slabbert, in argument before the Appeal Court.[8] He contended that the use of an IUD, which prevents implantation of the fertilised egg in the uterine wall, was not a factor in the case because ***in casu*** all the fertilised eggs had gone beyond implantation. The Legislature, in codifying common law took it over "as it was" and did not concern itself with the latest medical developments and knowledge.

But even if it is assumed that Parliament did know all the medical facts, Mr Slabbert argued, the Act "condoned" this type of abortion on social, medical and religious grounds. Alternatively, the Legislature might have regarded section 3 of the Act as not prohibiting the use of an IUD.

In line with these arguments, I would submit that where an IUD is used in good faith for birth control purposes it must be regarded as a *sosiaal-adekwate*[9] act, and therefore not unlawful, even if its use technically falls within the definition of abortion in terms of the Act.[10]

8 *Ibid*, 157-158.

9 The defence of social adequacy has enjoyed scant attention in South Africa but is known to legal science. We are here concerned with an act which, although *prima facie* in violation of a legal precept, should, on account of its social desirability be encouraged rather than discouraged. On the defence of social adequacy see H-H Jescheck *Lehrbuch des Strafrechts* (4th ed, 1988) 266 *et seq*.

10 L Hawthorne *The Crime of Abortion: A Historical and Comparative Study* (LLD thesis, Univ of Pretoria, 1982) 255, argues that where an IUD is inserted into a patient with the intention of causing an abortion, it is criminal. If, however, the intention is "to provide the patient with a contraceptive, even if the patient is pregnant and an abortion is caused, the *mens rea* requirement in terms of the Act is not fulfilled and criminal liability will not follow". (The use of the word "contraceptive" by Hawthorne in this context seems to be incorrect; conception has taken place at the stage when the egg was fertilised.)

PART X

Transsexualism

36 Transsexualism and the law

Introduction

About three decades ago, the syndrome of transsexualism was still referred to as "a truly untrodden, controversial and largely unexplored field of medicine".[1] Although the so-called "sex-change" operations have been performed with increasing frequency,[2] controversy has not ended. Despite important judicial pronouncements and some legislative enactments since that date, not all legal issues in this field have been settled.

For the purposes of this discussion it is assumed that the "transsexual" is a person who biologically belongs unmistakably to either the male or female sex,[3] but psychologically identifies himself (or herself) with the opposite sex. On account of this orientation he will probably have transvestite tendencies, although he cannot be considered a transvestite in the more general meaning of the word, i e a person who derives erotic pleasure from donning the clothes of the opposite sex. Nor is he a homosexual in the accepted sense of the word, although he might project himself upon members of his own biological sex.[4]

Transsexualism involves difficult problems of medicine, psychiatry, religion, ethics and law. This discussion will be confined to the law, but it must be observed that it is impossible to treat of the legal aspect of transsexualism *in vacuo*.

An unfriendly legal world

Although attitudes have changed during the past few decades, the legal world has proved to be an unfriendly one for the transsexual. In most, if not all, societies the law firmly entrenched the heterosexual outlook of the majority of citizens.

Transsexuals have been confronted with legal problems such as the following:

The wearing in public of clothes of the opposite sex could constitute a punishable offence in more conservative societies such as South Africa, if a court were to find that dressing in such a manner constitutes a disguise.[5] A surgical "change of sex" on the part of a spouse could entitle the other spouse to divorce. The mere refusal of sexual privileges on account of transsexual tendencies might have the same result.

1 Harry Benjamin *Clinical Aspects of Transsexualism in the Male and Female* (1963).

2 By 1970 the figure of known operations was estimated to exceed 1 000. See B v D van Niekerk 1970 *SALJ* 239 at 241.

3 This means that in the case of the male transsexual, e g, the following characteristics will be identified: the XY chromosome; male gonads (i e the presence of testes and the absence of ovaries); male external genitalia. The transsexual must therefore be distinguished from the hermaphrodite, who is characterised by the presence of both male and female sexual organs. In the hermaphrodite gonadal tissue typical of both sexes will be found. The transsexual must also be distinguished from the so-called pseudo-hermaphrodite whose sexual organs are so unusually formed that he is mistaken for a member of the opposite sex, but whose gonadal tissue nevertheless is typical of one sex only.

4 An interesting South African case study of "female-to-male" transsexualism is that of *Frederica* described in previous editions of this book. See the 2nd edition (1984) 264-274. The case study was also published in 1974 (3) *Forensic Science* 19.

5 In contravention of the Prohibition of Disguises Act 16 of 1969. See J R L Milton & N M Fuller *South African Criminal Law and Procedure* vol III (1971) 208-9.

Although the entry of sex of a newly born child upon his birth certificate in itself might be of little legal significance, a formal amendment of the sex indicated on the certificate might be refused by the authority concerned – an application for such an amendment would involve expense and formalities. So would the change of a name or names. A change of names or sex on other official or semi-official documents, such as school certificates, would likewise present difficulties. The validity of a marriage entered into by a transsexual who had undergone conversive surgery, would be questioned. Once "married", the possibility of bringing an action for divorce would be legally questionable. In some jurisdictions the question could arise whether a "converted" transsexual could be a party to an adulterous relationship. A person who posed as a member of the opposite sex could conceivably be charged with fraud. A change of sex could substantially affect the provisions of a will, e g a bequest by a testator to "my son", who in the meantime had undergone surgery to become a "woman". And it could affect typically male obligations by law, such as compulsory military training.

To the best of my knowledge the first country which endeavoured to legislatively create a friendlier legal atmosphere for the transsexual was Sweden. The Swedish Act of 21 April 1972[6] came to the rescue of persons who since their youth have felt a conviction of belonging to a sex other than that entered in the parish register and who for a considerable time have behaved accordingly and may be expected to continue living in such a sex role. Such persons may, upon application, obtain official recognition that they belong to the other sex. Applicants must be unmarried Swedish citizens of at least 18 years of age and must have undergone sterilisation or for other reasons be incapable of procreation.

The lawfulness of the "sex-change" operation

Of special concern to the transsexual as well as the surgeon performing the operation (and other specialists involved) was the question whether the "sex-change" operation was a lawful procedure.

Already in the 1960s it was argued that these operations had become so common that they had become socially and juridically accepted. But doubts regarding their lawfulness were nevertheless expressed from time to time.

In principle it would seem as though any drastic operation of a non-therapeutic nature is unlawful, unless a legally justifiable purpose is sought to be attained by it (e g a cosmetic improvement which will not substantially endanger the life or health of the patient, or the removal of tissue or an organ from a healthy person for the purpose of transplantation upon a diseased person). Did the objective sought to be achieved by conversive surgery fall within this category? The answer to this question depended upon a consideration of all the surrounding circumstances in a particular case, and evaluation of these in the light of public policy. It was clear that the consent of the patient could not *per se* afford justification, notwithstanding the superb skill with which these operations were performed. (Many of these operations, especially in the case of male to female conversion, produced astounding results judged by purely aesthetical standards.)

It was contended that the justification for this type of surgery lay in the fact that its true nature was therapeutic. The genuine transsexual, it was said, is a seriously disturbed person psychologically, who is unable to adapt himself to normal social relationships. Frequently he develops suicidal tendencies. Psychotherapy, so it was contended, was of almost no avail and the only remedy was for the surgeon to apply his skill and to convert the patient's "external" physiology to his psychological orientation, thereby bringing equilibrium.

6 The Swedish Act is discussed by A Cremona-Barbaro "Medicolegal Aspects of Transsexualism in Western Europe: A Comparative Review" 5 *Med Law* 89 (1986) 93.

But these views were seriously challenged by some. An official Dutch commission of inquiry[7] into the advisability of surgical sex-transformation came to the following conclusion in 1965: "There are insufficient grounds for treating transsexualism surgically in the sense of sex transformation. Where this is nevertheless undertaken, it must be realised that each operation is attended by a great and uncertain risk, not only in the somatic sense but also, and in particular, in the psychological sense, and there is no certainty whatsoever about its effect." In its report, the Dutch Commission complained of the lack of empirical data. It was pointed out that experience in the field of plastic surgery generally showed that the results were almost always disappointing. The fact also remained, the commission stated, that there could be no true conversion of sex, particularly in regard to the procreative function. All that could be attained through surgery was a skilful imitation of the desired sex. The conviction held by the transsexual that he belongs to the opposite sex was described as "a delusion". The best result that could be hoped for in conversive surgery was to cure the patient of this delusion. But in several cases, the commission found, the operation had brought no satisfaction; in one case a patient had even "reverted" to his original sex. Many transsexuals who had undergone surgery, sooner or later demanded further surgery. Although there might have been an initial alleviation of the patient's condition, his depression in many cases would reappear, sooner or later. The question remained whether sustained and patient psychotherapy would not eventually have brought a favourable result without physical mutilation. Physicians who undertook this type of surgery were accused by the commission of being too uncritical of their own work. Moreover, the commission held, no definitive scientific conclusions could be drawn unless there had been a follow-up of at least ten years.[8]

True as these objections might have been, it is submitted that they did not necessarily lead to the inference that conversive surgery was unlawful. In my opinion such an inference could only be drawn once it had been proved conclusively that the great majority of these operations were not only unsuccessful, but that they in fact led to harmful results for the patients.

At this stage of medical knowledge and experience there is at least some evidence that this type of surgery may be beneficial to a particular type of patient. There seems to be very little evidence that patients who have been operated upon may be in a worse psychological state. Would it be reasonable for the law to expect transsexuals to subject themselves to prolonged psychiatric treatment when there is no clear indication that such treatment may ultimately be successful? It is submitted that although the eventual beneficial effect of the "sex-change" operation may still be doubtful, the therapeutic objective aimed at, in the light of present-day knowledge of transsexualism, fully justifies this kind of surgery. Provided that the operation had been preceded by an exhaustive investigation and was performed with adequate skill and care, and provided that an informed consent had been obtained from the patient, the operation should be ruled as lawful. "Informed consent" in this context would imply that the patient be fully informed of the physiological hazards and implications; it should also be pointed out to the patient that although it is hoped the desired long-term psychological results will be brought about, this cannot be guaranteed.

Court rulings on the legality issue and statutory law

In one of the first cases involving a transsexual, *Anonymous v Weiner, etc*[9] (1966) an

7 *Gezondheidsraad: Rapport betreffende Plastisch-Chirurgische Geslachtstransformatie* (1965).

8 For a more recent – and more sympathetic – Dutch assessment, see A J Kuiper, P T Cohen-Kettenis, F van der Reyt "Transsexuality in the Netherlands: Some Medical and Legal Aspects" 4 *Med Law* 389 (1985).

9 270 NYS 2d 319.

American court refused to order the amendment of the birth certificate of a transsexual who had undergone conversive surgery. But the court did not rule upon the lawfulness or otherwise of the operation; the only point at issue was whether there was a proper exercise of an administrative function entrusted to the New York Board of Health, which had refused to amend the birth certificate.

A comparable decision was handed down by a German court in 1969.[10] In this case the applicant, a male transsexual who had undergone conversive surgery, unsuccessfully applied to court to have his birth certificate amended. Upon appeal the *Oberlandesgericht* of Frankfurt refused to interfere with that decision. The court held that this was an instance of transvestism, of which the court accepted the following definition: "an abnormal development of a person's personality, which at first only involves a psychological identification with the other sex but later also a physical identification (as the result of hormone treatment or an operation)." The court held that although there was the theoretical possibility that hormone and genetical factors may be involved in the causation of such a situation, they are not yet identifiable according to scientific knowledge presently available. Until medical science provides a generally acceptable explanation of the origin and the conditions for development of transvestism, a person of the said kind cannot be classified, legally, to the opposite sex after an operation has changed his appearance. Inherent in this decision, it was pointed out,[11] is the willingness at a later stage to reconsider the matter in the light of scientific developments in this field.

The 1966 case of *Dr Ricardo San Martin*[12] of the Argentine is one in which the lawfulness of a sex-change operation was directly at issue.

The accused, a medical surgeon, performed an operation upon the "victim", one F, in which he emasculated him. According to the court's findings, F was a homosexual, who did not manifest any feminine characteristics. "He was a man and would continue to be so until the day he dies. No female chromatin bodies were found in his cellular nuclei." The accused claimed in court that he had acted for strictly scientific reasons (removal for cancer of the penis), but this was rejected by the court. It was found that the accused had not requested a chemical examination beforehand. He had not preserved the parts removed, nor had he prescribed post-operative treatment. He had left an outward form of vaginal semblance (a "pseudo vulva"). The accused was criminally charged and convicted of assault.

In his review of the case, the *Fiscal da Camara* stated as follows: "There is no scientific reason for the removal of a healthy penis from a physically healthy man. No aesthetic reasons, nor the satisfaction of an unhealthy sociological interest, nor the desire to placate the perverted sexual craving of the victim can justify such a removal. The experience of qualified medical staff, the use of proper instruments and medical technique during the operation do not suffice to licitly condone the fact that it is a grievous bodily injury, recognised as a crime by the Penal Code...

"The consent of the victim does not alleviate the crime ... The perverted mind of the victim, whose mental age is 12 years, prevents him from rightfully disposing of his body, and even more so when there is evidence of wrongful intent ...

"[T]he accused is a doctor who has gone against the precepts of his profession: to not destroy the bodies of these sick people, but rather cure their minds ...

"The nature of the crime must also be considered because the act *per se* constitutes a grievous assault on the man in his capacity as a man, and, in more general terms,

10 1969 *Neue Juristische Wochenschrift* 1576. And see Van Niekerk *op cit* 239.

11 Van Niekerk *op cit* 240.

12 Through the kind offices of the Argentine Embassy in Pretoria, a photocopy of the record was supplied to me. I am much indebted to Dr Mary Catherine McDonald, professor in Spanish in the University of South Africa, for translation of the judgment into English. The case was noted in the Argentinian *La Ley*, 1 September 1966. See also *La Ley* of 8 August 1966.

an absolute disregard for the social [natural] law – the one law above all the norms of [positive] law and morality – that of the preservation of the species.

"Mankind would subsist although every man in this world were to have his arms cut off, were to lose his property, his honour and his fatherland. However, if an act such as this were allowed to go unpunished – if it were not severely punished – a gap would be opened into which the whole human race would fall.

"The action of the accused absolutely defies all that nature imposes. He knew he could not change a man into a woman; he attempted to simulate this. However far medicine advances, it can never violate the secrets of creation – procreation and death.

"Nothing can exonerate this physician, not even his unconfessed lack of faith in the possibility, now or in the future, of curing homosexuals, something that, we assert, can never benefit F. Do we know perchance, that F, in other hands, might not have been cured? San Martin has eliminated any such possibility.

"Again, the consent of the victim in this case is of little or no consequence to the accused, since it was not honestly motivated. The motive of F was induced through corruption ..."

Upon appeal, the *Poder Judicial de la Nación* confirmed the conviction, holding, *inter alia*, that "there is no justification whatever which mitigates the criminal liability for the act. The consent of the victim is not a defence. The act constitutes grievous bodily injury, and in view of the consequences, society cannot accept the consent of the victim, whose interests are protected by this Court. It cannot be submitted that the physician, who accepted this consent, was ignorant of the fact that the consent was invalidated by the mental incompetence of the victim whose perverted sexual craving distorted the real scope and significance of the operation; even supposing the best results F could not be somatically changed into a woman: the differences between body and mind could not be remedied by these means. Although it could be held that it were psychologically possible to give real relief to the craving of F, such a limited and incomplete solution could not justify the irremediable corporal harm caused, apart from the moral and social implications."

It is doubtful whether these views would be supported without reservation in courts of other Western countries. It may well be respectfully asked whether in convicting the surgeon the Argentine judges took sufficient cognisance of humanitarian considerations *vis-à-vis* the patient. The argument that the existence of mankind could be jeopardised if operations of this nature went unpunished, is bordering on the grotesque. Surely the law must take notice of the fact that only a very negligible minority of individuals have transsexual tendencies and that this "perversity" affords a very real psychological and almost existential problem to the individual concerned. It is true, however, that no court of law can ride roughshod over religious, ethical and sociological attitudes. The legal position of the transsexual and that of his surgeon present a challenge to thoughtful men generally – and to jurists in particular.

In the Belgian case of *Dr Fardeau et alii*[13] the accused were criminally charged after a transsexual had died as a result of a series of pulmonary emboli following conversive surgery. According to the evidence before the court, the patient was wearing female clothes when first he consulted Dr F. He was found to have had male genitals, but had female busts, a smooth skin and a general behaviour which was altogether female. He claimed that he was not a homosexual, but considered himself a female and was anxious to escape from the twilight world in which he existed. He was subjected to a thorough examination by a panel of physicians. A testicular biopsy led to a finding of hypoplasia. Excessive estrogen was also found to be present. The pros-

13 1969 *Journal de Tribunaux* 635. The author is much indebted to Dr R Dierkens of Ghent University, Belgium for supplying the text, and to Professor Johan Joubert of the University of South Africa, for translation thereof.

ecution contended that the accused could not rely on the defence of justification since they had not acted with a curative objective, there had not been a free and clear consent on the part of the patient, and they had committed an act of malpractice. It was further contended that the operation had been performed solely with the objective of placating the desire of the patient and not with the intent to bring about any cure.

The accused, however, claimed the surgery had been undertaken with the objective to restore the patient's psychological equilibrium and to facilitate his social re-acceptance, and that the operation was therefore legally justifiable. Upholding the defence contention, the court confirmed the view that the knowledge a judge possesses does not entitle him to interfere with medical theories and methods. The court referred to the conflicting views of medical experts regarding the nature of transsexualism and the efficacy of surgery as a cure, and held that it was not in a position to evaluate the respective theories where there was no reason to doubt the scientific competence and intellectual integrity of the experts concerned.

The court referred to the evidence of Professor Hastings to the effect that in the majority of cases in which he had operated, the patients had afterwards lived a far more harmonious life, that three of them had married, and that 20 out of 24 patients had experienced sexual gratification comparable to that of a normal woman. Professor Hasting also testified that surgical treatment had already been employed in Germany since 1933, and afterwards in Switzerland, Denmark and the United States of America. The court also dealt with the prosecution's contention that the accused had arrived at their diagnosis without subjecting the patients to a profound psychiatric and psychological examination. The court recognised the value of such an examination because "the highly exceptional and irreversible nature of the operation and its repercussions upon the entire future of the patient render it imperative that recourse should not be had to such an operation without as complete an examination as is possible".

In casu the court could nevertheless not come to the conclusion that such a psychiatric examination would have led to a different diagnosis. On the issue of consent, the court held that there was an informed and voluntary consent. The patient was quite an intelligent and balanced person (apart from his sexual maladjustment). The court rejected the prosecution's allegation that the operation amounted to a contravention of articles 12 and 17 of the European Convention on Human Rights whereby a person of marriageable age was entitled to marry and to establish a family. Finally, the Court rejected the allegation that the patient's death was caused by professional error on the part of the accused.

In December 1969 another case came before the Argentinian *Poder Judicial de la Nación*. The appellant was *Dr Francisco Defazio*,[14] who had been convicted of aggravated assault on three charges brought as a result of conversive surgery. The first charge concerned one M who was diagnosed as a pseudo-hermaphrodite. An examination brought to light that there was total atrophy of one testicle and partial atrophy of the other. The forensic physicians claimed the patient was a male (on the basis of chromosomes, chromatin, size and position of the testicles) although there was evidence of some female characteristics (female libido, female sex hormones). But they attributed the latter characteristics to prolonged and indiscriminate administration of estrogen which they claimed led to deliberate "chemical castration". There was no evidence, however, that the appellant had anything to do with this treatment. The court of appeal held that the operations performed by the appellant were not injurious to him. No useful organs were removed and both operations were intended to adapt the patient to his true psychological sex. The appellant's conviction was accordingly set aside.

14 The text of the judgment was kindly supplied to me by the Argentine Embassy in Pretoria and kindly translated by Dr Mary Catherine McDonald of the Department of Romance Languages of the University of South Africa.

The second case concerned one L (the brother of M), who had had normal external male genitals since early childhood. His behaviour had been that of a woman. The appellant claimed on the basis of a biopsy that there was ovotestis in the patient. The forensic physicians, however, contended that the patient was a male because XY chromosomes were found to be present. Defence physicians testified that the patient was an "intersexual" and that the operation successfully orientated him "bio-psycho-sexo-socially". There was also evidence of various symptoms of female dominance in the hair, voice and deterioration of the male genitals. A spermogram taken prior to the operation revealed azoospermia. While all this could be attributed to the administration of estrogen, it did not preclude other factors such as the endocrine factor.

The third case concerned one P, who had shown signs of feminity since childhood. He was subjected to male hormone treatment but without favourable results. He was found to have marked feminine characteristics, such as wide hips, lack of facial hair and a feminine bone structure but normal external male genitals. The appellant performed conversive surgery upon him and the first operation confirmed his diagnosis of hermaphroditism and ovotestis. According to hormone tests the patient had characteristics of both sexes. The appellant also testified that he had found in the inguinal canals a testicular formation on the left side and an ovary on the right. According to the appellant P was more of a woman than the brothers L and M. There was evidence before the court that the biopsy of a testicle revealed complete spermatogenesis. (This was found by the court not to be inconsistent with the other evidence because it referred to only one testicle.)

Considering the cases of L and P the court came to the conclusion that the convictions had to be quashed. Even if the court were to assume that the operations were injurious to the bodies and health of the patients, there was no proof of *dolus*, i e the intention to wilfully cause bodily injury, or the awareness of such possibility. The court (*per* Judge Victoria) pointed out that the conflicting views expressed by the prosecution and the defence, respectively, were understandable, as the subject-matter was difficult and one in which recent scientific discoveries had led to conflicting and rapidly changing criteria. Even if the appellant had committed an error in good faith, he was not criminally liable provided that he had studied the cases, analysed them and made a decision on the sincere conviction that he had definite reasons for it. "The physician is under a duty to proceed according to what he considers best for his patient and we as judges must be extremely cautious in passing judgment on this." The other judges concurred with these views. In his judgment, Judge Esteves observed that all surgical operations can be said to cause bodily injury of some sort or another and that criminal liability can only be based either on *culpa* or on *dolus*. Much had been made of the designation of the sex of the respective patients on their birth certificates; but male/female are the only designations accepted by the Registry and then they are based on external factors. It would be wrong for a judge to convict upon contradictory medical evidence. It is not simply a question of actions performed by the accused, but of very complicated scientific problems regarding diagnosis and therapeutics and it is not juridically feasible to solve a medical problem. Account must be taken of recent developments in the study of "intersexuals". According to these studies the influence of both sexes in one person is a biological fact. The greater internal influence of one factor in contrast with another external factor makes it difficult to diagnose the true sex of a person, and many eminent physicians differ on this. The appellant had diagnosed the various cases in the light of his knowledge and understanding of such phenomena. His decision to operate cannot be considered irresponsible since his specialised technical ability is highly recognised. The judge referred *inter alia* to the Belgian case of *Dr Fardeau et alii.*[15]

In England and South Africa court decisions were handed down on the validity of

15 *Supra.*

the marriage of a transsexual. These cases are discussed below. In none of these was the lawfulness of the "sex-change" operation as such at issue. As Kennedy and Grubb[16] have pointed out, however, the legality of this type of operation was probably established in *Corbett's* case[17] when the judge, Mr Justice Ormrod, made the following observation: "There is, obviously, room for differences of opinion on the ethical aspects of such operations but, if they are undertaken for genuine therapeutic purposes, it is a matter for the decision of the patient and the doctors concerned. The passing of the Sexual Offences Act 1967, s 1, seems to have removed any legal objections which there might have been to such procedures."[18]

In South Africa quite a number of "sex-change" operations have been performed during the past three decades. Teams consisting of gynaecologists, surgeons, psychiatrists, psychologists and social workers – all highly reputable practitioners – were involved. They discussed their procedures and results at professional meetings and published their views and findings in professional journals. Some of their patients "went public" and received considerable media coverage. Never, to the best of my knowledge, has there been any suggestion of a criminal prosecution of any of these professionals or a suit for damages brought on the basis of an alleged civil wrong. There can be no doubt that the performance of such an operation – or series of operations – in good faith is regarded in South Africa today as not being contrary to the *boni mores* (juristic notions of society) and, therefore, lawful. Support for the view that these operations are lawful, is to be found in the fact that in 1974[19] Parliament made express provision for the alteration of the description of sex in the birth register, of a person "who has undergone a change of sex".[20] The Director-General, Home Affairs, may do so on the recommendation of the Director-General, National Health and Population Development, and may for this purpose call for such medical reports and institute such investigations as he may deem necessary.

A 1971 decision of the German Federal Supreme Court[21] was – according to Giesen[22] – unfavourably inclined towards transsexual surgery, but the case was overruled on constitutional grounds by the German Federal Constitutional Court.[23] In consequence of this decision, the German legislature passed the *Transsexuellengesetz* ("Transsexual Surgery Act").[24] This Act makes provision, first, for a change of a person's given names so as to reflect his or her psychological gender, and secondly, for an official change, post-operatively, of the person's sex entries in all registers.

If it is assumed that the performance of conversive surgery upon transsexuals, subject to certain conditions, is lawful, not all juristic problems connected with transsexualism are solved. Evaluation of the juristic "status" of the transsexual involves considerations separate from the issue of the lawfulness of the operation. As far as matters such as formal amendment of sex in the birth registry, marriages by patients and the lawful wearing of clothes of the "opposite" sex are concerned, the legal position of the patient will in the final analysis depend on whether or not there was in

16 *Medical Law : Text and Materials* (1989) 136.

17 *Corbett v Corbett (otherwise Ashley)* [1970] 2 All ER 33.

18 As Kennedy & Grubb 136 point out, the judge's reference to the Sexual Offences Act "is, perhaps, a little curious since it legalises sexual intercourse between consenting male adults over the age of 21".

19 Act 51 of 1974 which inserted section 7B into the Births, Marriages and Deaths Registration Act 81 of 1963.

20 This provision was enacted shortly after the "re-registration" of the gender description of *Frederica* (the case referred to in note 4 *supra*).

21 BGH, 21 Sept 1971 (IV ZB 61/70) BGHZ 57, 63.

22 D Giesen *International Medical Malpractice Law* (1988) 332 n 116.

23 BVerfG, 11 Oct 1978 BVerfGE 49, 286, FamRZ 1979, 25, and see Giesen *loc cit*. In his *Arzthaftungsrecht – Medical Malpractice Law* (1981) 237 Giesen discussed this case in detail.

24 See E Deutsch *Arztrecht und Arzneimittelrecht* (1983) 172; and Giesen (as referred to in note 22 above).

fact a transformation of sex, or to phrase it perhaps more accurately, whether the patient post-operatively belongs to the sex to which he has orientated himself all along. This raises the problem: "What is sex?" It is not for a jurist to solve this problem. The courts must of necessity be guided by the opinions of experts in the field of medicine and psychiatry. It is sufficient to say that the view that sex is determined exclusively by somatic features, in particular chromosomal findings, is no longer unchallenged. There seems to be a growing body of opinion that a more important criterion is psychological orientation, especially where this is the dominant factor.[25] In the case of the transsexual this orientation may, to a very large extent, have been conditioned by physical and environmental factors. It is therefore not inconceivable that a court of law may be convinced by expert opinion that, despite the chromosomal finding, the person concerned does in fact now belong to the opposite sex.

Legal validity of transsexual's marriage

One of the first cases to deal with the legal status of a marriage entered into by a "converted" transsexual was the 1971 English case of *Corbett v Corbett (otherwise Ashley)*.[26] In this case the court based its decision entirely upon biological criteria. The applicant, a man who married a transsexual who had undergone a "sex-change" operation, applied to court for a decree of nullity, declaring that the ceremony of marriage was void *ab initio*, or alternatively, on the ground of non-consummation. It appeared that at the age of about 21 years the respondent had joined a troupe of male female-impersonators in Paris. By that time he was taking estrogen regularly to encourage the development of breasts and a feminine type of physique. Four years later he underwent conversive surgery, and subsequently had his name changed. Attempts to have his birth certificate amended were unsuccessful.

In the meantime the respondent became acquainted with the petitioner, a married man with transvestite tendencies. The petitioner obtained a divorce from his wife and he and the respondent subsequently went through a marriage ceremony at Gibraltar. A fortnight later the respondent left the petitioner permanently. According to the evidence before the court, there was general agreement among all the medical witnesses on the basic principles and the scientific facts. The court's conclusion was that the respondent was correctly described as a male transsexual, possibly with some comparatively minor abnormality. It was common ground between all the medical witnesses that the biological sexual constitution of an individual was fixed at birth (at the latest) and could not be changed, either by the natural development of organs of the opposite sex, or by medical or surgical means. The respondent's operation therefore could not affect his true sex. Since marriage was essentially a relationship between a man and a woman, the validity of the marriage in the present case depended upon whether the respondent was or was not a woman. Having regard to the essentially heterosexual character of the relationship which was called marriage, the criteria in the court's judgment had to be biological, for even the most extreme degree of transsexualism in a male or the most severe hormonal imbalance which could exist in a person with male chromosomes, male gonads and male genitalia could not reproduce a person who was naturally capable of performing the essential role of a woman in marriage. The court held that these (biological) criteria were decisive and not the psychological factor. For the purpose of determining sex any operation should be ignored.

The court's conclusion, therefore, was that the respondent was not a woman for the purpose of marriage, but a biological male and had been so since birth. It followed that the so-called marriage was void. On the matter of non-consummation of the mar-

25 Compare the note by D A R Green 1970 *New Law Journal* 210.
26 [1970] 2 All ER 33. For criticism of this case, see Van Niekerk *op cit*, Green *op cit*.

riage, the court ruled that the respondent was physically incapable of consummating a marriage because sexual intercourse with the respondent who had an artificial vagina could not possibly be described as *vera copula*. It was the reverse of what was ordinary and was in no sense natural.

In the 1970 South African case of *Jonker v Jonker*,[27] a man who had married a male transsexual who had undergone a series of "sex-change" operations, was granted a restitution order in an action for divorce. However, in view of the fact that the action was not contested, this cannot be regarded as a judgment to the effect that the marriage was legally valid. In fact, when the case was heard, the judge asked the plaintiff's counsel why an application for an annulment of the marriage had not been brought.

In 1976, however, the Witwatersrand Court in *W v W*[28] in a detailed judgment considered the marital status of a married transsexual. It was also an undefended action in which the woman sought a decree of divorce on the ground of the defendant's adultery with another woman. On the evidence adduced in the case, the court was satisfied that the defendant had committed adultery as alleged.

In her particulars of claim, the plaintiff was described as an "adult female". She testified, however, that she had been born and registered as a male. For many years, she said, she had felt herself to be a woman "encased in a male body". She was a homosexual in the sense that she was sexually attracted to persons of the male sex. In 1970, at the age of approximately 27 years, she underwent a "sex-change operation" on psychiatric advice. The purpose and effect of the operation was construction of an artificial vagina and the insertion of a prosthesis which gave her the appearance of having the enlarged breasts of a woman.

Since then she had regarded herself as a female and had passed in society as such. Her sex description in her birth certificate as well as her Christian names were altered. She testified that her husband, the defendant, had been aware of the operation. The marriage had been consummated and the parties had had normal sexual relations. According to her, the breakdown in the marriage was not due to any inadequacy on her part as a woman.

On these facts the court refused to grant a decree of divorce and ordered absolution of the instance. Mr Justice Nestadt held that the plaintiff's evidence did not show that the operation which she had undergone had converted her into a female.

"What it did was to artificially supply her with certain of the attributes of a woman, namely breasts and a vagina-like cavity. This, however, so it was argued, taking into account the fact that the plaintiff was (always) a transsexual and thus psychologically a woman, was sufficient, that in her post-operative state, and in particular, because of her ability to have sex with the defendant, she was capable of fulfilling the essential role of a woman in marriage (and this, despite her inability to procreate) and that it would be anomalous to classify the plaintiff as a male when she had the physical and psychological attributes of a female and was socially accepted as, and looked like, a woman."

The judge held that to accede to that argument would be to subvert the requirements of our law that a valid marriage requires the parties to be of the opposite sex. It seeks to overcome the impliedly admitted impossibility of changing one's sex by the argument that post-operatively the patient is no longer an effective male but is, on the contrary, now capable of having sexual intercourse with a male in the normal manner.

The judge said that the issue was not whether, after the operation, the plaintiff was an effective male, nor whether she looked like a female (which she did), nor whether society had accepted her as a female, nor whether she was capable of having sex with

27 For particulars of this case, see *The Star*, Johannesburg 26 February 1970; *Die Beeld* 1 March 1970; *Sunday Times*, Johannesburg 1 March 1970.

28 1976 (2) SA 308 (W). See also *Simms v Simms* 1981 (4) SA 186 (D).

a male; the issue was whether the plaintiff at the time of the marriage had been a woman.

"I find no justification, however desirable it may be, for finding that a person in the position of the plaintiff was a woman when she married the defendant where, on the evidence, she was a male prior to her operation but which the evidence does not reveal had changed her sex. Imitation cannot be equated with actual transformation. If what I may call this pseudo-type of woman is, for the purposes of the marriage, properly to be regarded as a female, then in the absence of medical evidence justifying such a finding, the intervention of the legislature would be necessary," the judge said.

The judge then referred to section 7B of the Births, Marriages and Deaths Registration Act[29] (which was introduced into the Act in 1974[30] to enable "converted" transsexuals to officially "re-register" as the opposite sex). It would appear that the Legislature does recognise the factual possibility of a change of sex, the judge observed, but added that how, if in fact, cases to come confirm that a change of sex is not possible, the section will be interpreted, lay beyond the scope of the judgment.

Granting absolution of the instance, the judge intimated that if the pleadings were properly amended, he would on the basis of his finding that the plaintiff was a male prior to the operation, annul the marriage.

Attention must be drawn to the fact that in *W v W* no medical evidence was adduced in court. The court was clearly influenced by the English judgment in *Corbett v Corbett (otherwise Ashley)*.

The question may be asked whether expert evidence on the psychological inclination of the transsexual might have led to a different verdict. In psychiatric literature the dilemma of the transsexual has been described in detail. The transsexual is no true homosexual. He is psychologically committed totally, often from early childhood, to the opposite somatic sex. The young child with the body of a girl already sees herself as a boy and does not wish to be anything else. As the years advance, it becomes even more difficult for her to assume the compulsory female role. Only after a series of operations which give her the physical appearance of a male, "he" feels properly adjusted to the social environment for the first time. Some converted transsexuals enter into a marriage which creates a lasting bond even in the absence of a possibility of procreation.

Regrettably, it must be observed with the necessary respect, the decision in *W v W* does not contribute to a solution of the dilemma of the transsexual, which quite clearly was the very objective sought to be achieved by the Legislature with section 7B of the Births, Marriages and Deaths Registration Act.

In contrast with *Corbett* and *W v W* an American court in the 1976 case of *M T v J T*[31] upheld a marriage between two biological males and required the "husband" to pay spousal support to the "wife" since the male spouse had become physically, psychologically and anatomically female. The court held that where a transsexual was born with the physical characteristics of a male, but successful reassignment surgery harmonised her gender and genitalia so that she became fully capable of sexual activity as a woman, such a transsexual became a member of the female sex for marital purposes. Her subsequent marriage to a male, accordingly was not void.

The *Corbett* court's approach to transsexualism was reaffirmed when the English Court of Appeal in 1983 in *R v Tan*[32] extended the legal determination of sexual identity as held in the former case to criminal law. The case concerned a criminal charge

29 Act 81 of 1963.
30 By section 1(1) Act 51 of 1974.
31 355 A2d 204 (NJ 1976), and see Giesen (as referred to in note 22 above).
32 [1983] 2 All ER 12 (CA); [1983] QBD 1953 (CA). The case is discussed by J Taitz "The Legal Determination of the Sexual Identity of a Post-Operative Transsexual Seen as a Human Rights Issue" 7 *Med Law* 467 (1989) 470.

brought against one Ms G for living on the earnings of prostitution, an offence which can be committed only by a male. G's defence was that she was a post-operative female. Applying the *Corbett* test, the court refused to uphold her defence and found that G was a male.

Conclusion

The changing outlook on transsexualism reflected in some of the court decisions and a few statutory provisions discussed above, hold the promise of a more favourable legal climate for transsexuals. But not all problems have been solved.

A good deal of scepticism about the eventual success of transsexual surgery remains. In August 1979 at Johns Hopkins Hospital in Baltimore, USA, doctors announced that they were abandoning the surgery for all but hermaphrodites (those born with male and female organs). The reason was that a new study had found no difference in long-term adjustment between transsexuals who go under the scalpel and those who do not. Dr Jon K Meyer, a psychiatrist connected with the hospital, expressed the opinion that "the surgery serves as a palliative measure ... [but] it does not cure what is essentially a psychiatric disturbance".[33]

I discussed this development with the Pretoria gynaecologist, Dr Meredith Botes, shortly before his untimely death in 1980. Dr Botes had treated a number of transsexuals and developed a special interest in the syndrome.[34] He told me that he regarded his success rate as high and could not agree with the latest outlook at Johns Hopkins.

But in 1981 Professor Max Feldman, psychiatrist of Johannesburg, expressed the opinion that except for the hermaphrodite, "so-called 'sex-change' operations ... in fact are not sex-change but *gender change* procedures". He seemed to be sceptical, and held the view that in the case of "gender change" in persons not of intersex, the abandonment of "mutilative surgery" was to be welcomed.[35]

In 1983 J Pellegrin and three collaborators of the Institut Regional de Medecine Legale et de Medecine Sociale in Montpellier, France, posed the question whether individuals who have undergone a surgical transformation and effected a change in civil status will acquire the balance they hoped for. Pellegrin *et al* are pessimistic and feel that the "psychism of an already traumatised individual" will be put under constraints that will be equally strong after the change in civil status, due to "a misleading mutilation" which, after all, will be "the outcome of a fraud".[36]

What is beyond doubt, however, is the legality of operations and medical treatment intended to assist the hermaphrodite to assume the desired gender identity.[37]

In ending this brief discussion of transsexualism I want to quote the views of two authors.

D A R Green,[38] in commenting on *Corbett's* case, posed the following questions: "What does it comfort any of us to insist that an individual shall be a man, when for all the purposes of ordinary life that individual can only be, and be recognised, as a woman? What pride can there be for a law which vetoes the attitudes dictated by ordinary humanity?"

And Jerold Taitz,[39] in discussing the legal determination of sexual identity of a post-operative transsexual seen as a human rights issue, had this to say: "The plight of

33 See *Time* magazine, 27 August 1979.
34 See his paper "Wat is Transseksualisme?" *Geneeskunde* of 26/8/1972 page 156.
35 See (1981) 98 *SALJ* 111.
36 J Pellegrin *et al* "Contribution of Medico-legal Expertise to the New Tendencies of the Jurisprudence with regard to Transsexualism" *Newsletter, International Academy of Legal Medicine and Social Medicine* No. 5, Dec 1983.
37 E Kahn "The True Hermaphrodite – Of No Sex" (1981) 98 *SALJ* 111.
38 See note 25 above.
39 See note 32 above.

transsexuals is a sad one. They undergo dangerous and mutilating surgery for therapeutic purposes, with the aim of becoming integrated and responsible members of society, only to find at the conclusion of the treatment that they are not recognised by the law as members of their post-operative sex."[40]

Adapted from a paper read at the Second World Meeting on Medical Law held in Washington DC, in August 1970. The author gratefully acknowledges the generous support of the Human Sciences Research Council and the University of South Africa which enabled him to attend the meeting. The paper in its original form was published in (1970) 3 CILSA *348.*

40 For other South African contributions to the debate, see J Taitz "Legal Consequences of a Sex Change – A Judicial Dilemma" (1980) 97 *SALJ* 65; P J Thomas "Can the Lawyer keep up with the Doctor?" (1980) 97 *SALJ* 77; P D Gilson *Gender Dysphoria Syndrome : Medical Aspects and Legal Consequences* (LLM thesis, Univ of Natal, 1985).

PART XI

Medical negligence, malpractice liability

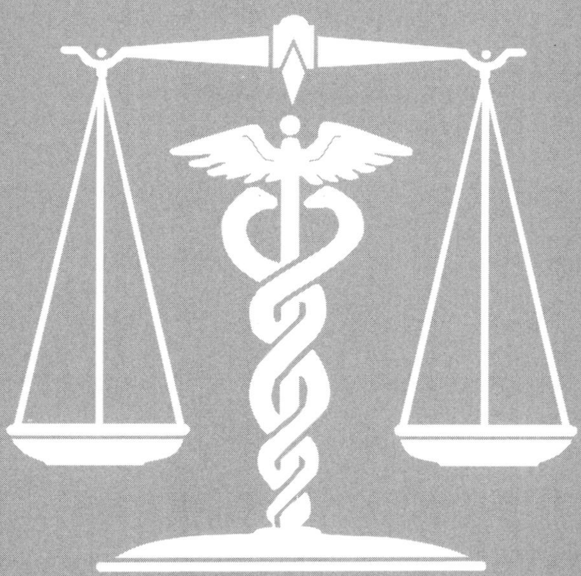

37 Medical malpractice liability: doctor, insure thyself!

The size and scope of the risk

The concept of medical malpractice liability is not narrowly confined to liability for damages flowing from professional negligence. It also embraces other causes of action, such as : liability for assault in the form of an operation performed properly and skilfully on a patient without his informed consent; liability for invasion of a patient's privacy by an unwarranted disclosure to outsiders of medical details pertaining to the patient; liability for the performance of an altogether unnecessary operation, although it was done with due care and skill; liability for breach of contract in failing to perform an operation agreed upon, which failure has caused financial loss for the patient.[1] In this section of the book, however, attention is directed in particular to medical negligence.

The increasing incidence of malpractice litigation in Western countries seems to be a trend of our time. Without a doubt, the unquestionable "leader" in the field is the USA. By 1964 one out of seven doctors in the US had already been sued; in California, it was said, the figure was one out of every four.[2] In 1983, the figure for the USA as a whole was said to be 16 out of every hundred doctors.[3]

The consequences are well known:

- soaring insurance premiums (some specialists in the USA allegedly pay up to $50 000 a year) being passed on to the patients;
- reluctance on the part of doctors to become involved in unknown cases of accidental injury;
- over-cautiousness on the part of doctors and time-consuming over-documentation of cases;
- some doctors refusing to attend lawyers or their families!

The situation in South Africa is not really comparable to that of the USA. A very small number of malpractice cases are brought to trial in our courts, but they represent only a minute percentage of cases in which attorneys are consulted by patients with real or imaginary complaints. Most claims pressed are settled out of court, the incentive to settle being very strong on both sides.

Yet the incidence of malpractice litigation in South Africa seems to be rising. According to figures supplied by K Simons[4] to the 1977 Medical Congress in Bloemfontein, the ratio of requests by South African doctors to the Medical Protection Society and the Medical Defence Union, for legal assistance in the period 1968 to 1976, rose from 1 per 522 doctors to 1 per 108 doctors – an increase of almost five times in eight years. In 1986 the relevant figures were 1 per 48 doctors and in 1988 1 per 22.[5] It should be mentioned that not all these requests for legal assistance relate to patient

1 See e g *Administrator, Natal v Edouard* 1990 (3) SA 581 (A). The case is discussed above 177.
2 This figure was supplied in 1964 by J C Steincipher "Survey of Medical Professional Liability in Washington" 39 *Washington Law Review* 704 (1964).
3 Spring and Tennenhouse "Radiology Malpractice Lawsuits : California Jury Verdicts" 1986 *Radiology* 159 : 811-814.
4 *De Jure*, April 1978, 123.
5 Personal communication to me by a MASA representative. See also 78 *S Afr Med J*, 226 (18 Aug 1990).

threats to bring suit for alleged malpractice. The protection societies advise doctors on professional legal issues in general as well as on complaints relating to alleged unprofessional conduct.

There is of course no evidence of increasing negligence on the part of doctors! On the contrary, medical standards are generally very high. By the very nature of their work, doctors are probably more careful than members of most other professions.

What then are the reasons for the increase?

Apart from the normal population increase, factors such as the following have been suggested:[6]

Medicine is a high-risk profession, like that of the airline pilot; a slight error may have disastrous consequences. Medical treatment directly involves the health and body – and sometimes the life – of the patient. A number of local cases may be cited of unfortunate results following alleged negligent treatment.

The man in the street has perhaps become conditioned to demand more from medicine. The mass media constantly offer him romanticised write-ups on the marvels of modern medicine. At the same time, the media give great publicity to medical mishaps. Reports on malpractice trials undoubtedly serve as a spur for other aggrieved patients to contemplate legal action.

We live in the age of human rights and the consumer society. Today's man in the street is more demanding about getting quality products and quality service – and if these fall short of his demands, he may sue.

In the past the doctor's social image was second to none. Today he must share the "glamour" of prestige with spacemen, nuclear scientists and film actors – not to mention pop stars.

The image of the doctor as the benevolent father figure has undergone change. In the eyes of many a patient he is seen rather as the impersonal super-technician, the kind of man whom you can call upon to account in court for his conduct if he has slipped. Medical paternalism is giving way to patient autonomy.

Legal services have been improved. Today there are big firms of attorneys who themselves have become super-specialists. Every respectable firm in this country boasts one or more Supreme Court specialists. In the big cities some advocates may even develop a specialised practice to some extent. Following the example of other countries, we have introduced into South Africa a meritorious legal-aid system whereby indigent persons are financially enabled to litigate.

The plaintiff – or at least his attorney – knows that the real defendant in the majority of cases is not so much the doctor who has allegedly erred, but an insurance company – "a giant of concrete and glass with millions at its disposal"[7] – or a protection society with a fistful of rands.

Yet there are special reasons why malpractice litigation in South Africa will probably never reach the pandemic proportions of the USA.

Our law has undeniably assumed a somewhat protective attitude towards the medical profession in general. If one reads the older reported decisions handed down against doctors, an almost apologetic note can be detected.

The 1924 decision of the Appellate Division in *Van Wyk v Lewis*[8] still stands unchallenged after almost seven decades. This is the case of the swab which was sewn up in a patient.

This celebrated ruling by a three-judge appellate bench has functioned as a protective shield as far as the doctor is concerned. It can indeed be described as the legal charter safeguarding the doctor against unduly stringent malpractice liability. With

6 See also S A Strauss "Geneesheer, Pasiënt en die Reg : 'n Delikate Driehoek" 1987 (1) *TSAR* 1.
7 To paraphrase the words of A Klass.
8 1924 AD 438. The case is discussed more fully *infra* 270.

a slender majority to two against one, the Appeal Court held in effect that the rule of *res ipsa loquitur* does not apply to medical situations. The Latin words quoted, mean: "the matter speaks for itself". Generally speaking, in the law of negligence this rule is a great boon to the plaintiff. If a motorist were to collide with a parked vehicle, it would raise an inference of negligence on the part of the motorist which he will have to disprove. The same fundamental notion underlies the rule in the law of contract that where a newly built house cracks, it is for the builder to convince the court that the cracks are not attributable to his defective workmanship.[9]

But even where a swab is post-operatively sewn up in a patient, there is no presumption of negligence on the part of the doctor, it was ruled in the *Van Wyk* case. "The maxim *res ipsa loquitur* has no application to cases of this kind," Mr Justice Kotze said. The onus therefore remains on the patient to prove his case on a preponderance of probabilities. The nature of the occurrence is an important element in deciding whether there was a lack of reasonable care and skill, but, said Chief Justice Innes, "it must be considered along with the other evidence in the case".

If ever the medical profession in this country were to erect a monument to the great men of medicine, the names of the two majority judges, Chief Justice Sir James Rose Innes and Appellate Judge Sir Johannes Wilhelmus Kotze, must be inscribed on it in golden letters!

Van Wyk v Lewis has been strongly criticised[10] but after all these years it still reigns supreme. In *Pringle's* case[11] (1988), a Witwatersrand judge once again held that there was no room for application of *res ipsa loquitur* in a medical negligence suit. "The maxim," said the judge, "could only be invoked where the negligence alleged depends on absolutes."

In the USA *res ipsa loquitur* has gained a strong foothold and has become a powerful tool in the hands of lawyers acting for dissatisfied patients. There it has developed into a "rule of sympathy" for the patient, used – so it has been said – to combat the so-called "conspiracy of silence" among doctors.[12]

Another difference between our system and that applying in American jurisdictions, is that the contingent fee is not allowed here. In those jurisdictions where the lawyer may render his services on a commission basis, he may contract with his client for a percentage of the award made by the court – e g one-third or one-half. If the case is won, the lawyer's cut may be a handsome amount.

In South African law, the *pactum de quota litis* is still a legal swear-word and the legal practitioner who makes himself guilty of it, may be disbarred.

The most powerful deterrent against litigation in South Africa is the risk that the plaintiff runs of an order of costs being made against him if his case fails. The general rule in our system is that the loser pays the costs, i e his own legal costs as well as the taxed costs of his opponent on the so-called "party and party" scale. The costs of a major Supreme Court trial may run into tens of thousands of rands.

It is a trite saying among lawyers that only the very rich or the very poor can afford the luxury of losing a lawsuit: the poor because they have nothing to lose.

The cost factor therefore constitutes a powerful incentive for settlement of cases out of court. The plaintiff may issue summons and take the defendant to the very doors of the court. But by that time the urge to settle gets stronger by the minute.

The defendant doctor may also be anxious to settle, if not because of the bad publicity, then to avoid the situation where he does obtain judgment in his favour, but

9 *Hughes v Fletcher* 1957 (1) SA 326 (SR).

10 See e g S A Strauss & M J Strydom *Die Suid-Afrikaanse Geneeskundige Reg* (1967) 279; Cynthia Birrer *The Medical Cop-out* (1976) 118-119.

11 *Pringle v Administrator, Transvaal* 1990 (2) SA 379 (W). Judgment in the case was delivered in 1988. The case is discussed in detail below 282.

12 C Morris "Malpractice: Medical – The Important Events of the Last Two Years" 30 *Insurance Counsel Journal* 44 (1963).

finds himself stuck with an order of costs in his favour which proves to be unenforceable against an impecunious plaintiff. This happened to the successful Dr Lewis of *Van Wyk v Lewis* fame. His victory was pyrrhic. Miss van Wyk had sued *in forma pauperis*[13] and claimed £2 000 damages. Dr Lewis was not insured against professional liability and had to pay his own legal costs which amounted to approximately £2 000 – the equivalent of perhaps R60 000 or more in today's currency value. (Insurance against liability would have cost him one guinea[14] in those days.)[15]

It is absolutely imperative for medical practitioners to obtain malpractice cover. Statistically the risk of an adverse court order is still very small. Moreover, our courts are relatively conservative in their awards for damages where the plaintiff succeeds in proving his case. The biggest court award on record is R93 482, made in 1988 in *Pringle's*[16] case, following the tearing of the vena cava in the course of a mediastinoscopy which resulted ultimately in the plaintiff losing her job. But medical protection society membership or insurance is perhaps of even greater importance to meet eventual legal costs. (The total costs of a major malpractice suit in Cape Town in the middle seventies were estimated at about R100 000: the unsuccessful plaintiff was liable for these.)

In 1979, in the case of *Blyth v Van den Heever*,[17] the Appellate Division reversed a favourable judgment handed down by the trial court, and ordered the doctor to pay the patient damages of R34 542 – a sum that must be paltry in comparison with the costs of the suit, which the doctor was likewise ordered to pay.

Membership of a medical protection society obtainable through the Medical Association of South Africa (MASA) currently (1991) costs R850 a year in the case of senior practitioners[18] and provides cover for an unlimited[19] amount of liability. This is low compared with premiums in some other countries and compared with insurance for certain other risks.

Incidentally: hospital employees should check on whether they themselves are covered in any way by the hospital's insurance scheme[20]. It is not always possible for an employee to hide behind the hospital authority. True, the latter will be vicariously liable for its employee's negligence, but that does not mean the employee may not be sued individually or jointly with the employer. Moreover, by law the employer has a right of recourse against the employee for any loss suffered on account of his negligence. There is also no guarantee that the employer will financially back up an employee in conducting his defence in court. Generally speaking, employers take *ad hoc* decisions on whether or not they will support an employee in this way. The State makes its decision in accordance with a set of fixed policy guidelines.

Because of the problems confronting a prospective plaintiff in proving the doctor was negligent, plaintiffs sometimes allege as an alternative cause of action – or even as the main cause of action – absence of informed consent, which involves simple fac-

13 This is the legal procedure whereby an impecunious person is enabled to sue.

14 A guinea was the equivalent of 21 shillings and a shilling became ten cents when we decimalised in 1961. A guinea of the early twenties would be worth about R30 or R40 in today's currency value.

15 Facts obtained from the paper by R Schaffer entitled "The Queenstown Swab Case 1923", delivered before the 1977 Congress of the SA Medical Association; a summary was published in the official *Summaries of Papers* (no 127).

16 See note 11 above.

17 1980 (1) SA 191 (A). The case is discussed below 257.

18 This is the membership fee payable by a medical practitioner as from his fifth year of practice. During internship (i e the first year of practice) the fee is R80, during the second year R175, the third year R315 and the fourth year R440. The hospital rate is R710. For senior dentists, the Medical Protection Society rate is R150 and that of the Medical Defence Union R320. The figures quoted are those applicable in February 1991 and were kindly supplied by the Medical Association of South Africa.

19 The cover provided is subject to the Society's articles of association whereby its council is given the right to restrict or decline indemnity in a case.

20 Registered nurses whose membership fees are paid up, are automatically covered by the SA Nursing Association's indemnity insurance scheme.

tual issues. Although most malpractice cases decided in South Africa in the last decade or two have been unspectacular from the point of view of the patient, the mere fact that such cases are being brought, reaffirms the absolute necessity for the doctor to make provision for professional indemnity.

Protection society membership or commercial insurance?

Before taking out commercial indemnity insurance – and abandoning membership of a mutual organisation – the doctor should take a good and sober look at the terms and conditions of the policy.

The system of medical indemnity offered by an organisation such as the Medical Protection Society (MPS) differs in material respects from that offered by commercial insurers. The MPS is a non-profit mutual organisation of doctors and dentists with almost 100 years' experience of medico-legal problems. The Society has no shareholders who seek a profit on their investments.

The cover provided by the MPS is unlimited for legal problems arising from medical practice. Commercial insurers, on the other hand, will normally provide limited cover only.

The small print of a commercial insurance policy may well exclude cover in respect of activities involving a contravention of criminal law. A classical case is that of *Lourens N O v Colonial Mutual Life Assurance Society Ltd*[21] : Mr V had taken out a life insurance policy with an accident benefit of R30 000 payable in the event of death resulting from injury caused by "a violent, external and visible accident". In terms of the policy the benefit was excluded, however, in respect of death "caused while the insured life was contravening the criminal law".

V died in a road accident when his car collided head-on with another vehicle. The collision occurred when he was overtaking a vehicle on a rise. His view of approaching traffic was restricted and he drove on the right hand side of a barrier line. In so driving he committed at least five contraventions of the Road Traffic Ordinance. The executor of V's estate sued the insurance company for payment of the R30 000 benefit, but was met with the defence that the company was not liable because V's death had been caused by injuries sustained "while he was contravening the criminal law".

On behalf of the executor it was contended that the company's defence would lead to an absurd result which would "be subversive of the whole purpose of the insurance effected by the policy". Counsel argued that the insured who negligently fails to pay his TV licence, or parks his car on a yellow line, or has an illegal number of crayfish in the boot of his car, and is accidentally killed while these "crimes" are committed, will not be covered by the policy. The use of the words "violent, external and visible", it was argued, would convey to the ordinary man signing the insurance document that, whatever else the policy might cover, he would be covered if involved in a road accident.

The provincial court nevertheless upheld the company's defence and the case went on appeal to the Appeal Court which (by a majority ruling of three judges against two) confirmed the provincial decision. It was held that the exception clause applied whenever the criminal law is contravened, irrespective of the relevance, nature and extent of the contravention. The deceased's estate could accordingly not claim the benefit.

Medical practice is affected by many statutory provisions as well as the common law, and many actions of a doctor which may result in civil liability or a disciplinary inquiry may also involve a contravention of criminal law. A prime example is medical negligence which results in the death of the patient and would constitute the criminal offence of culpable homicide. A clause of the kind in *Lourens's* case, in a professional

21 1986 (3) SA 373 (A).

indemnity policy, can accordingly have the effect that a commercial insurance company will deny liability – leaving the doctor without cover in the very situation where he desperately needs cover. The MPS, on the other hand, will invariably come to the rescue of the doctor in a case of medical negligence if he has taken out membership of the Society.

There is another aspect of major importance to doctors in considering taking out indemnity insurance. The question should be asked: "Supposing I have not renewed my policy and I am sued for an incident that occurred a year or two ago when my policy was still valid, will I be covered?" Commercial insurers may make cover conditional upon the policy still being valid *at the time the insured person is sued.* The Medical Protection Society, on the other hand, provides cover even if membership has lapsed, provided the membership dues were paid up at the time the incident which led to a claim, occurred.

It is to be noted that the MPS has ample funds in the Republic to cover the liabilities of its members. The subscription levels are not determined by what happens in the UK or the US; they are based solely on the claims experience in South Africa. Moreover, MPS members have access to a highly reputable firm of attorneys which has specialised for many years in medico-legal and ethical matters.

During the mid-1960s when professional liability insurance was provided by agreement with a commercial insurance company, the insurers summarily suspended operations after an adverse judgment required them to pay a large sum. No other South African insurers were prepared, at the time, to provide such a service and the MASA entered into an agreement with the medical protection societies which have since provided expert assistance to thousands of doctors working in South Africa. It is to be noted that the societies also provide legal assistance to doctors involved in SAMDC disciplinary inquiries.

38 "Mere" error of judgment may constitute negligence

Although judgments of the English courts generally do not constitute binding precedents for our courts, they have always had considerable persuasive force and are often cited by our judges. The 1981 decision of the English House of Lords in *Whitehouse v Jordan and Another*[1] is of special significance because it lays down the principle that it is not *per se* a defence for a medical practitioner, charged with negligence, to say that his act amounted to a mere error of judgment.

In this case the English Court of Appeal overruled a decision by a trial judge against a doctor. Finding in favour of the defendant, Lord Justice Denning (one of the three judges hearing the appeal), *inter alia* made the following statement: "We must say, and say firmly, that, in a professional man an error of judgment is not negligent."

The plaintiff took the case on further appeal to the House of Lords which affirmed the judgment of the Court of Appeal. However, the Law Lords who tried the final appeal, were critical of the statement by Lord Justice Denning quoted above. Lord Fraser of Tullybelton regarded it as an inaccurate statement of the law. "Having regard to the context," he said, "I think Lord Denning M R must have meant to say that an error of judgment 'is not *necessarily* negligent.'"

Lord Fraser continued: "Merely to describe something as an error of judgment tells us nothing about whether it is negligent or not. The true position is that an error of judgment may, or may not, be negligent; it depends on the nature of the error. If it is one that would not have been made by a reasonably competent professional man professing to have the standard and type of skill that the defendant held himself out as having, and acting with ordinary care, might have made, then it is not negligence."

The facts of the case will be of interest to general practitioners, and in particular to gynaecologists and obstetricians.

Mr J, a senior hospital registrar, took charge of a baby's delivery after the mother had been in labour for a considerable time. The notes made by Professor M, the consultant professor in charge of the hospital maternity unit, identified the pregnancy as likely to be difficult and noted that a "trial of forceps" delivery would have to be tried before proceeding to delivery by Caesarian section.

Having examined the mother, Mr J embarked on a trial of forceps delivery. He pulled on the baby six times with the forceps coincident with the mother's contractions, but when there was no movement on the fifth and sixth pulls he decided, some 25 minutes after the commencement of the procedure, to abandon it and to proceed to a Caesarian section. He then quickly and competently delivered the baby.

The child was found soon after the delivery to have sustained severe brain damage due to asphyxia. Legal action was brought on behalf of the child for damages for negligence on the allegation that Mr J had pulled too long and too hard on the baby's head, thereby causing the brain damage.

At the trial the mother gave evidence that she was "lifted off" the bed by the application of the forceps and although that description of what happened was rejected by the judge as being clinically impossible, on the suggestion of an expert witness he interpreted it to mean that the forceps were applied with such force that she was

1 [1981] 1 All ER 267 (HL).

pulled towards the bottom of the bed in a manner inconsistent with a properly carried out trial of forceps.

Mr J testified that when there was no progress on the fifth pull of the forceps he pulled once more to see if he could ease the head past what might have been only a minimal obstruction but as there was no further progress he decided to proceed to Caesarian section and he easily pushed the head slightly upwards to effect the Caesarian section. He denied that the head was wedged or stuck prior to the Caesarian section. The judge interpreted this evidence to mean that he had pulled too long and too hard, causing the head to become wedged or stuck.

Professor M was of the opinion that the mother had received correct and skilled treatment. However, in his report he referred three times to "disimpaction" of the head prior to the Caesarian section. At the trial the professor testified that he had used that term as meaning no more than that a gentle push of the head up the birth canal was needed before proceeding to the Caesarian section.

There was no unanimity of opinions among the other medical experts as to the meaning of the term "impacted" or whether it meant that there had been excessive or unprofessional traction with the forceps. The evidence of the medical experts made it clear, however, that the amount of force to be properly used in a trial of forceps was a matter of clinical judgment, although there should be no attempt to pull the foetus past a bony obstruction, and if the head became so stuck as to cause asphyxia, excessive force had been used.

The judge came to the conclusion that Mr J had pulled too long and too hard on the forceps so that the baby's head had become wedged or stuck, and that in so doing or in getting the head unwedged he had negligently caused the baby's asphyxia. A substantial amount of damages (£100 000) was awarded to the child.

However, the Court of Appeal reversed the judge's decision on the grounds that (i) if the judge's finding that the defendant pulled too long and too hard with the forceps was accepted, that amounted only to an error of clinical judgment and as such was not negligence in law, and (ii) in any event the judge's decision was based on an unjustified interpretation of the evidence.

As I have mentioned, the Appeal Court's decision was affirmed by the House of Lords, although not on exactly the same legal grounds as were advanced by the Appeal Court. But in essence the Law Lords supported the Appeal Court's finding that the evidence did not justify the inference that Mr J negligently pulled too hard and too long with the forceps.

The Law Lords ruled that the test whether a surgeon has been negligent is whether he has failed to measure up in any respect, whether in clinical judgment or otherwise, to the standard of the ordinary skilled surgeon exercising and professing to have the special skill of a surgeon.

The consensus of the Law Lords' opinion was that to "say that a surgeon has committed an error of clinical judgment is wholly ambiguous and does not indicate whether he has been negligent, for while some errors or clinical judgment may be completely consistent with the due exercise of professional skill, other acts or omissions in the course of exercising clinical judgment may be so glaringly below proper standards as to make a finding of negligence inevitable".

In an earlier English case, *Hatcher v Black and Others,*[2] the judge instructed the jury not to find a doctor guilty of negligence simply "because in a matter of opinion he makes an error of judgment".

In a 1957 South African case, *Esterhuizen v Administrator, Transvaal,*[3] a hospital authority was sued for damages in respect of injuries sustained by a youthful patient as a result of excessive radiological treatment administered for cancer. The defen-

2 QB case, 30 June 1954; a report of the case appeared in *The Times* (London), 2 July 1954.
3 1957 (3) SA 710 (T).

dant sought to advance the defence, *inter alia*, that if there had been any error on the part of the doctor, it was an error of judgment "in a matter of opinion". On the facts of the case, however, the court found that the patient's misfortune had not been occasioned by an error of judgment, but by actions on the part of the therapist which fell short of ordinary care and diligence.

In the 1988 case of *Pringle v Administrator, Transvaal*[4] in which the same hospital authority was sued for damages following the tearing of the patient's vena cava in the course of a mediastinoscopy, the question likewise arose whether the surgeon committed an error of clinical judgment. Referring to the *Whitehouse* case, the court pointed out that there was no suggestion that any act or omission of the surgeon was so glaringly below proper standards as to make the finding of negligence inevitable. The court found, however, that the amount of force applied by the surgeon was excessive and that he had acted negligently.

4 1990 (2) SA 379 (W). The case, which was decided in 1988, is discussed below 282.

39 Legal liability for a wrong diagnosis

A wrong diagnosis may result in a doctor being held liable for damages. In itself the wrong diagnosis can hardly render the doctor liable, but the diagnosis may be causally responsible for wrong treatment being given to a patient or the patient suffering injury in another manner.

Whether or not the doctor is liable for damages, will in the final analysis depend on whether the patient has succeeded in proving negligence on the part of the doctor. Moreover, the patient must show that the doctor's negligence was the proximate cause of the damage suffered by him.

A case in point is the 1938 Rhodesian case of *Rautenbach*.[1] A married woman consulted a doctor who made a diagnosis of venereal disease, of which he also informed the woman's husband at a later stage. (His diagnosis was subsequently disputed by another doctor.) The woman was then ill-treated by her husband and ultimately deserted by him. She claimed she had suffered damage in the form of ill-treatment and desertion by her husband as a result of the negligent diagnosis. The court held, however, that even if the doctor had in fact been negligent, such damage was legally too remote and could not be recovered from the doctor.

No inference of negligence can be made merely on the basis that the diagnosis was wrong. The courts have time and again pointed out how difficult it is to make a correct diagnosis. The language of the body is limited and the range of possible diseases almost limitless.

As long ago as 1914 the South African Appeal Court declared in *Mitchell v Dixon*[2]: "No human being is infallible: and in the present state of science, even the most eminent specialist may be at fault in detecting the true nature of a diseased condition. A practitioner can only be held liable in this respect, if his diagnosis is so palpably wrong as to prove negligence, that is to say, if his mistake is of such a nature as to imply an absence of reasonable skill and care on his part, regard being had to the ordinary level of skill in his profession."

This dictum still holds good today, although medical science has made tremendous strides since 1914 and today's technological aids are vastly superior to those in 1914. Despite the advances of our century, medicine still is not – and probably never will be – an exact science comparable to mathematics. Much depends on the skill and experience of the individual practitioner.

Moreover, the standard of care required of a doctor is not the highest possible degree of professional skill, but reasonable skill and care. This principle was again reaffirmed in a 1976 South African case, *Buls v Tsatsarolakis.*[3] The patient, a bricklayer, had injured his wrist. He went to hospital and was examined by the casualty officer on duty, who had X-rays taken but found no evidence of a fracture. Subsequently, the patient consulted a private specialist orthopaedic surgeon, who referred him for X-rays, and these revealed a fracture of the scaphoid bone of the right wrist. On the evidence the court held that the casualty officer could not be accused of negligence. Ac-

1 *Ex parte Rautenbach* 1938 SR 150.
2 1914 AD 519.
3 1976 (2) SA 89 (T).

cording to medical evidence his conduct was that which one would have expected from an ordinary casualty officer.

In a 1958 English decision, *Crivon v Barnett Group Hospital Management Committee,*[4] the judge made the following comment: "Unfortunate as it was that there was a wrong diagnosis, it was one of those misadventures, one of those chances, that life holds for people."

If a doctor were to fail in observing proper standards of care in examining a patient or if the doctor knows he is not properly equipped at all to make a proper examination, and fails to refer the patient to a colleague who is so equipped, the doctor may of course be held liable. A number of cases are reported where doctors were held liable because of such lack of care.[5] In a 1980 case, *Blyth v Van den Heever,*[6] a doctor was held liable for damages for having failed to diagnose an impending ischemia in the arm of a patient upon whom he had performed an operation.

It must also be pointed out that a doctor may be held liable for failure to inform a patient of the diagnosis, where the circumstances are such that it would be reasonably necessary to inform the patient in order to bring to his attention the need of taking certain precautions or to take certain positive measures to protect his health.[7]

4 *The Times* (London) 19 November 1959.
5 Cf S A Strauss & M J Strydom *S A Geneeskundige Reg* 292 *et seq.*
6 1980 (1) SA 191 (A). The case is discussed fully below 257.
7 Strauss & Strydom 295.

40 The doctor's liability for dangerous side-effects of penicillin

The following question was put to me:

"Recently I treated a child who was allergic to penicillin for a lung abscess with an oral antibiotic. The child was brought in by his mother who was always careful to mention the allergy. One Saturday afternoon, the child was brought in by a relative when no nursing staff was present. I was in a hurry to catch a plane and in the rush I completely forgot that the child was allergic and gave him an injection.

"Only when I was sitting in the plane did I realise that I had administered penicillin to a patient who was allergic. Since the patient's address was unknown to me, I had a most troubled weekend. Fortunately, however, there was no reaction, and the patient was brought in to me by the mother on Monday and she told me that the injection had done him a world of good!

"My question is this: will a doctor, acting in a harassed situation, with no records available, and not being cautioned by the patient (or by the adult bringing in a juvenile patient) be considered to be negligent, and in the event of death arising from such a situation, be held responsible for the patient's death?"

My answer is as follows:

The facts as described raise a number of interesting aspects. The first question to be considered is whether the doctor should have attended the child at all, that Saturday afternoon.

In the absence of an emergency there is generally no legal duty upon a doctor to attend a patient brought to him – even if he has treated that patient before – unless the patient is undergoing a form of treatment carried out over a period, in which case the doctor may not simply abandon the patient.[1]

If another doctor had been available, it would have been wise to refer the relative who brought in the child, to such doctor. (From the facts provided it is not quite clear whether another doctor was available – the address given indicates that the doctor practises in a country town.)

Assuming that another doctor was not available, the doctor consulted ought at least to have taken the precaution of ascertaining whether or not the child was allergic to penicillin. This he had to do either by checking his records or enquiring from the person who brought the patient.

Although I am mindful of the circumstances – in particular that the doctor was in a hurry to catch a plane – it must nevertheless be stated that the use of penicillin will today *prima facie* be considered negligent unless the doctor first makes a reasonable enquiry or check concerning allergy. What is more, if the doctor does in fact administer penicillin, he should make sure that he would be in a position to take remedial action should an adverse reaction set in. Legally his position may be untenable if he rushes off beyond reach immediately after administering the drug.

So far we have not had a case on penicillin tried in our courts, but there have been several overseas cases. On the basis of American decisions, Ficarra[2] (1966) postulated three "working rules":

1 See my comments above 3, 24.
2 B J Ficarra *Surgical and Allied Malpractice* (1968) 837.

1. Enquiry should be made about a previous penicillin reaction.[3]
2. It should be used only where specifically indicated (one decision was handed down against a doctor where penicillin was used in mumps). Another antibiotic, if equally effective, should be used especially in allergic or asthmatic subjects.
3. Give a skin test if the patient is suspected of possible allergy (most cases brought against doctors are based on fatal or serious reactions to penicillin allergy). However, Ficarra's statement regarding scratch tests for penicillin cannot be endorsed today. There is now sufficient ground to suggest avoidance of such tests, since even the minute test dose has in some instances been known to cause a near-catastrophic effect.

Writing on American law, Holder[4] (1978) makes the statement that "[w]here a drug allergy which is known to the patient or can be predetermined is overlooked and an adverse reaction occurs, the doctor will be liable". This is generally true of South African law as well, but the following riders must be added:

First, in this country doctors treat a large number of relatively unsophisticated patients. In enquiring from a patient or his guardian as to a known drug allergy, the doctor must take into consideration the level of sophistication and education of the person to whom the enquiry is directed. It is one thing to ask a man with a B Sc degree behind his name; it is a completely different matter to enquire from a man who comes from a tribal community.

Secondly, actual damage must be proved by the plaintiff where a legal action is brought for negligence. If the patient has survived the personal injury, his claim for damages may include a claim of compensation for pain and suffering. If the action is brought for assault – on the ground of intentional violation of the plaintiff's body, i e medical treatment resulting in bodily harm to which the patient has not given an informed consent – nominal damages may be awarded by the court, however.

Thirdly, where death was caused by negligence, a civil action for damages will lie on behalf of a relative only where he (the relative) was caused patrimonial loss by such death.[5] The plaintiff must, in other words, prove that he was deprived of his source of sustenance. Where a young child dies as a result of negligence, this can of course not be maintained by the parents. However, the fact that the aggrieved parents have no civil claim does not preclude the State from bringing a prosecution for culpable homicide against the negligent doctor.

Holder[6] makes the following statement which undoubtedly sums up the position for South African law as well, provided the plaintiff proves compensable damage: "Administration of a medication to which a patient has indicated a known allergy will impose virtually automatic liability as a matter of law." In this context she refers to the well-known American decision *Yorston v Pennel*[7] (1959), the facts of which were as follows: A patient had been sick on a prior occasion, had been given penicillin, and had developed a rash. His doctor warned him against ever taking the drug again. He gave the patient a note which the latter kept in his wallet indicating penicillin allergy. After involvement in a road accident he was brought to the emergency room of a teaching hospital. His history was taken by an intern and he told the intern of the allergy. He also handed the intern the note. The intern did not mention this on the chart. During surgery he remembered it and took the note to the door of the operating-theatre. He gave it to a nurse and told her to tell the surgeon, but she failed to do so. Penicillin was administered during surgery and again after the patient regained consciousness. He told the nurse who was about to administer another injec-

3 Compare the case cited by D Giesen *Arzthaftungsrecht – Medical Malpractice Law* (1981) 229.
4 A R Holder *Medical Malpractice Law* (2nd ed, 1978) 160.
5 R G McKerron *The Law of Delict* (7th ed, 1971) 151.
6 *Op cit*, 160.
7 153 A 2d 255 (1959).

tion that he had an allergy, but she insisted on giving it to him. Finally, after several days he flatly refused to be injected at all until he had seen the surgeon – who had not visited him since the operation – and told him about the allergy. The surgeon ordered immediate cessation of penicillin, but the patient had an acute and serious cardiovascular accident. The court held the surgeon liable for all the separate negligent acts of his subordinates.

Another American case to which reference may be made is *Campos v Weeks*,[8] (1966). In this case a patient had an infected finger. The doctor asked her if she was allergic to penicillin and she answered in the negative. She told him that she had taken it on prior occasions without problems. He gave her an injection and she dropped dead of anaphylactic shock. Since he had used all known means to determine allergy, he was not held liable.

It is to be noted that where the skin test is administered in regard to a substance such as tetanus antitoxin, the proper time must be allowed to elapse before the skin is observed. Failure to wait long enough after the test before administering the injection will afford clear evidence of negligence.

8 53 Cal Rptr 915 (Cal 1966).

41 Volkmann has yet another sequel in court

In 1962 in the case of *Dube v Administrator, Transvaal*[1] a patient successfully sued a hospital authority for damages caused by Volkmann's ischemic contracture, negligently brought about, which resulted in the loss of his arm. (The amount of R6 000 was awarded by the court.)

The Volkmann again featured prominently in the case of *Blyth v Van den Heever*[2] (1977-1979) and the final judgment again went against the doctor. The trial court's verdict was against the patient, but was reversed on appeal to the Appellate Division. The decision highlights a number of features of medical malpractice law in South Africa.

The plaintiff was injured on a Sunday in 1971 during a polo match when his horse fell on him. He sustained a simple transverse fracture of the ulna, and a fracture of the radius, which was allegedly a comminuted fracture. He was treated and operated on by the defendant, a general practitioner. The operation, an open reduction, was performed on the same day, some three and a half hours after the accident.

During the course of treatment complications set in. Notwithstanding intensive medical care, involving at a later stage attendance and surgery by specialists as well, the patient's forearm was in the course of time reduced to what the trial judge in his judgment described as "a shrunken, claw-like appendage of extremely limited functional value".

The patient sued the doctor for R112 123 damages. The plaintiff's case was that due to the defendant's negligence he sustained acute vascular embarrassment in the forearm which caused extensive muscle necrosis and nerve lesion, or which devitalised the forearm to such an extent as to render an extensive virulent and destructive attack of sepsis in the forearm possible.

The defendant, however, denied that he was guilty of any acts of negligence. He also denied that the patient manifested any signs of significant ischemia during his treatment, and contended that the only discernible and diagnosable complication while he was treating the plaintiff, was sepsis in the forearm. He conceded that the sepsis was a particularly virulent invasive infection, but disputed the suggestion that infection of such a nature could only have taken place if the forearm had been devitalised by significant ischemia.

The judgment represents the most comprehensive analysis by a court of law of the issues surrounding a Volkmann, yet recorded in South Africa.

There were material differences of opinion on a number of points in the evidence of expert witnesses who testified for the respective parties, and this played a major role in the assessment of the plaintiff's claim. The trial judge reiterated the fundamental principle that the onus of proof is on the plaintiff.

The trial judge found that the doctor had indeed been negligent in a number of respects, namely:

- the cast applied to the forearm or the underlying wrapping was not suitable and too tight, and should have been split shortly after the operation;

1 1963 (4) SA 260 (T).
2 1980 (1) SA 191 (A). The judgment of the trial court, in 1977, was not reported.

- the doctor should have realised that the omission to do so might contribute to the build-up of pressure and induce ischemia;
- the doctor should not merely have instructed the staff to split the cast and apply a crepe bandage; he should himself have checked on this and should have examined the arm and have done all the necessary tests;
- after the splitting of the cast the doctor should have seen that the wool beneath the cast had not been cut and was constrictive.

However, the vital finding of the trial court was that on the basis of the facts before the court and in particular the expert evidence led on behalf of the defence, "it cannot be taken to be more probable than not that plaintiff at the relevant time sustained significant ischemia". There was accordingly no basis for a finding that the negligent intromission in any way had contributed to the final catastrophe.

It must be mentioned that the trial judge on several associated issues (e g the fact that the doctor operated although X-rays had not been taken; and the fact that the doctor did not involve the aid of a specialist) found that the defendant had not been negligent.

In the course of his judgment the judge observed that it would be prudent for a doctor who intends to hand over a patient to another practitioner, to give him a written case history.

Of special significance was the judge's comment on the attitude of the doctor towards the patient and his mother at the stage when it became evident that the destruction of most of the plaintiff's forearm was complete: "It seems to me to be most surprising that the doctor did not at once tell plaintiff's mother about it ... Here was an example of lack of consideration for the family ... If defendant was unfortunate in having been landed in this litigation, I feel that the intromission in point may well have played a signal role in the view taken by the family, and he has himself to blame for that."

The patient took the judgment on appeal to the Appellate Division. The Appellate Division's judgment was delivered by Mr Justice Corbett; his four colleagues on the five-judge appeal bench concurred with his judgment. Among them was the Chief Justice, Mr Justice Rumpff.

As the Appeal Court saw it, the case resolved itself into three main questions:

- What factually was the cause of the ultimate condition of the patient's arm?
- Did negligence on the doctor's part cause or materially contribute to this condition in the sense that by the exercise of reasonable professional care and skill he could have prevented it from developing?
- If liability on the part of the doctor be established, what amount should be awarded to the patient by way of damages?

As far as the question of causation was concerned, Mr Justice Corbett made the following observations: "Fractures of the nature sustained by the patient, if properly and timeously treated, do not usually have the dire results that these fractures did. They usually heal with little or no adverse after-effect. What went wrong in this case?"

The judge of appeal pointed out that in determining what had caused the virtual destruction of the patient's arm the court must make its finding on a preponderance of probability. Certainty of diagnosis is not necessary. If it were, then in a field so uncertain and controversial, a definitive finding would become an impossibility.

In the final analysis, the judge said, the issue as to whether the patient had suffered a serious and generalised ischemic condition must be determined by putting in the balance, on the one hand, the probabilities favouring such a diagnosis, and, on the other, the probability against such a diagnosis flowing from the evidence concerning the passive extension of the patient's fingers.

Having carefully considered the evidence, the judge came to the conclusion that there was a substantial preponderance in favour of the patient's case. The court found it was more probable than not that the patient had suffered a severe and generalised ischemia in his right forearm, that this ischemia so devitalised the muscle tissues that it was possible for the staphylococcal infection to become a massive and invasive one, and that as a result there was a large-scale destruction of muscle and nerve tissue and ultimately a fairly typical Volkmann's contracture.

As regards the issue of negligence, the inquiry was limited to the doctor's post-operative care of the patient. It was clear, Mr Justice Corbett said, that the reasonably skilled and careful medical practitioner – the notional "reasonable man" of the law – in the position of the defendant doctor would have been aware of the danger of an ischemic condition developing in the patient's forearm.

He would have known that this danger was a dual one, i e it could arise by reason of arterial occlusion or embarrassment or because of the development of a compartmental syndrome.

In view of various factors – the site and nature of the patient's fractures, the degree of trauma involved as a result of not only the accident itself but also the manipulative and surgical procedures applied, and the application of a circumferential (unsplit) plaster cast – the reasonably skilled and careful practitioner would have realised that the development of a compartmental syndrome was a special risk in this case.

This would have placed upon him a duty to be especially careful to watch for any untoward signs that might point to the development of an ischemic condition and to act immediately if any such signs became apparent.

The judge held the view that the immediate splitting of a circumferential plaster is a safe and prudent practice, but that he would hesitate to say that a doctor who fails to do so is necessarily negligent. But if he does not do so, the situation casts upon him a duty of especial vigilance. He must then watch the patient, or ensure that he is watched, very carefully, for signs of a threatened ischemia.

A reasonable, skilled and careful doctor in the position of the defendant would have realised on the Monday – the day after the operation – that there were symptoms which, even if they did not demonstrate a developing ischemia, raised the real suspicion that one might be developing. He would have been alerted when he first saw the patient at 08:00 that morning, first by the patient's persistent pain and discomfort and, secondly, by the notations on the bed-sheets (on which had been noted, at 02:30 that the patient's fingers were "very stiff", with entries in regard to pain and the analgesics administered). These suspicions would have been strengthened, if not confirmed, when later that morning the doctor was telephoned by two nursing sisters and told that the patient's arm and hand were abnormally swollen.

The remedial action the notional reasonably skilled and careful doctor could and should have taken, in essence amounted to this, the judge said: The very first step would be to remove the plaster or at any rate split it completely and expose the skin. This in itself has two advantages: If the plaster is constricting the arm, removal or splitting will bring relief. Secondly, removal or splitting enables the practitioner to examine the arm and to see what is occurring underneath all the dressings. The doctor is then able to see whether the arm itself appears swollen or whether from the appearance of the skin there seems to be swelling and compression within the fascial compartments. Furthermore, the usual tests for ischemia, designed to detect "the five p's"[3] and the passive extension tests, would be performed. Thereafter the patient's condition would be carefully watched, and if the adverse symptoms persisted,

3 The classical symptoms of an impending ischemia as described by the court are known as "the five p's": pain, pallor, pulselessness, paralysis and para-anaesthesia (loss of sensation over and below the ischemic area).

the more drastic step of a fasciotomy would have to be considered, and, if necessary, performed.

On the evidence as a whole, the judge was of the opinion that it established as a matter of probability that had the doctor been alerted as was indicated, and taken the appropriate remedial action, the severe and generalised ischemic condition with concomitant tissue necrosis would have been avoided. This would have prevented the staphylococcus aureus infection from spreading in the way it did; it would have been sealed off and localised by the body's natural defensive responses. The patient might have had two unpleasant abscesses in the region of the surgical wounds, but there it would have ended. More probably than not the fractures would have healed satisfactorily and the patient would have regained the full use of his arm.

It was clear, the judge held, that the requisite remedial action had not been taken by the doctor. This was partly because he did not diagnose an impending ischemia or suspect the possibility of one developing. In failing to do so, he was, therefore, negligent in that he failed to display the skill and care reasonably to be expected from him. Another reason why he failed to make the appropriate diagnosis was because he had not maintained the necessary vigilance (he allowed 24 hours to elapse between visits during this vital period) and when he was telephoned by the sisters and told of their concern, he did not go to see things for himself.

"That was the stage *par excellence* when he should have hurried to the hospital, removed the plaster and commenced the remedial procedures," the judge said. In failing to do so and in particular in leaving the splitting of the plaster to the nursing staff he failed in his duty towards the patient and was negligent. Consequently the plaster was not properly split on the Monday and even on the Tuesday when the plaster was split, the padding was not cut. In the result the court held that the doctor's negligence was causally connected with the damage ultimately sustained by the patient.

As far as the amount of damages was concerned, the court of appeal found that there was a distinct possibility that the patient might at some stage in future be compelled to have an amputation and obtain an artificial arm. Whether he continued with his present disablement (with the possibility of slight improvement as a result of reconstructive surgery) or opted for amputation and an electronic arm, he would be severely handicapped as a farmer. The court further considered that the pain and suffering attributable to the ischemia, the invasive sepsis, the virtual destruction of his forearm and the various remedial procedures must have been very considerable. Having a suppurating, septic arm for about four months must itself have been a very unpleasant experience.

Accordingly an amount of R34 542,30 damages was awarded, made up as follows: medical expenses to date, R673,70; estimated future hospital and medical expenses, R2 868,60; costs of electronic arm (and amputation), R3 500; reduction in earning capacity, R7 500; and general damages for pain and suffering, disability, disfigurement and loss of amenities, R20 000.

The case undoubtedly was the biggest malpractice action ever tried in South Africa up to 1979, from the point of view of the duration, the amount of damages awarded and the costs of action. An attorney with experience in civil actions estimated the total costs – legal expenses as well as the qualifying fees of the five eminent medical experts who testified – in the region of R300 000. There were four advocates involved, a senior and junior on either side. The Appellate Division allowed the appeal with costs, which means that in accordance with our law, the defendant doctor became liable for his own costs as well as the patient's taxed costs (which were probably the bulk of the latter's costs). My information is that the doctor was a member of a medical protection society, and therefore covered as far as the award for damages and costs were concerned.

The case illustrates how agonisingly slow the wheels of justice may turn at times. From the moment that the plaintiff post-operatively first complained that his fingers were stiff, until the verdict of the Appeal Court was announced, took 8 years, 4 months and 3 days. But the case also highlights the painstaking care which goes into a judgment of the highest court of the land: the written reasons for the judgment ran to 141 typed, foolscap pages.

42 Compartment syndrome resulting in loss of leg: hospital held liable for premature discharge of patient

In a 1989 case, *Soumbasis and Another v Administrator of the Orange Free State and Another*[1], a hospital authority was found to be guilty of negligence in respect of premature discharge of a patient. The orthopaedic surgeon who had attended to the patient, a 17-year-old male, was found not to have been negligent.

The patient, a first-year medical student in Bloemfontein, was kicked on the left lower leg by a member of the opposing team during a football match at about 19:45 one Wednesday evening. He fell down and the immediate sensation was one of tremendous pain. He was brought to the casualty section of the defendant hospital in Bloemfontein where he received a pain-relieving injection and was X-rayed.

Later in the evening the defendant doctor, an orthopaedic surgeon, Dr L, diagnosed a fracture of the tibula and fibia, and having telephonically obtained consent from the patient's father, performed a standard reduction at about 23:00. He put on a plaster of Paris cast from the upper part of the leg to the foot, leaving the toes open.

The patient later testified in court that he had experienced intense pain throughout the night and early the next morning. He was given pain-relieving tablets, but the pain did not abate. He could not recall that the doctor came to see him that morning. At about 12:25 he was discharged from the hospital after his parents had arrived with a pair of crutches. He travelled with his parents to the family home in Welkom.

The next day the pain in his leg was still there and became intense. On the Saturday morning the pain became unbearable. By 13:00 that day, the patient was seen by Dr Z, an orthopaedic surgeon practising in Welkom. He bi-valved the plaster cast, which he did not regard as being too tight. He performed a fasciotomy and found a haematoma.

It was common cause that the patient had suffered a complication of the fracture in the form of a compartment syndrome. As a result of this it became necessary for his left leg to be amputated below the knee some four months later. The patient, assisted by his father, sued Dr L and the hospital authority for damages in the amounts of R71 363 and R476 526, respectively, on the ground of alleged negligence. The essence of the allegations against the doctor was that he had failed to administer proper post-operative care. As concerned the hospital authority, it was alleged that the nurses *inter alia* had failed to alert the doctor to his condition when he complained of pain, that they had discharged him prematurely and that they had omitted to give him proper instructions in regard to possible complications.

It appeared in the course of trial that a student nurse had made an entry on the hospital's official "progress report" form at 03:00 on the Thursday morning reading: "For discharge today". She testified that she had done so because either Dr L or someone from the casualty department had told the nursing staff that the patient would be discharged. Dr L, however, testified that he had authorised the patient's discharge only at a later stage.

According to Dr L he visited the patient after 06:30 that morning. The patient was awake, with his leg elevated. He said that he felt "all right", although his leg had been sore during the night and he had been given pills. The plaster cast fitted well and

1 1989 OPD, unreported.

there was no abnormal swelling, according to Dr L. He looked at the patient's toes and felt them. The colour was normal. He tested the sensation in the toes. He told the patient everything looked all right and that he could find nothing wrong. He told the patient that he thought he should stay for a further day, but the patient said he wanted to go home. Dr L told the patient the pain should get better and that he should go to his family doctor if it got worse.

On the evidence before it, the court found that Dr L had not been negligent. Sister F who took charge of the day staff at 07:00 also did not detect any abnormality. Had she noticed any abnormality she would have contacted Dr L. There was no reason for Dr L to think the patient would not have consulted the family doctor should any danger signs have developed. Two specialists who testified for the patient accepted that the warning Dr L said he had given to the patient was adequate.

The court found, however, that the nursing staff had been negligent. Mr Acting Justice Farlam accepted the patient's evidence that he had told Sister J early on Thursday morning that he had severe pain. She gave him pain-relieving pills at 09:00. At 10:00 and again at noon – when he was discharged – the patient still complained of "lots of pain".

Sister J was negligent in two respects, the court found:

- ❑ she should have reported the apparent change in the patient's condition to Dr L before physically discharging him;
- ❑ she gave an inadequate warning to the patient.

The judge ruled as follows: "It is clear that a nurse must not *undo* the warning given by the doctor and that she must see to it that a proper warning is given when it is clear to her that the doctor has not given a warning *or the patient is not aware of it.*"

The court rejected the contention that there was contributory negligence on the part of the patient, in that he allegedly had failed to carry out the instructions of Dr L or the nurses and had failed to call in medical advice timeously.

The court accordingly held that the hospital authority was liable for damages. The latter was ordered to pay legal costs, including the doctor's legal costs.

It is understood that the plaintiff and the hospital authority agreed on the *quantum* (amount) of damages but that an application was lodged by the latter for leave to appeal against the finding and order of the court made against the hospital.

Since the incident that resulted in this claim occurred, it has become general practice at hospitals in the Orange Free State to give written instructions to patients setting out the signs to look for and to report increasing or persistent pain, swelling, discolouration, etc.

43 Patient burnt by earth plate of cautery: who is liable?

The following question was put to me:

"It has occurred more than once that during an operation, while the patient is under an anaesthetic, he was burned by the earth plate of a cautery. This has the result that the patient after such an electric burn, apart from pain and suffering, must undergo plastic surgery; moreover, the patient may be permanently disfigured.

"Clearly the patient cannot be held responsible for the burns which he sustained. Who must actually bear the responsibility – the theatre staff, the anaesthetist, the surgeon or the hospital?

"Such a burn may of course be caused by a defect in the cautery or because the earth plate has not been properly attached."

My answer is as follows:

To say that in modern medicine apparatus and instruments play an increasingly important role is to state the obvious.

Should apparatus in the course of its use become defective, causing some or other ill-effect to the patient, it is the manufacturer or supplier who in the first instance may be held legally liable.

In South African law, delictual liability (i e liability for compensation of damage caused wrongfully) is based upon fault, which will ordinarily consist of negligence. This means the aggrieved party must prove that a reprehensible lack of foresight on the part of the defendant caused his harm. Our courts apply the test of the reasonable man: would the reasonable man have foreseen the possibility of harm being caused to another on account of the defendant's act or omission, and would the reasonable man have taken measures to prevent such harm?

"Strict liability" in respect of products, i e that the manufacturer (or supplier) of a product will be held liable *ex delicto* to compensate the party who suffered loss irrespective of the fault of the manufacturer, etc, is not known in our law.

Proof of negligence on the part of the manufacturer or supplier may be facilitated by the principle of *res ipsa loquitur*. This is a legal principle whereby an inference of negligence is drawn in the absence of explanation by the defendant, if injury was caused by a thing under the control of the defendant and the nature of the occurrence was such that it would not have happened if proper care had been exercised. In South Africa the principle has been applied for negligent services involving e g an exploding boiler in a power station,[1] and where a woman's hair was scorched during a "perm".[2]

In the two cases mentioned, the liability of the person in control of the defective object was at issue and not that of the manufacturer. There seems to be no reason, however, why the principle should not be applied to a manufacturer. As Schmidt[3] has indicated, *res ipsa loquitur* is not a mystical doctrine : the maxim is often resorted to where the court is asked to draw an inference of negligence from the circumstantial evidence.

Apart from the manufacturer or supplier, a technician responsible for the main-

1 *Clair v Port Elizabeth Harbour Board, Kennedy v The Same* 5 EDC 311 (1887).
2 *Mitchell v Maison Libson* 1937 TPD 13.
3 C W H Schmidt *Bewysreg* (3rd ed, 1989) 163.

tenance of the apparatus, or a doctor or nurse who handles it, may be held delictually liable. In the Free State case of *Blore v Standard and General Insurance Co*,[4] a mechanic in a garage failed to properly repair the defective steering mechanism of a car. Shortly thereafter the vehicle was involved in an accident in which the plaintiff was injured. The court held that the garage's omission constituted a potential danger to all road users, and by allowing the car to go on to the road without warning the owner, a source of danger was created by the garage. In the result a cause of action was stated against the garage owner.

In each case the liability of the party concerned will depend on proof of his or her individual negligence. A hospital authority may be vicariously held liable for the negligence of its staff, i e its employee(s), in operating the device.[5]

The doctor's liability will depend on whether he was aware, or ought reasonably to have been aware, of the defect in the apparatus. The more obvious the defect, the more readily negligence on his part will be inferred. However, the device may be so complicated that the doctor may be "externally" *au fait* with its functioning and operation only; this will ordinarily be the case with sophisticated devices maintained by the supplier or by the manufacturer's agents.[6]

In such a situation the doctor will of course not invariably be held liable for injury caused to a patient as a result of a latent defect of the device. To what extent the doctor may be expected to be familiar with the defect, and particularly with its dangerous propensities, is a factual issue which depends largely on the complexity of the instrument. The same principles apply to nursing staff.

There have been numerous cases involving liability for injuries caused to patients by defective devices. In South Africa a doctor who was not a radiologist, but had practical experience of X-ray work, was held liable for burns sustained by a patient as a result of a "Coolidge" tube in a new X-ray apparatus having been so placed that it was too close to the patient. The court held that there had been a duty on the doctor to see that the apparatus was safe, even though it had been installed by an electrician: *Dale v Hamilton*.[7]

In another South African decision, *Mitchell v Dixon*,[8] again the Appellate Division refused to hold a doctor liable for injuries caused to a patient by the breaking of the needle of a syringe used during exploration of the chest cavity for suspected pneumothorax. The court came to the conclusion that although the needle could have had a latent defect, no sign of it was visible at the shoulder of the instrument.

So far we have not had any reported court case in South Africa on burns caused by a cautery. In the USA, however, decisions have been handed down on liability in such cases, and the approach of the courts in these may well be followed by our courts.

In the American case of *May v Broun*[9] a cautery which had malfunctioned during an earlier operation was used during a haemorrhoidectomy. The patient was burned on the chest where the electrode had been placed. In finding that the surgeon was not negligent, the court pointed out that the hospital owned the machine and that the theatre nurses, not the surgeons, were trained to operate it. In this case it was held that when technical equipment and personnel to man it – which are furnished by a hospital – cause injuries due to malfunction, the hospital will be solely liable.

4 1972 (2) SA 89 (O).
5 On vicarious liability, see below 299 *et seq.*
6 In *S v Lombard and Another* (Pretoria magistrate's court, 1979) a specialist anaesthetist was charged with culpable homicide after the death of an 11-year-old boy. The patient died after the oxygen-pipe of a Boyle machine had been wrongly – and inexplicably – connected to the carbon dioxide connection of the gas tank, which resulted in a flow of carbon dioxide to the patient instead of oxygen. Evidence was led that the connections were so designed that they could not be wrongly coupled. The accused was held to be blameless and was acquitted.
7 1924 WLD 184.
8 1914 AD 519.
9 492 P 2d 776 (Oregon, 1972), quoted by A R Holder *Medical Malpractice Law* (2nd ed, 1978) 208.

However, where the doctor is an active participant in directing the use of the machine or positioning the patient on the table, he may be liable for his own negligence: *Holloway v Hauver.*[10]

Where a patient received severe leg burns from the contact plate on an electrosurgical machine, it was held that the hospital was vicariously liable for the improper placement of the plate by the nurse. However, she had asked the surgeon to check the placement and he had done so, and it was accordingly held that these facts disclosed a cause of action against the doctor as well: *Monk v Doctor's Hospital.*[11]

I am not going into the contractual rights of the purchaser (or lessee) of equipment which is latently defective, to sue the seller (or lessor) for damages. Suffice it to say that our law provides adequate remedies to protect the aggrieved party.

Note: After publication of this article in the *SA Medical Post* in December 1978, I received a letter from Mr R G Nelson, marketing director of the firm Medical Equipment and Maintenance Services (Pty) Ltd, in which he made several interesting comments (published in full with his kind permission):

"I am confused at the USA Court decision in 1968 (*Monk v Doctor's Hospital*) in finding a measure of negligence on the part of the surgeon in the placement of an indifferent electrosurgical plate on the leg of a patient and which resulted in thermal burns to that patient, because substantially, only two criteria could have caused such trauma:

1. insufficient surface area of such plate;
2. damage to the cords, resulting in short-circuits through the patient, etc.

"I find it very hard to credit that any experienced surgeon would countenance the use of a patient plate which might be mildly suspect as far as surface area is concerned because the hazards of such procedure have been too well and too long, publicised and emphasised.

"If either cord has been damaged, active or negative (I refer to the macroscopic cracks which appear in the normal 'permanent' cords carrying a heavy layer of rubber isolation and which tend to become brittle because of the vulcanising effects of autoclaving), thereby giving rise to the hazard of current leakage, the surgeon could not be expected to accept responsibility for such defective material as the damage is usually invisible unless under very close scrutiny, which should be the responsibility of the hospital authorities, as the product, its sterilising and its maintenance is solely the property and responsibility of such hospitals.

"Some years ago in a Japanese hospital, a paediatric patient who was undergoing minor surgery, suffered what resulted in a leg amputation because of minute cracks in the active cord. I doubt those hospital authorities have made their final payment to the parents under public liability! Which just goes to prove how negligence can be seen by various courts."

10 322 A 2d 980 (Maryland, 1974), quoted by Holder *op cit* 208.
11 403 F 2d 580 (CA DC 1968), quoted by Holder *op cit* 228.

44 Can a failure to adequately inform the patient constitute negligence?

It is a well-known principle of our law that consent, in order to operate as a defence, must be a real consent, based on knowledge of the material facts allegedly consented to by the plaintiff.[1] In this context the expression "informed consent" is used nowadays.

In *Richter and Another v Estate Hammann*[2] the plaintiff, a young married woman, had fallen on the sharp edge of a chair and for the second time injured her coccyx. The defendant, an experienced neuro-surgeon, gave her an injection known as a phenol block of the lower sacral nerves, which had the most unfortunate consequences for the patient, namely, loss of control of the bladder and bowel, loss of sexual feeling and loss of power in the right leg and foot. The plaintiff alleged that the doctor was negligent in failing to warn her of the possibility of these consequences ensuing.

The judge drew attention to the fact that the plaintiff's case was not based on assault (i e that she had not consented to the treatment at all). The allegation was that the doctor had been negligent in failing to warn the patient.

"A doctor whose advice is sought about an operation to which dangers are attached – and there are dangers attached to most operations – is in a dilemma," Mr Justice Watermeyer said. "If he fails to disclose the risks he may render himself liable to an action for assault, whereas if he discloses them he might well frighten the patient into not having the operation when the doctor knows full well that it would be in the patient's interests to have it."

The judge continued: "It may well be that in certain circumstances a doctor is negligent if he fails to warn a patient, and if that is so, it seems to me in principle that his conduct should be tested by the standard of the reasonable doctor faced with the particular problem. In reaching a conclusion a court should be guided by medical opinion as to what a reasonable doctor, having regard to all the circumstances of the particular case, should or should not do. The Court must, of course, make up its own mind, but it will be assisted in doing so by medical evidence."

All three of the neuro-surgeons who testified at the trial had expressed views on this point. Dr A thought that when the doctor has won the patient's confidence he should discuss the risks with him, and if his complaint is bad the doctor should tend to emphasise the possible relief and minimise the risks, whereas if the complaint is trivial, the doctor should be perfectly frank and possibly even over-emphasise the risks.

Dr B thought that the doctor's assessment of the risk was all-important, and applying it to the circumstances of the case expressed the view that there was no need to mention the risks.

Dr C was of much the same opinion. He felt that a doctor should always tell a patient of consequences that he knows will ensue, such as that the patient will have a stiff knee after an arthrodesis of the knee joint, but where there is only a remote possibility of complications – as in this case – he did not think it necessary to warn the patient.

1 See S A Strauss & M J Strydom *Die Suid-Afrikaanse Geneeskundige Reg* (1967) 211 *et seq*.
2 1976 (3) SA 226 (C).

According to the evidence of the doctors who testified during the trial, the likelihood of the plaintiff's present complications occurring was extremely uncommon. In these circumstances, the court held, the fact that the defendant had not mentioned the possibility of complications to the plaintiff, did not constitute negligence. It is respectfully submitted that the judge was quite correct in holding that there is no duty on a doctor to inform a patient of potential consequences which are remotely possible. However, his remarks on negligence, in this connection, deserve further attention.

It is to be noted the court did not conclusively decide that failure of the doctor to adequately inform the patient would in fact constitute negligence. If this were to be decided, a new principle would be introduced into our law. Traditionally our courts have dealt with non-compliance of doctors with the duty to obtain an informed consent on the basis of assault. It is submitted that to consider failure to inform as negligence would not be in accordance with the Roman-Dutch concept of *culpa* which until now has been defined as the failure to foresee the damaging consequence and to take reasonable measures to avoid it. The essence of negligence in the medical context is unskilful treatment.

In England, in the 1981 case of *Chatterton v Gerson and Another*,[3] it was held that a failure to inform a patient adequately can constitute negligence. The facts of the case were almost on all fours with *Richter's* case. The plaintiff suffered chronic pains in a post-operative scar and was sent to a pain clinic where the defendant doctor administered an intrathecal injection to block the sensory nerve. The pain returned, however, and she underwent a return operation ten months later. As a result she lost sensation in her right leg and still experienced such acute agony in the scar area that she could not bear clothing in contact with it, and could only move with a stick.

The patient sued the doctor for damages on the basis of trespass – i e that there was no real consent on her part; and negligence, in that the defendant had failed to give her an adequate explanation of the nature and implications of the proposed operation. On the negligence issue, the court held that the plaintiff must prove not only the breach of a duty to inform, but that had the duty not been broken, the patient would not have chosen to have the operation. The court intimated – obiter, it would seem – that a failure to go into risks and implications is negligence.

On the facts of the case, the court held that the plaintiff had been under no illusion as to the general nature of what a nerve block would be and that "her consent was real". There was therefore, no question of liability for trespass on the part of the doctor. As to the alleged negligence, there is no obligation on a doctor to canvass with the patient anything other than the inherent implications of the operation envisaged. He must warn of what may happen by misfortune if there is a real risk of misfortune inherent in the procedure. *In casu* there was no real risk that her leg and foot would be deprived of sensation or control. Moreover, there was no proof that anything done in the course of the second operation had caused that result. Accordingly the plaintiff's claim of negligence also failed.

There are also American judgments which indicate that a failure to inform a patient adequately is tantamount to negligence. I would submit that these precedents and the ruling in *Chatterton's* case should not be followed by our courts. Where there has been no consent to a medical procedure – or what is legally the same, where the consent in fact given was so "uninformed" as to the nature of the procedure or consequences thereof that may well manifest themselves, that it cannot be said that there was a "real" consent – the patient will have an action based upon assault. This was the approach of the court in *Esterhuizen v Administrator, Transvaal*.[4]

The issue of a failure to adequately inform constituting negligence was also

3 [1981] 1 QB 432.
4 1957 (3) SA 710 (T).

raised in an older decision of our Appeal Court, *Lymbery v Jefferies*[5] (1925), but not conclusively decided.[6]

5 1925 AD 235, at 240.

6 F F W van Oosten *The Doctrine of Informed Consent in Medical Law* (LLD thesis, Univ of South Africa, 1989) 452 holds the view that where the medical intervention was performed with due care and skill, but the undisclosed risk of danger materialised, the negligence action is appropriate. If the patient, had he been properly informed of the risk, would nevertheless have consented, negligence liability would, however, not lie.

45 The missing swab and the theatre nurse's legal liability

Legally speaking, the number one risk for the theatre nurse seems to be the swab that remains behind in the patient after an operation. Judging by legal actions brought by dissatisfied patients, this constitutes a major headache to hospitals, surgeons, nurses and insurance companies – rare as such a mishap may be.

One of the most important cases ever brought for alleged medical malpractice in South Africa concerns the missing swab. The case is *Van Wyk v Lewis*,[1] which was decided by the Appellate Division in Bloemfontein in 1924. It was a landmark case in all respects. In its judgment the court laid down certain principles which have guided other courts to this day. The decision is as relevant today as it was then, and after more than six decades it is entirely appropriate to dust off the case, as it were, and to have a fresh look at it.

In the case, civil action was brought by the patient against a surgeon. The facts were as follows:

The patient, a woman, was in a critical condition of appendicitis and an immediate operation was decided on. It was found that the appendix was inflamed and adherent and was accordingly removed. The surgeon also found the gall-bladder in a state of acute inflammation and decided to drain it. He packed off the field of the operation with swabs, made an incision and inserted a tube with some difficulty. There was a rush of septic matter to be dealt with and the surgeon put in more packing to prevent the spread of sepsis.

At this stage he was warned by the anaesthetist that the patient should be taken off the operating table as soon as possible. The surgeon removed all swabs he saw or felt, and being satisfied that they were all accounted for to the satisfaction of the sister, proceeded to stitch up.

The patient made a rapid recovery, but some time after the operation the wound opened slightly and there was an oozing of pus. She also informed the surgeon that several gallstones had come through the opening. Some months afterwards she evacuated a piece of muslin, the shape and size of a small-sized packing swab, with tape attachment.

The patient sued the surgeon for £2 000 damages (sounding in today's money, the equivalent of perhaps R60 000) on the ground that he had been negligent in failing to remove the swab. According to the evidence it was generally the duty of the theatre sister or nurse in charge to keep a number of swabs available and to hand them to the surgeon as he needed them. The small swabs he threw away after use, but the packing swabs remained in the wound until the conclusion of the operation.

According to the evidence, removal of swabs – saturated with blood and packed into a small space – was not so much a matter of surgical skills as of careful search, conducted under critical conditions. Evidence was given of the various devices used to keep a check on the swabs, but it was testified that as yet no check had been devised which was infallible.

According to the evidence the task of checking on the swabs was that of the theatre sister. She kept a mental record, checking against the number of swabs left on the

1 1924 AD 438.

table. At the conclusion of the operation the sister informed the surgeon whether the number was correct, and the surgeon then sewed up the patient while the sister made the count. If any discrepancy was revealed, even at that final stage, the stitches would be taken out and a further search made.

The court refused to hold the surgeon liable. It held that although there had been a duty upon him to search diligently for the swabs (which he had done), he was entitled to rely on the sister regarding the final count. The court made the following remarks on the duties of the theatre sister: "The theatre sister, though her work is largely mechanical, also has important duties to discharge. She sees to the preparation of the theatre, the sterilizing of instruments, the laying out of swabs and other details. She stands ready to anticipate or to supply the needs of the operator, and she undertakes the counting and checking of the swabs. She is as a rule – and she was in this instance – not only a duly certified but a highly experienced nurse, upon whom during the period of her instruction and training the importance of keeping a correct tally has been authoritatively impressed. In a general sense she is under the orders of the surgeon, but she also has independent duties to discharge, and checking the swabs is one of the most important."

The conclusion of Chief Justice Innes was: "I am unable to say that a surgeon who leaves that task to a competent sister is on that account guilty of negligence."

The case was also of great significance because in its judgment the Appeal Court held that the principle of *res ipsa loquitur* ("the matter speaks for itself"),[2] whereby an inference of negligence can be drawn in the absence of an explanation by the defendant, did not apply to cases of that nature.

It must be pointed out that it was the doctor who had been sued and not the nurse. The court was accordingly not called upon to decide whether or not the nurse had been negligent. Had the sister also been cited as a defendant, the court might have come to that conclusion. What is more, if a similar situation were to occur today, the patient would in all probability sue the hospital in whose employ the nurse is. It is a principle of our law that a hospital authority is vicariously liable for the negligence of its professional employees.[3]

A very well-known nursing personality in South Africa, Dr Ann Latsky, at a nurses' conference in Pretoria in 1978, related to the audience the episode of a theatre nurse who had had a sleepless night after an operation on a patient in the hospital. She (the nurse) was convinced that a swab had been sewn up in the patient on account of a mistaken count made by her. The next morning she decided to tell her superiors. The patient was opened up again, and, sure enough, the swab was found inside him. The hospital authority was urged to take stern disciplinary action against the nurse, but Dr Latsky's point of view was: "For Heaven's sake, don't punish her; give her a medal!" I fully agree with that view.

If a mistake has been made, it should be reported immediately, so that remedial action can be taken without delay. Surveys have shown that prompt and sympathetic action to cure the ill-effects of medical negligence may prevent lawsuits against the parties involved. In 1978 there was a case in Johannesburg, reported in the newspapers, of a patient who had had a clamp sewn up inside her body. Her mother told reporters that she had no hard feelings towards the doctors and intimated that legal action would not be brought – because of the anxious concern of the professional staff to remedy the situation forthwith.

2 See also above 283.
3 See below 302.

46 Radiological mishaps

Excessive amount of contrast medium administered

The decision of the Appellate Division in *S v Bezuidenhout*[1] originated in a tragic event that had happened some four years earlier.

The accused, Dr B, who practised as a radiologist, performed a radiological examination on a six-week-old baby boy who had presented with a urological problem. An intravenous contrast medium, Urografin, was administered and a number of X-rays were taken. Shortly afterwards the child developed convulsions that would not cease. He was taken back to the children's ward of the hospital where he was treated for convulsions. Later that day he was transferred to an intensive-care unit in a nearby city, where he died five days later.

Dr B and the radiographer who had assisted him were charged with culpable homicide. The regional court found that an overdosage of the contrast medium had been administered, that this had been the cause of the convulsions and that the administration of the overdosage was attributable to the negligence of the accused. They were convicted of culpable homicide. On appeal to the Supreme Court, the radiographer's conviction was set aside but that of Dr B was confirmed. Dr B then appealed to the Appellate Division.

It was conceded on behalf of the radiologist that the child's death could be attributed to the administration of the contrast medium. It was contended, however, that the prosecution had failed to prove that an overdosage had been administered.

Evidence was adduced that the recommended dosage of a child with the bodily mass of the deceased was 6 to 12 ml of the substance. A radiologist who gave expert evidence at the trial stated that the maximum amount which should have been administered to the deceased should not have exceeded 30 ml. This evidence was never contested. The danger connected with the substance was to be found in the fact that it was a fluid with high osmolarity and that an overdosage could affect the patient's central nervous system.

After the radiological examination, Dr B sent a report to the referring urologist in which he mentioned *inter alia* that the patient had been dehydrated before the examination and that he regarded it as imperative that a relatively large quantity of the contrast medium be administered; that was done over a period of about two hours.

On the day of the examination Dr B, according to the evidence of his partner, Dr V, had told V that he regarded it as reasonable to administer more than the normal amount of contrast medium. According to what B told V, about half a bottle (i e approximately 125 ml) was administered when the child started getting convulsions.

Before the Appeal Court counsel for Dr B argued, on the basis of the evidence of one of the witnesses, that the convulsions could have been caused either by (a) an overdosage, or (b) hypersensitivity, or (c) a congenital inclination to epilepsy. It was contended that in the event of any of the latter two possibilities, the administration of even a normal dosage of the contrast medium could cause convulsions.

According to a pathologist who testified for the defence, the baby's convulsions

1 1985 AD (unreported).

were attributable to one of the last-mentioned two factors. His opinion was based on the view, *inter alia*, that an overdosage of some 125 ml would have interfered with the electrolytes in the deceased's blood, which in fact were normal after the radiological examination. In the light of other evidence, counsel for Dr B conceded, however, that the first ground of the pathologists' opinion was not based on an accepted substratum.

The pathologist further testified that pulmonary oedema would have developed had the child been administered 125 ml or more of the contrast medium. There was no evidence of such symptoms and according to him the child could therefore not have received that amount of the contrast medium.

The State pathologist who performed the *post mortem* examination was of a contrary opinion, however. According to him intravenous administration of the substance would stimulate the kidneys and cause an increased excretion of fluid. There would accordingly not be signs of overhydration.

In his judgment, Mr Justice van Heerden of the Appellate Division pointed out that it was important to bear in mind that the two doctors who had treated the baby a short while after the radiological examination, had been confronted with an emergency. One of them testified that it had been wellnigh impossible to determine clinically whether the baby had been overhydrated.

The court found that it was unlikely that Dr B would have conveyed to his partner wrong information as to the amount of contrast medium administered to the child. It was held that the State had in fact proved that approximately 125 ml had been administered.

The court rejected the argument that there had possibly not been a causal connection between the overdosage and the convulsions. One of the expert witnesses testified that she had administered contrast medium to approximately 2 400 babies over twelve years and not one of them had been allergic to it.

As concerns a congenital tendency to convulsions, doubt had never been cast on the State pathologist's evidence that if in this case the intake of a normal dosage of Urografin had acted as trigger for an epileptic attack, it would have been of short duration and controllable.

Lastly, the court rejected the contention that it had not been proved that Dr B had been responsible for the overdosage and that the radiographer could have decided to administer a larger dosage than the normal. There was uncontested evidence, however, that the quantity and tempo of administration of such a contrast medium were determined by the radiologist.

The Appeal Court accordingly confirmed the radiologist's conviction.

Death following pyelogram not proven to have been caused by negligence

In *Pearce v Fine and Others*[2] the widow of a patient who died in the course of a radiological examination, brought action for damages against radiologists practising in partnership on hospital premises.

The deceased was a 54-year-old male who had experienced problems with micturition. His doctor, suspecting prostatitis (inflammation of the prostate gland) referred him to the defendants for a radiological examination of his kidneys, bladder and urinary tract. Such an examination is known as an intravenous pyelograph: The patient, while lying on an X-ray table, is injected with a chemical substance called a contrast medium. Thereafter X-ray exposures are taken at intervals of approximately five minutes of the area of the body containing the organs mentioned. The object of injecting the contrast medium into the bloodstream is to enable better pictures to be taken of the internal organs of the body.

2 1986 DC & LD (unreported).

The procedure was commenced by G, a radiographer, taking control X-ray photographs for comparison at a later stage. Having perused the developed photographs, Dr L injected the contrast medium, after the usual explanation and test dosage. When the solution was injected, the patient experienced a hot flush, an alien taste and a feeling of nausea (common reactions experienced by patients undergoing this test). Within minutes, Dr L left the X-ray room. G then proceeded to expose the required series of X-ray films. When this had been done, she left the patient and took the X-ray films to the darkroom for processing. The darkroom is approximately eleven paces from the door of the X-ray room. She left the film with the darkroom attendant and returned to the X-ray room.

When G returned, she found the patient unconscious and breathing stertorously, i e with a snoring sound. She hurriedly summoned Dr L and an emergency team from the hospital's intensive care unit. Resuscitative measures were applied to the patient without success, and he died.

The court accepted G's evidence that when she left the patient she did so in the *bona fide* belief that his state of health gave no cause for alarm and that she was absent from the X-ray room for less than two minutes. Dr L testified that when he examined the patient after being summoned by G he diagnosed cardiac arrest. He immediately started resuscitation procedures. The intensive care team applied defibrillation (delivering an electric shock to "restart" the heart). The very first shock produced normal sinus rhythm but the heart relapsed in ventricular fibrillation (an irregular quivering contraction of the lower chamber of the heart). A second and third shock were delivered with the same result. The fourth shock was without avail.

Expert witnesses were in agreement as to the probable cause of death: The injection produced a drop in the patient's blood pressure (caused by the patient's anxiety or by the toxic effect of ingredients of the contrast medium, or by both these factors). The deceased's heart was unable to pump sufficient blood and went into ventricular fibrillation which could not be effectively reversed.

It was alleged that Dr L had been negligent in that he had left the patient without satisfying himself that it would be safe to do so, or in that he had failed to take steps to ensure that G would remain with the patient until it was safe. It was further alleged that G had been negligent in that she had left the patient unattended before it was safe for her to do so.

The court found that it was unnecessary to make any finding on the question of negligence. Even if there were negligence, it was not established that such negligence had been causally connected to the patient's death. On a conspectus of the evidence relating to causation, the court was of the opinion that the plaintiff had failed to establish on a balance of probability that the patient's life would have been saved had he been kept under constant observation and had resuscitation commenced as soon as he displayed symptoms of distress. There was evidence that the patient's heart had been overweight by some 30 to 80 grams. The fact that the heart is overweight usually means that there is some disease of the heart. An expert witness was of the opinion that the deceased might have suffered from cardiomyopathy, which is a weakness of the muscle of the heart. There was also some atheroma in the coronary artery. Atheroma is a deposit of fatty tissue inside the artery which usually causes some degree of narrowing of the artery.

There was expert evidence that all in all the chances of survival of a cardiac arrest are very poor. It is not the experience that if one starts resuscitation early one can bring the patient round and he will survive the episode. Starting resuscitation at the first wave of ventricular fibrillation does not guarantee a successful result. Even under the best circumstances, however early one gets there, one is dealing with a very lethal condition. The death rate where defibrillation is administered within the first four minutes is between 86 per cent and 92 per cent. The difference in the survival rate between treatment in minute one and minute four after cardiac arrest is very slight, according to one observer (in the order of approximately 13,5 per cent as compared with approximately 6 per cent).

The case illustrates how difficult it may be to prove a causal nexus between an alleged medical omission and the death of a patient in these cases. It may be observed that the risks connected with the use of contrast media are so slight and the potential benefits to patients so substantial, that the procedure can in no way be regarded as wrongful *per se*.[3]

3 See J P de V van Niekerk & S A Strauss "The Conventional versus the New Radiological Contrast Media – Cost-benefit Analysis and Medicolegal Implications" 70 *S Afr Med J* 799 (20 Dec 1986).

47 Anaesthetic mishaps

Surgeon not liable for anaesthetist's negligence

In some American jurisdictions, the so-called "captain of the ship" doctrine[1] was applied in the field of medical malpractice, particularly in respect of mishaps occurring in the operating theatre. The doctrine embodies the notion that a surgeon is responsible for the actions of all persons assisting him in the theatre, in the same way that the captain of a ship assumes responsibility for all souls on board. The surgeon can, therefore, be held legally liable for the acts and omissions of persons who are not his employees, including hospital personnel – the so-called "borrowed servants".

This doctrine found some acceptance in a Transvaal case early in the century but was rejected in no uncertain terms by the Appeal Court in the case of *Van Wyk v Lewis*.[2] In consequence of that decision, a doctor can be held liable only on the basis of his own negligence, unless the catastrophe was caused by the negligence of an employee of the doctor, acting within the scope of his (or her) employment, in which event the doctrine of vicarious liability would apply.

The rule that a doctor is not in principle or automatically liable for the negligence of someone assisting him was reaffirmed in the recent case of *S v Kramer and Another*.[3] In that case a 10-year-old girl underwent a tonsillectomy and adenoidectomy. Dr K performed the duties of a surgeon and Dr X those of an anaesthetist.

Having examined the patient in the theatre, Dr X administered atropine, fabantol and scolene. Pure oxygen was thereafter administered through a face mask for a few minutes. X then chose an endotracheal tube which he inserted through the nose into the trachea with the aid of a laryngoscope and McGil forceps. The theatre sister connected the tube to the Boyle machine and secured the connections. The patient was ventilated manually for some time. K then asked for permission to proceed with the operation.

A mouth gag was put in and K started curetting the adenoids. That having been completed, K started to remove the left tonsil. As he was doing so, he noticed an excess of bleeding. The blood was dark in colour and the patient was also showing signs of waking up. It was obvious that the patient was cyanosed. K removed the left tonsil, sucked the blood in the throat away and, with the aid of a laryngoscope, came to the conclusion that the tube was not in the trachea. He immediately ordered further doses of fabantol and scolene to be administered, removed the tube and reintubated the patient with another tube.

The patient was ventilated and her colour improved. She suddenly became cyanosed again and as no pulse was palpable, cardiac massage was started. Attempts were made to stimulate the patient's heart with a defribrillator, but to no avail. The patient died in the theatre.

K and X were both charged with culpable homicide and convicted. They appealed to the Supreme Court. K's appeal succeeded, but X's conviction and sentence were confirmed. The court held that there was no evidence that there had been a duty on

1 On this doctrine, see below 302.
2 1924 AD 438.
3 1987 (1) SA 887 (W).

K to check that X had correctly placed the tube. Nor, on the evidence, was there anything which had occurred prior to the operation that should have alerted K to the danger that the patient was not receiving an adequate supply of oxygen – even though X, at the time of the operation, was relatively inexperienced in the field of anaesthesia. When faced with an emergency, K acted swiftly and in a reasonable manner.

As far as X was concerned, the court found that the evidence adduced by the prosecution was consistent with the tube not having been inserted correctly. The incorrect placement or displacement of the tube must have continued for a couple of minutes during which X should have detected it, had he performed his duties properly.

In the course of his judgment, Mr Justice van der Merwe made the following observations:

"If a mishap should occur during the operation it is of importance to ascertain who was responsible for the mishap and to what extent any other member of the operating team can be held liable for the actions of that person.

"In the present case it was never suggested that any of the two nurses was responsible for the mishap or that the accused were liable as a result of negligence on the part of any of the nurses.

"I am of the opinion that, in general, neither the surgeon nor the anaesthetist is liable for the other's negligence. This general rule will, however, be subject to exceptions, for example, where the surgeon knew that the anaesthetist was incompetent or not in a fit condition to perform his duties."

Acute sequential awareness with pain during anaesthesia : patient's claim denied

An important judgment was handed down recently by an English court in the case of *Ludlow v Swindon Health Authority*.[4] A female patient brought a claim against a hospital authority for damages in respect of pain suffered during a Caesarean section, on the ground that she had not been properly anaesthetised.

The hospital conceded that the patient had at some stage been aware of what had been happening. The central issue before the court was whether the patient had proved that during a period of some ten minutes ending with the birth of the baby the anaesthetic mixture she had been receiving had *not* contained 0,5 per cent of a volatile anaesthetic agent called halothane.

It was the patient's second Caesarean and she had actually requested an epidural anaesthetic, but the procedure was then less common in the hospital concerned and an anaesthetist with the required skills was not available, so it was arranged that she should have the operation under general anaesthetic.

The patient later described how she had had some premedication, how the anaesthetist (Dr D) reassured her and having inserted a needle into a vein, put her to sleep with a familiar instruction to count back from 100. She thought she got to about 95 before becoming unconscious. The next thing she remembered was a searing pain across her stomach, so terrible that she wanted to die. She was conscious of the endotracheal tube in her throat. She could feel her stomach being parted and was aware of extreme pain in two parts. She became aware of a machine making a constant bleeping noise. At about this time she heard a baby crying and a "constant babble" in the background. She then became unconscious. At no stage could she move, open her eyes or speak.

Expert evidence was adduced that it was common practice to include in the anaesthetic mixture a small portion of a volatile agent such as halothane. However, a belief existed at the time that, even at low concentrations, this substance could be

4 1989 QBD (unreported).

productive of haemorrhaging after birth, and accordingly many anaesthetists would cease using it at the moment of birth.

An expert anaesthetist, Professor R, who testified for the patient, said that in a study of world literature he had found no case of acute sequential awareness of pain where 0,5 per cent halothane was given with nitrous oxide. He concluded that the only explanation of the patient's experience was that she had not in fact been receiving halothane, though the anaesthetist believed the contrary; the reason for this in the circumstances of the case must have been that the reservoir of the vaporiser was empty.

Professor A, an expert anaesthetist who testified for the defendant, accepted a published figure that examination of 2 500 cases of Caesarean section showed that even where nitrous oxide at 50 per cent and halothane at 0,5 per cent was used, a small proportion – 0,35 per cent of cases – experienced awareness. He himself had interviewed more than 20 patients and two had been conscious and had recall of pain.

He did not accept Professor R's view that the patient's account was one which indicated consciousness at the time of the initial incision lasting through until after birth. He regarded it as highly probable that she awoke towards the end of the operation, when halothane had been discontinued. In his opinion the sensations of pain she described were caused by swabbing of the wound and, possibly, pressure to extrude surplus blood and to ensure that the uterus was contracting as it should.

Dr H, a consultant anaesthetist at another hospital, testified the normal practice was that at the beginning of the day, a check would be made and the reservoir of the vaporiser filled if necessary. Dr D, while not purporting specifically to remember doing so for this operation, said that it was his invariable practice to check all the anaesthetic equipment, including the vaporiser. An anaesthetic nurse testified that she invariably checked, "and was confident that she would have done so on this occasion".

The judge disagreed with the submission that there was "no evidence" that the halothane reservoir was full. "Very often a person who performs a routine task on occasion when nothing occurs to fix that occasion in his memory will, years afterwards, not be able to *remember* doing that; and will rely on his practice. Such evidence can be extremely cogent."

The judge found it unnecessary to have recourse to the doctrine of *res ipsa loquitur* whereby evidence of the occurrence of an unexplained catastrophe can lead to an inference of negligence. If the reservoir had been empty when the operation began, he said, there must have been an elementary failure by two – probably three – skilled professional people, which was improbable. Moreover, there was evidence that halothane had been used in the last Caesarean section operation two days before. Given the quantities of the drug needed in one operation, ample would have remained in the reservoir on the morning of the later operation.

An analysis of the patient's evidence satisfied the court that – although she was an entirely honest and straightforward witness – her recollections were far from unequivocally attributable to the halothane phase. It was possible that contrary to her belief, she had been unconscious for a spell and again awoken. The noise of the machine, the babble of voices, the abdominal pain – all these were explicable on the basis of things happening in the final phase of the operation. Of significance were several things that she did *not* remember. The crying of the baby could be referable to a period just after birth but it could also have occurred considerably later. Moreover, the patient was under the influence of powerful drugs and it reflected not at all on her *credit*, the judge said but must cause one to doubt the *reliability* of her recollections.

In the result the court – with "considerable sympathy for her" and "with a feeling of some regret" – came to the "inexorable conclusion" that liability had not been established.

It is to be noted that in this case the anaesthetist involved, Dr D, was described by a colleague who also testified, as "highly competent and above average" although he was relatively inexperienced as an anaesthetist. The judge found that Dr D had maintained a full, clear and meticulous anaesthetic record and that his management of the case was not in any material respect open to criticism.

48 Failure of general practitioner to call in specialist gynaecologist to assist in problem case

In *S v Nel*[1] Dr N, a general practitioner, was attending to a woman when she gave delivery to her third child. Immediately after the birth, Dr N experienced problems with the removal of the placenta from her uterus. The patient bled profusely and died later the same evening from loss of blood and shock.

It appeared that the patient had been admitted to a maternity home at about 11:45, that day, for her confinement. By 17:45 the doctor was called to the maternity home. He regarded it as necessary for the purposes of the confinement to apply surgery and carried out a left lateral episiotomy (a cut through the labia). The baby was delivered at 18:45.

Complications set in, however, in that the placenta of the patient remained behind in the uterus. Dr N tried by application of the Brandt-Andrews method to deliver the placenta, but had no success. He proceeded to make several attempts to remove the placenta by hand, but these were also in vain.

The patient's husband, H, was present and observed that the doctor was apparently experiencing serious problems and that, in the meantime, his wife was suffering tremendously. Subsequently H testified in court that shortly after the birth, Dr N had pushed his hand into the patient's vagina and pulled on the umbilical cord so that it broke and blood splashed all over a nursing sister. A heated argument between the doctor and the sister followed. Thereupon the doctor twice inserted his hand into the patient's vagina up to his elbow and kept it there on each occasion for approximately 30 seconds.

This was to no avail and by 19:00 Dr N left the maternity ward. Mr H learnt from the matron that there was a specialist on the premises. H came across Dr N outside the maternity ward and told him of the specialist. Dr N's reaction, however was to tell H that he was "not a monkey" and that he would call in a specialist should he be in need of one.

Between 19:00 and 19:20 H was informed by Dr N that he had called in an anaesthetist. The anaesthetist arrived at 19:40 and noticed that there had already been a massive loss of blood. He established that no blood specimen had been taken, that no blood plasma had been ordered and that no intravenous infusion of fluid had been done.

The anaesthetist immediately took the patient's blood pressure, commenced an intravenous infusion and administered anaesthesia by means of pentothal (sodium thiopentone). Only at this stage did N at the request of the matron agree to call in a specialist, Dr S, with the remark that "a second opinion would do no harm". To the knowledge of Dr N, Dr S had already been in the maternity home since about 19:00 and had been available should N have required his assistance.

Accordingly it was only at a relatively late stage, at 20:10, that Dr S arrived in the maternity ward and started attending to the patient. He removed the placenta by hand with ease. Then he removed the placenta tissue and began to suture the episiotomy incision which had remained unsutured up to that stage. Before he could complete this, the patient died at 20:20.

1 1987 TPD (unreported).

Dr N was charged in the regional court with culpable homicide. The court found that he had been negligent in several respects. Among other things he had failed to take proper blood-pressure measurements, to do a necessary intravenous infusion before endeavouring to remove the placenta by hand, to take a blood specimen and to order blood, to call in a specialist obstetrician despite a request by the patient's husband, and to rub the uterus to let it contract. He had made unsuccessful and unskilful attempts to remove the placenta while valuable anaesthetic time had been lost, and he had left the maternity ward at a critical time. The court held that the accused's negligence had been the cause of the patient's death.

On appeal to the Transvaal Provincial Division of the Supreme Court, it was contended that it had not been proved beyond a reasonable doubt that an omission on the part of Dr N had been the cause of the patient's death. A specialist anaesthetist had testified during the trial that the administration of pentothal and halothane by the anaesthetist could have caused the patient's death. However, the court rejected this argument with the following comment: "This sort of statement is not of real value. Anything *can* happen. One sometime reads that the taking of aspirin *can* cause death. That does not say a thing."[2]

What the witness ought to have done according to Mr Justice Eloff, if he had wanted to make an objective scientific contribution to the court's task, was to explain how real the possibility had been that administration of these substances could have caused death. It is difficult to avoid the impression, the judge observed, that the expert witness "simply took a shot in the dark" to try and help the accused. The court accordingly confirmed the magistrate's verdict.

However, the court held that the sentence imposed by the regional court – five years' imprisonment, of which three years were conditionally suspended – was excessively heavy. The accused's failure to call in a specialist was no more than a reprehensible error of judgment and did not constitute recklessness. The facts of the case pointed rather to clumsiness and a lack of skill. A sentence of a fine of R5 000 with the alternative of a sentence to two years' imprisonment, coupled with a suspended sentence of two years, was accordingly substituted. (The Appeal Court subsequently refused to grant the doctor leave to appeal.)

2 My translation.

49 Superior vena cava torn during mediastinoscopy

The case of *Pringle v Administrator of the Transvaal*[1] resulted from a bronchoscopy followed by a mediastinoscopy performed on a 63-year-old woman by a senior registrar, Dr S, who had been employed by the defendant hospital authority. The patient had had a history of carcinoma and had undergone a mastectomy 29 years earlier. She presented with opacity of the right lung and an investigation of the lung was necessary.

A bronchoscopy is an examination of the bronchi (air passages within the lungs) by means of an instrument. A mediastinoscopy is an examination of the mediastum by means of a tubular instrument permitting direct inspection of the tissues in the area. The mediastum is the mass of tissues separating the two lungs.

In the course of the mediastinoscopy, the patient's superior vena cava was torn, in consequence of which torrential bleeding occurred. (The superior vena cava is the venous trunk draining blood from the head, neck, arms and hands, and chest.) The mediastum was packed. The patient lost approximately two litres of blood, and a right thoracotomy (a surgical incision in the wall of the chest) was performed to repair the damaged vena cava. On the day following the operation she went into acute renal failure and required haemodyalisis (i e purification of the blood by means of a machine).

The patient suffered brain-damage as a result of the operation which she claimed had resulted in permanent damage to her eyesight and permanent inability to work. She also underwent personality and character changes. She had been employed by a business firm for general office work and to control the switchboard. She was responsible for the payment of wages, banking, post, ordering and was a general factotum. She had had a record of complete reliability, trustworthiness and competence. After the operation, however, her employment was terminated summarily by her employer.

The patient alleged that the surgeon and his assistants had been negligent in a number of respects, and claimed damages in the amount of R97 228 in respect of her loss of earnings and general damages for pain and suffering, shock, loss of amenities of life and disablement.

Inter alia the patient averred that the procedure adopted, namely the mediastinoscopy was neither correct nor appropriate. At the trial there was no unanimity among the medical experts in regard to which procedure should have been followed. The doctors agreed, however, that the type of operation to be performed is a matter of personal choice.

Dr M, a thoracic surgeon called by the patient as an expert witness said in his report that "an accident as occurred in this case, is one of the dangers of mediastinoscopy, and it could come about in the hands of the most experienced operator". He testified that on the basis of the pre-operative X-rays, he himself would have performed a bronchoscopy, but if in the face of the X-rays the results were normal, he would have proceeded to have done a limited thoracotomy.

The court held that on the basis of Dr M's evidence, the plaintiff had not dis-

1 1990 (2) SA 379 (W).

charged the onus of proving that the procedure had been incorrect or inappropriate, even though Dr M might have preferred the limited thoracotomy.

Dr S testified that the decision to perform the bronchoscopy and mediastinoscopy had been a departmental decision, taken after consultation. Dr K, who was called by the defendant as an expert witness, was also of the view that the mediastinoscopy was preferable, because, among other considerations it had a lower morbidity ("sick rate").

Another ground of alleged negligence on which the plaintiff relied was that once the haemorrhaging had occurred during the mediastinoscopy, the doctors failed to immediately proceed with sternotomy or right thoracotomy to stabilise and prevent further or recurrent bleeding. (Sternotomy is the operation of cutting through the sternum or breastbone.) The emphasis fell on "immediately" since it was common cause that a thoracotomy had in fact been performed approximately 75 minutes after the mediastinoscopy procedure had concluded.

This aspect was thoroughly canvassed by the expert witnesses. Decision of this issue turned *inter alia* on the fact that Dr S had arranged for emergency X-rays to be taken prior to performing the thoracotomy, by reason of the patient's previous medical history. (She had presented with two etiological incidents of heart disease, namely she was a smoker and had some hypertension.) As soon as the X-rays were available, Dr S was aware of the fact that the bleeding was still continuing and that the bleeding was in the pleural cavity.

Dr M testified he would have opened the chest and sutured the vena cava, since being the major vessel in that area, that was the likely source of danger. He was of the opinion that if the delay had not occurred, it was unlikely that the blood pressure would have dropped. Dr S however, testified that at the stage when he had ordered emergency X-rays the blood pressure (which he himself had constantly monitored) had dropped, but it had never been unrealistically low. He did not think at the time that the bleeding had been into the pleura and thought that the X-rays would show that the bleeding had been in the mediastinum but had been controlled.

Dr K was of the opinion that there had been no undue delay between the two procedures and that it would have been unwise to proceed to a thoracotomy immediately. He regarded it as imperative first to have X-rays done so that a proper diagnosis could be made; thoracotomy is a major operation and should not be undertaken unless it is inevitable.

On the evidence before her, the judge, Miss Acting Justice Blum, was not satisfied that the plaintiff had shown on a balance of probabilities that if the doctors had proceeded to do a thoracotomy immediately, the damage would not have been done. It was accordingly not proved that the delay which occurred through waiting for X-rays before making a diagnosis was unreasonable and therefore negligent. Certain other allegations of negligence had likewise not been proved, the judge held.

The court did find, however, that Dr S had been negligent in tearing the superior vena cava, while attempting to biopsy the lymph-node in the gland adjacent thereto. (A biopsy is removal of a small portion of tissue from an organ for microscopic examination with a view to diagnosis.) When, in cross-examination, it was put to Dr S that the tearing of the vena cava was negligent, he replied that an event such as this had happened in the hands of the most experienced surgeon, and that such a complication could not be called a mistake or negligence. His expert witness, Dr K, supported the view that there was no question of negligence in the management of the case.

In cross-examination it was also put to Dr S that he had "tugged" at the lymph-node and pulled the vena cava. His answer was: "In retrospect I would say that I tugged too hard." He also conceded that "there must have been excessive force because the event occurred; I am more experienced and it makes a similar event unlikely".

The judge said that in assessing the foreseeability of harm, the court must guard against "the insidious subconscious influence of *ex post facto* knowledge". "Negligence is not established," she said, "by showing merely that the occurrence happened ... or by showing after it happened how it could have been prevented.

"I am mindful too of all the pressures and the tensions which operate on a surgeon at a time like this," the judge continued. "However, in the light of all the evidence and the only possible explanations as to how the perforation of the vena cava and the mediastinal pleura occurred, I am driven to find that on this particular aspect, and by using the 'excessive force' which he concedes, Dr S did not apply that skill and diligence possessed and exercised at the time by the members of the branch of the profession to which he belonged."

Damages of R92 483 were awarded to the plaintiff. In assessing the amount of damages the court took into account that the plaintiff had reached the age of 67 ½ at the time of the trial, without further incident, and that her life expectancy had not been reduced as a result of the incident. It is of interest to note that the amount awarded by the court was only some R4 000 short of what the plaintiff had claimed. This is unusual; in lawsuits for damages plaintiffs often claim far more than they hope to recover eventually and, if successful, are awarded a fraction of what they have sued for.

The judgment reaffirmed the view taken in the 1924 case of *Van Wyk v Lewis*[2] that there is no room in this type of case for application of the doctrine of *res ipsa loquitur* ("the thing speaks for itself") which may in practical terms lead to an inference of negligence being drawn from the mere fact of an unexplained catastrophe. Observed Miss Justice Blum: "The maxim could only be invoked where the negligence alleged depends on absolutes."

2 1924 AD 438. The case is discussed above 270.

50 Plastic surgery: medico-legal aspects

The medico-legal risks connected with plastic surgery are generally considered to be high. "In no other surgical speciality is the doctor so apt to be sued than in the field of plastic surgery," says Ficarra[1] in writing on American law, and, adds he: "The plastic surgeon stands in the forefront of vulnerability because the products of his labour are usually more visible than that of any other speciality."[2]

Yet, although the risks may theoretically be high, relatively few cases involving cosmetic surgery have been reported, even in the USA which has an extremely high overall incidence of malpractice litigation.

Cases

In South Africa there has been no reported case, so far, on litigation involving plastic surgery. By "reported" I mean a judgment of the Supreme Court reported in the *South African Law Reports*. But claims against doctors have been brought in this country which have either been settled out of court or abandoned by the patient. The following are cases which have come to my attention:

- A 48-year-old woman had contracted poliomyelitis as an infant from which she fully recovered subsequently. But in her middle forties she noticed that she had more loose skin on the right side of her face than on the left, giving her face a lopsided appearance. She was operated on by a specialist plastic surgeon who administered injections of a substance to ease the flow of blood to enable him to work more freely. Allegedly as a result of the injections she developed deep and most unsightly erosions on both her cheeks and on her neck, which necessitated expensive further surgery. The doctor denied any negligence on his part and blamed the mishap on the drug used. The manufacturer, however, claimed that the drug was well-tried and faultless. The patient could not obtain expert evidence supporting the allegation that the drug was defective and ultimately abandoned her claim.
- A 23-year-old unmarried female was unhappy with the size of her breasts and with the fact that one breast was bigger than the other. She approached a general practitioner, who had apparently undertaken plastic surgery on a large scale, for a breast reduction. Following the operation the right areola and nipple complex became black and necrotic, without sensation and also septic. Antibiotic treatment was of no avail. The nipple, areola and ducts in the left breast were also allegedly destroyed as a functional unit. The patient then consulted a specialist plastic surgeon, who attributed the mishap to the general practitioner's negligence. A series of corrective operations was subsequently embarked upon. The patient sued the doctor and the matter was ultimately settled out of court.
- The third case involved the same general practitioner. This time the plaintiff was a 37-year-old married woman who went to the doctor for a reduction of her buttocks and thighs which she regarded as flabby. Two weeks after the operation

1 B J Ficarra *Surgical and Allied Malpractice* (1968) 469.
2 *Ibid* 470.

ulcer craters appeared in her thighs, through which bone was visible. The doctor attempted further surgery, transplanting fat from her breasts to her buttocks with disastrous results. The patient ended up with deep depressions in her badly scarred thighs and complained of constant pains. A plastic surgeon consulted by her, attributed negligence to the general practitioner and the patient sued. The patient claimed that the doctor had "guaranteed" that "no dimples would develop in the thighs". The case was settled out of court.

The only reported case in South Africa which peripherally touches on cosmetic "surgery" is *S v Van der Merwe*[3] in which it was held that a person not registered as a medical practitioner who practised as a tattoo-remover had contravened the Medical, Dental and Supplementary Health Service Professions Act, 1974[4] because a tattoo mark is regarded as a physical defect, and the Act proscribes *inter alia* the treatment by an unregistered person of "any physical defect" for gain. The accused had removed tattoo marks by means of cauterisation after his "patients" were given a local anaesthetic, procaine.

In 1975 DeMere[5] reported that qualified plastic surgeons in the USA had had very few successful malpractice suits against them. He ascribed this to the fact that plastic surgeons know that the danger of lawsuits exists which has the effect that they take more care to prevent such suits. Says he: "A ship that sails between the reefs will keep a closer look-out than one in 'safe waters'."

Although, then, plastic surgery may be regarded as a relatively low-risk area in comparison with other fields of medicine, there are nevertheless substantial medico-legal risks of which the practitioner should be aware at all times.

Basic principles

Traditionally the law has favoured therapeutic procedures. In the case of non-therapeutic procedures, the requirements of the law are decidedly more stringent.

Where the objective is neither the healing of the patient nor that of another (e g by means of organ transplantation), a "medical" procedure would not be considered lawful merely because the patient has consented to it. A further requirement must be met, namely that a legally justifiable objective is sought to be attained by it. It is a principle of our law that consent only operates as a defence if it is not *contra bonos mores*,[6] or, as it is sometimes put, against public policy.

To use an extreme example: where a young man gets a doctor to surgically amputate his perfectly healthy and normal right hand so as to enable him to evade military duty, there is no doubt that the doctor would be guilty of aggravated criminal assault, even if the operation is performed with the utmost degree of skill. The patient's consent clearly is *contra bonos mores*.[7]

It seems to be generally accepted today that the interest in beauty constitutes a legally justifiable objective.[8] There is a rider to be added however: where the sole purpose with the operation is to improve the patient's appearance, it should not entail a serious risk to the life or health of the patient.

3 1977 (3) SA 747 (T).
4 Act 56 of 1974.
5 M DeMere "The Plastic Surgeon and Legal Matters" in 1975 *Legal Medicine Annual* 293, 294.
6 S A Strauss & M J Strydom *Die Suid-Afrikaanse Geneeskundige Reg* (1967) 184; J C van der Walt *Delict: Principles and Cases* (1979) par 34; Neethling, Potgieter & Visser *Law of Delict* (1990) 89. But see E M Burchell & P M A Hunt *South African Criminal Law and Procedure* vol 1 (*General Principles*) (2nd ed, 1983) 371.
7 As to the question whether the "patient" can sue the doctor for damages in a situation such as this, see my remarks below on plastic surgery on a fugitive criminal to shield him from justice.
8 An interesting project in the USA revealed that plastic surgery performed on gaol prisoners is a substantial factor in the reduction of recidivism. See Ficarra 471.

But where the objective primarily is to alleviate a serious psychoneurotic condition in the patient which stems from disfigurement or even from a subjective aversion towards a particular physical feature, it is submitted that even relatively drastic surgical procedures must be regarded as lawful.

Fugitive from justice

What about plastic surgery performed upon a fugitive criminal with the exclusive purpose of shielding him from justice? Pope Pius XII ruled that this motive would render the operation illicit.[9] There can be no doubt that in this country such a motive would be regarded as *contra bonos mores.*

Logically this would lead to the conclusion that the operation must be held to be unlawful notwithstanding the fact that the patient was a consenting party in the fullest sense of the word, in that he urgently beseeched the doctor to carry out the operation.

It seems doubtful, however, to say the least, that a court would allow a patient to recover delictual damages from the doctor on the ground that the operation was unlawful![10] But if the operation was unsuccessful because of the doctor's negligence and the patient ends up looking like Frankenstein's monster, an arguable case for damages might be put forward.

It goes without saying that a doctor who knowingly performs plastic surgery on a criminal with the object of shielding him from justice will not be entitled to sue for his fee.[11] Another point that should be considered by the doctor who is approached to perform the operation is that he will most probably make himself guilty of defeating or obstructing the course of justice. This is a criminal offence which essentially consists in unlawfully doing any act which is intended to defeat and obstruct the due administration of justice.[12]

An interesting case of a woman who underwent plastic surgery to evade the law was reported upon by the South African media[13] in the late 1980s. She was sought by the Police on a charge of fraud and a photograph of her appeared on the television programme, "Police File". She was given a "new face" but her efforts were in vain. When it came to the attention of the plastic surgeon that his ex-patient was wanted by the Police, he reported her and she was subsequently arrested.

Contractual issues

Ordinarily the contract entered into by doctor and patient assumes the form of a tacit agreement whereby the doctor undertakes to diagnose the patient's complaint and to treat him for it in the usual manner. In the case of the patient who desires plastic

9 Ficarra 470.

10 Although surgery performed on the basis of a consent which is legally inoperative, in these circumstances may be said "technically" to amount to an assault, it can hardly be said that the patient suffered damage (other than perhaps nominally). Even if it can be said that there has been a violation of a legal right of the plaintiff in such a case, it would be tantamount to an abuse of rights to allow the plaintiff to recover damages. The plaintiff, being a party himself to a socially reprehensible contract, does not approach the court with "clean hands". The "clean hands doctrine" has been recognised in our law of contract in the maxims *ex turpi causa non oritur actio* (from a base consideration no action arises) and *in pari delicto potior est condicio defendentis* (in a case of equal wrong (delict) by both parties the defendant is in the stronger position), to prevent plaintiffs from benefitting from illegal transactions. See E Kahn *Contract and Mercantile Law through the Cases* (1971) 176 *et seq* and cases quoted. It is submitted that there is no reason why these principles should not be applied to delictual actions as well.

11 The "clean hands doctrine" applies: see preceding note.

12 See P M A Hunt *South African Criminal Law and Procedure* vol III *(Common-law Crimes)* (2nd ed, 1982, by J R L Milton) 143.

13 See *Die Burger* 10/3/87.

surgery, there is usually a slight variation of this situation. The patient has already made the diagnosis himself and he has also decided on the cure: he is unhappy with his physical appearance and desires it to be improved by surgery.

By undertaking a case, a doctor does not guarantee that the patient will be cured of his complaint. He undertakes no more than to treat the patient with the amount of skill, competence and care which may reasonably be expected from a practitioner of his branch of medicine.[14]

If a doctor departs from the patient's express instructions or fails to treat him in the manner tacitly agreed on, the doctor will be guilty of breach of contract and may be sued for damages. Should the doctor be so bold as to guarantee a cure, he assumes a special risk of liability in the event of him being unable to fulfil his guarantee.

It would be particularly unwise for the plastic surgeon to guarantee the patient "full satisfaction". This type of patient usually enters the doctor's consulting rooms with a psychological hang-up and particularly high expectations.

Moreover, as Holder[15] has pointed out, plastic surgery presents psychological problems usually absent in other types of surgery: "Some of the persons who seek to have cosmetic surgery are generally unhappy about their social life and consider themselves unattractive solely as a result of their physical problem."

If the surgery does not prove to be a panacea for these problems, says Holder, it may well be that this type of patient would have serious adjustment traumas when he realised that his difficulties were caused by more factors than his looks. This type of emotional reaction not infrequently leads to allegations that the doctor, not the patient, is at fault.

Warns Holder: "When personality problems of which the patient is presumably unaware are blamed on a cosmetic deficiency, removal of the deficiency may actually increase the extent of the problem. This sort of patient is the one who may be quite hard to please under any conditions, and if there is any excuse for doing so, can become quite litigation-minded with little difficulty."

As Ficarra[16] has pointed out, the plastic surgeon will be courting disaster if he shows his prospective patient, who is unhappy with the shape or size of his nose, photographs of handsome people and asks the patient which he prefers. Similarly, to retouch a photograph of the patient in order to demonstrate how the surgical end result will look is equally hazardous and foolish.[17] These actions might well be interpreted legally as amounting to an express undertaking or guarantee to produce a particular result, and, as I have said, if that result is not accomplished, an allegation of breach of contract may be made.

There is one redeeming feature, however, as far as our law is concerned, and that is that the object of an action for damages for breach of contract is to compensate the aggrieved party for actual pecuniary loss suffered. The patient will therefore have to prove a calculable economic loss: no damages of a purely sentimental or punitive character and no nominal damages will be awarded.[18]

In theory this is conceivable, for example a prospective film star alleging that she has failed to secure a highly profitable role in a movie because cosmetic surgery did not improve her looks as was guaranteed by the doctor. But in actual practice she would most likely be confronted with the almost insurmountable obstacle of proving a causal nexus.

14 Cf the judge's remarks in *Buls and Another v Tsatsarolakis* 1976(2) SA 891 (T).
15 A R Holder *Medical Malpractice Law* (2nd ed, 1978) 115.
16 Ficarra *op cit* 469.
17 As P F Swanepoel & I Eisenberg "Current Concepts in Cosmetic Rhinoplasty" 1981 *S Afr Med J* 536 at 544 point out, films and television have played dominant roles in establishing the criteria of beauty. The Hollywood plastic surgeons, they say, are in no small way responsible for setting the fashion to be followed by the rest of the world.
18 Wille & Millin's *Mercantile Law of South Africa* (18th ed, 1984 by J F Coaker and D T Zeffertt) 146.

A more practical aspect of the doctor's failure to fulfil his guarantee will be that he may be unable to recover the fee agreed upon or a substantial part of it.[19]

Informed consent

Apart from legal liability for medical negligence (see below) the single most important potential ground for liability is the absence of informed consent.

Because of the difficulties confronting an aggrieved patient to prove negligence on the part of the doctor, there is a clear tendency in some countries for plaintiffs to resort to a lack of informed consent as a cause of action. This trend has also manifested itself in South Africa.

There is a positive duty on the doctor to inform the patient of the nature of the treatment and its likely side-effects,[20] and if it is of importance in "ordinary" therapeutic medicine, it is of even greater importance in relation to cosmetic surgery of the "luxury" kind, where the practitioner cannot rely on the excuse of therapeutic privilege.

The doctor is not required to inform the patient of every conceivable risk attached to the procedure envisaged. In particular there is no duty on the doctor to inform the patient of highly unusual complications that might set in.[21]

In the field of plastic surgery, experience has taught that the initial procedure decided upon may necessitate further operations to endeavour to achieve the best cosmetic end-result. It would obviously be wise for the doctor to apprise the patient of that possibility. Like any major surgery embarked on in a non-emergency situation, it would be unwise to let the patient rush into it. After the initial surge of enthusiasm the patient might have second thoughts. It would clearly be advisable for the doctor to allow for a "cooling-off" period to enable the patient to calmly reconsider.

There are two different schools of thought on the best way to take a consent. The one school holds that a detailed written consent should be taken; the other holds that there should be no written consent at all and that the doctor can rely on the patient's tacit consent.[22]

There is obviously no necessity to insist on a formal written consent in respect of minor procedures. Much of the work done by ordinary dentists, such as the fitting of a crown, also has a "cosmetic" component, yet a written consent is almost never taken.

The more drastic the procedure is, the more advisable it is in my opinion, from a legal point of view, for the doctor to take a fairly detailed written consent,[23] in which the essential character of the operation is described in simple terms understandable by the layman. The patient should also consent to incidental procedures such as anaesthesia. A consent form is a useful document in which to include a statement by the patient that the doctor has fully explained the surgery, that the patient understands it, and that the doctor has given no guarantee of success or satisfaction. [24]

Golan and Ben-Hur[25] have drawn attention to the fact that it is technically almost

19 See *Sutherland v White* 1911 EDL 407 where a doctor was denied recovery of his fee for ill-fitting dentures supplied.

20 See e g *Richter and Another v Estate Hamman* 1976 (3) SA 226 (C).

21 *Ibid.* See also *supra* 9–10.

22 M DeMere "The Plastic Surgeon and Legal Matters" in 1975 *Legal Medicine Annual* 293 at 296 makes the observation that "[one] of the finest medical centres in the world, the Mayo Clinic, has never had a written consent form to this day and had no difficulty with 'informed consent'". However, he himself makes use of a written consent, which he quotes in full in his article.

23 DeMere's suggested consent form (see preceding note) mentions no specific operation but merely authorises "whatever operation, operative procedure, treatment, or technical procedure (the doctor) may deem necessary". He claims that his form has twice been tested in court and upheld. In my respectful opinion, however, authorisation in that form is too general to be legally valid.

24 In these respects, DeMere's form is satisfactory.

25 J Golan and N Ben-Hur "Informed Consent in Plastic Surgery" 2 *Med Law* 113 (1983), 115.

impossible to remove tattoo marks without scars remaining. The patient should be told of this to avoid dissatisfaction afterwards.

A high percentage of patients seeking plastic surgery are married women. Must the husband's consent be insisted upon? In our law the husband generally[26] has no say over what medical treatment the wife should or may undergo, and vice versa. Each spouse may therefore consent independently irrespective of whether the spouses are married in or out of community of property. In not obtaining a husband's consent the doctor therefore does not expose himself to a delictual claim.

But in the absence of the husband's consent, the doctor may be unable to hold him liable for his fees. As far as medical services are concerned, a husband's marital duty to provide his wife with household necessaries stretches no further than reasonable medical care. What is reasonable depends among other things on the couple's social and financial status.[27] Thus, while the wife of a salaried municipal worker clearly does not have the capacity to bind the husband contractually for expensive plastic surgery to convert her into another Bo Derek, an aging actress wedded to a millionaire might well do just that!

Professional negligence

The law on medical negligence is simple to state: the doctor must exercise reasonable care and skill. What is reasonable in a particular situation, is essentially a matter of expert medical evidence. It is the medical profession which lays down what the appropriate standard of care is. The courts do not make findings *in vacuo*, but strictly on the facts before them.

Because of the profits to be reaped from a successful practice of plastic surgery, some general medical practitioners have been tempted to become engaged in this type of work, without prior specialised training. In this country at least one such general practitioner set himself up as plastic surgeon and established a large practice; sad to say, the quality of some of his work was appalling; this resulted in several lawsuits brought by aggrieved patients for alleged malpractice.

If a practitioner ventures beyond his own area of training, expertise and skill, he should realise that he is skating on thin ice, legally speaking, because the law will hold him to reasonable standards applying to the field into which he ventures. An ancient legal principle warns: *imperitia culpae adnumeratur* ("lack of skill amounts to negligence").[28] A general practitioner who practises plastic surgery must therefore be expected to be judged by the standards set by specialist plastic surgeons.

The mere fact that an adverse result has set in does not lead to an inference of negligence. In this country the evidential principle of *res ipsa loquitur*[29] ("the thing speaks for itself") would not readily be applied to the medical situation – unlike a number of American jurisdictions where the principle has become a "rule of sympathy" on which aggrieved patients suing their doctors rely heavily.

In South Africa the *onus* lies on the shoulders of a plaintiff suing for damages to convince the court that there was negligence and that he has suffered damage in consequence thereof. As was illustrated by the above-mentioned case of the woman whose face was lopsided as a result of polio, the proof of a causal connection between

26 See above 5. A possible exception to this general rule is abortion. See above 211.
27 Thus in *Johnston v Powell* (1909) 19 CTR 86 it was held that artificial dentures are a medical necessity for a woman whose husband has a reasonable income. *Brudo v Chamberlain* 1912 TPD 131 held that dental treatment was a household necessity although the husband earned only £10 a month (the 1991 equivalent of about R600 or R700?).
28 On the principle see T J Scott's essay in *Petere Fontes: L C Steyn – Gedenkbundel* (D J Joubert, ed, n d) 124 *et seq*.
29 See *supra* 245.

an allegedly negligent act and the ultimate catastrophe will sometimes present serious difficulties to the plaintiff.

Violation of privacy

A few words should be said about legal liability for violation of the patient's privacy. The plastic surgeon runs no special risk in this respect as compared to practitioners in other fields. But this type of surgery frequently involves the face of the patient. Photographs may be taken of the patient in the course of treatment by which he may be identified, and the plastic surgeon should be on his guard not to display photographs that might cause embarrassment to the patient, without the latter's consent. Should the surgeon wish to make use of these photographs for the purposes of illustrating a publication, or lectures given by him, he would be well-advised to obtain a written consent.

Records

Lawyers have often stressed the importance of keeping adequate records. In the event of a lawsuit or a disciplinary inquiry these will often be the doctor's first line of defence. In plastic surgery, documentation of a case should go beyond the keeping of notes by the practitioner. It is advisable for the plastic surgeon to take photographs of the patient before and after surgery. The photographs should be shown to the patient and he should sign a statement on the back thereof – attested to by an independent witness – that the photograph is an accurate likeness of him when it was taken. Such photographs will constitute an important part of the surgeon's records and may afford incontestable evidence should a dispute arise at a later stage as to the quality of his professional work.

Talking about medical records: in this country they are still regarded as the exclusive property of the doctor, and the patient has no access to them except if permitted by the doctor, and then only on the doctor's terms.[30] According to our law, in a civil suit disclosure of records can only be enforced by means of the procedure known as discovery, after the pleadings have been closed, which may take place weeks or even months after the plaintiff issued summons. Our courts will not allow a person contemplating litigation against another, to get access to the latter's documents for the purposes of a "fishing expedition".

It may nevertheless be advisable for a doctor who is threatened with legal action to give the aggrieved patient a copy of his records. Such a decision is best taken after the doctor has taken legal advice in a specific instance. As Bromberg and Hirsh[31] have warned, by refusing to release records to a patient, the doctor is only inviting the patient to file an action and to obtain access by procedural means: "the refusal will only serve to arouse the patient to a state of paranoia".

Based upon a paper read at the congress of the Association of Plastic and Reconstructive Surgeons of South Africa, held at Sun City, Bophuthatswana, October 1980.

30 See *supra* 110 *et seq.*
31 J Bromberg & H Hirsh "Medical Records and Hospital Reports" (1982) *Medicine and Law* 253 at 255.

51 Legal liability for defective drugs

Introduction

In this chapter attention is directed primarily to potential liability towards the ultimate consumer of drugs, i e the patient, for injury or other harm sustained as a result of the use of defective medicine.

I do not propose to go into the statutory requirements pertaining to the development, registration, and marketing of drugs. Suffice it to say that, in South Africa, we have detailed legislation regulating the control of medicines in the form of the Medicines and Related Substances Control Act.[1]

This Act has created the Medicines Control Council, the main function of which is to approve medicines for registration in the register of medicines. The Council exercises strict supervisory powers in regard to, among other things, the quality of medicines and the distribution of medicines in general.

The present discussion is confined essentially to delictual liability for a defective drug. It is not intended here to deal with a claim based on negligent misrepresentation of the qualities of a drug which is not inherently defective.[2]

Liability for fault

According to the South African common law of delict, liability of a person for damage unlawfully caused to another rests primarily on the issue of fault. Fault may take the form either of intent to cause damage, or negligence.

It is difficult to conceive of any responsible pharmaceutical firm, medical practitioner or chemist being guilty of the deliberate distribution, administration, prescription or dispensing of a defective drug. If this were proved, there would, of course, be a clear case for delictual and even criminal liability on the part of the firm, practitioner or chemist.

I mention intent as a form of fault merely to draw attention to the fact that intent need not necessarily take the form of a direct volitional act on the part of the wrongdoer, but may assume the form of what lawyers term *dolus eventualis*. This is present when the wrongdoer foresees the possibility of his act resulting in harm to another, but proceeds regardless of whether or not such harm ensues. It is not too difficult to conceive of situations relating to the distribution of drugs in which this form of intent may be present.

However, the present discussion need not go beyond an assessment of liability based upon negligence. According to our law, negligence is the (reprehensible) failure to take such care as is reasonably demanded from the defendant, considering all the circumstances of his case. This may result in the wrongdoer failing to foresee that his conduct may harm another and to take such action as would be necessary to prevent that harm.[3]

1 Act 101 of 1965.
2 See e g *Bayer South Africa (Pty) Ltd and Another v Viljoen* 1990 (2) SA 647 (A) in which a pharmaceutical manufacturer was sued for damages resulting from its alleged incorrect misrepresentation that a product was suitable for use as a systemic fungicide for the control of a certain plant disease.
3 J Neethling, J M Potgieter and P J Visser *Law of Delict* (1990) 111.

The manufacturer

It is to be noted that other systems of law have moved away from the notion of fault liability for defective products, and have introduced the concept of no-fault or strict liability as regards the manufacturer.[4]

Thus, in the USA, it was held[5] that a manufacturer is strictly liable when he sells a product with the knowledge that it is to be used without inspection for defects, if it is proved that the product has a defect which causes injury to human beings.

Strict liability is a form of consumer protection: the manufacturer, by marketing his product, virtually assumes the role of insurer of consumers who are harmed by the product. (Incidentally, there is a school of thought in the USA favouring extension of the principle of strict liability to professional services.[6])

Our law, however, still stands firmly on the principle of fault liability, and, what is more, holds that the onus of proof is on the aggrieved person, the plaintiff in a lawsuit.

It may be extremely difficult for a patient who alleges that a prescribed drug was defective, to prove that his damage is attributable to the negligence of the manufacturer. The doctrine of *res ipsa loquitur* may perhaps, to a certain extent, alleviate the burden of proof for the patient.[7] This doctrine enables a court to draw an inference of negligence, in extreme circumstances, from a catastrophic result, in the absence of a convincing explanation on the part of the causer of the catastrophe. But, needless to say, the apparently simple issue of proving a causal connection between the use of the drug and the patient's injury in itself may present the patient with an insurmountable obstacle.[8]

Moreover, as De Jager[9] has pointed out, the mere fact of registration of a medicine under the Medicines etc Control Act will probably be regarded by our courts as a strong indication that the manufacturer has not been negligent in the design of his product. After all, extreme caution was built into the statutory machinery to ensure that only safe and efficacious medicines are sold to the public,[10] and then only with appropriate warnings and directions regarding their ultimate use.

As De Jager has indicated, manufacturers' liability for injuries to patients caused by defective medicines will probably be limited to the following types of cases:

- when there has been a negligent deviation from the formula submitted for official registration;
- when the manufacturer has failed to warn against adverse side-effects, or to give directions for use as prescribed by the Medicines Control Council;
- when registration of a medicine was cancelled and the manufacturer has failed to withdraw his product from the market within a reasonable time.[11]

Apart from delictual liability, a person who is harmed by a defective product sold to him by a manufacturer may have a claim based on breach of contract, irrespective of the proof of negligence. I shall have more to say on the merchant's liability when dealing with the pharmacist, below.

The doctor

If it is difficult for a patient who has suffered bodily harm, allegedly as a result of the

4 D M Davis "Products Liability in South African Law" 1979 *CILSA* 206.
5 *Greenman v Yuba Power Products Inc* (1963) 59 Cal 2d 57, 13 ALR 3d 1049, quoted by Davis *op cit.*
6 On the Scandinavian attitude, see the remarks made by N E Siegerfors in his paper presented to the First World Meeting on Medical Law, reproduced in *Jus Medicum* (1969) 235.
7 On this doctrine generally, see *supra* 245. See also *Bayers* case *supra* 661 G-H.
8 See the example quoted *supra* 285.
9 F J de Jager "Defective Pharmaceutical Products" 1980 *Businessman's Law* 234.
10 *Ibid.*
11 *Ibid.*

use of a drug which is defective, to sue the manufacturer successfully, it would seem to be considerably more difficult to hold the doctor liable *ex delicto.*

As is the case with the manufacturer, the doctor's liability rests squarely on the postulate of proof of negligence. Moreover, even if the patient succeeded in proving negligence on the part of the manufacturer, such negligence cannot be transferred to the doctor without more proof. The doctor's liability will depend on the extent to which he could have foreseen the ultimate catastrophe, in the light of what can reasonably be required from him in his particular circumstances.

We have had several cases[12] in South Africa in which a doctor was held legally liable for drug damage, but these cases invariably involved over-prescribing or over-administration – on account of ignorance or carelessness on the part of the doctor – of drugs that are quite safe when used in accordance with the manufacturers' directions.

In the case of a drug which was properly designed, developed, tested, registered and distributed and which was prescribed in conformity with the statutory standards, and which is now alleged to be potentially hazardous to patients, proof of negligence on the part of the doctor may wellnigh be impossible.

If registration as such is regarded as a strong indication that there was no negligence on the part of the manufacturer, this factor will weigh even more heavily in the favour of the doctor. The doctor may, in the absence of very special circumstances, certainly rely on the fact that the Medicines Control Council has been fully satisfied as to the safety of the product before allowing the manufacturer to market it and, in particular, that exacting clinical trials have been performed and that all reasonable measures have been taken to identify potentially harmful side-effects so that contra-indications can be specified. Yet, it is not inconceivable that, in exceptional circumstances, a doctor may be held liable for a defective drug.

First, there is the possibility that a drug, despite all the precautions taken to ensure its safety, turns out to be unsafe. The thalidomide disaster immediately comes to mind, but other examples in recent pharmaceutical history may also be cited. Without a doubt, there is a duty upon a doctor to keep himself adequately informed on developments in the pharmaceutical field in so far as his profession is affected. If, for example, a doctor were to prescribe or administer a drug despite the fact that its risks – newly discovered – have been fully described in a medical journal circulating in his area of practice, an inference of negligence can clearly be drawn. This will also be the case where a manufacturer has withdrawn a drug, the safety of which has become suspect, and has given wide notice of its decision.

Secondly, there is the possibility, in the case of doctors who do their own dispensing, or even in the case of a doctor who gratuitously hands pharmaceutical specimens to a patient, that that particular batch has become unsafe or ineffective (due to contamination or a chemical reaction). The doctor's liability in this respect is the same as that of the chemist which will be dealt with next.

The pharmacist

As is the case with the manufacturer (and the doctor) the chemist will ordinarily be able to seek legal refuge in the fact that the drug has been developed in accordance with the statutory requirements. As I have indicated, this is not altogether conclusive on the issue of negligence, but it is a powerful indication that there has not been negligence.

The cases which we have seen in South Africa involving pharmacists, almost without exception relate to the negligent dispensing of drugs that are ordinarily safe.[13]

12 See e g *R v Van der Merwe* 1953 (2) PH H124 (W); *R v Van Schoor* 1948 (4) SA 349 (C); *S v Mkwetshana* 1965 (2) SA 493 (N).

13 See e g *R v Hosiosky* 1961 (1) SA 84 (W).

As far as potentially defective drugs are concerned, the chemist can, of course, not rely blindly on the assumption that what he has received from the manufacturer (either directly, or indirectly through a wholesale distributor) is invariably in a safe condition.

The pharmacist is an expert in his own right and must, at the very least, keep himself informed – in so far as is reasonable for members of his profession – of pharmaceutical developments, and in particular of occurrences such as the *ex post* discovery of the fact that a drug, thought to be safe, has serious side-effects. This also applies in particular to a reported withdrawal of a drug because its qualities have become suspect.

Finally, there is the aspect of a perfectly safe drug becoming patently unusable or unsafe on account of its limited shelf-life, or for whatever other reason. This is one area in which the pharmacist cannot shelter behind the manufacturer or the doctor who has prescribed the drug.

The prudent chemist should always be on his guard against the possibility of drugs arriving from the manufacturer or the wholesale distributor in a patently defective condition. Similarly, he should be on his guard against drugs deteriorating on his own shelves. The crucial stage is that of dispensing: at that stage, if not before, the drugs should be properly examined. Before a substance is dispensed, the pharmacist should check the expiry date as indicated by the manufacturer. The dispensing of medicine which has expired will constitute unprofessional conduct.

If the pharmacist has failed to ensure that the patient receive safe and effective medicines, he may be held delictually liable for harm suffered by the patient.

Quite apart from delictual liability, however, the patient would be entitled to sue the chemist on the ground of breach of contract. This might involve a claim for consequential damages brought about by a *latent* defect in the drugs sold. The chemist will probably be regarded as a "merchant [publicly] professing skill and expert knowledge in relation to the kind of goods sold"[14] for the purposes of the consumer's action. If a farmer who has bought a defective pesticide from a co-operative society can sue for the loss of his crop[15] (and not only for return of the purchase price), the potential liability of the pharmacist towards a patient who was not cured of his ailment because of a defective drug assumes staggering prospects in the legal mind!

14 Wille & Millin's *Mercantile Law of South Africa* (18th ed, 1984) 235.
15 *Kroonstad Westelike Boere-Koöperatiewe Vereniging Bpk v Botha and Another* 1964 (3) SA 561 (A).

PART XII

Hospital liability, superintendents and employees

52 Hospital liability for delicts committed by professional personnel

Introduction

The principle of indirect or vicarious liability, i e liability for the wrongful act of another by virtue of the doctrine of *respondeat superior*[1] is well established in the modern law of delict. First, a person can be held delictually liable if he has ordered or authorised another to commit a wrongful act.[2] Thus a doctor who has instructed his professional assistant to perform an unlawful operation cannot later seek refuge in the excuse that he did not perform the operation with his own hands.

As far as liability for negligence is concerned, authorisation to perform a negligent act will probably seldom occur. The question of vicarious liability will ordinarily arise in those cases where a person employs another to perform a lawful activity, and the servant then does not proceed with the required or expected measure of skill and care, and causes harm to others. As far as the medical situation is concerned, the potential liability of the doctor for the negligence of his professional assistants and nurses he employs is relevant, as well as the possible liability of a hospital authority for the negligence of doctors, nurses, paramedics and other personnel it employs.

Relationship of employment

The general principle is that there must be a relationship of employment whereby one person (the master or employer) stands in a position of authority *vis-à-vis* another (the servant or employee) in terms of which the former is legally capable of exercising control over the latter's actions.[3] Partners do not stand in such a relationship. Legally they are equals, even though the one may be more senior than the other. It is nevertheless generally accepted that one partner is vicariously liable for the wrongful act of another when such act falls within the scope of partnership business.[4]

A person is not vicariously liable, however, for the wrongful act of an independent contractor engaged by him. Such a contractor undertakes a specific job and in the execution thereof acts in accordance with his own judgment, in particular as concerns the method applied.[5] He is not a servant but is "his own master". In the medical context, the anaesthetist who collaborates with the surgeon performing an operation,

1 Hospital liability for negligence may according to American law be based on another ground as well, known as the "corporate negligence" theory – i e negligence which occurs when the hospital furnishes defective equipment or supplies, selects or retains incompetent personnel, maintains its premises in a negligent fashion, etc. See Health Law Centre *Problems in Hospital Law* (1968) 116. See also M Nesterowicz 6 *Med Law* 553 (1987) 560. This form of liability falls outside the scope of this chapter.

2 R G McKerron *The Law of Delict* (7th ed, 1971) 89; N J van der Merwe & P J J Olivier *Die Onregmatige Daad in die Suid-Afrikaanse Reg* (6th ed, 1989) 521; J M Burchell "Liability of Hospitals for Negligence" 1977 *BML* 109; W E Scott "The Theory of Risk Liability and its Application to Vicarious Liability" 1979 *CILSA* 44, at 60.

3 McKerron 91; J Neethling, J M Potgieter & P J Visser *Law of Delict* (1990) 313.

4 *Lindsay and Others v Stofberg N O* 1988 (2) S A 462 (C), 467 E–F; D Giesen *International Medical Malpractice Law* (1988) 42.

5 McKerron 91. There may be exceptional circumstances in which a person who has engaged the services of a contractor to do a specific job for him may be liable for *his* (the employer's own) negligence. See below 305.

ordinarily is such an "independent contractor",[6] as is the case with the specialist to whom a general practitioner refers his patient or who is called in on the case.[7] Provided that the surgeon (or general practitioner) on reasonable grounds believes that the anaesthetist (or specialist) is professionally competent to do the job, there is no question of liability on the part of the former. If the practitioner who refers the patient is not so convinced, he may be held liable on account of his own negligence. (This principle is reminiscent of the ancient Roman form of vicarious liability, *culpa in eligendo* – fault through a poor choice of servant.)

An independently practising doctor who "hires" an operating theatre in a hospital, is not an employee of the hospital. The hospital can, therefore, not be held liable for his negligence. But the hospital may incur direct liability for its own negligence, e g where a patient operated on by such a doctor suffers harm caused by defective theatre equipment, which is the hospital's property.

The doctor or nurse who is a member of the staff of a hospital, i e occupies a firm and fixed position, is a servant of the hospital authority, and the latter will be delictually liable for acts of professional negligence committed by the servant within the scope of his or her employment.

In England, the courts in earlier years held the view that a hospital authority was not liable for the acts of members of the staff performed in the execution of their professional – as opposed to purely administrative – duties.[8] This "archaic cleavage", as Martin[9] has called it, was based mainly on the idea that hospitals were charitable institutions for the sick and needy, and that medical staff who visited and treated patients without payment, were part of the charitable conception. Moreover, the theory was that in the execution of their professional functions, staff members were not subject to orders or to detailed control. With the advent of nationalised hospitals, however, a new approach manifested itself. In 1942 in *Gold v Essex County Council*[10] it was held that a hospital authority was liable to a patient on account of the negligence of a radiographer who was in the full-time employ of the hospital.

In later English decisions hospital authorities were held liable for the negligence of nurses, resident medical officers, interns and even part-time anaesthetists.[11]

Developments in the United States in the field of hospital liability are comparable to those in England. Early decisions in New York State and elsewhere adopted a rule that where a doctor was employed by a hospital, the hospital was liable for his administrative acts but not for his medical acts.[12] In 1957, however, this rule was abandoned in New York and it was held that a hospital may be held liable for the negligence of an employee even if the act charged is of a "medical" nature.[13] This seems to be the general rule in the USA today. It is of significance that decisions were handed down by the courts in which it was held that a hospital may even be liable for the conduct of doctors who render their services exclusively through the hospital, although they are not paid a salary by the hospital.[14]

6 B D Hirsch "Consent to Medical Treatment", 5 *Trial Lawyers Guide* 59 (Nov 1961) 64, n 75 and cases cited; J H Harland "Anaesthetic Malpractice in Canada" 10 *Cleveland-Marshall LR* (1) 19 (1961) 25.

7 *Lymbery v Jefferies* 1925 AD 236, 241. Compare Harland 25. In *Rockwell v Stone* 173 A 2d 54 (1961), however, it was held that the doctor who had performed the operation could be held liable for the anaesthetist's negligence; in this case the doctor and the anaesthetist agreed that the latter was under the control of the former.

8 *Hillyer v Governor of St Bartholomew's Hospital* [1909] 2 KB 820.

9 C R A Martin *Law relating to Medical Practice* (1973) 380.

10 [1942] 2 KB 293.

11 See in particular *Cassidy v Ministry of Health* [1951] 2 KB 343, and compare Lord Nathan *Medical Negligence* (1957) chapter 5.

12 C R Morris and A R Moritz *Doctor and Patient and the Law* (5th ed, 1971) 389.

13 *Ibid.*

14 As Morris and Moritz 387 put it: "The modern trend is toward imposing more and more liability upon the hospital for negligence in the delivery of health care within its walls, regardless of the status of the person performing the act."

South African cases

The older English doctrine that a hospital authority could not be held liable for negligence of its employees in the performance of professional duties, was also applied in earlier South African decisions, notably *Hartl v Pretoria Hospital Committee,*[15] *Byrne v East London Hospital Board*[16] and the Natal case of *Lower Umfolosi District War Memorial Hospital v Lowe.*[17] In the last-mentioned of these cases it was held that the placing of a hot-water bottle in the bed of a patient who had been under the effects of an anaesthetic was a "professional duty", for negligence in the performance of which the hospital authority could not be held liable. Reviewing case law in England, the USA, Canada and New Zealand, Price[18] in 1953 strongly criticised the South African judgments, urging the courts here to follow the more recent trend in England and elsewhere.

In later cases, the Transvaal court did in fact depart from the older line of cases. In 1957, in *Esterhuizen v Administrator, Transvaal*[19] Mr Justice Bekker, without dealing explicitly with earlier rulings, held that a hospital authority was liable for the unskilful professional acts of a doctor employed by the hospital (excessive X-ray treatment of a patient suffering from a sarcoma, resulting in necrosis which necessitated the amputation of both her legs and the left hand). Six years later, in *Dube v Administrator, Transvaal*[20] the Witwatersrand Local Division held that the hospital authority was liable for negligence on the part of two plastermen and a doctor in the service of the hospital, in regard to the treatment of a patient's broken forearm, which resulted in a Volkmann's contracture (on account of the plaster having been applied too tightly, and subsequent failure to notice this; ultimately the patient's arm had to be amputated). Mr Justice Trollip in his judgment referred to "negligence on the part of the hospital", and drew attention to the fact that it was not disputed in the case that "the Hospital was liable for any negligence by those of its servants who treated and attended to the patient". In this judgment too, there was no reference at all to the earlier South African decisions referred to above.

The issue of vicarious liability of a hospital was again expressly raised in South Africa in 1975 in the Natal case of *St Augustine Hospital (Pty) Ltd v Le Breton.*[21] A 92-year-old patient with a fractured arm had been admitted to a hospital, but due to the negligence of the nursing staff, the sides of her cot were not erected at night and she fell out, or fell in getting out of bed, fracturing a leg. This resulted in a greatly prolonged stay in hospital. The case was tried by a single judge, Mr Justice Fannin, who referred to the 1937 Natal case of *Lower Umfolosi District Memorial Hospital.*[22] The judge observed that it seemed probable that if the Natal court in that year had had before it the subsequent English decisions, the result in that case might well have gone the other way. That case was decided by a Full Bench (two judges, at the time) of the Natal court, which came to the conclusion that the law in South Africa was in accordance with English decisions. By virtue of the precedent system a single judge cannot overrule a previous judgment by a Full Bench, and that being so, Mr Justice Fannin was constrained to hold that "in the absence of any special term in the contract between the hospital and the patient, the ordinary contract between patient and hospital does not cast upon the hospital an obligation to do more than take reasonable steps to assure itself of the professional competence of the nurses it employs to attend to the patient". In the result the patient could not hold the hospital liable for the neg-

15 1915 TPD 336.
16 1926 EDL 128, at 142, 158.
17 1937 NPD 31.
18 I Gordon, R Turner & T W Price *Medical Jurisprudence* (3rd ed, 1953) 179 *et seq.*
19 1957 (3) SA 710 (T).
20 1963 (4) SA 260 (T).
21 1975 (2) SA 530 (D).
22 *Supra.*

ligence of its nursing staff. The judge added *(obiter)* that had he been free to do so, he would have been disposed to accept as more in accordance with South African law the later English decisions, and to have applied the law as applied in the later Transvaal rulings. In 1989 a Full Bench of the Natal court in *Mtetwa v Minister of Health*[23] finally overruled the case of *Lower Umfolosi District Memorial Hospital* so that the legal position relating to hospital liability, is now uniform for the whole of South Africa.

What is a servant?

The modern rule clearly is far more equitable than the earlier approach. In so far as there is a choice, there are certainly powerful arguments to be advanced in favour of vicarious liability to be on the broad side rather than being too narrow. To mention only a single consideration from the point of view of public policy: the consequences of a simple act of negligence may be of catastrophic dimensions to the patient and apart from injury to his body and disfigurement, may take the form of a substantial pecuniary loss. When that runs into tens of thousands, or even hundreds of thousands of rands, the patient's chances of recovery against a hospital authority may be far better than against the negligent doctor or nurse, who in legal phraseology may be "a man of straw".

It cannot be argued that the modern rule is casting the net of liability too wide. The courts have over the years laid down a number of common-sense limitations on vicarious liability. Thus the courts have generally been at pains not to unduly broaden the concept of what a "servant" is.

It was held in the Transvaal that a doctor who at the request of a hospital authority renders gratuitous services to the hospital, is not a servant thereof.[24] So too, nurses or doctors who are employees of a hospital and who render assistance to an independent doctor performing an operation in the hospital theatre, were held in South Africa not to be the servants of the doctor. (In England, the view is taken that the hospital authority will remain vicariously liable for the negligence of its servants in such a case, notwithstanding that they are temporarily under the control of the independent doctor.[25] In the USA, however, the courts have ruled that the visiting doctor – and not the hospital[26] – is liable for such "borrowed servant", by virtue of the "captain of the ship" parallel,[27] but this doctrine, although receiving initial support in South Africa,[28] was emphatically rejected by the Appellate Division in its 1924 decision in *Van Wyk v Lewis.*[29])

In the USA the situation in regard to hospital liability has become somewhat com-

23 1989 (3) SA 600 (D).

24 *Hartl's* case, *supra* 340.

25 Nathan, *op cit* 68; J M Burchell *op cit* 110. Nathan states the qualification that negligence on the servant's part will not be established if he faithfully and carefully followed the doctor's instructions. I submit, however, that this qualification is only valid where the latter did not instruct the servant to perform an act which was manifestly negligent, also to the servant's knowledge. See also S R Speller *Law of Doctor and Patient* (1973) 83, and the Scottish judgment cited by him.

26 Health Law Center *Problems in Hospital Law* (1968) 122. But "routine acts" performed by the nurse, even on orders from a doctor, are nevertheless considered as falling within the scope of the hospital employment, and could render the hospital liable: *ibid.*

27 *McConnell v Williams* 65 A 2d 243 (1949). The "captain of the ship" doctrine has evoked strong criticism, however. See C Morris "Malpractice Medical – The Important Events of the Last Two Years" 30 *Insurance Counsel Journal* 44 (1963) 56; A H McCoid "The Care required of Medical Practitioners" *12 Vanderbilt LR* (1958) 599–605. According to Giesen 41, the doctrine is now on the retreat.

28 In *Hartl's* case, *supra.*

29 1924 AD 438. In this case it was held that a visiting surgeon was not liable for the failure of a nurse to perform an independent duty. Compare Gordon, Turner & Price *op cit* 183; see also *Hewat v Rendel* 1925 TPD 679, 685.

plicated by the fact that emergency-room medicine is becoming a distinct speciality. What is the position of the hospital where its emergency service is run, not by doctors full-time in its employ, but on contract by an "outside" partnership? Strictly speaking, the outside doctors would seem to fall within the category of "independent" contractors. Most American courts initially held that the negligence of such "contract" doctors will not render the hospital vicariously liable.[30] However, these decisions are being questioned. More and more states are beginning to realise that contract doctors for emergency rooms are in the public mind employees of hospitals, and this has led to decisions in some states whereby the hospital authorities were held liable.[31]

No South African court has as yet been confronted with this problem. Here, emergency medical services are almost exclusively provided by state hospitals and not by private hospitals. Private hospitals ordinarily make their operating theatres available on an *ad hoc* basis to doctors who operate on their (the doctors') own patients, the hospital providing nursing staff only. Should the situation develop in South Africa that a private hospital as such provides an emergency service rendered by "outside" doctors on a contract basis, a court will probably rule that because the hospital authority has neither actual physical control over the actions of the contract doctor, nor the right to so control the doctor, the hospital cannot be held liable.

Scope of employment

The notion of "scope of employment" today is wider than before. The emphasis seems to have shifted from actual control, in the form of instructions to and actual supervision of the servant's actions to the *right* of control. According to some authorities it is sufficient to establish that the servant is a member of the "organisation" of the employer. The question must be asked, so it has been suggested, whether the employer exercised control over the "where" and the "when", rather than the "how".[32] The test which a court will apply in this regard, in the ultimate analysis depends on considerations of public policy. The American view in regard to the contract doctor in the emergency room goes very far and would seem to imply that "course of employment" also includes the impression of that concept prevailing in the mind of the general public. It is doubtful whether a South African court will go so far. In 1978 the Appeal Court[33] ruled (not in a medical context, though) that "the element of control has always been regarded as a factor of prime importance in determining the existence or otherwise of a master and servant relationship ...", but the court appears to have been satisfied in this case that the master would be liable if the alleged servant in the *"manner"* of performing the act in question *"could* lawfully receive directions" from his superiors.[34]

In *Mtetwa's* case[35] the court emphasised that the degree of control exercised by persons in authority over him is not the sole criterion "to determine whether someone is a servant or something else". The deciding factor is the intention of the parties to the contract, which is to be gathered from a variety of facts and factors. Control is merely one of the indications.

The South African courts have so far clearly guarded against the notion of scope of employment – although already very wide in modern industrial society – being

30 A R Holder *Medical Malpractice Law* (2nd ed, 1978) 213.
31 *Ibid.*
32 W H Neff "Liability of Surgeon for the Negligent Acts of Servants" 64 *Dickinson L R* 180 (1960), 184; J G Flemming "Developments in the English Law of Medical Liability" 12 *Vanderbilt LR* 633 (1959), 653; Harland *op cit,* 25–27; R Bryce-Smith "Malpractice Actions involving Blood Transfusions" 9 *Defense L J* 54 (1961), 16–17; McKerron *op cit* 91–92; Gordon, Turner & Price *op cit* 178–183; Scott *op cit* 60 *et seq.*
33 In *Mhlongo and Another NO v Minister of Police* 1978 (2) SA 551 (A) 567–568.
34 *Ibid,* 570A (italics supplied).
35 *Supra.*

broadened to such an extent that it becomes a meaningless fiction. There is no indication that our courts are moving towards absolute or strict liability, i e the notion whereby a hospital authority would automatically be liable for the negligence of any professional, whether employed or not, who makes use of its facilities.[36]

There are some indications in decided South African cases that the question whether the employee has acted within the scope of his employment may be judged on the basis of the creation of a risk of harm by the employer.[37]

What is the position of the non-paying patient or the patient in a State hospital? Will the hospital authority be vicariously liable for negligence on the part of an employee? In South Africa it was held that the patient need not be a paying patient in order to have a right of recovery.[38] The hospital involved was a State institution. This is also the position in England.[39] In the USA there have been decisions to the effect that a non-profit hospital was immune against liability in the case of non-paying patients, but the more recent trend is clearly in favour of liability.[40] It has also been held in the USA – on the basis of the ancient principle that "the King can do no wrong" – that a State hospital cannot be sued, unless it has waived its immunity.[41]

Statutory exceptions have been made in the case of federal hospitals and in a number of states.[42]

Direct hospital liability

I have drawn attention above[43] to the possibility of a hospital authority incurring direct liability for its own negligence, i e not via the conduct of an employee. Hospital liability on the basis of "corporate negligence" does not fall within the ambit of this chapter.[44] It is convenient at this point, however, to draw attention to the notion of "direct liability".

As Giesen[45] has observed there is a clear trend towards greater hospital accountability in both Common Law and Civil Law jurisdictions. "The development of a new approach to the liability of hospital authorities," he says,[46] "has probably deprived of most its practical significance the point of whether in a given case a hospital may be held vicariously liable for the negligence of staff or independent contractors operating on its premises." He draws attention to a 1986 English decision,[47] in which the opinion was expressed that there is "no reason why, in certain circumstances, a health authority could not be directly liable to a plaintiff if it failed to provide sufficient or properly qualified and competent medical staff for the unit". He also cites a 1980 Australian case[48] in which the view was taken that a case could be made that the hospital in question was an institution which, by admitting a patient, undertook to render complete medical services through its staff. As Giesen[49] remarks, on this basis it makes no difference whether an independent contractor (a specialist, a visiting con-

36 This seems to be the tendency in the USA and Canada. On the position in Canada, see J E Magnet "Aspects of Hospital Liability in Common-Law Canada" *Reports, 5th World Congress on Medical Law* (1979) vol II 367.
37 Neethling *et al op cit* 315. See *Feldman (Pty) Ltd v Mall* 1945 AD 733, 741; *Minister of Police v Rabie* 1986 (1) SA 117 (A), 234.
38 *Dube's* case, *supra*, 266H.
39 Nathan, *op cit* 12.
40 Morris and Moritz, 387 *et seq;* Giesen 54.
41 Morris and Moritz 391.
42 *Ibid.*
43 See *supra* 300.
44 See *supra* 299, note 1.
45 *Op cit* 55.
46 *Ibid* 59.
47 *Wilsher v Essex AHA* [1986] 3 All ER 801 (CA).
48 *Albrighton v Royal Prince Alfred Hospital* [1980] 2 NSWLR 542 (CA).
49 *Op cit* 60.

sultant or a concessionaire) can be brought under the traditional head of "servant" or not.

It is certainly not inconceivable that a South African court could arrive at the conclusion that a particular hospital authority undertook to provide such an all-embracing service. But whether there has been breach of contract or negligence, will depend on all the circumstances and the evidence before the court in a given case. An assessment whether the care given fell short of what is reasonable, will involve consideration *inter alia* of the availability of human, physical and financial resources, the demands made of staff, the patient load, etc.

Although a person is not vicariously liable for the wrongful act of an independent contractor engaged by him, the circumstances may be such that an actionable duty may arise for the employer himself to take steps to prevent harm to members of the public, e g where the owner of a building engages a contractor to do work on the building, and harm to passers-by is foreseeable unless the area of operations is cordoned off or warning signs erected.[50] This is, strictly speaking, not vicarious liability; the employer is held liable on the basis of his own negligence – liability is, therefore, direct.

Exclusion of liability

May a hospital authority exclude or limit its liability *ex ante* in respect of potential vicarious liability? Some private hospitals make use of an exemption form to that effect which is signed by the patient as a condition of admission to the hospital.[51] Several jurisdictions in the USA have declared agreements of this nature invalid.[52] The South African courts, however, are not at liberty to do so and will give effect to an exemption clause if it is couched in unequivocal terms.[53] However, the patient may still sue for damage caused by intentional misconduct or grossly negligent conduct on the part of the hospital staff.[54] (As far as is known, however, there have been no reported cases specifically involving hospitals.) The patient clearly is in a disadvantageous position and it may be argued that from the point of view of public policy[55] the validity of exemption clauses is an undesirable feature deserving of the attention of the South African Legislature.

Adapted from a paper read at the Fifth World Congress on Medical Law, held in Ghent, Belgium in August 1979. The author gratefully acknowledges the generous support of the Human Sciences Research Council and of the Association of Law Societies which enabled him to attend the Congress.

50 *Langley Fox Building Partnership (Pty) Ltd v De Valence* 1991 (1) SA 1 (A); *Minister of Community Development and Another v Koch* 1991 (3) SA 751 (A)

51 Burchell, *op cit.*

52 *Ibid.*

53 *Ibid.*

54 *Ibid.*

55 S A Strauss & M J Strydom *Suid-Afrikaanse Geneeskundige Reg* (1967) 324 *et seq* argue that where such an agreement of waiver is entered into by a *doctor* with his patient, it ought to be regarded as null and void as being contrary to public policy. In my opinion the same considerations ought to apply in the case of hospitals in respect of personal injury to the patient. After all, it is the interest in his bodily inviolability (the *persoonlikheidsgoed*) that is at stake here and not merely his patrimonial interest.

53 The legal liability of a hospital superintendent

The following questions were put to me: "In terms of the Ordinance a medical practitioner must be in charge of a provincial hospital. Does that mean that the superintendent, as part of his functions, is also responsible for all hospital finances – regardless of the fact that it is not a prerequisite for his appointment or a condition of his employment that he must have any knowledge of bookkeeping?

"It is generally accepted that an employer must largely assume responsibility for his employees. Does that mean that the function delegated by a superintendent to a doctor, i e the treatment of patients, would officially render him liable as employer for malpractice or negligence on the part of a doctor?

"Would the superintendent also be exposed to disciplinary action against him on the part of the SA Medical Council? Will the Council, for instance, be able to suspend a practitioner on account of the negligence of one of the members of his staff?"

My answer is as follows:

In terms of the Transvaal Hospitals Ordinance,[1] the superintendent of a provincial hospital – who must be a medical practitioner – is the person in whom the "local control and management" of the hospital vests. The Ordinance further provides that the superintendent is subordinate to the Director of Hospital Services, and is responsible to the latter "for the efficient control and management" of the hospital.

The Ordinance goes on to provide that "any power, right, function or duty conferred or imposed on [the] superintendent ... in terms of the provisions of the Ordinance or the regulations made thereunder, shall be exercised subject to such directions as the Director may give and are not inconsistent with the provisions of this Ordinance or the regulations made thereunder ..."

The Director of Hospital Services, in turn, is by virtue of the Ordinance subject to the direction and control of the provincial Administrator and responsible for the efficient management and control of the Department.[2]

The Ordinance and the regulations framed thereunder, give no indication what "the local control and management" of a hospital does or does not entail. In the absence of any statutory definition or limitation of that concept, it will in my opinion clearly include the finances of the hospital concerned.

The fact that the superintendent is required to be a medical practitioner, and need not necessarily have any knowledge, experience or qualifications in the field of bookkeeping, accountancy, etc, does not make any difference. In other organisations doctors and other professionals who have no such expertise, are in a variety of managerial posts where their functions include financial control of the body concerned. The actual bookkeeping, accounting and auditing are generally done by experts, but control in the form of ultimate financial responsibility forms part of the responsibility of the manager – who in a provincial hospital is the superintendent.

A superintendent will in my opinion incur liability in his personal capacity for the negligence or other unlawful act of an employee of the hospital, in highly exceptional

1 Ordinance 14 of 1958 (T), section 6.
2 *Ibid*, section 3.

circumstances only. By "liability" I mean civil liability for damages or criminal liability, in the form of a conviction of culpable homicide or some other offence.

As I see it, doctors and nurses are not employees of the superintendent; they are employees of the hospital owner or authority, which is the provincial administration.[3] Having consulted a number of works on English, American and Canadian medical law, I could not find any authority for the proposition that a hospital superintendent – or his "opposite number" in those systems – is to be regarded as an employer for the purposes of vicarious liability. Nor am I aware of any court ruling or any other authority in South Africa that tends to support such a view. In all the countries mentioned, it is invariably the hospital authority that is held liable. In England express provision is made in section 13 of the National Health Service Act of 1946 that the hospital's "board" or "committee" must be sued in civil actions.[4]

It is the employer who incurs vicarious liability for professional negligence of employees. A superintendent will, it is submitted, be held liable only if he was in fact a co-perpetrator (or "joint wrongdoer") of a particular unlawful act.

That would be the case, for example, if he personally assisted with medical treatment or a medical operation performed in a negligent manner; or if he negligently gave an order to a subordinate member of his staff to perform a task which is contrary to modern medicine or to accepted procedures of treating patients; or if he actively associated himself with an unlawful operation, such as an illegal abortion.

In these cases, it is invariably a matter of personal fault on the part of the superintendent. The issue will always be: could he, in respect of actions of hospital personnel which were found to be negligent, have prevented harm to an individual patient by taking reasonable precautions? Did he in respect of intentional acts, knowingly and actively associate himself with the unlawful act of a subordinate employee of the hospital?

Where a superintendent has exercised reasonable care to ensure that all hospital procedures are conducted in a proper and orderly manner and that all available facilities are utilised, and a patient nevertheless suffers injury or damage in consequence of the negligence of a subordinate, and the circumstances are such that it cannot be said the damage could reasonably have been prevented by the superintendent, there is no question of the latter being held liable delictually.

In my opinion the same principles apply to the superintendents of private hospitals, whether or not they are qualified medical practitioners. The owner of such a hospital, e g a company, is legally the employer of the nursing and administrative staff and other employees. If a superintendent who is a non-medically qualified person, were to issue instructions of a medical nature he would obviously run the risk of being accused of negligence if his instructions were not based upon sound medical advice which he had previously obtained.

As far as a possible contravention of the Medical and Dental Council's code of ethics is concerned: The Council is vested with wide disciplinary powers. Even apart from those ethical contraventions expressly circumscribed in the code, the Council may find that a particular act charged, amounts to improper or disgraceful conduct. However, the Council's disciplinary action is primarily directed towards the accused's own, personal fault. As long as a superintendent performs his duties in a proper manner and does not act negligently and does not associate himself with the negligent conduct of others or with unlawful or unethical practices, it is difficult for me to conceive of any ground on which disciplinary proceedings might be instituted against him.

3 *Cf* Health Law Center *Problems in Hospital Law* (1968), 6.
4 S R Speller *Law of Doctor and Patient* (1973), 175.

54 Patient insists on leaving hospital too soon after operation

The following question was put to me: "In our hospital, which is a big institution, we occasionally have 'difficult' patients who refuse to stay in the hospital until they are formally discharged. Recently we had a case of a man who had undergone a kidney operation. Before he had recuperated fully, and while he still had drainage tubes inside his body, he insisted on going home. The hospital staff refused to allow him to leave, pointing out that it was dangerous in his condition. The patient would not listen to any reason and simply walked out of the hospital. The staff members in attendance were unsure whether they were entitled to restrain the patient forcibly. The patient refused to sign any discharge papers and went home. Is there any legal risk involved for the hospital or staff in this type of situation?"

In my opinion a patient is not entitled at any stage convenient to him, to insist on being allowed to leave a hospital. A hospital can only function properly if its procedures are adequately regulated, either by fixed rules or at the very least in accordance with standing instructions issued by the superintendent from time to time. In addition to these there are of course common usages which have evolved in hospitals through the years.

A hospital authority would be fully entitled to lay down a rule that patients may be discharged only if authorised by the attending doctor, by the hospital's medical personnel, or by the superintendent, and that discharge shall only take place during reasonable hours, e g between 07:00 and 20:00. Should a patient insist on leaving the hospital at an inconvenient hour, such as one o'clock in the morning, the hospital staff would in my opinion be fully entitled to refuse to discharge him formally.[1]

Where a patient flatly refuses to abide by the hospital rules and manifests an intention to leave the hospital immediately, I would nevertheless not advise the hospital staff to restrain him by forcible means. The proper course would be to warn the patient of the medical risks to which he would expose himself should he leave. If possible, the staff should persuade the patient to sign a document to the following effect, before departing: "I hereby acknowledge that I have been warned by the staff that it would be dangerous for me to leave the hospital in my present condition. Despite such warning I have insisted on leaving the hospital forthwith. I do so voluntarily and at my own risk, the hospital staff having refused to discharge me formally. It is understood that I shall not be entitled to hold the hospital authority or individual members of its staff liable for any damage that I may suffer on account of my refusal to remain in the hospital any longer."

The date, exact time and circumstances of the patient's departure should then and there be recorded by the staff members confronted with the situation. This is of particular importance if the patient refuses to sign a document with the content suggested. The patient's doctor should be informed without any delay and the matter should of course be reported to the superintendent at the earliest opportunity.

Physical restraint of the patient would in my view be legally safe, however, if the

1 There is, in fact, a serious medico-legal risk for a hospital in discharging a patient too soon and without the doctor's approval. This was well illustrated in the case of *Sambousis and Another v Administrator of the Orange Free State and Another* (1989 OPD, unreported), which is discussed in detail above 262.

patient ostensibly is *non compos mentis* and the case presents itself as one of dire emergency. In such a case the hospital would undoubtedly be able to rely on the legal doctrine of *negotiorum gestio* (unauthorised administration) if reasonable force is applied to restrain the patient in his own interest. It may even be argued that there is a legal duty on hospital staff to restrain the patient in these circumstances, if that can be done without danger to the staff members themselves.

It is to be noted that my remarks apply only to patients in "ordinary" hospitals. Different considerations apply to patients in mental hospitals. The Mental Health Act[2] makes provision, *inter alia,* for involuntary detention of patients in certain circumstances, and clearly envisages the possibility of definite restraints on the freedom of patients to leave an institution, within the limitations provided for in the Act and the regulations thereunder.

2 Act 18 of 1973.

55 Liability of hospital or staff for loss of patient's property

Because a patient sometimes presents at the hospital with valuable personal effects on him, such as money, credit cards, jewels, a watch, the hospital authority should consider its potential liability towards the patient in so far as the hospital may have assumed responsibility as a depositary.

It is a question of fact whether the hospital has in fact agreed to be a depositary and has not merely allowed the patient to bring valuable property with him into the hospital room or ward. Deposit is a contract whereby one person delivers a thing to another for the purpose of safe custody and the latter gratuitously or for reward undertakes to take care of the thing and restore it on demand. To constitute the contract of deposit there must be an undertaking to retain and have charge of something, not merely passive willingness "that something may be left somewhere".[1]

If the thing deposited is lost or damaged through the depositary's negligence while it is in his custody, he is liable in damages to the owner; it is for the depositary to prove that the loss or damage is not due to his own fault.

The depositary is not liable, as a rule, if the thing is lost or damaged as a result of fortuitous accident (such as a violent storm) or the wrongful conduct of a third party (such as a burglar who breaks open a safe and steals the thing).

A hospital authority which has accepted the custody of a patient's valuables may limit its liability, by the incorporation into its conditions of admission of an "owner's risk" clause. Such a clause will exempt the hospital from responsibility for loss or damage resulting from ordinary negligence on the part of the hospital or its employees, but not from gross negligence or intentional harm.[2]

State and provincial hospitals ordinarily accept responsibility for the property of a patient only in accordance with their official regulations. Thus hospitals of the Transvaal Provincial Administration accept goods subject to the following condition only: "No liability will be accepted by the Hospital in respect of effects and valuables belonging to patients unless such effects and valuables shall have been entrusted to the hospital authority for safe custody and a receipt obtained therefor. Effects and valuables accepted for safe custody will be returned against surrender of the safe custody receipt only."[3]

It is to be noted that there is no obligation on a nurse or other member of the hospital staff to accept responsibility for valuables a patient brings to the ward. It would be unwise for a nurse or other ward staff to undertake to look after patients' valuables; patients should be advised to deposit these with the reception desk or to entrust their valuables to their relatives.

Aged and debilitated patients, in some cases neglected by their relatives, are sometimes inclined to make gifts of money, jewels or other valuables to hospital staff who care for them with kindness or devotion. Hospital regulations may forbid the acceptance of gifts that are of substantial value. But even in the absence of an express prohibition, it may be unwise for staff members to accept gifts of considerable value,

1 D H Bester in Joubert's *Law of South Africa* vol 8, (1979) pars 68 *et seq.*
2 *Essa v Divaris* 1947 (1) SA 753 (A).
3 See Administrator's Notice No 649 of 29/8/58 (Transvaal) under the Hospital Ordinance 14 of 1958.

because relatives of the patient may afterwards claim that the donation was null and void in that the patient was *non compos mentis* when the gift was made.[4] A staff member may, in accepting a valuable gift, even expose himself to a malicious charge of theft made by a jealous relative of the patient at a later stage.

It goes without saying, however, that a hospital doctor or nurse need not offend a patient or his relatives by refusing the kind of small, acceptable social gifts often made by grateful people, such as a bottle of wine, a box of chocolates, a book or a bottle of perfume.

4 Compare the well-known case of *Preller and Others v Jordaan* 1956 (1) SA 483 (A) in which it was held that a proper cause of action for setting aside a transaction was stated where an elderly patient averred that he had been unduly influenced by his family doctor, at a time when he was sick and bodily and mentally weak and exhausted, to give and transfer four farms to the doctor.

56 Suspension of a hospital doctor for misconduct

The powers and obligations of the Transvaal Director of Hospital Services in regard to the suspension for alleged misconduct of a medical officer on the staff of a provincial hospital, formed the subject of a court decision in *Director of Hospital Services v Mistry.*[1]

The applicant, a medical practitioner, was serving on the staff of a provincial hospital as acting head of the casualty section.

The Hospitals Ordinance of Transvaal[2] provides that a hospital officer is guilty of misconduct, *inter alia* if he commits a criminal offence. The procedure to be followed in a case of misconduct is set out in the Ordinance.[3] The Ordinance provides that the Director may charge the officer in writing in the manner set out. The Director is empowered before or after the officer has been charged, to suspend him from duty. An officer who is suspended is not entitled to any emoluments for the period of his suspension. (The Administrator of the province may, however, in his discretion order payment to the officer of the whole or portion of his emoluments.) The Ordinance finally provides that if no charge is preferred against an officer who has been suspended from duty (or if a charge is withdrawn) the officer must be allowed to resume his duty and must be paid his full emoluments for the period of his suspension.[4]

Dr M was arrested by the Police and told to appear in court on a date in August 1976 on criminal charges arising out of his employment. He was not asked to plead to any charge, nor was he informed of the precise nature of the charges but he was advised by the investigating officer that the charges concerned fraud and forgery. The case was remanded until August 30.

A week or so later, Dr M received a notice signed by the Director of Hospital Services to the effect that he was suspended from duty and that he would not be entitled to any emoluments during the period of suspension. The person who served the notice informed him that his suspension arose from the matters which had given rise to the criminal charges against him. Dr M was further informed that having been only suspended and not discharged, he was precluded from taking any other employment as a medical doctor.

The case in the magistrate's court was not heard on the date to which it had been remanded, but was again postponed several times until it was finally set down for trial on 19 January 1977. Through his attorney Dr M made unsuccessful requests to the prosecutor for a copy of the charge sheet. The case was not heard on the appointed date, and Dr M was informed that it would not be possible for the case to be heard for at least two or three months. (There were several reasons for the delay. One of these was the fact that the Police had not yet completed their investigations.)

Six months after his suspension, the doctor instituted proceedings in the Supreme Court against the Director of Hospital Services, for his reinstatement on the hospital staff and for certain ancillary relief. He submitted that he was being harshly penalised for his alleged criminal conduct in that he had not only received no emoluments and

1 1979 (1) SA 626 (A). The case was decided in November 1978.
2 Ord 14 of 1958.
3 Section 53.
4 *Ibid.*

no annual bonus, but he was also precluded from taking other employment while he was under suspension. He denied his guilt and said that, regard being had to the consequences of his suspension, he was entitled to have the matter determined as expeditiously as possible. He declared that the Director was obliged to act in such a manner as to ensure that any charges against him were determined with a minimum delay. When he learned in January 1977 that the trial could not proceed, the doctor averred, he formed the view that the Director had not acted promptly or expeditiously to ensure that his guilt or innocence was determined with a minimum of delay.

Dr M alleged in his papers that his attorney had unsuccessfully tried to interview the Superintendent of B Hospital, who referred him to an employee of the Director in Pretoria. Another employee ultimately informed the attorney that the matter could not be discussed. The doctor contended that sufficient time had elapsed for his trial to have been concluded and for an administrative inquiry into his alleged misconduct to have been held.

The Director's defence was that there was *prima facie* evidence to justify a charge of fraud and forgery against the doctor, involving an amount of R9 274. The Director stated that after the criminal trial he would take action in terms of the Ordinance and he further gave reasons why the investigations could not be completed and the trial not held. The Director denied that he could be held to blame for any delay. The Police officers also explained that the delay was in no way attributable to the conduct of the hospital authorities.

The trial judge held that although the Ordinance did not indicate any time within which an officer who was suspended for alleged misconduct must be reinstated if no charge is preferred against him, the words "within a reasonable time" must be read into the provision concerned.

The judge further held that the fact that the Legislature allowed the Director to await the result of a criminal trial, indicates that the officer involved must convince the court that the Director was responsible for the delay in the bringing of the criminal charge. The judge found that prior to 15 April 1977 there had been no unreasonable conduct on the part of the Director; neither he nor his officials were guilty of any negligence. However, the Director failed to show that subsequent to 15 April, steps had been taken to exert pressure on the Police to bring the case to trial. The Director's failure to take action after that date justified the conclusion that he was no longer interested in a prosecution of the doctor, the judge said. Alternatively, the doctor's explanation might have satisfied the Police. The court accordingly ordered the Director to reinstate Dr M.

The Director appealed against the trial judge's order and the Appellate Division set aside the judgment. The appeal succeeded primarily on procedural grounds. On behalf of the Director it was contended that the crisp point for decision was whether at the date when the action was launched by the doctor – i e 24 February 1977 – the Director had delayed unreasonably in charging the doctor with misconduct. What may or may not have happened after that date, or at the latest after the date when the Director's opposing affidavit was filed (13 April 1977), was not relevant. The Appellate Division upheld this contention, basing its decision on the ancient principle that a judge in civil proceedings must resolve the dispute on the issues raised by the parties and confine the enquiry to the facts placed before the court; he must not have regard to extraneous issues and unproved facts.

It is to be noted that although the final judgment went against the doctor, the decision is authority for the proposition that administrative action by the Director of Hospital Services against a hospital officer for alleged misconduct must take place within a reasonable time, and where such action depends on the outcome of a criminal charge against the doctor, the Director must take all reasonable steps within his power to ensure expeditious finalisation of the criminal trial.

57 Handling of hospital strikes

Only actual strikers may be dismissed and dismissal may not be retrospective

The case of *Tshabalala v Minister of Health*[1] highlights the proper procedure to be followed by a hospital superintendent in handling an illegal hospital strike.

This case originated in an unfortunate clash between student nurses and the authorities of B hospital. The dispute arose after a delegation of student nurses, at a monthly meeting, raised a number of grievances with the chief matron of the hospital. The matron referred them to the chief superintendent. The students' delegation reported back to the student body that the grievances had not been considered by the matron. The students were upset at receiving that report and violence erupted, involving the students and the hospital security guards. The following day some of the students failed or refused to report for duty at the hospital. The deputy superintendent drew the attention of the student body to the fact that the Nursing Act declared a strike by nurses to be unlawful and criminal. He warned the students that they would be contravening the law if they failed to return to work within 30 minutes. The strike action of the student nurses created a crisis in the hospital to the extent that members of the SA Defence Force Medical Services were called in to care for the needs of more than 1 600 patients in the hospital.

A meeting with a student delegation was arranged a few days later. At the meeting the chief superintendent informed the students that their services had been terminated as from a date five days before the date of the meeting. A list of student nurses so dismissed was handed by an administrative officer of the hospital to an attorney representing them. It appeared that this list contained the names of all student nurses, who were more than 900 in number. It also appeared that the administrative officer at that point was in fact not in a position to provide a list of all the dismissed students, as their identity – i e of those who had gone on strike – had still to be ascertained. No further notice of dismissal was given.

Two of the student nurses and a pupil nurse brought an urgent application to the Supreme Court for an order declaring their dismissal unlawful. The superintendent relied on a provision in the Hospitals Ordinance entitling the superintendent to summarily discharge a hospital employee whose conduct in his opinion has been "unsatisfactory".

The court held that a nurse or student nurse whose employment is subject to the provisions of the Nursing Act and who goes on strike, is guilty of conduct rendering her subject to summary discharge. Section 40 of the Act makes any strike by such a person a criminal offence.[2]

However, the chief superintendent could only dismiss those student nurses who had participated in the strike action. From the evidence of the superintendent it was clear that he had been able to ascertain which of the students had so acted. But, before attempting to do so, he had intimated to the student delegation at the meeting

1 1987 (1) SA 513 (T).

2 See also below 429 *et seq*.

referred to above, that the employment of all students had been terminated with retrospective effect, i e the day prior to any strike action having been taken.

Mr Justice Goldstone observed: "That action by the chief superintendent was quite clearly improper. In the first place, he had no right in law to dismiss any but the striking students, and in the second place, he could only dismiss them from the date upon which any or more of them went on strike. I would add that there is no evidence that all the students conspired to go on strike ..."

The exercise of the power to dismiss, the judge said, is one which clearly affects very important rights of the students or pupil nurses concerned. Apart from affecting their monetary interests, in many cases it would affect their future careers in the nursing profession.

"Accordingly, the decision to terminate the employment of such a person is a matter of concern, requiring the careful and *bona fide* consideration of the person to whom the discretion is given by the ordinance." The chief superintendent is required to satisfy himself that the person concerned is guilty of the conduct charged, and that such conduct is unsatisfactory.

The court found that when the chief superintendent purported to dismiss the students, he had not applied his mind to all the relevant questions in relation to any of the individuals with whom he was concerned.

"The question in the cases before him was not so much whether unlawful strike action was unsatisfactory conduct – that is obvious ... The question was which of the students were guilty of such conduct. By his own admission, he knew then that it was not all the students and pupil nurses. He was therefore obliged to consider each individual case, and in doing so afford such person the right to be heard." He had not done so, and for that reason alone he had not validly exercised the discretion conferred on him by the Ordinance.

Moreover, it is trite law that a decision to terminate a contract must be communicated to the other party. The notice to terminate was not given by the superintendent clearly or unambiguously to any of the students. He was not entitled to issue a general order terminating the employment of all students and leave it to those who participated in strike action to determine for themselves whether the termination applied to them or not. The fact that the termination was stated to be retrospective made it worse. None of the students failed to report for duty until the following day.

The judge stressed that the chief superintendent was obliged to give careful and *bona fide* consideration to the case of each individual in respect of whom he was considering dismissal. He had to give each such person the right to be heard.

In the event the court found that the notice of termination was invalid in respect of all the students. In respect of one of the applicants who had been unlawfully dismissed, the court ordered that she remain in the hospital employment and was entitled to remain in occupation of her room at the hospital's hostel.

In respect of an applicant who admitted to have participated in the illegal strike, the court refused to order reinstatement. That applicant had "not come to the Court with clean hands". As a matter of public policy a court should not order reinstatement in such circumstances. Illegal strike action by a student nurse "subverts the very purpose and being of the profession which such person is seeking to join".

It is to be noted that the Medical, Dental and Supplementary Health Service Professions Act[3] makes it a criminal offence for any medical practitioner or other person registered in terms of the Act, to strike. The considerations stated in *Tshabalala's* case would in equal measure apply to a strike by doctors employed by a hospital.

In his judgment, Mr Justice Goldstone had the following to say on strikes by nurses: "The nursing profession is a venerable and noble one. The services it renders very properly can be described as essential services in the sense that if they are with-

3 Act 56 of 1974, section 55A.

held, the lives of many people may be endangered. It is no doubt for that reason that the Legislature has seen fit to render strike action unlawful and punishable by the criminal courts. Similar legislation in respect of essential services is by no means peculiar to this country, and may be found on the statute books of most Western nations. A strike by members of the nursing profession, apart from being a repudiation of their contract of employment, undermines the very fundamental ethic of their calling and constitutes a material breach of contract." But, said the judge, the added responsibility places a very important reciprocal duty on employers to ensure that nurses' conditions of employment are fair and proper.

No absolute right to terminate employment by way of notice

In *Langeni and Others v Minister of Health and Welfare and Others*[4] a large number of hospital workers refused to work in consequence of a dispute with the administration of a provincial hospital following the dismissal of a co-employee. The workers were given an ultimatum to return to work within 30 minutes, which they ignored. The next day they were given 24 hours' notice of their dismissal.

In terms of their written agreement, the workers' services could be terminated by 24 hours' written notice on either side. Provision was also made in the agreement for summary dismissal by a hospital superintendent in cases of insubordination or misconduct, or absence without leave.

Four of the workers who were fired approached the court for an order reinstating them. They claimed their employment was unlawfully terminated for the sole reason that they had not been given a hearing prior to the decision to give them 24 hours' notice. It was argued on their behalf that natural justice demanded that the principle of *audi alteram partem* – "hear the other side" – should have been observed.

In its judgment, the court drew attention to the fact that the notion of a "legitimate expectation" had been afforded some recognition in South African law. This notion involves the concept that even in the absence of a legal right or interest, a person affected by an administrative decision, may have a "legitimate expectation" or a "legitimate claim of entitlement" which would make an arbitrary decision concerning that expectation both unfair and unjust.[5]

In the present case the termination of the workers' employment had not taken place in consequence of alleged misconduct. The Administration relied purely on the agreement as to 24 hours' notice. The court held that the situation of the workers was not a "pure case of master and servant". Their employment was by a public administration and was governed both by the terms of their individual contracts and the terms of the relevant statute and regulations.

The court held that the workers were employed from the first day in the knowledge that they could be dismissed on 24 hours' notice. They clearly had no right or legal interest to remain in their employment after the expiration of a notice period of 24 hours. Moreover, they did not have a legitimate expectation that their employment would continue indefinitely unless there were good reasons for termination. The fact that in some cases the employment had continued for many years, in no way conferred an additional right, interest or legitimate expectation on the employee. The

4 1988 (4) SA 93 (W).

5 The doctrine of legitimate expectation was accorded full recognition by our Appeal Court in *Administrator, Transvaal and Others v Traub and Others* 1989 (4) SA 731 (A). In that case a provincial director of hospital services refused applications by certain doctors for appointment or reappointment to posts at provincial hospitals. The doctors had been parties to a published letter severely criticising the Provincial Administration's attitude to conditions in a hospital. The court set aside the director's refusal, holding that, in the circumstances of the case, the applicants had a legitimate expectation that their applications would be granted and/or that a departure from past practice would not occur without a fair hearing being given prior to such decision.

employees had not been entitled to a hearing and accordingly their claim for reinstatement was refused.

Mr Justice Goldstone was of the opinion, however, that the position would have been different in the case of a public official who, for instance, would become entitled to a substantial pension benefit if he remained in his job for a future 12 months. In terms of the agreement with his employer, his employment may be terminated with six months' notice. Although he has no legal right to remain in his employment for any period after such notice, he might have a legitimate claim of entitlement to remain in such employment in the absence of some good and sufficient reason to dismiss him. It would, therefore, be unfair and unjust to dismiss him without giving him the right to be heard, the judge said.

Interestingly enough, such a situation came before the same judge shortly afterwards in *Mokoena and Others v Administrator, Transvaal.*[6] In this case, temporary hospital workers employed by the same provincial administration were likewise dismissed by means of a 24 hours' notice, apparently because of some involvement in a go-slow strike of which the object was to induce the administration to recognise a trade union.

In *Mokoena's* case the workers involved, although temporary staff members, belonged to a pension fund of which membership was compulsory. They had been employed for many years (one of them for about 20 years) and had been members of the pension scheme for some nine or ten years. The most senior of the workers would have been 60 years of age and, if still employed by the administration, would have qualified for retirement with full pension benefits.

In this case, the court held, the administrative authority to give 24 hours' notice clearly affects the workers' pension rights and involves legal consequences to them. "That", the judge said, "is sufficient to have entitled them to have been heard before such action was taken against them and the official concerned would have been obliged to give honest and *bona fide* considerations to any representations made by them. Failure to have done so would have vitiated such a decision." In any event, the judge said, there was no doubt that the workers had had a legitimate expectation that they would not be deprived of their right to qualify for a pension without good or sufficient or reasonable cause. That would have entitled them to a hearing before the decision was made to terminate their employment.

In the event, the *Mokoena* court found that the dismissal of the workers had been wrongful.

The effect of these two rulings is that an employer who wants to dismiss an employee may not be able to rely merely on a simple notice-of-termination clause in the agreement between the parties.

It is to be noted that State or provincial employees do not fall under the Labour Relations Act[7] which affords special protection to employees against unfair dismissal.

6 1988 (4) SA 912 (W).
7 28 of 1956.

PART XIII

Death, death certification, dying and euthanasia

58 Death and the moment of death: some reflections by a lawyer

Death as a juristic fact

Death has always been an important juristic fact, a *regsfeit;* it is an event to which the law attaches a variety of consequences. As jurists we are inclined to have regard to the consequences of death rather than to the concept of death itself. An anecdote which is told of the late Professor Mortie Malherbe of Stellenbosch, a very well-known legal luminary of yester-year, illustrates this statement very well. One day, it is said, he was conducting an oral examination on the law of succession and he put the following question to the student: "How does a person die?" The hapless student desperately searched his brains for the precious little medical knowledge stored in them, and began by saying that the heart stops beating, that the person stops breathing, that the body temperature starts falling, etc. But Professor Malherbe in his customary curt fashion, cut him short, saying: "No man, you're on the wrong track; a person dies with or without a will!"

A major part of our common law concerns the law of succession with all its fascinating ramifications. If one looks at Johannes Voet's treatment of the law of succession in his 29th to 33rd books, one hardly comes across any reference to the death of the testator – although that, of course, is the most important implied condition for succession to take place. If, again, one looks at Voet's treatment of homicide under the title of *Lex Cornelia de Sicariis* in book 48, one finds a comprehensive discussion of almost all aspects of death – *inter alia* the problem of causation – without any reference to the question when the victim can be said to be dead. Here too, death as a fact is a tacit prerequisite for criminal liability in respect of homicide.

The question of *when,* i e the precise moment at which death occurs, may nevertheless juridically be of the utmost importance, particularly in the light of modern resuscitation techniques. Several examples may be given. First, the moment of death may be of cardinal importance in the law of succession. I usually give my students the example of the tycoon who has become estranged from his wife, without divorcing her though. He and his wife have six children. He also has a mistress with whom he lives; in his will he has bequeathed his entire estate to her. One day he and his mistress go for a ride in his Cadillac. They are involved in a collision and both are critically injured, but still living when the ambulance brings them to the hospital. The question is now which of them may or should be kept alive for some time. If the man dies before his mistress, even if it is a matter of minutes, it has the practical effect that the mistress as sole testamentary heir will inherit his entire estate,[1] and upon her death, shortly afterwards, his estate of millions together with her estate which is worth a few rands, will devolve upon her heirs (who may be her hippie brother, a ne'er-do-well). If, on the other hand, the mistress dies before her millionaire lover, the legal position is that the sole heir mentioned in his will has not fulfilled the first and foremost prerequisite for succession, viz that she should have lived at the mo-

1 Subject, of course, to the provisions of the Matrimonial Property Act 88 of 1984 and the Maintenance of Surviving Spouses Act 27 of 1990, in terms of which the deceased's surviving spouse will have certain claims against the estate.

ment of *delatio*. In the result, his entire fortune will go to his intestate heirs – who are his virtuous wife and six children.

The moment of death may also be of the utmost importance in the law of insurance. One thinks of the clause invariably inserted into the small print of life insurance policies, whereby the policy will become null and void if the insured person were to die in consequence of suicide, within two years after the policy has been issued. It may be that, unaware of this condition in his policy, the insured attempts to commit suicide a short while before the two years' period expires. He injures himself critically, but is brought to hospital in a still living condition. If the doctors can manage to keep him alive for a brief period so that he may cross the two-years' border in a living state, it may make a huge difference for his heirs, who will now receive the proceeds of a policy worth tens of thousands.

The moment of death may further be of great importance in fiscal law, where the termination or transfer of rights may entail advantages from the point of view of taxation.

The moment of death and criminal law

Lastly, the moment of death may be of vital concern to the criminal law when issues of liability for alleged murder or culpable homicide must be solved. Questions such as the following may arise: Whose act was the true cause of the deceased's death? Was the deceased still alive when the second assailant joined in the assault? – in which case the latter may himself be guilty of murder, a capital offence, and not merely of attempted murder if the deceased had already expired (as was held in *S v Thomo and Others*[2]). Where a critically injured person is connected to a heart-lung machine by hospital doctors, who is causally responsible for his death: the wrongdoer who assaulted him, or the doctor who ultimately switches off the machine? According to most theories of causation, the original actor will undoubtedly be judged to be causally responsible for the death of the victim, at any rate where the wound was of a serious nature. By application of a narrow causation theory, however, the doctor's act may in such a case be held to be the *causa causans* of death. In several American cases the allegation has been made that the real cause of the victim's death was the removal of his heart, for transplantation purposes, by surgeons. According to press reports in 1972 the relatives of one Bruce O'Tucker, the donor in the world's 16th heart transplant, brought civil action for damages against the surgeons. The deceased had been "kept alive" on a heart-lung machine until his heart was removed. Unfortunately the result of the case is not known to me. In a 1977 homicide case, again, *State of Kansas v Ronald Shaffer*,[3] the accused claimed that it was not the gunshot wounds to the deceased's head, inflicted by him (the accused) that had caused the death, but the kidney transplant by a doctor who had turned off the respirator in order not to prolong life. The court rejected this defence.[4] A comparable case came before a South African court. In *S v Williams*[5] (1986) the accused, who was charged with murder, raised the defence that the shot he had fired had not been the cause of the deceased's death, but that disconnection of the respirator, which – it was contended – constituted an *actus novus interveniens*, had. The court likewise refused to uphold this defence.

2 1969 (1) SA 385 (A). See also *S v Khoza* 1982 (3) SA 1019 (A) and *S v Motaung and Others* 1990 (4) SA 463 (A).

3 574 P 2d 205 (Kan 1977), quoted by J E Cook & L Hirsh "The Legal Implications of Brain Death" (1982) 1 *Medicine and Law* 135 at 139. Compare the two cases quoted by M L Norton *et al* "Organ Transplantation: Medico-Legal Considerations" (1983) 2 *Medicine and Law* 291 at 301–302.

4 In several American cases not involving transplantation it has likewise been alleged that the cause of death was not a wound, but the certification of brain death and/or disconnection of the respirator. See Cook & Hirsch *op cit* 139 *et seq.*

5 1986 (4) SA 1188 (A). Compare the English cases of *R v Malcherek, R v Steel* [1981] 2 All ER 422 (CA) and *Mail Newspapers plc v Express Newspapers plc* [1987] FSR 90.

Even if in a case such as the latter, the original wrongdoer were still to be regarded as having caused the victim's death, the possibility cannot be excluded that the doctor may according to some theories of causation be considered as being causally co-responsible for his death. The doctor's liability will then depend *inter alia* on the elements of unlawfulness and fault *(mens rea)*. Thus the question may be posed – as was done in *R v Makali*[6] – "whether the deceased would have died *when he did* but for the appellant's unlawful act. If this inquiry gives an affirmative answer, the appellant is responsible for the death because he caused it to take place when it did, that is to say because he hastened it". As Russell[7] put it: "[T]he person wounded does not die simply *ex visitatione Dei,* but his death is hastened by the hurt which he received." Death is caused by some or other intervening human action, either the original wounding by the assailant, or the medical act subsequently performed. Juridically, the hastening of death may be tantamount to the causing of death. According to the theory of *conditio sine qua non* the hastening of death will invariably amount to the causing of death.

In considering the question of unlawfulness in criminal law and the law of delict, the question arises of when the doctor will be entitled to switch off the resuscitation apparatus. Can we as lawyers give a conclusive answer to that? I am doubtful. In my opinion the best we can do is to indicate a method which might be employed in trying to find an answer.

The doctor's dilemma

In this connection, I want to refer to what George P Fletcher[8] of Washington had to say in a note under the heading *Legal Aspects of the Decision not to Prolong Life*. Having considered several aspects of the question, he stated as follows: "Thus the analysis leads us along the following path: the doctor's duty to prolong life is a function of his relationship with his patient and in a typical case that relationship devolves into the patient's expectations of the treatment he will receive. Those expectations in turn are a function of the practices prevailing in a community at the time. And on what do these practices depend? Practices in the use of respirators to prolong life are no more and no less than what doctors actually do in the time and place. Thus, we have come the full circle. We began the inquiry by asking: is it legally permissible for doctors to turn off respirators used to prolong the life of doomed patients? And the answer after our tortuous journey is simply this: it all depends on what doctors customarily do. The law is sometimes no more precise than that."

It seems somewhat ironic that the answer to a legal question is made to depend on medical opinions and practices. But this is in accordance with recognised legal tenets. The jurist does not claim that his discipline has all the answers. Sometimes the answer to a question of law will depend on societal attitudes, on how custom is evolving, and the point Fletcher makes is that in respect of resuscitation procedures, a new norm must be sought on the basis of what is medically customary.

As Fletcher indicated, there is an even more difficult question, viz: "Does this patient *deserve* prolongation of life?" Here, already we have an antecedent decision on the part of the doctor. In this situation the doctor may be confronted with a difficult conflict of interest. Two patients with more or less the same type of injury are brought to the casualty department of a hospital, in a comatose condition. There is a single heart-lung machine available and the resuscitation process must be put into operation immediately. Which of the patients must be kept alive? Inevitably the doctors must exercise a choice. But is this really a new problem? What about the dilemmas

6 1950 (1) SA 340 (N), 344.
7 *Russell on Crime* (9th ed) 381.
8 203 *J Amer Med Assoc* (1968), 65.

of doctors on the battlefield or on the scene of an air-crash or a train disaster or an earthquake, or even in the casualty ward when a number of seriously injured patients are brought in simultaneously and only a single doctor is on duty? In all these cases, the question arises: which of the patients is to be treated first? This question is particularly difficult where the factual circumstances are such that the one who is not attended first, will surely, or almost surely, die.

As I have said, this dilemma is not new to the medical profession. The dilemma presents itself in another situation as well, which likewise is not unusual, and that is when an operation is contemplated on a patient who is gravely ill and whose chances of survival are slim. The patient's ailment and the operation proposed are of such a nature that the doctors may with almost total certainty predict that in a specified percentage of cases the operation will be unsuccessful and the patient's death will be hastened. The question is now: When is the doctor going to operate? Will it be this morning, this afternoon or tomorrow? His decision is decisive for the moment of death of the patient in the event of the latter being one of those unfortunate persons whose demise is accelerated by the operation. By taking the decision, the doctor in a way of speaking determines the moment of death – which may be decisive for the existence or non-existence of the rights of others, as we have seen.

Medical "power"

In all these cases, we have in the words of J H van den Berg,[9] of Leyden, a problem of *medische macht en medische ethiek* (medical power and medical ethics) which, incidentally, is the title of his monograph in which he argues a qualified case for euthanasia. The theme of Van den Berg's book is that the phenomenal developments in the medical field in our century have vested the doctor with a tremendous power which poses difficult problems of medical ethics. I think we are here confronted with one of those problems.

It is clear that none of the numerous problems arising in relation to the moment of death and life-sustaining procedures may be answered by means of neat and simplistic little legal formulas. If questions such as I have posed were to come before a court of law by way of actual cases, the court as interpreter of the juristic notions of society, the *regsgevoel*, would endeavour to decide the case to the best of its ability. In so doing, the court would probably be guided by what is considered to be socially acceptable, *sosiaal adekwaat,* and would hand down a judgment which reflects, among other things, contemporary religious attitudes, current societal attitudes and current opinions in the field of medical ethics and medical practice. (In this regard it may be pointed out that medical practice is sometimes several steps ahead of expressly enunciated medical ethics.)

The principles formulated in regard to the defence of necessity may possibly in some cases be resorted to – even if it is merely by way of analogous application – particularly where the dilemma of life-saving, in those cases where a selection of one life must be made in preference to another, is involved. This dilemma and the grim choice which it entails, are as old as the hills. To refer to only one or two of these cases in legal history: there are the well-known shipwreck cases of the *Mignonette* and the *William Brown,* and the 1972 South African case of *S v Goliath.*[10]

Defining death

I want to return now to the definition of death. Being lawyers, we are anxious for the sake of legal certainty to work with fixed principles, formulas and definitions, and in so far as that is possible, it is of course a sensible policy. If one were to look at death

9 *Medische Macht en Medische Ethiek* (10th ed, 1969).
10 1972 (3) SA 1 (A).

purely as a biological fact within the realm of natural science, one might perhaps maintain that it is capable of being expressly defined by Parliament in a statute. After all, in South Africa we have defined "nuclear hazard material", which is a concept of natural science, in an act of Parliament. I am referring to our Nuclear Energy Act.[11] It would be possible to give other examples of scientific concepts being defined in statutory law.

After the first dramatic heart transplant in 1967, some jurists insisted that a legally acceptable definition of death be formulated. But the fact of the matter is that we were somewhat simplistic in our outlook. Since that time we have been persuaded by the doctors that death does not necessarily take place at a specific moment, but that it should rather be regarded as a process. Sometimes the process occurs very rapidly; at other times it is a gradual process. Moreover, death can be looked at from more than one point of view. In a narrow sense one may refer to physical or somatic death. In this connection reference is sometimes made to vegetative or metabolic death. Opposed to this is death of the intellect or of the mind. (I suppose we should avoid talking of "spiritual death"; we may find ourselves in difficulties with the theologians. It is perhaps better to speak of "social death".) The medical men have also persuaded us that the determination of death is based largely on personal, clinical impressions of the doctor in a situation where his experience may be decisive. This led Professor Chris Barnard to make the following terse statement when testifying before the Select Committee of Parliament in 1969, when consideration was given to the Anatomical Donations and Post Mortem Examinations Bill: "A person is dead when the doctor says he is dead."[12]

These are some of the considerations which in South Africa prompted us not to endeavour to include in our Anatomical Donations and Post Mortem Examinations Act of 1970 (and in its successor, the Human Tissue Act of 1983) a definition of death. Other states, however, have introduced laws pertaining to the criteria to be employed in determining whether death has taken place.[13] But in our country the question whether or not death has taken place, is for the purposes of the Act a purely medical matter. Our Act requires death to be established – except in certain cases – by two medical practitioners (who may not be members of the transplant team). One of the doctors must be relatively senior in that he is required to have had at least five years' practical experience.

In the *Williams* case to which I made reference above,[14] the trial court found that, according to traditional medical standards, the moment of death is when brainstem death sets in. The Appeal Court held, however, that it was not necessary to decide whether this criterion was also to be accepted in law. The moment of death therefore remains an open question in South African law.

The mysteries of life and death

As Chief Justice Rabie has intimated in the *Williams* case, determination of the moment of death is not within the exclusive province of medical science. This is in line

11 Act 92 of 1982.

12 *Report* of the Committee SC 11–'68, par 2. See also par 40. Professor Barnard's brother, Professor Marius Barnard, however, came out strongly in favour of a statutory definition of the criteria to be applied in determining death, in the course of radio debate (in which I also participated) in 1983.

13 In 1988 it was reported that about half the states of the USA had by statutory enactment recognised brain death. Some of these statutes recognise both brain death and the "traditional" concept of death (failure of cardiac function, etc). Other statutes recognise brain death only when traditionally defined somatic death cannot be determined. Yet another type of statute makes provision for brain death as the sole criterion. See D Giesen *International Medical Malpractice Law* (1988) 613; compare Cook & Hirsh 137. According to Giesen, five European countries have statutory criteria for determining death, namely Finland, Greece, Italy, Norway and Spain.

14 See 151 and 322.

with the views of a prominent Swedish physician, Gunnar Björk,[15] expressed at the First World Congress on Medical Law, held in Ghent in August 1967, shortly before Professor Barnard performed the first heart transplant: "The concept of death is the negative image of the concept of life. In that concept we all have a share. Therefore we also have a share in the concept of death. After all, death is the end of the early existence of each of us." As Björk observes, life is a many-splendoured thing. Lawyers experience problems even in trying to define the beginning of human life. The concept of life simply would not allow itself to be confined within the formal dialectics of jurisprudence. "We can look at a living object and say: this is life. We can look at a dead object and say: that is not life, it is dead. But we may be mistaken: a seed from a Pharaonic tomb may still be able to develop into a plant a thousand years later; a bull's sperm, immobile, in the frozen state, may ultimately propagate the father's genetic message to innumerable calves in another hemisphere," says Björk.

According to a news report soil samples were taken from deep below the surface of Antarctica and frozen bacteria discovered in these may be between ten thousand and a million years old. When the exterior of these specimens was sterilised with a blowtorch (please note!), and the bacteria incubated, not only did they "return" to life, but they also reproduced! As I have said, life is a concept full of wonder, and every human being is entitled to have his own view on what life is and what it is not.

Likewise, death is something full of mystery to man. One man sees in it the violent severing of the line of life, and intensely fears it. In art, death has been depicted as something terrible. Thus Albrecht Dürer depicted death as a skeleton in full armour on horseback with lance in hand, dealing destruction – Death, the Tyrant. Another man sees death as the passage to a peaceful, dreamless sleep. In the art world there are many depictions of this concept of death. Some people are looking forward to the fulfilment of the promise of heavenly bliss which they believe will follow death, or to reincarnation in a different form upon death. Many people view the notion of the hereafter as pure delusion and are fearful merely of the transmission from a state of consciousness to unconsciousness and oblivion.

Views on what death is are highly individual. To some a loved one never dies. One is reminded of the Portuguese king who had had the body of his deceased wife embalmed and seated next to him at his table so that he could see her every day. A more recent example is the body of Lenin which lies in the *sanctum sanctorum* of the communistic credo, the Kremlin, for all to see. In 1982 there was a news item in the press[16] of an English woman who slept beside her dead husband for almost a year. Police discovered the corpse only after other tenants in the block of flats complained of the smell. At the inquest the woman told the Police: "My husband's asleep in bed. I think he's getting better."

The ancient Egyptian custom of embalming has a modern counterpart in cryobiology: the practice of deep-freezing the body of a person who has just died, in the hope that scientists of the future may discover a remedy which will bring about his revival. In a specially designed deep-freeze compartment in Phoenix, Arizona, lies the body of Professor James Bedford, medical researcher. He died of incurable cancer in 1966, but before his death he had given instructions that his body was not to be allowed to decay, but had to be preserved (at minus 195^{0} C) to await a cure for cancer.

Cerebral death

If I as an individual, and not necessarily as a lawyer, were to select a standpoint in regard to this highly personal question of what death means, I would support the no-

15 "Second Thoughts on Life and Death", paper read at the First World Congress on Medical Law, held in Ghent, Belgium in August, 1967.

16 *Rand Daily Mail* 5 June 1982.

tion of the so-called brain death or cerebral death. After all, the brain is *par excellence* the seat of human individuality. My feeling is that the point where resuscitative techniques may be terminated, is when the prospect of future restoration of at least partial consciousness has finally become impossible or, for that matter, highly unlikely. When irreversible or irreparable brain damage has occurred and this can be ascertained with a reasonable degree of certainty, the doctor would therefore in my opinion be entitled to disconnect the patient from the resuscitation apparatus. The distinction made by H A H van Till-d'Aulnis de Bourouill[17] in her book on medico-legal aspects of the end of human life, is significant. She defines cerebral death as "the complete and irreparable cessation of the brain function, including the function of the brain stem".[18] This she regards as the only juridical criterion for the end of human life. Irreversible coma, on the other hand, she defines as "a very deep unconsciousness, with some brain function, but without a discernible reaction to external stimuli".[19]

In her opinion, irreversible coma is not yet death, and the doctor may accordingly not deal with the body in the same manner as he would be entitled to do in the case of a corpse; he may not dissect the body and remove organs. But, says Van Till, from both the ethical and the juridical point of view, irreversible coma may be considered as an argument in favour of terminating resuscitative treatment, because the conclusion is that the patient's dying process has already advanced far and may be allowed to be completed.

The period of time elapsing between irreversible coma, on the one hand, and the cessation of the brain function on the other, may sometimes be very brief. But where cerebral death has set in, one may perhaps speak of "a corpse with a beating heart", from which organs may be removed. As a conditional supporter of euthanasia, Van den Berg[20] goes further than his compatriot, Van Till, by maintaining unequivocally that human life *may* be terminated. He says: "It is stated so cruelly: the doctor may kill the patient. It sounds unusual. It seems to be improper. But what is improper, is to allow the totally disabled, long defeated, dying and already dead [patient] to continue vegetating. That must be unusual. That, at any rate, is cruel."[21]

Establishing irreversible coma and irreparable brain damage in a particular case is not without problems. The electro-encephalograph is an important instrument used to measure the absence of brain activity. If for 20 minutes and at normal body temperature, or somewhat below that (but not lower than 34^0 C), no brain activity can be measured, it is generally accepted that brain death has occurred. But cases have been described of patients in whom brain death was diagnosed and who nevertheless recovered fully or almost completely, afterwards. (Van Till[22] describes two such cases.) For that reason more sophisticated tests or combinations of tests are required. Among other things, use is being made of an angiogram to establish whether blood is still flowing to the brain. But that is a procedure which is not altogether without risk. At a conference in Washington in 1970 I listened with interest to a harmless experimental method being described by H P Müller[23] of Switzerland: the use of ultrasonic sound waves (by means of echo-cinematography) to establish whether there is still a flow of blood to the brain in the carotid artery. According to him that test may be supplemented by analogous tests for the vertebral artery.

From a practical point of view, doctors in certifying death are guided by criteria

17 *Medisch-Juridische Aspecten van het Einde van het Menselijk Leven* (1970), 121–2.
18 My translation.
19 *Ibid.*
20 *Op cit* 48.
21 My translation.
22 *Op cit* 155.
23 H R Müller "Ultrasonic Techniques as an Aid in Assessing the Diagnosis of Brain Death" in *Jus Medicum* (1973) 189.

for brain death suggested by professional bodies, such as the British Transplantation Society (in 1975),[24] the British Royal Colleges (1979),[25] the German Gesellschaft für Chirurgie (in 1968).[26] But it would seem that the last word on cerebral death is yet to be spoken.

The "right to die"

Sometimes objections are raised to the application of utilitarian considerations *pro* or *con* a particular view of what death is. As jurists we are entitled to allow ourselves to be guided by such considerations up to a certain point. Numerous examples may be cited of specific legal rules based on expediency rather than on pure logic. Although cerebral death in my opinion is acceptable on the basis of general ethical considerations, it must nevertheless be pointed out that doctors hold that organ transplants, as opposed to tissue transplants, will be made more difficult if heart death is applied as the criterion. Doctors emphasise that the removal of an organ before blood circulation has ceased, has a major advantage, the advantage being that the period of ischemia (degeneration of the organ on account of inadequate "nutrition" with blood) where minutes are important, is shortened. If the test of heart death is applied, the surgeon who removes a still beating heart from a body in which all brain activity has already ceased, will legally speaking be a murderer. In fact, he will be a "double murderer", because in removing the recipient's heart to make room for a new heart, he invariably brings the activity of the heart removed to an end.

In conclusion: today there is strong support for the notion that the individual has a qualified "right to die". True, our common law does not recognise the principle that the individual is *dominus membrorum suorum* (owner of his own bodily members), but it certainly recognises the principle that a person who is capable of validly expressing his will, may refuse medical treatment. Even where such an expression of a will is no longer possible, those who are "totally disabled, long defeated, dying and already dead", in the words of Van den Berg, ought to be allowed, without further medical aid – however well intended – to take the final step into eternity.

Adapted from a paper delivered at a symposium on The Moment of Death *held at the Faculty of Law, University of the Orange Free State, Bloemfontein, in May 1974. The paper was first published in Afrikaans in 49* S Afr Med J *976 (1975).*

24 Giesen *Arzthaftungsrecht – Medical Malpractice Law* (1981) 246.
25 Mason & McCall Smith *Law and Medical Ethics* (2nd ed, 1987) 214.
26 Giesen (note 24) 246.

59 "DOA" (dead on arrival) certificates

It would seem there is some confusion surrounding the legal status of "Dead on Arrival" (DOA) statements issued by hospitals. In particular, there is the question whether registered nurses are legally entitled to sign a DOA statement as they have done in certain hospitals in the past.

It is clear that the DOA statement essentially serves a twofold purpose:

- It places certain important facts relating to bodies brought to a hospital formally on record for the hospital itself, should any question subsequently arise in relation to a particular case handled by hospital staff.
- It constitutes *de facto* notice to the Police for the purposes of the Inquests Act,[1] section 1, which imposes a duty on the public in general to report suspected non-natural deaths to the Police.

In my opinion the law does not regulate DOA statements *per se* and such a statement is not, strictly speaking, a death certificate as required by the Births, Marriages and Deaths Registration Act,[2] section 20 (still-born children), section 23 (where a doctor was not in attendance but issues a certificate to "the best of his knowledge and belief") and section 24 (other deaths, where a doctor was in attendance). As far as Act 81 of 1963 is concerned, it should be observed at this point that only a doctor or a midwife may issue death certificates in the case of still-born children (by virtue of section 20), and only a doctor in other cases (by virtue of sections 23 and 24).

In particular it must be emphasised that DOA statements are not governed by section 212(7) of the Criminal Procedure Act.[3] Perhaps it would be more correct to say that this subsection was not intended or designed to regulate the issue of DOA statements used in the hospital context.

The purpose with section 212, as its heading[4] indicates, was to make provision for the proof of certain facts, in criminal proceedings, by way of affidavit. The usual principle is that evidence in criminal proceedings must be adduced by means of *viva voce* (oral) evidence. Because certain types of evidence of a more formal (and often scientific) nature are seldom contested in a court of law, section 212 facilitates proof of certain facts by making provision for the evidence to be put before a court in written form by means of a sworn statement. The statement amounts to *prima facie* proof which, if not contested, can become conclusive proof. In practice the application of section 212 saves an endless amount of time for expert witnesses, prosecutors, defence counsel and presiding officers.

A DOA statement may be used by the prosecutor – or for that matter, the defence – in criminal proceedings if made by way of affidavit. To that extent DOA statements are affected by section 212. It may certainly be useful to the Police or the Attorney-General if there is a DOA affidavit in the docket of a case which eventuates in a criminal trial.

Paragraph 9.1 of the SA Police Special Force Order (General)[5] provides that a

1 Act 58 of 1959.
2 Act 81 of 1963.
3 Act 51 of 1977.
4 "Proof of certain facts by affidavit or certificate."
5 5A of 1990.

body may not be admitted to a Police mortuary "unless it is certified dead or unless the condition of the body is such (e g decomposed or beheaded) that it can be accepted with certainty that the person is dead". This provision is in the nature of a directive to the *S A Police* and is not applicable to doctors, nurses or hospital staff in general.

It is a sensible directive, because it sets out to avoid the tragic situation where a (living) person who happens to be in a deep coma – where there is medically still a possibility of resuscitation – is mistakenly taken by policemen with a limited medical knowledge to be a corpse and put into the mortuary.

Cases of a mistaken diagnosis of death occur occasionally: In 1969 a 36-year-old woman was declared dead by a doctor in Sweden, but found alive in the infirmary mortuary 90 minutes later by two policemen.[6] An almost identical case occurred in South Africa in 1990 when a 58-year-old woman certified dead by a doctor later "woke up" in a mortuary in Natal.[7] Compare an Indian case: the apparently lifeless body of a boy was left in a congested crematorium during a cholera epidemic after the local doctor had certified him dead; he regained conciousness after his relatives had left.[8] And then there is the case of a 19-year-old Frenchman who took an overdose of barbiturates, intending to commit suicide. He was found by hunters a day later and pronounced dead by a medical team. A morgue attendant was about to place his body in the iceroom when he noticed that the man was still breathing. He was taken to a hospital where he recovered.[9] It is to be noted that in all these cases doctors made the diagnosis of death.

It is clear that under paragraph 9.1 of our Police Special Force Order, the Police have a discretion, in regard to the requirement of death certification, because the condition of the body may be such that even a layman can see that the person is dead beyond any doubt. Obviously the Police on duty at mortuaries would prefer to receive a death certificate by a doctor, nurse or other medical expert in cases where there may be room for doubt. The provision quoted, however, does not require certification by a medical practitioner. The typical DOA statement, even where it has not been made under oath or by a doctor, but by some other knowledgeable person, can serve as certification for the purposes of this subsection. The view of the Police that the document they require need not necessarily be issued by a doctor but also by a "suitably qualified person", is an altogether practical and reasonable approach.

The Human Tissue Act[10] requires that for the purpose of removing tissue (except eye tissue) from the body of a dead person for transplantation to living persons, or for other scientific purposes, the death of the person concerned must be established by two doctors, one of whom must have been practising for at least five years. This provision applies for the purposes of that Act only and has no bearing on DOA statements as such.

There is, therefore, no requirement in statutory law that DOA documentation may be performed only by registered medical practitioners. If that were to be insisted upon, it might present practical problems where a body is brought to a hospital and a doctor is not available to make a diagnosis of death. It would, in my view, be acceptable and not contrary to any law if a registered nurse were to perform this function. I deal with this aspect in more detail below.

A *caveat* must be sounded, however, in this connection: A hospital authority may incur legal liability by common law if a wrong diagnosis of death is made negligently by that authority acting through its employees. Assuming that a "borderline case" is brought in (e g hypothermia, electrocution, deep coma after barbiturate poisoning)

6 *Rand Daily Mail* 14 August 1969.
7 *The Citizen* 29 December 1990.
8 *The Star* 19 November 1968.
9 *The Citizen* 4 November 1989.
10 Act 65 of 1983, section 7(2).

and an erroneous diagnosis of death is made so that the person is not given treatment which would have saved his life or would have prevented serious brain damage, the person's dependants (or personal representative in the case of brain damage) may bring a lawsuit for very substantial damages against the hospital authority and the professional person(s) involved.

For such a suit to succeed, the plaintiff(s) will have to prove negligence, at the very least. It is trite law that the standard of negligence is that of the reasonable man. The question would be whether the reasonable man – *in casu* the reasonable hospital authority who, it may be assumed, would be guided in its actions by professional medical advice – would have foreseen the catastrophic consequence and would have taken measures to guard against it. There is also the possibility of a prosecution for culpable homicide. The onus of proof in criminal cases (guilt beyond a reasonable doubt) is heavier than in civil cases (persuasion on a preponderance of probabilities).

It would therefore be advisable for a hospital authority to ensure that in all "borderline" cases, i e where there may be doubt as to whether or not the person brought in, is in fact dead, the diagnosis of death should be made by a doctor, or where this would be impossible or extremely difficult because of a shortage of staff, by a registered nurse or paramedic who has been given expert training concerning the diagnosis of death.

All such cases should be carefully documented (i e the diagnostic procedures applied and the reasons for the ultimate diagnosis recorded). A hospital authority should safeguard its own interests by giving written instructions to all professional staff members.

It goes without saying that the possibility of a claim for damages may only arise in "borderline" cases and not in cases where the condition of the body is such that no-one would doubt that the person is dead. There are cases in which even a three-year-old child can tell that a person is dead.

In my view the entire matter of DOA statements may be adequately dealt with by a hospital authority by way of "in house" regulation and no legislation is required. All that is necessary is that the legal status of a DOA statement be properly understood and that clear instructions be issued by hospital authorities to staff. The risk of delictual or criminal liability in relation to DOA "certification" in general seems to me to be absolutely minimal if simple procedural safeguards are maintained.

It is also comforting to staff employed by the State, the provincial administrations and local authorities to know that statutory indemnification is provided by section 58 of the Health Act.[11] In terms of that section no legal proceedings shall lie against the State, a person in the service of the State, a provincial administration, a person in the service of a local authority (or any person generally or specially authorised by the State, etc, to perform any function in terms of the Act) for anything done in good faith under the Act. This section will protect staff in cases of *bona fide* errors of judgment, although it will clearly not provide indemnity where a staff member is manifestly negligent or fails to apply his mind to the matter at hand.

Can it be argued that a nurse who makes a diagnosis of death in a DOA "certificate" will be acting beyond the legitimate scope of nursing practice?

Prior to 1984 the scope of nursing had not been statutorily defined. In the event of a dispute arising, a court of law or the S A Nursing Council would have had to settle the issue on the basis of fact, i e evidence as to what is customarily the work of a nurse.

There is little doubt in my mind that since time immemorial nurses, as trained health-care workers, have taken it upon themselves, particularly in the hospital context, to make a simple finding (or "diagnosis", to use more professional terminology) that a patient has died. Take the everyday situation of a nurse on night duty in a hospital ward. A critically ill or injured patient's condition has deteriorated over days (or

11 Act 63 of 1977.

weeks) and ultimately the patient expires at 02:00. The nurse in attendance, who is experienced and has often been at a bedside when a patient has died, makes this observation and records the fact of death on the patient card. In the overwhelming majority of cases the nurse would certainly not think of telephoning an overworked doctor at that time of the night to seek his confirmation of the fact that death has occurred or even to merely inform him of that fact.

Likewise, in the usual hospital situation where a person is brought in who is ostensibly dead, a nurse who observes this will certainly not hesitate to make a statement to that effect, be it orally or in writing on a hospital record. Such recording cannot in my view be said to be formal "certification" in the sense envisaged by sections 23 and 24 of the Births, Marriages and Death Registration Act, which is statutorily "reserved" for doctors in express terms.

In Government Notice R2598[12] the Minister exercised the power granted to him by the Nursing Act[13] to make regulations relating to the scope of practice of registered nurses. (The regulations were amplified in 1987[14] to provide for the scope of practice of registered midwives.)

These regulations are of a fairly general nature and it is doubtful whether they were intended to constitute an exhaustive definition of nursing. They serve a practical purpose, first, to give an indication of what acts would constitute illegal practising of nursing for gain, in contravention of the Act,[15] and secondly, to serve as guidelines to the S A Nursing Council as to conduct on the part of a nurse which would be improper or disgraceful because it exceeds the bounds of legitimate nursing.

The regulations do not contain any express reference to the making of DOA statements or assessments of the fact of death, but in my view such action would by necessary implication fall within the ambit of item (t) of the regulations, viz "care of the dying patient and the care of a recently deceased patient within the execution of the nursing regimen". I cannot see how a nurse can at all times perform that nursing function unless she would be entitled to make an assessment that a patient is dying or dead, without necessarily seeking confirmation on the part of a medical practitioner.

At this point it is appropriate to mention that the ethical rules of the S A Nursing Council expressly provide in general terms for certification on the part of nurses.[16]

It might perhaps be argued that making an assessment (or diagnosis) of death is an act specially pertaining to the profession of a medical practitioner, in terms of section 36 of the Medical, Dental and Supplementary Health Service Professions Act,[17] and *ergo* criminal if done for gain by a non-medical (unregistered) person.

I do not think, however, that there is any substance in that argument. Section 3 of the Inquests Act enables a policeman, and section 23 of the Births, Marriages and Deaths Registration Act, the Registrar of Births, Marriages and Deaths, to form the opinion that a person is dead. These provisions militate against the view that making an assessment that a person is dead, is within the exclusive province of a medical practitioner.

The traditional role of the nurse to make such an assessment as part of her nursing functions, which I have described above, likewise militates against such a conclusion. There are, no doubt, other situations in which persons such as paramedics, soldiers and firemen may – and sometimes, must – make on-the-spot decisions in their line of duty that someone is dead.

12 Of 30 November 1984 (*Government Gazette* 9513).
13 Act 50 of 1978, section 45 (1) *(q)*.
14 By Government Notice R1469 of 10 July 1987 (*Government Gazette* 10818).
15 Section 27.
16 See rule 14, headed "Certificates", contained in Government Notice R387 of 15 February 1985 (*Government Gazette* 9589).
17 Act 56 of 1974.

To sum up:

- Although it is preferable that a doctor should make the DOA "certification" in cases where there may be a reasonable doubt as to whether the person brought in is dead, it can be done by any professional person who has had adequate training in the diagnosis of death when a doctor is not available.
- A registered nurse who has had adequate training in the diagnosis of death may, where a doctor is not reasonably available, perform the DOA documentation.
- Section 212(7) of the Criminal Procedure Act is relevant to DOA "certification" to the extent only that a DOA *affidavit* is rendered admissible as *prima facie* proof in criminal proceedings.
- The ward diagnosis and notification of death as done by registered nurses traditionally, is legally acceptable and within the scope of their practice.

60 Certification of death in cases of sudden cot-death

There is, apparently, a difference of opinion in medical circles on what the correct procedure is in cases of sudden cot-death. How should a practitioner handle such a case? Must he report it to the Police? If he is acquainted with the family that has experienced such a disaster, may he issue a death certificate to the effect that the death is attributable to unknown, natural causes? Must there be a *post-mortem* investigation? What does the Inquests Act[1] stipulate?

This Act prescribes that anybody with reason to suspect that somebody else has died and that the death was attributable to other than natural causes, must accordingly make a report to a police officer as soon as possible, unless he has reason to suspect that a report has been or will be made by somebody else. Failure to make a report in this manner constitutes a criminal offence.[2]

The Act makes further provision for a police officer who has reason to suspect that someone has died from causes other than natural causes, to investigate this or cause it to be investigated,[3] and for a magistrate to whom the death is reported "if he deems it expedient in the interests of justice" to cause it to be examined.[4]

In the first place, in considering the position of a *practitioner* to whom a sudden and unexpected cot-death has been reported, I would always advise him not to issue a death certificate stating that the infant died from unknown natural causes, unless there was a clinical picture of which the practitioner, on the grounds of previous investigation and/or treatment, was aware.

I find it impossible to see how a practitioner can issue such a certificate in the classic case of a cot-death where the baby, according to all available observations, was ostensibly perfectly healthy and normal; in my opinion a practitioner who certifies in this manner would expose himself to possible criminal prosecution. I respectfully agree with the view expressed by Schwär, Loubser and Olivier in their book *Die ABC van Geregtelike Geneeskunde*:[5] "Although the sudden, unexpected-death-syndrome is a known phenomenon, it cannot, because the cause is not known, be certified to the best of the practitioner's knowledge and belief that the death occurred exclusively as a result of natural causes; therefore the death must be reported to the magistrate."[6] In my opinion this is a perfectly clear and legally correct opinion.

As far as the position of the *policeman* is concerned, I believe that in the absence of medical information to the effect that the death is attributable to natural causes (whether known or unknown), he would not be entitled, as a layman in the medical field, to come to the conclusion that a sudden infant-death can be attributed to natural causes. Should this occur, however, there is no criminal sanction applicable to such a misdirection on the part of the policeman. Erroneous handling of a case of death may, however, lead to administrative sanctioning.

As far as the magistrate is concerned: if a report is made to him, he may within

1 Act 58 of 1959.
2 Section 2.
3 Section 3 (1).
4 Section 3(2).
5 (1984) 312.
6 The translation is mine.

his discretion decide whether he considers a *post-mortem* examination expedient "in the interest of the administration of justice". A magistrate should in accordance with common law exercise this discretion in a judicial manner, i e on the basis of thorough consideration of the factual information laid before him.

In my opinion, a magistrate would misdirect himself if he were to fail to instruct that an unexpected infant-death be the subject of a *post-mortem* examination, unless a certificate by a medical practitioner is furnished to him stating that the cause of death (known or unknown) is attributable to natural causes.

The magistrate is also a layman in the medical field, and would misdirect himself if, on his own initiative, he were to form an independent opinion on the matter. The only corrective for such a misdirection would be for the Supreme Court, on application by an interested party, to issue a *mandamus* (mandatory order) in terms of which a magistrate is ordered to direct that a *post-mortem* examination take place.

61 The euthanasia debate: a South African view

"All that live must die"

Life is perhaps the most self-evident quality of man and the preservation of life – survival – is his most basic instinct. In a graveyard in Surrey, England, there is a century-old stone on which these striking words are inscribed:

"If life were merchandise that men could buy
The rich would live and none but poor would die."

Even primitive Neanderthal man forty thousand years ago buried lumps of bloodstone (haematite) with his dead, probably associating the red substance with the essence of life, and hoping – if not believing – that it might restore life to the deceased.

Men who had been faced with violent death and who came back to tell their stories, have often related that they had felt no fear and that in a split second many happy memories of their lives had flashed through their minds like scenes from a newsreel. Psychologists explain that this is a reminder to the man in mortal danger that life has been a worthwhile experience and that it is worth clinging to with all the power at his disposal.

Even serious injuries inflicted with violence have brought no pain where the victim was face to face with death. David Livingstone, the great 19th century missionary-explorer of Africa, told of an attack on him by a lion which sprang upon him and caught his shoulder, crushing it. "The shock", he wrote, "produced a stupor similar to that which seems to be felt by a mouse after the first shake of the cat. It caused a sort of dreaminess in which there was no sense of pain nor feeling of terror, though conscious of all that was happening."

No wonder that the hallmark of Western civilisation – if not always upheld in practice – is respect for life. Perhaps the preoccupation with the sanctity of life in our civilisation has in recent times largely shifted from sheer preservation of life to the *quality of life.* This has manifested itself in particular in the legalisation of abortion in our century, where the emphasis has increasingly been put on consideration of the woman's interests relating to the quality of her own life, rather than on preservation, at all costs, of the incipient life – *die wordende lewe* – in her womb.

It is almost impossible to discuss euthanasia in cold, unemotional terms. We are all too much part of life, and "all that live must die" (Shakespeare). We find ourselves here in an area where the cold rhetoric of law and the dispassionate vocabulary of medicine are of little avail. Almost any stand on euthanasia will be affected by one's own impressions of the death of a beloved, by some uneasiness, perhaps subconsciously, on one's own dying "one day", by an abhorrence of human suffering in general, by one's deepest religious beliefs in the eternal destiny of the soul, by one's sense of propriety.

Conflicting views of euthanasia

On the one hand there are those who on religious or ethical grounds find the notion of mercy-killing altogether unacceptable. Thus to Bernard Ficarra,[1] the euthanasia

1 B J Ficarra *Surgical and Allied Malpractice* (1968) 808 *et seq.*

issue is part of the conflict between two systems of thought: the system which recognises its obligation to God and His Law, and the other system which claims that man need have no higher motive than the gratification of his own desires. Ficarra accuses the proponents of mercy-killing of "flirting with moral insanity"; when we adopt euthanasia in any form, he says, we are on the path back to the jungle.

In his book *Medische Ethiek* (1960) G A Lindeboom, professor of medicine in the Free University of Amsterdam, discussed euthanasia from the Christian-Protestant point of view.[2] Although he concedes that euthanasia does occur in medical practice, he maintains that it is rejected almost universally by the Christian conscience and ethics. He quotes Karl Barth in support of the statement that it is for God and God alone to put an end to the life of a human being; man can only be a collaborator at God's specific and clear command. Concludes Lindeboom: "Neither the difficulty in drawing a border, nor the very distinct possibility of an undesirable extension and wrong or criminal application, nor the principle of the respect for life, but solely his belief in God's sovereign order, prohibits the Christian from accepting euthanasia, even if more and more voices are heard pleading for it."[3]

On the other hand there are those who on humanitarian grounds advocate legalisation of euthanasia. According to Glanville Williams[4] the manifold arguments against euthanasia "contrast with the simple humanitarian argument for it". The absolute interdiction of suicide and euthanasia involves for him the "impossible assertion that every life, no matter what its quality or circumstances, is worth living and obligatory to be lived". If it is true that euthanasia can be condemned only according to a religious opinion, he says, this should be sufficient at the present day to remove the prohibition from the criminal law: "The prohibition imposed by a religious belief should not be applied by law to those who do not share the belief, where this is not required for the wordly welfare of society generally." Nevertheless, argues Williams, according to the usual view of Christian religion, the greatest of all commandments is to love, "and this surely means that euthanasia is permissible if performed truly and honestly to spare the patient and not merely for the convenience of the living".

What is described by the Leyden psychiatrist, J H van den Berg,[5] as *medische macht,* the power of modern medicine, has given a new dimension to the euthanasia debate. Van den Berg's eloquent plea for legalised euthanasia is essentially a treatise on a series of tragic cases of vegetating human beings who are the victims of that power. To him, the exercise of medical power results in cruelty and he appeals to the medical profession to put an end to this cruelty.

There is no denying that the mere continuation of life by artificial means in cases of hopelessly ill, dying patients can result in unnecessary suffering and distress, not only for themselves but also for their next of kin. "The medical profession should not be a slave to medical techniques and neither should it enslave patients in these techniques", says G C Oosthuizen,[6] the Natal theologian. The famous heart surgeon, Dr Christiaan Barnard,[7] argues that life should be allowed to continue only when it is enjoyable. Why, he asks, should modern medicine try to prolong the process of life when it cannot be enjoyed any more? "In fact we are not prolonging the process of life; in this way we are actually prolonging death."

J D van der Vyver,[8] the lawyer and human-rights champion, believes man has "a sacred right" to die peaceably and with dignity, and that a person who is ready to do so, should be permitted to meet his God at the right time: "The artificial perpetuation

2 *Op cit* 123 *et seq.*
3 *Ibid* 132 (my translation).
4 Glanville Williams *The Sanctity of Life and the Criminal Law* (1958) 277 *et seq.*
5 J H van den Berg *Medische Macht en Medische Ethiek* (1969).
6 G C Oosthuizen in *Euthanasia* (eds Oosthuizen, Shapiro & Strauss) (1978) 62.
7 C N Barnard in *Euthanasia (op cit)* 197.
8 J D van der Vyver in *Euthanasia (op cit)* 115.

of the life of a person whose death, within the immediate future, has become inevitable may therefore in particular circumstances infringe the will of God."

The latter three views reflect the consensus of opinion in South Africa today. In a way, South Africa is a microcosm of the world. People of many nations in the world have made it their home. Several great African peoples such as the Zulu, the Xhosa, and the Sotho dwell here. There are representatives of many other nations which live elsewhere on the African continent. There are people from every corner of Western Europe and the British Isles, from Eastern Europe and Asia and the Near East, from Malaysia, from China and from India. In a society which is so heterogeneous, one must expect differences of opinion and clashes of interest – sometimes even violent conflicts. But on many important issues of life and of law we are *ad idem.* Mercy-killing is one of them.

In 1977 a national symposium on euthanasia was held in Durban in which all major national groups and religions were represented.[9] On one point there was agreement, namely that euthanasia in the sense of active mercy-killing was unacceptable. One possible exception, *de lege ferenda,* was raised by a geneticist, T Jenkins,[10] who felt that perhaps the time had come to seriously consider legalising selective euthanasia of the defective newborn. Although Jenkins presented a well-reasoned paper, it seems doubtful that this suggestion will receive much support in South Africa.[11] Generally speaking, our society is a conservative one. And apart from all other considerations, South Africans are all too aware that the eyes of the world are constantly focussed on our country.

The traditional Black African view of life does not favour euthanasia either. Although, as in all other societies, the killing of defective newborn children is not unknown, it certainly is not the rule. It was sometimes asserted by historians and writers on Bantu life, that the aged, when they reached the stage of helpless senility, were taken out to the bush and left to die, or to be devoured by wild beasts. J H Soga[12] has pointed out that if this custom exists – as it possibly may among a few degraded tribes – it is by no means common to the great majority. Among the Xhosa, he says, the old and decrepit were carefully tended. He describes a custom amongst these people: When a man or woman was no longer able to take the ordinary food, an ox or cow was slaughtered, and the inner lining of the skin, the dermis, was peeled off and pegged down to stretch and dry. It was afterwards dressed or curried till soft and pliable, and then sewn into a small bottle-shaped article, open at the one end. Into this container, called *utishwa,* was poured milk, either curdled or sweet according to taste, and the aged person either fed himself, or was fed by someone detailed for that duty, much as a European child is bottle-fed.[13]

In South Africa, indigenous African law is still widely applied in the various Black communities, particularly in fields such as matrimonial relationships and succession. The criminal law, however, is essentially modern "European" law. South Africa is one of the few countries in the world in which Roman law still applies. It is of course not pure Roman law, but the Roman law as received in Holland up to the beginning of the 19th century, and "transplanted" to the Cape of Good Hope by the Dutch who first settled at the Cape in 1652. From there it spread all over Southern Africa. In due course, with the spreading of English political influence across the subcontinent, the Roman-Dutch law was substantially modified by English principles and procedures.

9 The proceedings of the symposium are recorded verbatim in *Euthanasia* (eds Oosthuizen, Shapiro & Strauss) (1978, Oxford University Press, Cape Town).

10 T Jenkins in *Euthanasia (op cit)* 173.

11 As is pointed out above 199, withholding of medical treatment from a grossly defective neonate to allow it to die a natural death, will probably not be regarded as unlawful. But Jenkins argues that there is morally no difference between that and active euthanasia in the form of selective infanticide.

12 J H Soga *The Ama-Xhosa; Life and Customs* (1931) 317.

13 See also the comments of V Z Gitywa "A Traditional African Viewpoint" in *Euthanasia (op cit)* 60.

It is clear that notwithstanding eloquent support by prominent members of society to euthanasia movements, the general feeling against euthanasia is still very powerful. No doubt the current sentiments of the general public in South Africa overwhelmingly reject any suggestion of active euthanasia being legalised. Ficarra's views on mercy-killing and those of Lindeboom are for all practical purposes identical to Christian-ethical attitudes prevailing in South Africa. On more than one occasion our courts have held that intentional killing at the request or by consent of the victim constitutes murder. Examples are *R v Peverett*[14] (suicide pact) and *S v Robinson and Others*[15] (insured person consenting to be shot). The motive which leads the victim to request his death is irrelevant as far as the court's verdict is concerned. Accordingly active euthanasia must be regarded as murder. In deciding on a proper sentence, however, the motive with which the wrongdoer acted, may be relevant.

South African criminal law

Modern South African criminal law is unequivocal in its rejection of active euthanasia. The following are some of the cases that have come before our courts:

R v Davidow (1955):[16] The accused's mother was suffering from an incurable disease on account of which she suffered unbearable pain and was in a constant state of despair. Davidow loved his mother dearly and did whatever was in his power to obtain medical attendance and to have her cured, if possible. When all his attempts proved to be of no avail, he requested a friend – in a moment of despair – to kill his mother by means of a fatal injection. His friend flatly refused. The evidence which was later led at his trial, indicated that Davidow at the time had been in a state of extreme tension. Sometimes, in discussions with others about his mother, he burst out in tears. It was also observed that he sometimes wept in his sleep. Evidence was led that his mother often in his presence expressed the wish that she could be dead, and that she could no longer bear the excruciating pain. Finally, Davidow decided to relieve her from further pain and suffering. He visited her in hospital, and during a severe emotional outburst, shot her in the head with his revolver, killing her.

A staff nurse later testified that when she had heard the shot, she hurried to the deceased's bed, where she found the accused in a totally hysterical state, crying out: "God, forgive me! Staff nurse, forgive me! I have killed my mother." In a letter which the accused had written to his brother the previous night, he told the latter of his intention to relieve their mother of her suffering, "without causing her pain, however", to which he added: "I do not have the courage to kill myself. That I will leave to the law to do." (According to South African law, at the time, the death sentence was mandatory for intentional murder in the absence of a finding of extenuating circumstances.)

Davidow was duly charged with murder. On his behalf, psychiatric evidence was adduced to the effect that the accused had developed an obsession to "help" his mother, and that this obsession induced an irresistible impulse in him to kill her. When he committed the act, the psychiatrist concluded, he acted automatically and involuntarily. A psychiatrist, called by the prosecution, contested the finding of irresistible impulse, but nevertheless agreed with the conclusion at which the defence psychiatrist arrived. The accused was acquitted by the jury which tried him.[17]

S v De Bellocq (1968):[18] The accused, a young woman, and her husband were immigrants from France. Her husband was employed by the Council for Scientific and

14 1940 AD 213.
15 1968 (1) SA 66 (A).
16 WLD June 1955, unreported, discussed by H P van Dyk in 1956 *THRHR* 286.
17 As a matter of historical interest, it may be noted that the jury system was subsequently, in 1969, abolished by the South African Legislature; the *Davidow* case, however, had nothing to do with that; abolition of the jury was sought to be justified on general policy considerations.
18 The case was first reported and commented on by the author in 1969 *THRHR* 385.

Industrial Research in Pretoria in connection with the search for oil. He and the accused were newly married and when they had arrived in the country some months earlier, she was pregnant. A month later, Mrs de Bellocq gave birth to a premature child. She was very pleased to have had this child, and nothing could be seen wrong with it for the first three weeks or so. But the child had to be kept at the nursing home although she was discharged, because it had to be put in an incubator for a while and had to be given treatment. After three weeks, on a visit to the nursing home, she found that the child had been taken to a hospital. A few days later she ascertained that the baby had had a lumbar puncture and that the diagnosis was that the child suffered from toxoplasmosis.

Mrs de Bellocq had been a medical student in Paris for some four years and knew what this disease was and what the prognosis was – that the child was in effect already an idiot. It could not drink and had to be fed with a tube through the nose into the stomach. There was practically no chance of the child living for any length of time. During her trial, a prominent paediatrician testified for the prosecution and said *inter alia* that if it had been his child, he would not have treated it medically.

The child was kept at the hospital for some weeks and nothing more could be done for it. She took the child home. In bathing the child she suddenly decided it would be best to end its life, and drowned it.

She was charged with murder and her counsel contended that her conduct amounted to culpable homicide (manslaughter) and not murder. The judge found it could be accepted that she had been in a highly emotional state and that "she was in a puerperal state when a woman is inclined to be more emotional than the normal person". Nevertheless, from her own confession she had intended to kill the child, and it could not be said that her emotional state had reduced that intention to anything less than an intention to kill. "The law does not allow any person to be killed whether that person is an imbecile or very ill. The killing of such a person is an unlawful act and it amounts to murder in law." However, on the facts of the case and the clear extenuating circumstances, the judge held that there would be no object in sending the accused to prison, nor would a suspended sentence be appropriate. The sentence accordingly was that the accused was discharged and was required to enter into recognisances to come up for sentence within six months after the date of sentence, if called upon; she was not required to deposit any amount of money in connection with the recognisances. (The accused was never called upon to come up for sentence, so that in actual fact no sentence was ever imposed.)[19]

S v Hartmann (1975):[20] The accused was a medical practitioner practising at Ceres, Cape Province. His father, an 87-year-old gentleman, had for a number of years been suffering from a carcinoma of the prostate. This condition had spread to other parts of his body, and secondary cancer manifested itself in his bones and more particularly in the ribs. He was being treated in Pretoria up to a stage, and was then induced to come to Ceres, some 1 500 km distant, where he entered the hospital as a private patient of his son, Dr Hartmann. At that stage he was on symptomatic treatment, and there was no longer any question of a cure. On admission he was completely bedridden, very emaciated, incontinent and suffering great pain for which pain-killing drugs were administered.

After being in hospital for some days he suffered a pulmonary embolism and a laryngeal stridor. He appeared to be dying, but on receiving treatment, revived for a short time. After a day or two he was put on intravenous food because he was unable to swallow without choking. Some days later it was apparent that he was in a critical state and soon was moribund. He was suffering pain and was given morphine by a nursing sister. An hour after a dosage of morphine, the accused placed another ½ gr

19 The case is also reported in the *South African Law Reports*, 1975 (3) SA 538 (T).
20 1975 (3) SA 532 (C).

of morphine in the drip. A few hours later, the accused injected 250 mg of pentothal into the drip and within seconds the patient died.

From the medical evidence adduced at Dr Hartmann's trial for murder, it was clear that the deceased at that stage had been in such a critical condition that he may very well have died as little as a few hours later. The court held that the accused was guilty as charged because "the law is clear that it nonetheless constitutes the crime of murder even if all that an accused has done is to hasten the death of a human being who was due to die in any event".

In considering a proper punishment, the judge observed that punishment served the public interest in the sense of discouraging a repetition of the offence by the offender and the prevention of like offences by others. The circumstances of this case were so unique, the judge said, that it could be accepted that the chances of the accused repeating his offence were negligible. "In how far is a deterrent necessary to prevent other medical men from taking similar action in regard to patients who are their close relatives or to their patients generally?" the judge asked, and gave this answer: "Regard being had to the known commitment of members of that profession to preserve life, I would think that such a deterrent has not a great role to play ... This was a case, if ever there was one, in which, without having to be unfair to society, full measure can be given to the element of mercy." The judge accordingly sentenced the accused to imprisonment for one year; however, he was to be detained only until the rising of the court and the balance of the sentence was suspended for one year, subject to the condition that during that period the accused was not to commit an offence involving the intentional infliction of bodily injury.

S v McBride (1979):[21] The accused killed his wife whom he dearly loved, in the following circumstances: Over the years her health had deteriorated drastically, and this affected him severely. At different times in the past she had nursed her sister and mother, both of whom died in painful circumstances of cancer. Both the accused and his wife believed that she too was dying of cancer. Simultaneously with the deterioration of his wife's health, the spouses experienced a deterioration in their financial position. After a series of depressing events, the accused decided to take his wife's life and then his own. He shot and killed her, but before he could kill himself, was saved through the intervention of others. Ironically, the *post mortem* examination of his wife's body showed that she did not have cancer. The spouses' fears would probably have been dispelled if she had been willing to submit to a proper and full medical examination, but she had resolutely refused to do so. The accused was found not guilty by reason of mental illness and declared a State President's patient. The judge recommended that the earliest possible consideration be given to the accused's release.

S v Marengo (1990):[22] The accused, a 45-year-old unmarried woman intentionally killed her father by shooting him twice in the head with a pistol he had kept next to his bed for self-protection. The deceased was 81 years of age and suffering from cancer. The accused pleaded guilty to a charge of murder. She told the court that her actions had been motivated by her desire to end her father's terrible suffering "and to end the mental and physical deterioration brought about, both to myself and to my father by his constant pain and the hopeless and helpless position he was in". She was convicted and was sentenced to three years' imprisonment, suspended in its entirety for five years, subject to the usual conditions. The judge found that she was a victim of extreme circumstances which would never be repeated. Imprisonment he said, was not called for in her case as it could totally destroy her. A factor in the case was that as a young girl she had been totally isolated by her mother from other people. According to psychiatric evidence the accused had numerous traits of an obsessive,

21 1979 (4) SA 313 (W).
22 WLD October 1990. See reports in *The Citizen* 8 December 1989; 16 and 18 October 1990.

compulsive personality. She was incapable of making friends and her entire life existed of going to work as an insurance clerk, and going home to her flat where she locked herself in. She had been told by doctors that her father's condition could continue for many years, while she felt that she could not go on for "even days, never mind years".

Do we have criminal "non-law"?

It may be noted that Dr Hartmann was subsequently charged before the South African Medical and Dental Council with unprofessional conduct and his name was struck off the roll, which is the most severe punishment the Council is legally entitled to impose. (After a certain period of time he was reinstated.) Judging from comments in the press, his action generally evoked sincere and strong compassion. There was very little open condemnation, yet almost no one was prepared to advocate an amendment of the law in such terms as would have enabled him to have lawfully terminated his father's life. The court's judgment was generally regarded as inevitable and the sentence as laudatory.

In the public's mind, then, the law as it is applied to mercy-killing would seem to be ideal. Brand the mercy-killer a murderer. But do not punish him at all (*De Bellocq's* case) or, if the law says murderers shall be punished, impose a sentence which is nominal only, e g imprisonment until the rising of the court (*Hartmann's* case) or a suspended prison sentence (*Marengo's* case). Thereby the law registers society's disapproval in the strongest terms, and yet it is largely symbolic only, because the law then extends the utmost leniency.

One may well ask whether it is still criminal law which is applied when we say that murder is our most serious crime, that capital punishment, *sub condicione,* is in fact the prescribed punishment, but that we recognise a class of murderers whom we do not want to punish at all. Have we not thereby transformed the criminal law into criminal "non-law"? Be that as it may, it must of course be stated that the matter does not end there, at least not for the medical practitioner. Where a doctor is involved in euthanasia, it does not concern the criminal law only. Professional ethics also become relevant. Would the Medical Council have struck Dr Hartmann's name off the professional roll if the court's verdict were that he was not guilty because his act of killing was an act of extreme mercy? So, perhaps Hillel Shapiro[23] is right when he says: "There may be dangers in trying to create some sort of statutory framework ... The art of government is to refrain from legislation sometimes, and this may well be the situation here."

"Passive" euthanasia: let the doctor decide

In concluding this brief paper, I want to make one or two observations concerning the deliberate decision not to treat a patient, and discontinuation of life-preserving methods applied to a particular patient.

In its classical origin the word "euthanasia" probably referred to a certain attitude towards death: a happy and, if possible, also honourable death – *felici vel honesta morte mori.* It was only in the 19th century that the word came to be used in the sense of aid to the dying and the destruction of so-called "worthless" lives (Erhardt).[24] Today it is widely used as a synonym for active mercy-killing.

Whatever the correct meaning of the word, in talking about euthanasia we should try to define the ambit of our discussion. In my opinion we should not confuse the issue by bringing within its scope the decision of a doctor – taken in conjunction with the relatives of a terminal patient, and possibly the patient himself – not to initiate a

23 H A Shapiro in *Euthanasia (op cit)* 241.
24 H Erhardt *Euthanasie und Vernichtung "Lebensunwerten" Lebens* (1965) 7.

new form of treatment, because it would be meaningless and would only prolong the patient's agony. Through the ages doctors have taken the decision not to treat and were respected for it and trusted. Moreover, what has now been termed "passive euthanasia" – i e discontinuation of treatment which was started but no longer serves a meaningful purpose – does not seem to stand on a different footing. In the juridical context neat arguments may be advanced on whether or not such action on the part of the doctor amounts to an omission or a commission, and whether or not it can be said that it has legally caused the death of the patient. But in those cases where a doctor *bona fide* decides to discontinue such treatment, these issues in my opinion can hardly arise. We are here dealing with medical actions which are eminently *sosiaaladekwaat.*[25]

Although the means used by the doctor and his equipment were less spectacular in the past, doctors have through the ages assumed the responsibility of deciding when to terminate treatment. In my opinion they should be free to continue doing so.[26] A decision taken *mala fide* may be punished by the law as it now stands. It is highly unlikely therefore that the need will ever arise in South Africa for a court application similar to that brought in the tragic American case of Karen Quinlan.[27] If such a decision were brought, however, the judgment would undoubtedly be the same as in that case.

I have started by referring to man's overwhelming desire to live, his instinct for survival. Perhaps it is only fitting to end by saying that pain and suffering may torment a man until his desire is to live no more and to receive no further medical treatment. That desire we should also respect.

Adapted from the author's contribution to an international symposium on euthanasia held at Hebrew University, Jerusalem, Israel, in April 1979.

25 See also the remarks by Jennett and Teasdale in their book *Management of Head Injuries* at 312, quoted by Mr Justice Claassen in *Reyneke v Mutual and Federal Insurance Co Ltd* 1991 (3) SA 412 (W) 415.

26 Compare the remarks of A Rall "The Doctor's Dilemma: Relieve Suffering or Prolong Life?" (1977) 94 *SALJ* 40, at 52.

27 *In re Quinlan* 70 NJ 10,355 A 2d 647, 429 US 922 (1976). For the facts of the case see: R M Veatch *Death, Dying and the Biological Revolution* (1976) 137 *et seq;* K Bai "Around the Karen Quinlan Case: Interview with Judge R Muir" (1979) 1 *International Journal of Medicine and Law* 45; Ellison Kahn "Murder as a Fine Art" in *The Sanctity of Human Life* (ed E Kahn) Senate Special Lectures, Witwatersrand University (1984) 24 at 25.

62 The "Living Will" and the "right to die"

The modern physician has to a large extent become master over life and death. What might have been regarded as a hopeless case a few decades ago, may now be viewed as a still treatable case. The doctor has at his disposal techniques and instruments which belonged to the realm of science fiction not so long ago.

The voluntary euthanasia movement which has adherents in many countries, represents a concrete expression of the attitude that the patient should have the conclusive say on whether or not he should be the subject of life-prolonging procedures – a decision which, on account of the circumstances of a terminal patient, is frequently taken by the doctor or the patient's next of kin.

It is significant that medical men and nurses have played an active role in the voluntary enthanasia movement. The South African Living Will Society – its acronym is SAVES – was founded in 1974 by a nursing sister, Mrs Sylvia Kean. Its current president is Professor Harry Grant-Whyte, emeritus professor of anaesthetics at the University of Natal, and one of the best-known medical personalities of this country. The Society's membership in this country has grown steadily and in 1991 exceeded 20 000.

The society distributes the so-called "Living Will" for execution by its members. The document contains a declaration directed to the signatory's family and physicians that reads as follows: "If the time comes when I can no longer take part in decisions for my own future, let this declaration stand as the testament to my wishes. If there is no reasonable prospect of my recovery from physical illness or impairment expected to cause me severe distress or to render me incapable of rational existence, I request that I be allowed to die and not be kept alive by artificial means and that I receive whatever quantity of drugs may be required to keep me free from pain or distress even if the moment of death is hastened."

Is the Living Will a legally valid disposition?

The Living Will is of course not a will in the technical, testamentary sense of the word. Legally it is a declaration in which a person *in anticipando* by way of an advance directive[1] refuses medical attention in the form of being kept alive by artificial means.

In principle every person is legally entitled to refuse medical attention, even if it has the effect of expediting his death. In this sense the individual has a "right to die". All that is required is that the declarant at the time when making his refusal known, is *compos mentis*. The declaration remains valid even though the declarant may at a later stage become *non compos mentis* as a result of physical or mental illness, or for any other reason.

If a man in a concrete situation, where it is proposed that he should immediately be subjected to a particular form of treatment, is entitled to refuse that treatment, there is in my opinion no reason why he would not be entitled to express a "standing" refusal at an earlier stage. Such a refusal, if properly recorded, would then stand until revoked by the person who has made it. It should be seen as nothing but a statement to the following effect: "I am stating here and now that I am not consenting to medical procedure X being performed upon me, should this at any stage be proposed." Nat-

1 The term "advance directive" is of American origin.

urally such a statement remains freely revocable, but unless revoked, remains legally effective.

In my opinion, doctors and hospital staff must respect the declarant's statement of refusal. Should a doctor disregard it and keep the patient alive by artificial means, the doctor will in my opinion be "technically" guilty of an assault, both from the point of view of civil law and criminal law. In the words of Annas *et al,*[2] the Living Will is "a legal statement of the patient's; there is no public policy against the terminally ill patient refusing treatment". This statement, made in the American context, is in my opinion of equal validity for South African law.[3]

It is immaterial what the signatory's motive is, be it fear of prolonging his suffering when terminally ill or critically injured, a desire to spare his next of kin the agony of watching him over a long-drawn period of illness, or a desire to save his estate the major expense involved in lengthy treatment in a hospital's intensive care unit.

It is not necessary to discuss here the practical difficulties in enforcing the Living Will. Obviously, if a doctor or hospital staff were to disregard the fact that a terminal patient has signed a Living Will, nothing much can be done about enforcing the patient's rights, unless someone, e g a relative, were to intercede on behalf of the patient. In my opinion, if there is such a disregard, the court may be approached for appointment of a *curator ad litem* for the patient, in order to bring an application for an interdict against the doctor.

As regards the part of the Living Will in which the patient requests that "I receive whatever quantity of drugs may be required to keep me free from pain or distress even if the moment of death is hastened", the situation is not without problems in our law.

According to a South African judgment, to hasten death is in fact to cause it. In *R v Makali*[4] the court declared: "The true enquiry is whether the deceased would have died when he did but for the [accused's] unlawful act. If this enquiry gives an affirmative answer, [the accused] is responsible for the death because he caused it to take place when it did, that is to say because he hastened it."

This seems to be the general point of departure in English law as well,[5] but there is some authority for the proposition that a medical practitioner may by the administering of pain-relieving drugs lawfully shorten the life of a patient. (This situation is sometimes referred to as "indirect euthanasia".) In the prosecution of Dr John Bodkin Adams[6] in 1957, the judge instructed the jury in the following terms: "If the first purpose of medicine, the restoration of health, can no longer be achieved there is still much for a doctor to do, and he is entitled to do all that is proper and necessary to relieve pain and suffering, even if the measure he takes may incidentally shorten life." According to the judge this does not amount to causing death; the disease must be regarded as the cause.

Glanville Williams,[7] a foremost English criminalist, is of the opinion that a physician's conduct is not unlawful in the following instances: A patient is suffering from an incurable disease accompanied by excruciating pain. The physician administers the minimum dosage of drugs necessary to make the pain endurable knowing that such minimum dosage will probably also cause death. A patient is suffering from a painful and incurable disease and a drug is administered. Because of the resistance consequent upon the habitual administering of the drug, steadily increasing doses

2 *The Rights of Doctors, Nurses and Allied Health Professions* (1981) 221.

3 See also E Deutsch, in E Deutsch, H Kleinsorg and J G Ziegler *Das Patiententestament* (1983) 61. As Deutsch observes elsewhere (63) the human desire for a quick and painless death is primeval and should be obstructed by neither ethics nor law.

4 1950 (1) SA 340 (N) 344.

5 See Glanville Williams *The Sanctity of Life and the Criminal Law* (1958) 289.

6 Quoted by Williams *op cit* 289.

7 *Op cit* 285 *et seq.*

have to be administered. This means that unless the patient dies beforehand due to another cause, a point must be reached when the dosage becomes lethal.

I would respectfully support Williams's views. However, the situation in which a pain-relieving substance is administered, hastening the death of a terminal patient has so far not been the subject of a decision in South Africa. But in the well-known case of *S v Hartmann,*[8] where a doctor administered a fatal dosage of pentothal to his aged and ailing father, the court held that the doctor was guilty of murder. Mr Justice Van Winsen pointed out that pentothal is not an analgesic but used in anaesthesia. The learned judge said: "It is true that the deceased was in a dying condition when this dose of pentothal was administered and that there is evidence that he may very well have died as little as a few hours later. But the law is clear that it nonetheless constitutes the crime of murder even if all that an accused has done is to hasten the death of a human being who was due to die in any event. See *R v Makali,* 1950 (1) SA 340 (N). Here the State has proved that but for the accused's action the deceased would not have died when he did. That such action, if wilfully undertaken, constitutes murder is also the law of England, as appears from a number of decisions in the English Court, cited by Hart and Honoré in their work *Causation in the Law* at pp. 307–8."

On the face of it, it would appear that the *Hartmann* ruling does not apply to pain-relieving treatment administered in good faith by the doctor. As Ellison Kahn[9] has pointed out, "[t]he doctor who, in genuinely and reasonably attempting to relieve the pain of his patient, indirectly hastens the death of his patient, is not guilty of murder, because his conduct was not unlawful". That, he says, is trite law. I would respectfully associate myself with this view. Even if the causing of the patient's death were to be regarded as fulfilling the *Tatbestand* of murder, and therefore *prima facie* unlawful, it would in accordance with legal principle not in actual fact be unlawful, because what the doctor did was altogether *sosiaal adekwaat,*[10] and therefore justified in law. Moreover, there can be no question of either intent to kill which is required for a conviction of murder, or of negligence, which would be a requirement for the lesser verdict of culpable homicide.

As H J J Leenen[11] has observed, the doctor's aim in this situation is not to terminate life, but to alleviate the patient's suffering. "The administration of the pain-alleviating method can be qualified as an act with double effect," he argues. "It must not be defined according to its side-effect, the unavoidable shortening of life, but according to its aim, which is to combat the pain of which the patient is suffering. Many medical acts and drugs have side-effects, but nobody will define them from the viewpoint of these side-effects. The same is true for pain-killing."

That stipulation of the Living Will which expresses the patient's desire to receive whatever quantity of drugs may be required to keep him free from pain or distress, even if his death is hastened, therefore seems to be legally unassailable. As long as the doctor acts in good faith using the usual pain-relieving substances, in reasonable quantities, with the intent to relieve pain and not to kill, there will be no question of criminal or civil liability on his part.

An aspect of the Living Will which seems to require some attention is its possible implications in the field of life-insurance law.[12] For a patient to insist that he be given

8 1975 (3) SA 532 (C). The case is discussed *supra* 340.

9 "Murder as a Fine Art", in *The Sanctity of Life* (ed E Kahn) Senate Special Lectures, University of the Witwatersrand (1983) 24 at 25.

10 "Social adequacy" as a defence in criminal law has so far been accorded very little attention in South Africa, but is recognised in the science of criminal law. It involves an act which although *prima facie* unlawful, must be approved of rather than disapproved, because of its social usefulness. See H-H Jescheck *Lehrbuch des Strafrechts* (4th ed, 1988) 226 *et seq.*

11 In a paper on "The Definition of Euthanasia" (1983, unpublished) kindly put at my disposal. Professor Leenen is professor of law in Amsterdam.

12 I am indebted to an expert in the field of insurance law, Mr Lionel Hodes, formerly of the Faculty of Law, University of the Witwatersrand, for the benefit of his views on this subject.

pain-relieving drugs that may hasten his demise, might be regarded by insurers as tantamount to suicide. This may have the effect of invalidating the policy under the "suicide clause" (which usually specifies that the policy will become null and void if the insured commits suicide within two years after he has taken out the policy).

But can the mere refusal by a patient of medical treatment, or to be kept alive artificially, be regarded as suicide? I do not think so.[13] However, it may be argued that the fact that a person has signed a Living Will may affect the risk to be undertaken by the insurer. It will therefore clearly be advisable for a person who has signed the Living Will and who subsequently proposes to take out life insurance, to inform the company of that fact when he makes the formal insurance proposal. *Uberrima fides* – good faith in the highest degree – is required as between insurer and insured.

The Living Will, in the form of an advance directive to be allowed to die without medical treatment in the event of the signatory becoming mentally incompetent, began to receive the attention of state legislatures in the USA by the middle of the 1970s. The first of these statutes was the California Natural Death Act of 1976.[14] By the end of 1987, 38 states and the District of Columbia were reported to have enacted similar statutes which can broadly be described as "Living Will laws".[15] In 1983 the California legislature passed the Durable Power of Attorney Health Care Act[16] which enabled persons to appoint an attorney to make health-care decisions for the principal should the latter become unable to give an informed consent himself. Other states have followed suit with statutes that collectively became known as "enduring power of attorney" laws.[17]

It is of interest to note that even in the absence of legislation on the validity of Living Wills, American courts have given recognition to directives embodied therein.[18]

Attention may also be drawn to the World Medical Association's *Declaration of Venice* (October 1983) on terminal illness. The declaration reaffirms the duty of the doctor to heal and, where possible, to relieve suffering. It states, however, that this principle does not preclude application of the following rules: "The physician may relieve suffering of a terminally ill patient by withholding treatment with the consent of the patient or his immediate family if unable to express his will. Withholding of treatment does not free the physician from his obligation to assist the dying person and give him the necessary medicaments to mitigate the terminal phase of his illness. The physician shall refrain from employing any extraordinary means which would prove of no benefit for the patient."[19]

Adapted from a paper with the same title, read in the University of the Witwatersrand Senate Special Lecture series entitled "The Sanctity of Human Life", August 1983. The paper was first published in The Sanctity of Human Life *(ed Ellison Kahn) (1984). Reproduction here in this form is by kind courtesy of Professor Kahn.*

13 See also Deutsch *op cit* 60.

14 I Kennedy & A Grubb *Medical Law: Texts and Materials* (1989) 1123. See also P B Solnick 4 *Med Law* 1 (1985) at 6.

15 Kennedy & Grubb 1117.

16 *Ibid* 1145.

17 *Ibid.*

18 See in particular *Re Saunders* 492 NYS 2d 510 (1985) quoted by Kennedy & Grubb 1121. In the following cases courts accorded *obiter* recognition to Living Wills as advance directives not to be medically treated: *Re Conroy* 486 A 2d 1209 (1985) and *John F Kennedy Memorial Hospital v Bludworth* 452 So 2d 921 (1984), (quoted by Kennedy & Grubb at 1119 and 1120, respectively).

19 The World Medical Association's 1990 statement on the care of patients with severe chronic pain in terminal illness does not deal with the withholding of treatment but goes into detail on the clinical management of pain.

PART XIV

Alcohol abuse and drunken driving

63 The alcoholic and the law

A court "regular"

The alcoholic is a frequent visitor to our criminal courts and presents a difficult problem in our system of criminal justice. By the term "alcoholic" I understand a person who has developed a manifest dependence on alcohol. Before dealing with him specifically, it is necessary to say a few words on the problem of alcoholism in general, as concerns the law.

The abuse of alcohol generally presents serious problems to the law enforcement agencies and in particular to our courts. If the alcoholic – the person dependent on alcohol – is a frequent visitor to our courts, it must be observed that his cousin – the heavy or excessive drinker – is there more often. I am in this context referring to the man who cannot be classified as an alcoholic because he has not yet reached the stage where he is firmly dependent on alcohol. But he may be a man who is already well on the way to becoming an alcoholic, either because he enjoys regular drinking bouts as part of his social life, or because he is completely reckless in his use of alcohol.

This is the type of person who will appear in our courts on a charge of drunken driving or on a charge of a violent crime, ranging from common assault through public violence, rape, assault with the intent to cause grievous bodily harm, culpable homicide or even murder.

It is perhaps a simplistic view to say that the drinking habits of this "cousin", as I have called him, the excessive drinker, are a grave causative factor in crime. Often we are dealing here with a man who has a latent tendency to behave or respond violently, and this tendency is aggravated by the use of alcohol. He may or may not be a psychopath. Or we may be dealing with a person who, although not violent by nature, has a low level of social responsibility which becomes dulled by the abuse of liquor. At the other end of the spectrum is the person who is perhaps basically responsible, but who unintentionally – often in a mood of over-exuberance or depression – over-indulges, and when driving home in an intoxicated state becomes involved in an accident. Therefore, in my opinion, abuse of alcohol should rather be described as a triggering stimulus in the causation of crime.

Intoxication as a defence

The problem of the courts is, what to do with the man who is charged with a crime in which intoxication has played a role, and who pleads for mercy. Should he be treated more leniently, or more severely, or should the fact that he was drunk at the time of the commission of the offence be regarded as irrelevant and therefore ignored? It is very interesting to consider the attitude of the courts to the intoxicated man over the centuries in Roman-Dutch law.[1] We need not go into that now, except to say that intoxication was generally considered a mitigating feature. Occasionally, however, the lawgiver lost patience and prescribed sterner punishment. Thus

1 There is an excellent dissertation on the subject, by J L Snyman *Dronkenskap as Verweer in die Strafreg* (LL M thesis, University of South Africa, 1977).

Charles the Fifth in the year 1545 ordained that no mitigation was to be extended for homicide committed during fairs or within three days after a fair![2] Some 400 years later, in 1955, the South African Parliament also endeavoured to make intoxication an aggravating feature. Act 29 of 1955[3] stipulated that where it is proved that a person convicted of an offence was under the influence of liquor or a narcotic drug when he committed the offence, the court could in determining the sentence regard that fact as an aggravating circumstance.

This provision had little or no effect, however,[4] and was finally repealed in 1977.[5] The position was then that intoxication in principle would often constitute a mitigating feature. A severe degree of intoxication could lead to a clouding of the mind which precluded the wrongdoer from forming an intent.[6] This had the effect that he could not be convicted of a crime of which intention is an element. A typical example was murder. It is an everyday occurrence in our country that a person is killed in the course of a drunken brawl. The wrongdoer is charged with murder – a capital offence – but the evidence establishes that he was so drunk when he dealt the fatal blow that he was incapable of forming an intent.

He was accordingly convicted of culpable homicide, for which only a finding of negligence is required, and a relatively lenient punishment was imposed, say two or three years' imprisonment. Where drunkenness was a constituent element of the crime itself, the accused could not advance intoxication as a defence. A typical example was drunken driving.[7] Likewise, a wrongdoer could not rely on that defence if he deliberately drank himself drunk in order to muster courage to commit his deed.[8]

What about the man who has imbibed to such an extent that his mind virtually goes blank? In his drunken stupor he perpetrates an act of serious violence. Can he escape criminal liability on the ground that his act was altogether involuntary? In view of the basic legal principle that criminal liability presupposes at the very least a voluntary act, our courts have devoted special attention to alcohol-induced involuntary conduct. Up to 1981 our courts took the view that this type of wrongdoer could not be equated with the somnambulist or the epileptic and that he could not escape criminal liability altogether; in crimes for which "specific intent" was a requirement, however, his intoxication would have the effect of "reducing" his offence to a lesser one.[9]

But in 1981, in the landmark case of *Chretien,*[10] the Appeal Court adopted an entirely new approach. If a person was so paralytically drunk that he was unaware of what he was doing and commited an involuntary action, he could not be held liable.[11] Even if his intoxication fell short of that extreme degree but was so severe that he did not know what he was doing or did not realise that his act was wrongful, he would not be punishable, on account of a lack of criminal capacity. Mr Justice Rumpff, the Chief Justice, who handed down the court's judgment, in this connection referred to the substantial disintegration of the wrongdoer's inhibitions ("wesenlike verkrummeling van die dader se inhibisies").

2 Snyman 5. As Snyman notes, there was an even earlier enactment (1531) of Charles V to the effect that no leniency was to be shown to persons who in a drunken state committed homicide or an assault.
3 Section 51, which inserted section 357*bis* into the Criminal Procedure and Evidence Act 31 of 1917. The latter section became section 350 of the Criminal Procedure Act 56 of 1955.
4 See Snyman 173 *et seq.*
5 When the 1955 Criminal Procedure Act was repealed by the new Criminal Procedure Act 51 of 1977, section 350 of the old Act was not re-enacted.
6 See *Chretien's* case, below, at 1103 A–C.
7 See *S v Kelder* 1967 (2) SA 644 (T). There are other examples as well. See Snyman 183 *et seq.*
8 The so-called *actio libera in causa.*
9 See *S v Johnson* 1969 (1) SA 201 (A).
10 *S v Chretien* 1981 (1) SA 1097 (A).
11 Compare *S v Stellmacher* 1983 (2) SA 181 (SWA). It is not quite clear whether the accused's acquittal was based upon an involuntary act or upon lack of criminal capacity.

This decision, however, did not affect the principle of antecedent liability. By virtue of the latter principle the question must be asked, where the death of a human being was caused by the drunken conduct of another, whether at the stage when the wrongdoer brought the first glass to his lips, it was reasonably foreseeable that he could cause the death of another, should he become drunk. In these cases the wrongdoer will be convicted of culpable homicide because of his voluntary act of drinking and negligence at the stage when he was still sober, i e criminally responsible.[12] An example: A schoolbus driver leaves his bus full of cheerful children parked outside an hotel, in order to have a couple of "quick ones for the road" in the bar. In due course he becomes hopelessly drunk, but still manages to reach the bus, to start the engine and drive for a small distance. He then collapses in a drunken stupor and the bus collides with a tree. A child is killed in the accident. Although his final action may have been involuntary, the driver can nevertheless be convicted of culpable homicide.

Although it was an example of sound logical reasoning, the *Chretien* judgment did not find favour with the powers that be. It was also regarded as unacceptable by the general public that the drunker an offender was, the more likely his chances would be to escape criminal conviction and punishment.

In 1988 the Legislature, through enactment of the Criminal Law Amendment Act No 1 of that year, endeavoured to nullify the effect of *Chretien* whereby voluntary intoxication could constitute a complete defence.

Section 1 of the Act reads as follows:

(1) "Any person who consumes or uses any substance which impairs his faculties to appreciate the wrongfulness of his acts or to act in accordance with that appreciation, while knowing that such substance has that effect, and who, while such faculties are thus impaired, commits any act prohibited by law under any penalty, but is not criminally liable because his faculties were impaired as aforesaid, shall be guilty of an offence and shall be liable on conviction to the penalty, except the death penalty, which may be imposed in respect of the commission of that act.

(2) If in any prosecution for any offence it is found that the accused is not criminally liable for the offence charged on account that his faculties referred to in subsection (1) were impaired by the consumption or use of any substance, such accused may be found guilty of a contravention of subsection (1), if the evidence proves the commission of such contravention."

These provisions have the effect that where the wrongdoer was not criminally responsible on account of voluntary consumption of liquor or some other substance he will not be acquitted but may be convicted of a criminal offence under the section itself, and may be sentenced in the same manner as he might have been if it were not for his drunkenness (except that the death sentence cannot be imposed). The same would seem to apply where the wrongdoer was so drunk that his conduct became involuntary (alcohol-induced automatism, in other words). But the section does not refer to the situation where the accused, although criminally responsible, lacked the required intention to commit an offence as a result of his intoxication. This seems to be an omission on the part of the Legislature, which means that in such a case the accused will, by virtue of the ruling in *Chretien,* still go scot-free if the crime is one for which intention is a requirement.

It is assumed that the section does not apply where the accused has been forced to take liquor against his will. It goes without saying that there should be clear proof of that.

It should also be noted that there cannot be any doubt that intoxication will still be a complete defence where it has caused a pathological condition of mental abnor-

12 Chretien's conviction of culpable homicide in respect of the person he had killed, was clearly based on this principle.

mality such as ***delirium tremens.*** The accused will then be treated as a mentally abnormal offender,[13] with all the implications attaching to that, the most important of which is that he may be declared a so-called "State President's patient" and be detained in a mental institution for treatment.

Can intoxication still operate as an extenuating circumstance? Section 2 of the 1988 Act reads as follows:

"Whenever it is proved that the faculties of a person convicted of any offence were impaired by the consumption or use of a substance when he committed that offence, the court may, in determining an appropriate sentence to be imposed upon him in respect of that offence, regard as an aggravating circumstance the fact that his faculties were thus impaired."

This provision is reminiscent of the 1955 law to which reference was made above. The subsection confers a discretion upon the court to impose a heavier sentence because of the fact that the accused had imbibed excessively prior to the commission of the offence. On the other hand, it does not do away with the principle that the court may take intoxication into account in mitigation of sentence. It is doubtful whether the subsection will make any difference in practice: even by common law a criminal court may regard intoxication as an aggravating factor in an appropriate case.[14]

The chronic alcoholic

I want to return to the true alcoholic, to whom reference was made at the outset, and to deal with the special legal provisions pertaining to him. The idea behind these provisions is that the chronic alcoholic is a sick man and should be treated, not punished. This is of course no absolute notion, because alcoholism is not readily accepted by the man in the street as a ground which may exonerate an alcoholic in all circumstances for a foul deed committed by him. Within specified limits, and subject to societal interests, however, treatment may be substituted for punishment.

Our courts are generally reluctant to let a man go unpunished for a serious crime because he is an alcoholic. The person who deliberately kills another in a fit of alcoholic depression, short of a pathological state of mental abnormality, will probably be sentenced – at the very least – to a fairly long period of imprisonment. Likewise the alcoholic who over a long period systematically embezzles a large sum of money to keep himself supplied with liquor can hardly expect to escape a prison sentence.

However, certain pronouncements by our courts indicate an awareness of the alcoholic's need for rehabilitation. Thus, in *S v Popo,*[15] an attorney described by the court as a "very able" practitioner, was sentenced by a magistrate to imprisonment for a year in consequence of his conviction for theft for having stolen more than R6 000 from his trust account. The trial court in its judgment expressed concern about the possible effect of imprisonment on the accused's rehabilitation and the lack of facilities for a person of his type, but considered that a wholly suspended sentence would be inappropriate, even though the accused was a first offender. The judge was of the opinion that for an offence of that nature imprisonment could only be dispensed with if the circumstances were "so exceptional that, in effect, the accused can be said not to be really responsible for what he has done". However, on appeal to the Appeal Court in Bloemfontein, the sentence was wholly suspended. The Appeal Court pointed out that the commission of the offence was clearly to be attributed to irresponsibility arising from addiction to alcohol and not to any innate dishonesty. Imprisonment would in this instance operate more severely than is generally the case.

13 Snyman 118.
14 Act 1 of 1988 has been the subject of a good deal of comment in the law journals, much of it highly critical. See e g : J I Welch 1990 *SACJ* 268; T F Coetzee 1990 *SACJ* 285; "De Wet" 1990 *SACJ* 298.
15 1978 (1) SA 476 (A).

Amongst other considerations the Appeal Court concluded that the accused's rehabilitation – treatment had already begun before the trial – would be jeopardised.

In another case, *S v Heyns,*[16] the court was confronted with the problem of what to do about the person who habitually offends against the law penalising public drunkenness. If he fails to heed a series of fines and warnings of more severe steps, must he ultimately be sentenced to imprisonment – which would have the effect of him losing his work and of depriving his family of their main source of sustenance? The judge held that punishment for public drunkenness must be imposed with understanding of this human weakness and a measure of compassion for the unfortunate accused. A court ought not to impose a long period of imprisonment, he said, which would have the effect of putting the accused among hardened criminals and which would make him lose his work. If an offender persists in his conduct to such an extent that it appears that he has become an alcoholic, he ought to be referred to an institution for rehabilitation of inebriates rather than be incarcerated for long periods.

In *S v Fraser*[17] the court considered the position of an alcoholic who had repeatedly been convicted of drunken driving. The court held that there was no rule that an alcoholic should receive a lighter sentence or that a sentence of imprisonment should not be imposed. The possible effect of imprisonment on the accused's rehabilitation as an alcoholic should be taken into account, and the courts should endeavour not to impose a sentence which would prejudice such rehabilitation. The accused should, however, be willing to receive and to co-operate in any treatment given for his condition.

Institutional rehabilitation

This subject – i e institutional rehabilitation – is governed by the Abuse of Dependence-producing Substances and Rehabilitation Centres Act[18] (popularly known as the "Drugs Act" or the "Hippie Act").

This Act[19] makes provision for inquiries by a magistrate into the circumstances of, *inter alia,* alcoholics, with a view to making an order that the person concerned be committed to a rehabilitation centre. It is provided that whenever a declaration is lodged with a public prosecutor that a person "is dependent on alcoholic liquor or dependence-producing drugs and in consequence thereof squanders his means or injures his health or endangers the peace or in any other manner does harm to his own welfare or the welfare of his family", the clerk of the court must summon the person concerned to appear before him. The mere fact that the person is an alcoholic does not seem to entitle the prosecutor to initiate the inquiry. The Act expressly stipulates the further circumstances of squandering of his means, or jeopardising the welfare of his family, etc. It is further provided that the prosecutor may not request the clerk of the court to issue the summons unless he has first obtained from a social worker a report as to the social circumstances of the person who is the subject of the inquiry.

The magistrate before whom the person is brought must then in the presence of that person enquire whether he is a person such as I have described.[20] The magistrate may at the inquiry summon to his assistance a social worker, doctor, psychiatrist or clinical psychologist to sit with him as assessor(s). The Act contains all the usual procedural safeguards in favour of the subject, such as the right to be represented by his attorney or advocate.

It is to be noted that the statement to the prosecutor, which sets the "machinery"

16 1978 (1) SA 399 (E).
17 1987 (2) SA 859 (A).
18 Act 41 of 1971.
19 Section 29. See also the article by J L Snyman in 1978 (June) *TRW* 32.
20 Section 30.

for an inquiry into motion, may be made by a social worker or by any person, such as a relative or friend of the subject, a policeman or even a complete stranger.

The necessity or advisability of such an inquiry may also become evident in the course of a criminal trial. For that reason the Criminal Procedure Act[21] provides that if it appears to the judge or magistrate that the accused is an alcoholic (such as I have described), he may with the consent of the prosecutor, given after consultation with a social welfare officer, stop the trial and order that an inquiry be held instead. However, an accused who is tried on a charge for which the death sentence may be imposed may not be dealt with by this procedure.

Since the making of an order of committal to a rehabilitation centre is drastic, in the sense that the period of detention is indefinite, magistrates are legally empowered to postpone an order, subject to the conditions that the person concerned submit himself to supervision by a social worker and undergo prescribed treatment.

The question may be asked whether the committal procedure is in fact used often enough in cases where rehabilitation is urgently needed. A problem is that alcoholics who have committed a criminal offence would usually choose to go to prison for a fixed period, e g three months, rather than go to a rehabilitation centre for an indefinite period. On the other hand, it may be that although the alcoholic himself is anxious to undergo treatment and applies for an inquiry, the nature of his crime was such that the magistrate may consider he should not be allowed to escape his just deserts in the form of a prison sentence. Particularly in cases of drunken driving, prosecutors are sometimes reluctant to consent to conversion of trials into inquiries, for the simple reason that the "Hippie Act" does not contain a provision whereby a driver's licence may be suspended or cancelled. Moreover, that Act itself makes provision for a convicted person, who is serving a prison sentence, to be transferred to a rehabilitation centre.[22]

Based upon the text of a talk broadcast by Radio South Africa as part of a series on Alcoholism, *in the programme "University of the Air", October–November 1978.*

21 Section 255.
22 Act 41 of 1971, section 36.

64 The taking of blood samples in drunken driving cases

The following questions were put to me by a doctor: "If a suspect is brought to a doctor by the police, may he refuse to have a blood sample taken? If he refuses, can he be forced to give a blood sample? If he is forced, is this not tantamount to assault?

"If the doctor finds that the suspect is not incapable of driving a car and yet his blood-alcohol content is excessive, what is the position?

"Recently, a lady who never in her life had alcohol, was brought to me from a wedding reception. She had had half a glass of champagne and was absolutely drunk. Her blood-alcohol content was far below the statutory limit, yet I maintained that she was 'under the influence'. What will the position be here?

"Can a doctor refuse to take blood, or must he do so just because a policeman requires it, even where the doctor strongly feels that a blood test is not indicated?

"Must the policeman be in my private consulting room when I examine the patient?"

My answer is as follows:

In terms of section 37 of the Criminal Procedure Act of 1977[1] any medical officer of any prison or any district surgeon or, if requested thereto by any police official, any registered medical practitioner or registered nurse, may take such steps, including the taking of a blood sample, as may be deemed necessary in order to ascertain whether the body of a person arrested upon any charge (or of an arrested suspect who has been released on bail or on warning) has any characteristic or distinguishing feature or shows any condition or appearance.

The section further provides that if any registered medical practitioner attached to any hospital, on reasonable grounds is of the opinion that the contents of the blood of any person admitted to such hospital for medical attention or treatment may be relevant at any later criminal proceedings, the doctor may take a blood sample of such person or cause it to be taken.

It is clear that in the circumstances outlined above, an independently practising doctor (or a registered nurse) is authorised to take a blood sample. Secondly, a hospital doctor may in the situation described, take such a sample.

The statutory authorisation for taking a blood sample, presupposes the power to do so against the will of the suspect (provided, of course that he was lawfully arrested[2]). In fact, the policeman and/or doctor involved may without a doubt use a reasonable amount of force so that the doctor can take the blood sample, and this will not constitute assault.[3]

In his textbook on criminal procedure, Hiemstra[4] expresses the opinion that in the

1 Act 51 of 1977.

2 See my comments below 361.

3 V G Hiemstra *Suid-Afrikaanse Strafproses* (4th ed, 1987) 71. Hiemstra nevertheless states that the blood specimen may be taken against the will of the accused. But he cautions that the right to use force should be exercised with "good judgment".

4 It has been held that mere (passive) refusal on the part of a suspect to allow a doctor to take a blood sample does not constitute the crime of defeating the ends of justice (*S v Oberbacher* 1975 (3) SA 81 (SWA)). This judgment has been criticised, however. See C R Snyman *Strafreg* (2nd ed, 1986) 386 n. Compare *S v Gaba* 1981 (3) SA 745 (O).

case of suspected intoxication there may be other ascertainable indications and that a blood sample is not indispensable.

I would submit with respect, however, that the penalisation of an excessive blood-alcohol content by the Road Traffic Act[5] would largely be rendered nugatory unless our courts recognise as a matter of principle that the taking of a blood sample – even against the will of the suspect – is always a reasonable step "deemed necessary" (in the wording of the Act) in drunken driving cases. As was held in *R v Cawood* [6] the consent of a suspect is not necessary, because that would exclude the best evidence of intoxication, viz that of a doctor.

The provisions of section 37 are discretionary as far as the doctor is concerned and not peremptory, as is indicated by the use of the word "may". In my opinion, the doctor may in proper circumstances refuse to take a blood sample. However, this discretion should obviously be exercised in a reasonable manner and a doctor would clearly be acting improperly if he were to refuse taking a blood sample where *prima facie* the suspect seems to be under the influence of liquor or where there is information indicative of an excessive blood-alcohol content.

It is to be noted that the criminal offence of driving a vehicle while the blood-alcohol content of the driver is 0,08 or more, is a completely different one in law from "being under the influence". For the former offence (blood-alcohol) it is not necessary to show that the accused was intoxicated in the usual sense of the word. For the latter offence, again, it is not necessary for the State to prove that the driver's blood-alcohol content exceeded the statutory limit. It is not even necessary to prove that the driver was drunk and incapable. It is sufficient to show that the liquor the driver has imbibed has influenced him to such an extent that "the skill and judgement normally required in the manipulation of a car is obviously diminished or impaired".[7] Even an "exuberant or over-optimistic frame of mind" which causes the driver to take risks may constitute intoxication for the purpose of the law.[8]

There is nothing in the Criminal Procedure Act which gives the policeman the right to be present at the examination of the suspect by the doctor, but it would clearly not be improper for the doctor to allow the policeman to be present. It will sometimes be necessary for the policeman to assist the doctor in restraining the suspect.

It is to be noted that a suspect should be allowed to request his own doctor to be present at the examination and to be examined by him. The suspect should be informed, as soon as is reasonably possible after his arrest, that he is so entitled.[9]

5 Act 29 of 1989, section 122 (2) *(b)*.
6 1950 (4) SA 91 (E).
7 *R v Lloyd* 1929 EDL 270.
8 *R v Spicer* 1945 AD 433.
9 See W E Cooper *Motor Law* vol 1 (1982) 556 and cases cited.

65 Blood-alcohol: must the specimen taken be representative of the driver's blood generally?

The text of the uniform Road Traffic Act of 1989[1] on blood-alcohol (section 122) reflects a series of legal battles waged over a number of years, and which resulted in amendments being incorporated into the provisions of the uniform Road Traffic Ordinance[2] which preceded the Act.

The changing provisions on penalisation of excessive blood-alcohol in drivers present a fine example of the never-ending process of interaction – some observers would prefer to call it a duel – between the lawgiver on the one hand, and the legal practitioner on the other. Critics of the legal profession would be inclined to scoff at the whole process as "cunning phrase-mongering" or "devious loophole-seeking". But in actual fact the hypercritical scrutinising of penal laws by lawyers and the courts underlines the principle of legality which is a cornerstone of a democratic legal system.

In the 1970s the battle raged over the question whether or not a blood specimen taken from a driver can be said to be representative of the driver's blood generally.

In 1974, in *S v Vis,*[3] the Orange Free State court ruled that a person is only guilty of a contravention of section 140 (2) of the uniform Road Traffic Ordinance if he drives a vehicle on a public road while the percentage of alcohol in his blood, "taken as a whole" is not less than the statutory minimum (which now is 0,08 g per 100 ml – at the time when Vis drove his car the limit was still 0,15).

Additional evidence is required, the judge held, that alcohol, after consumption, is evenly diffused in a person's blood, before it can be said that the accused's blood as a whole contained the prohibited percentage of alcohol.

In this case the sample of blood of the accused taken by the doctor, on analysis, was found to contain 0,24 per cent of alcohol. After taking the sample, the doctor threw away the syringe and its container. The accused had made no request to the doctor to retain these objects for analysis by the defence. The court held that because of that fact it could not in any way be said it was irregular for the doctor to have destroyed the syringe and container.

The court further held that the evidence tendered by the State "by implication" proved that the blood drawn from the accused was representative of his blood as a whole. This the court inferred from the use of the word "specimen" by the doctor when he testified on the sample taken by him.

The Ordinance was subsequently amended to substitute the words "percentage of alcohol" (in blood) with "concentration of alcohol". Nevertheless the Free State court in 1975 in *S v Iveson,*[4] following the general principle laid down in *Vis*, quashed a conviction on the grounds that there was no evidence before the court that the blood specimen drawn by the doctor was representative of the accused's blood taken as a whole. Two further Free State decisions followed in which this view was sup-

1 Act 29 of 1989.
2 Ord 21 of 1966.
3 1974 (2) SA 437 (O).
4 1975 (3) SA 90 (O).

ported.[5] The Transvaal[6] and Cape[7] courts, however, refused to follow the Free State ruling.

In 1977 the question came before the Appellate Division in *S v Francis.*[8] Chief Justice Rumpff refused to follow the Free State decisions. Said the Chief Justice: "I do not know what the statement that the blood specimen must be representative of the 'blood as a whole' means. Is it the total of the blood in the arteries, veins, heart, brain, liver and other possible places in the body? Must of this 'blood as a whole' an average be obtained in order to obtain a 'specimen' in the same sense of 'part of the whole'?"

The judge referred to expert texts on acute alcoholic intoxication from which it could not be said that it was generally known that medical experts differ on the question whether blood drawn from a certain place was representative of the "blood as a whole".

In the result, the judge held, it could never have been the intention of the Legislature that specimens of blood had to be drawn from the arteries, veins and all possible organs of the body. Nor was it necessary to lead medical evidence that the specimen taken was representative of the blood as a whole.

It is to be noted that even before the *Francis* case was decided, the uniform Road Traffic Ordinances had been amended in 1975. Section 122 (1) *(b)* of the Act now provides that it is an offence for a person to drive a vehicle (or to occupy the driver's seat of a motor vehicle, the engine of which is running) while the concentration of alcohol "in any specimen of blood taken from any part of his body" exceeds the statutory limit of 0,08.

Yet another loophole in the legislative wall against drunken driving has been closed!

5 *S v Van den Berg* 1975 (3) SA 354 (O) and *S v De Waal* 1976 (2) SA 289 (O).
6 In *S v Jubelius* 1976 (2) SA 70 (C).
7 In *S v Francis* 1976 (2) SA 70 (C).
8 1977 (1) SA 643 (A). The translation in the text is mine.

66 Drunken driving and "breathalyser" tests: some legal problems

Without a doubt the abuse of alcohol is a factor in the high incidence of road accidents in the Republic. However, as Shapiro[1] has observed, this factor ought not to be overemphasised in relation to fatal traffic accidents.

In combating drunken driving on our roads, the traffic authorities are confronted with two problems which have *inter alia* difficult legal implications:

- Bringing to bay motorists who are under the influence of liquor, so as to take potential causers of accidents off the road.
- Adducing convincing evidence in a court of law that a motorist who was apprehended for suspected drunken driving, had been under the influence of liquor.

Regarding the first of these aspects, the majority of drunken drivers brought before the courts have so far undoubtedly been detected, either because they were involved in traffic accidents, or because they drove negligently and in so doing came to the attention of police or traffic officers, or because they were "smelt out" by coincidence at police road-blocks.

Lately, however, the traffic authorities have increasingly made use of road-blocks specifically set up in order to catch drunken drivers in the act. At these road-blocks the "breathalyser" type of alcohol breath-tester plays an important role. How effective is this apparatus for the purposes of law enforcement?

Unlike the position in regard to blood-alcohol, for which the "0,08 limit" was built into the Road Traffic Ordinances,[2] and reaffirmed in the Road Traffic Act of 1989[3] which superseded the Ordinances, no provision has been made in South Africa for penalisation of motorists merely on the basis of the alcohol content of breath.

Notwithstanding the fact that we apply a blood-alcohol criterion, there is from a practical point of view no possibility of mass-testing of motorists for blood-alcohol by traffic authorities.

True, the statutory provisions which are in force today are more strict than ever before, but it is simply not practicable to stop motorists *en masse* and to subject them to blood-tests. Apart from any other considerations, such a practice would offend against basic democratic notions that are respected in our society. Legally, a blood specimen may only be taken of someone who has already been lawfully arrested, or who voluntarily submits to the taking of a blood specimen.

The Criminal Procedure Act[4] vests a policeman with the power of taking such steps as he may deem necessary in order to ascertain whether the body of the person he has arrested has "any ... characteristic ... or shows any condition or appearance",[5] but the Act further expressly provides that a police official may not himself take a blood sample of the person concerned. That may lawfully be done only by a medical

1 H A Shapiro *Medico-Legal Mythology and Other Forensic Contributions* (ed I Gordon) (1975) 105, 231.
2 The uniform Road Traffic Ordinances 21 of 1966, section 140 (2).
3 Act 29 of 1989, section 122.
4 Act 51 of 1977.
5 Section 37 (1) *(c)*.

officer of a prison or a district surgeon, or if requested thereto by a police official, any other registered medical practitioner or nurse.[6]

If the motorist, not having been arrested, is willing to accompany a police official in order to have a sample of his blood drawn, he need not – as I have mentioned – be formally arrested in order to achieve that. However, it may be assumed that if motorists were to be stopped *en masse,* very few of them would be willing to so submit to the taking of a blood sample.

Even when it comes to effecting an arrest with a view to obtaining a blood sample, the police official is confronted with a legal problem. Legally he may arrest a suspected offender without a warrant only if the offence of drunken driving was clearly committed in his presence, or if – at the very least – he has a reasonable suspicion that the offence (or another, relatively serious type of offence) has been committed.[7] Our courts interpret these powers of arrest strictly and a police official who arrests arbitrarily and without reasonable grounds for suspicion, exposes himself and his employer – the State, the province or a municipality – to a civil action for wrongful arrest that may assume serious proportions.

The required reasonable grounds may arise from a variety of circumstances, e g the reckless manner in which a driver has been driving his car, the driver reeking of alcohol, the driver's speech slurring, bloodshot eyes, drunken aggressiveness, a staggering gait, etc. It is precisely in this regard that the breathalyser can be employed usefully.

Several types of apparatus are available on the market, and the manufacturers claim that when a person breathes into the apparatus, it will give a fairly reliable indication of the amount of alcohol consumed by him. As is generally known, a person whose blood-alcohol level exceeds the statutory limit of 0,08 will not necessarily display any of the usual signs of intoxication. He may appear to be as sober as a judge, but on the breathalyser – so it is claimed – his breath will invariably betray the fact that he has recently consumed a substantial quantity of alcohol.

The value of the breathalyser, therefore, primarily lies therein that it affords an aid to the police official in forming a reasonable suspicion of intoxication,[8] on the ground of which he may then arrest the motorist; once there has been a lawful arrest, a blood sample may be taken from the motorist – if need be against his will.

As far as is known, the breathalyser has not yet been "tested" by the Supreme Court, but judging from the claims made by manufacturers, it appears to be probable that a judge might be convinced that in the hands of a trained police official, the reading on the apparatus may at least be so reliable that it could lead to a reasonable suspicion that the person who is being tested, is "under the influence" for the purposes of effecting a lawful arrest. As Shapiro[9] has correctly pointed out, there is no simple and constant correlation between breath-alcohol and blood-alcohol. However, it is not a requirement for an arrest on the ground of suspected drunken driving that there must be a reasonable suspicion that the suspect has a minimum blood-alcohol content of at least 0,08. It is a well-known fact that a person whose blood-alcohol is less than that percentage may be distinctly under the influence of liquor, and even drunk in the generally accepted meaning of that word.

A legal problem which exists in connection with the breathalyser, is that no person can legally be compelled to breathe into it against his will – at any rate not before his arrest. There is no provision in either the Criminal Procedure Act or the Road Traffic Act which authorises that. Moreover, breathing or blowing into a breathalyser is a

6 Section 37 (2) *(a).*

7 Criminal Procedure Act, section 40 (1) *(a)* and *(b).*

8 *Cf* Shapiro, *op cit* 65, who refers to the limited value of the breathalyser test as a "screening test to establish qualitatively whether there is alcohol in the breath".

9 *Op cit* 64. *Cf* I Gordon, H A Shapiro & S D Berson *Forensic Medicine: A Guide to Principles* (3rd ed, 1988) 409.

deliberate and positive act – and how do you compel a man, even if he is under arrest, to blow into the apparatus if he does not want to blow?

If a motorist refuses to blow into the breathalyser, that in itself can surely not constitute a ground on which a policeman may form a reasonable suspicion that the motorist is "under the influence", or even that the motorist has consumed any alcohol. There are a number of reasons, apart from a guilty conscience, which may impel a man to refuse to blow.

The breathalyser can accordingly be of limited use only in the apprehension of potential drunken drivers. The experience so far has nevertheless been that many motorists who are stopped at road-blocks do in fact voluntarily blow into the apparatus when requested to do so by the police, and in this manner a number of drivers who had in fact consumed liquor were arrested and subsequently were subjected to the taking of blood samples which after analysis produced a positive result – and a successful prosecution.

So far we have paid attention to the value of breath testing by means of the breathalyser as part of police "dragnet" action. However, proof in court of the blood-alcohol content, or even of the mere fact of intoxication, is a completely different story. The courts apply extremely strict standards of proof to be observed by prosecutors in drunken-driving cases. Considering the present state of development of this type of apparatus, it seems to be highly improbable that it would be possible by means of a breathalyser reading of *breath-alcohol* to render proof beyond a reasonable doubt that the accused's *blood-alcohol* level reached or exceeded the prescribed limit of 0,08.

But when it is merely endeavoured to prove that the accused was "under the influence", evidence of a high reading on the breathalyser may of course be adduced by the prosecutor together with other evidence. Because it involves the proof of a fact by means of processes of natural science which requires scientific knowledge, it will clearly be necessary for an expert to interpret the reading obtained on the breathalyser, particularly where the defence challenges the evidential value of the reading. However, an expert's certificate may serve as *prima facie* proof in terms of the Criminal Procedure Act.[10]

10 Section 212 (4) *(a)*.

67 Some problems of proof relating to excessive blood-alcohol concentration

Decisions of our courts time and again illustrate the demanding standards set by our courts for proof of excessive blood-alcohol concentration in charges of drunken driving. Examples from the law reports:

In *S v Melamu*[1] the accused was convicted by a magistrate of "statutory" drunken driving, i e that his concentration of blood-alcohol exceeded the 0,08 limit. From the evidence it appeared that the process of sealing of the blood specimen taken from the accused may have been tampered with in some unknown manner. The district surgeon who had taken the specimen, testified that he had sealed the container with sealing wax, tape and string. The police-sergeant who mailed the specimen to Johannesburg for analysis, however, said under cross-examination that there was no string round the container when he dealt with it. On this evidence the court found that the sample of blood which was sent to the analyst and received by him was not in the same condition as it was when it was handed over by the district surgeon to the Police. It was held that as all reasonable possibility of a mistaken finding had not been excluded, the conviction had to be set aside.

In *S v Pretorius*[2] the defence took the point that the prosecution had failed to prove that the substance used to sterilise the skin of the accused before the taking of his blood-specimen did not itself contain alcohol. The evidence had been that the substance used was acetone which is provided in a "brandy-sized" bottle by the State. Upon receipt the content is invariably analysed and the certificate on the bottle indicates that it is pure acetone, without alcohol.

The district surgeon testified that the bottle was continuously being used and the court held that there was absolutely no indication that the contents could have been other than acetone, without alcohol. The defence had accordingly not succeeded in rebutting the result of the analysis. The judge observed that it is an everyday occurrence for people to use all sorts of products including medicines, on the strength of the manufacturer's label. On proof that the supplier is reliable, one would expect that this description can be relied upon. To require over and again independent proof of contents could render the administration of justice so difficult that it could be defeated.

There have been several cases in which the correctness of gas chromatography tests used in establishing the percentage of blood-alcohol concentration was challenged.

In *S v Strydom*[3] the court on appeal set aside a conviction when it appeared that the analysis of the accused's blood had been made with a Perkin-Elmer gas chromatograph machine, that the machine had been tested for accuracy against another type of gas chromatograph machine, and that the evidence of the expert witness – "honest and expert as he was" – could not be accepted as proof beyond reasonable doubt that the analysis of the accused's blood by this machine had been accurate. The judge held that this was not a case where judicial notice could be taken of the accuracy of

1 1978 (1) SA 421 (O).
2 1978 (4) SA 197 (T).
3 1978 (4) SA 748 (E).

a machine. "The machine and the process which it carries out, cannot be compared, so far as general knowledge and general acceptance of accuracy are concerned, with, for example, the use of an assized scale, tape-recording, X-rays, photography, or stop-watches which have been checked."

In *S v Terblanche* [4] evidence was led on behalf of the prosecution that the expert who had tested the blood had made use of two gas chromatograph machines and that he had compared their results. The court of appeal held that this did not constitute an adequate check. Both machines might have been defective. The expert further testified that the use of the apparatus was subject to his control. However, in the opinion of the court, that did not prove that in registering the impulses he had been in a position to ascertain whether it was done correctly. The expert explained that he applied an "internal standard" in order to ensure proper functioning of the machine. That in itself did not demonstrate the accuracy of the device, the court held. In the event the accused's conviction and sentence were set aside.

In *S v Burger*,[5] however, the court was satisfied that the analyst – the same expert who testified in the preceding case[6] – had applied adequate checks in ensuring the accuracy of the gas chromatography machines. There was evidence that the expert had first used the ordinary chemical method and then used the gas chromatographic method. In comparing the results, it was found that the latter method produced a somewhat lower reading, which was attributed to a different method employed with the pipette in obtaining blood for the analysis.

The reliability or otherwise of gas chromatography finally became the subject of a decision of the Appellate Division in *S v Dickenson*.[7] In this case the appellant attacked his conviction on the basis of the judgment in the *Strydom* and *Terblanche* cases, respectively. The Appeal Court distinguished these cases, however, by pointing out that all the evidence which it had before it *in casu* might not have been before the court in the two earlier cases. In *Dickenson* there was evidence that the expert and his colleagues had over a period of two years found that the analyses made of alcohol solutions by means of the purely chemical method and the gas chromatographic method had given results which were practically identical. The methods used in ensuring that the apparatus was functioning correctly, were adequate. In particular there was evidence of the expert's "external standards", which indicated that analysis by means of the gas chromatograph, measured by a criterion which is prepared in accordance with a purely chemical method, did not amount to using the apparatus in order to test its own accuracy. Although it could not be denied that two machines can have the same fault, the use of two machines nevertheless dimishes the possibility of error, the court said. On the evidence before it, the Appeal Court accordingly found that the accused's conviction was legally justified. From the decision it is clear that where the correctness of a forensic report is challenged in court, the expert witness will have to make sure that every relevant fact demonstrating the accuracy of the machine and the reliability of the test be put before the court.

In terms of the Road Traffic Act[8] there is a presumption that if it is proved the percentage of blood-alcohol was not less than 0,08 at any time within two hours after the alleged offence, the percentage was not less than that at the time of the offence. This presumption can be rebutted by the accused on a balance of probabilities. In *S v Van der Merwe* [9] the district surgeon, in giving evidence, made the following statement: "Many factors are involved in absorption of alcohol into the blood stream. I can give

4 1981 (1) SA 791 (T).
5 1980 (3) SA 1219 (T).
6 *Burger's* case was decided before *Terblanche's* case, but was reported after the latter case was reported.
7 1982 (3) SA 84 (A).
8 Act 29 of 1989, section 122 (3).
9 1982 (1) SA 313 (O).

no facts and figures on absorption as such. It is therefore very difficult to say precisely how quickly alcohol would be absorbed by a specific person."[10] On appeal it was held that the doctor's concession that the accused's blood-alcohol at the time when he drove his car might possibly not have been the same as that indicated in the forensic report, was insufficient to rebut the presumption. The accused's conviction was confirmed.

10 I have translated, and somewhat transcribed, the district surgeon's statement.

PART XV

Disciplinary proceedings

68 Medical Council disciplinary inquiries: some do's and don'ts

Great expectations

As opinion polls have indicated, the image of the medical profession in the public mind has never been higher. At the same time, the level of expectation of patients in regard to medical services has probably never been higher. This may be attributable not only to the high quality of medical services to which the public has generally become accustomed, but also to the spectacular advances in medicine constantly being reported upon by the media.

But there is a negative side to this as well. Some patients are inclined to demand from their doctors a quality of performance, and in particular an availability, which they would not expect from other providers of services – not to mention what they themselves are prepared to render in the line of occupational duty.

When the services demanded by the patient do not meet his subjective standards, the result may be a complaint against the doctor. Judging by letters appearing in newspapers' correspondence columns from time to time, and by the regular flow of sensational news stories about doctors and hospital services, doctor-baiting has become a kind of national sport.

This attitude is also reflected in some of the complaints made to the SA Medical and Dental Council (SAMDC). My impression is that there are patients who run too readily to the Council. Apart from the bedevilling effect which an ill-conceived complaint may have on the doctor-patient relationship, there is a legal danger to the patient of which many seem to be unaware.

Eyeball to eyeball

A half-baked, unfounded complaint made to the Council may expose the patient to an action for defamation. An allegation of professional incompetence or negligence or a reflection upon the honesty and integrity of a doctor will *prima facie* constitute defamation, and unless the person who made the allegation can advance a recognised defence, such as truth and public benefit, he may be sued for damages. Moreover, many a patient who drafts a complaint in the heat of the moment, exaggerating the facts, does not realise that at an eventual disciplinary inquiry, he may be vigorously cross-examined on it.

The sensible thing for a patient to do, is first to put his grievance directly, in person, to the doctor. There is nothing like an unemotional "eyeball to eyeball" to clear the atmosphere, and the wise doctor will not avoid such a confrontation, unpleasant as it may be. Surveys in the USA have indicated that many a malpractice suit would never have been brought, had the doctor displayed a more sympathetic attitude towards a dissatisfied patient. It has come to my attention that exactly the same thing has happened in some malpractice cases in this country.[1]

If a patient persists in his complaint and is convinced that it is genuine, I would advise him to consider taking legal advice before he writes to the Medical Council.

1 See e g the remarks made by the trial judge in *Blyth v Van den Heever* 1980 (1) SA 191 (A), quoted *supra* 258.

Consulting an attorney at this stage has a twofold advantage. First, while the patient's view of the facts may be clouded by an emotional involvement, the attorney will look at the matter with unemotional eyes and will be able to make a cold, "clinical" assessment of the complaint. He may well persuade the patient not to pursue the matter because of a lack of factual information. Secondly, if the decision is to proceed with the complaint, the attorney will assist the patient in drafting a complaint in legally unassailable terms which is based upon fact and would not unnecessarily expose the patient to a claim for defamation.

"Please explain" letter

When a complaint in writing is made to the Medical Council, the registrar may do one of three things:

- call for further information from the complainant
- inform the doctor of the nature of the complaint and to ask him for an explanation
- refer the case to a committee of preliminary inquiry of the Council.[2]

The registrar's letter to the doctor invariably contains a warning that any explanation given by the doctor may be used in evidence against him. This "please explain" letter,[3] as it is known in medical circles, with its somewhat formal, legalistic terms, may have a different effect upon different people. If the complaint comes out of the blue, it may produce shock, despondency or anxiety. Some doctors simply do not know how to react to it, and try to ignore the letter, in the vague hope that the problem will vanish of its own accord. Some recipients become enraged to such an extent that they compile an angry, emotional reply on the spot – sometimes in terms highly abusive of the complainant or doubtful of his sanity – and send it off to the registrar. That is the worst possible reaction.

My advice to a doctor who receives a complaint through the registrar, would be not to reply to it off his own bat, but to seek legal advice forthwith.

Apart from the emotional relief it would bring to the doctor burdened by a complaint, to discuss it with someone who is not emotionally involved, and whose job it is to counsel people who find themselves in trouble, an experienced lawyer's assessment of the matter may be of inestimable value to the doctor in the correct handling of the situation.

Legal aid

Doctors who are members of a medical protection society – membership is obtainable through the Medical Association of South Africa (MASA) – can obtain legal aid through the society's secretariat at the MASA offices. The protection societies have retained the services of a reputable firm of attorneys and the matter will be attended to by lawyers who are highly skilled and experienced in the handling of this type of case. Furthermore, the protection society will in an appropriate case[4] pick up the bill for these services.

A doctor who has not taken out protection society membership, must make his own arrangements with an attorney. In deciding on a lawyer, it is advisable to engage one with sound trial experience.

2 See the regulations relating to the conduct of inquiries held in terms of section 41 of the Medical, Dental and Supplementary Health Service Professions Act 56 of 1974, contained in Government Notice 2303 of 28 September 1990 (*Government Gazette* 12759), reg 3.

3 On the status of this letter and the rights of the doctor thereanent, see *Tucker and Another v SA Medical and Dental Council and Others* 1980 (2) SA 207 (T).

4 In terms of its membership rules the society has a discretion. Apart from cases involving provable conduct of a serious criminal nature, such as illegal abortion, the society will almost always provide legal assistance.

In attending to the matter, the attorney will delve into the facts which led to the complaint. He will assist the accused in drafting a suitable reply. Depending on the nature of the charge and its surrounding circumstances, the lawyer may well advise the doctor not to reply at all. This may be a difficult decision which can only be arrived at by the lawyer in consultation with the doctor after a thorough exploration of all facets of the complaint and its background, as well as its future implications for the doctor.

In many cases, the doctor's explanation will be the end of the matter. The Council's committee of preliminary inquiry will routinely consider it together with the information supplied by the complainant and, possibly, facts obtained through the committee's own investigation, and may come to the conclusion that the complaint even if substantiated, would not constitute improper or disgraceful conduct. The doctor will in due course be notified accordingly.

A fool for a client?

If it appears to the committee of preliminary inquiry, after such investigation as it may deem necessary, that an inquiry should be held into the conduct of the doctor, it will direct the registrar to arrange for the holding of a disciplinary inquiry.[5] The registrar will then issue a notice addressed to the doctor stating where and when the disciplinary inquiry will be held and enclosing a charge.[6]

If the doctor has up to this point not taken legal advice, he would be well advised not to hesitate a moment longer to seek the services of an attorney. This is particularly important where the doctor feels that the allegations against him are false or unfounded or exaggerated and that he wants to defend himself against them. In the legal profession there is a saying that "a lawyer who defends himself has a fool for a client", and certainly this is true not only of lawyers.

So much may be at stake for the doctor that it would be foolish for him to try and take care of his own defence. The charges may be of a very serious nature or the facts may be complex. In some cases the attorney consulted by the doctor will recommend that counsel be instructed to appear on behalf of the doctor. The attorney and advocate will then work together on the case in preparing the doctor's defence.

"Admission of guilt" fines

If the SAMDC on reasonable grounds is of the opinion that it will impose a fine of not more than R500 in the event of the practitioner eventually being convicted after an inquiry, a summons with an "admission of guilt" endorsement may be issued. The practitioner involved will then have to pay the fine within 14 days.[7]

The advantage of admission of guilt is that the accused doctor will be able to avoid appearing at an inquiry – and all the publicity attendant on a public hearing. The media always display keen interest in disciplinary inquiries involving professional people.

But a word of warning must be sounded. Depending on the nature of a charge against a practitioner, admission of guilt may have serious consequences for him if he is the defendant in a civil suit for damages brought against him by an aggrieved patient. The fact of such an admission – if it becomes known – will without a doubt be used by the legal representatives of the patient to bolster the case against the doctor. It will decidedly be in the interest of an accused doctor, who is faced with a claim of damages for alleged professional negligence, to seek legal advice before paying an admission of guilt fine.

5 Reg 3.
6 Reg 9.
7 Act 56 of 1974, section 42 (8).

If the committee decides not to charge

If the committee of preliminary inquiry resolves that a complaint even if substantiated, does not constitute improper or disgraceful conduct, or, for any other reason should be withheld from an inquiry, it must take such action as it may think fit and report its action to the SAMDC.[8]

This is not necessarily the end of the matter. The complainant, believing that he has a strong case, may feel aggrieved by the committee's decision and may approach the Supreme Court for an order to compel the SAMDC or the committee to direct an inquiry to be conducted.

What would the aggrieved complainant's chances of success be if he were to bring such an application to court?

In *Veriava's* case[9] the court underlined the fact that the SAMDC is "truly a statutory *custos morum* of the medical profession, the guardian of the prestige, status and dignity of the profession and the public interest in so far as members of the public are affected by the conduct of members of the profession to whom they had stood in a professional relationship". Although the Act[10] and the regulations thereunder confer an enabling power on the SAMDC, the court held that there may be circumstances which may couple the power with a duty to exercise it. In the circumstances of the case, the court held that both the inquiry committee and the Council in performing their administrative functions had erred on a matter of fact in concluding and resolving that there was no new evidence to support the charges and complaints and/or that the evidence did not disclose *prima facie*[11] evidence of improper or disgraceful conduct in a professional respect. Alternatively, they had misdirected themselves by not applying their minds properly or at all to the charges and complaints. All this had led to both the committee and the Council wrongly passing the resolutions turning down the charges and complaints. In the event the court ordered the inquiry committee to arrange for an inquiry to be conducted.

It is clear from this case that the court will overrule a decision of the committee not to direct that an inquiry shall take place, in exceptional circumstances only.

A pretrial judicial remedy?

Where a notice to appear has been issued and served on a doctor, it would be an understandable reaction if the doctor were to think along these lines, especially if he feels that the complaint is unfounded: "Is there no way in which I can avoid being hauled before the disciplinary committee and tried in public? Can I not obtain a court interdict against the Council to prevent it from pursuing the matter?"

It can be categorically stated that a court will be prepared to interfere with the proceedings at this stage in highly exceptional circumstances only. By virtue of the general principles of administrative law, the Supreme Court would be entitled to review the decision of a domestic tribunal on grounds such as *mala fides* or bias on the part of the tribunal or failure to apply its mind to the matter before it.[12] But where only an intermediary step or ruling has taken place, the attitude of the court, if approached for relief, would probably be that the applicant must first exhaust his domestic remedies, i e must fight his case before the disciplinary committee and if

8 Reg 7.

9 *Veriava and Others v President, SA Medical and Dental Council and Others* 1985 (2) SA 293 (T).

10 Act 56 of 1974.

11 The old (1976) rules referred specifically to "*prima facie* evidence". Although the new (1990) rules do not contain this phrase, it is submitted that this would make no difference as far as the result of the decision in *Veriava's* case is concerned.

12 *Divisional Commissioner of SA Police, Witwatersrand Area, and Others v SA Associated Newspapers Ltd and Another* 1966 (2) SA 503 (A) 510H.

found guilty, put his case to the Council itself,[13] unless the Council states that it is prepared to wage a forensic battle at this early stage.

The Supreme Court has ruled that in effect the Council is the sole repository of the power to decide what is ethical and what is unethical in medical practice.[14] The court would accordingly be unwilling to intercede at this stage and order the Council not to pursue a matter which on the face of it is clearly an issue of professional ethics. Thus, the court has refused, in the cases of *Pretorius*[15] and *Meyer,*[16] respectively, to restrain the Council from trying disciplinary cases in which an opthalmologist allegedly had supplied spectacles to a patient in a town in which an optometrist was available, in contravention of a Council ruling.

A trial in every sense

The disciplinary committee is for all intents and purposes a court. Its procedure is akin to that of a court of law, although it is not quite as formal and the rules of admissibility of evidence are not applied quite as rigidly. To the accused doctor, a disciplinary inquiry is a trial in every sense of the word. An experienced attorney or advocate acts as so-called *pro forma* complainant and conducts the prosecution energetically. If the doctor himself testifies, he is subject to cross-examination by a skilful lawyer. The accused's conduct is scrutinised closely by his peers who serve on the disciplinary committee.

It is not necessary for the accused doctor to attend the inquiry. If he is not present, the inquiry will be conducted in his absence. The accused may by letter notify the registrar before the hearing that he pleads guilty to the charge or charges against him. If the accused refuses or fails to plead to a charge, a plea of not guilty is entered on his behalf.[17]

It goes without saying that where a doctor who has been charged wants to establish his innocence, it will almost always be in his interest to attend the hearing and to be legally represented. In such a case he will naturally enter a plea of not guilty. His legal representative can then challenge the evidence adduced by the *pro forma* complainant and can cross-examine witnesses. In many cases, cross-examination is undoubtedly the most useful method of uncovering the weaknesses in the prosecution case and in bringing home the accused's defence.

Plea in mitigation

Even where an accused doctor admits the charge against him and intends entering a plea of guilty, it may definitely be in his interest to attend the hearing and to avail himself of the services of a legal representative in pleading in mitigation of sentence. The services of an attorney or advocate may be of great help in identifying mitigating circumstances, in cross-examining witnesses – where *viva voce* evidence is adduced – in order to highlight such circumstances and to lead evidence in mitigation. The doctor, finding himself in the unfortunate and often humiliating position of being in the dock, may be unable to present a coherent defence or plea in mitigation.

An accused doctor's self-confidence is not likely to be strengthened when he learns that disciplinary proceedings are ordinarily[18] conducted in public. Newspaper

13 *Liassou v Pretoria City Council* 1979 (3) SA 217 (T).
14 *Meyer v SA Medical and Dental Council* 1982 (4) SA 450 (T) 455 H.
15 *Pretorius v SA Geneeskundige en Tandheelkundige Raad* 1980 (2) SA 354 (T).
16 See note 14 *supra*.
17 Reg 10 (1) (*b*).
18 Reg 16. Any decision of the disciplinary committee may be arrived at *in camera*. Evidence adduced during the inquiry may on good cause shown in the discretion of the committee be heard *in camera*. The committee may also prohibit the publication of information which would probably reveal the identity of any particular person other than the accused practitioner.

reporters are almost always present at the hearings. The late Professor Hillel Shapiro, one of the most senior and respected members of the Medical Council, described these inquiries as "a procedure whereby the publicity accorded to the evidence led ... virtually throws the reputation of an accused person to the journalistic lions in the arena of a Colosseum, to make a Roman holiday for the seekers after sensation".

I have often seen people handling their own cases in court or before a domestic tribunal, turn embarrassingly speechless. Not all persons are equally eloquent or assertive. And this is where the professional pleader – the lawyer – who comes to the tribunal with a carefully prepared case, can come to the rescue of the accused. Every word spoken in a trial court and a seemingly unimportant line of questioning or reasoning may make or break a case. The art of the advocate and the significance of good advocacy must never be underestimated.

No reasons given

Disciplinary inquiries conducted by the Medical Council's disciplinary committee generally do not last very long. The duration depends on the nature of the charges and the complexity of the issues raised by them and by the accused's defence. It may also depend on the extent to which the proceedings may be shortened by means of admissions made on behalf of the prosecution and the defence. Undefended cases may be over in less than a hour. Even strenuously defended cases may be conducted within a matter of hours rather than days.

After the parties have been given the opportunity of presenting their respective cases in full, the disciplinary committee will deliberate on its verdict *in camera.*[19] Upon the resumption of the hearing, the chairman of the committee – who will often be the president of the Medical Council himself – will announce the verdict in brief terms, without giving reasons for it.

It is at this stage, following a conviction, that evidence and/or argument in mitigation must be presented, and when this is concluded, the committee will once again sit *in camera* in order to deliberate on sentence. When its members have reached consensus, which ordinarily does not take long, the session will be resumed and the sentence announced.

In terms of the Medical, Dental and Supplementary Health Service Professions Act,[20] no penalty imposed by the disciplinary committee, other than a caution or a reprimand (or both) takes effect until the Medical Council itself has confirmed its imposition. It is therefore customary, where the recommended penalty takes the form of a suspension from practice (whether conditional or otherwise), removal from the register or a fine,[21] for the chairman of the committee, when he announces the recommendation, to draw the accused's attention to the fact that it will come before the Council.

Final power

The Council has the final power to impose a sentence of suspension, removal from the register or a fine: it may accordingly alter the sentence recommended by the disciplinary committee.[22] Only in exceptional circumstances will the Council exercise its discretion to increase the sentence.[23] The Council also has the power to refuse to confirm the disciplinary committee's verdict and/or recommendation on sentence.

19 Reg 16.
20 Section 11 (5) and see also reg 10 (2).
21 Fines were introduced as a possible form of penalty in 1990. The maximum fine is R10 000.
22 Reg 15.
23 *Volschenk v President, SA Geneeskundige en Tandheelkundige Raad* 1985 (3) SA 124 (A).

A doctor who was found guilty by the disciplinary committee and who was not merely cautioned or reprimanded is entitled to make written representations to the Council regarding the committee's verdict or recommendation as to sentence.[24] I would advise a doctor who feels himself aggrieved by the verdict or sentence, and who is desirous of making representations to the Council, to be closely guided by his legal adviser as to, a) whether representations should be made at all, and b) if representations are made, what form they should take. Representations will not invariably be to the advantage of the doctor.

Clumsily worded representations might at a meeting of the full Council create the impression that the case was even more serious than it was regarded by the disciplinary committee. In this respect too, the doctor's attorney may be able to make a more objective assessment than the doctor himself.

It is to be noted that where a penalty has been imposed and, where necessary confirmed by the Council, the registrar is statutorily obliged to publish in the *Government Gazette* the name of the doctor and the essential details of the charge(s) upon which he was convicted, as well as the penalty imposed.[25] Even where the inquiry itself was not reported upon by the press, newspapers will often pick up these details when they appear in the *Gazette.*

A sentence of suspension or removal of a doctor's name from the register, when confirmed by the Council, takes immediate effect and cannot be postponed until a later date.[26]

Case closed?

There is no appeal against the Council's ultimate finding in a disciplinary matter.[27] It is nevertheless not altogether a case of *Roma locuta, causa finita* – "Rome has spoken, case closed" – because there is still the possibility of taking the matter on common-law review to the Supreme Court. However, the grounds upon which such a review can take place are extremely limited and difficult to prove, such as malice or bias on the part of the disciplinary committee or serious procedural irregularities resulting in a failure of justice.[28]

A decision to go on review should never be taken lightly, and in this respect, too, the aggrieved doctor should be carefully guided by his legal adviser. Running hastily to court with a review may involve the doctor in considerable expense – and may prolong his agony indefinitely.

Finally, mention should be made of the fact that a doctor whose name has been removed from the register may at a later stage approach the Council to have his name restored. Such an application should of course be brought after a "decent" period of time has elapsed, and should be well-substantiated.[29]

24 Reg 10 (5) (*g*).
25 Reg 15 (3).
26 *SA Geneeskundige en Tandheelkundige Raad v Van Rensburg* 1982 (2) SA 745 (T).
27 Section 20 and section 42 (6) of Act 56 of 1974 were repealed in 1976. For the history of the legislation, see the previous edition of this book (1984) 425–7.
28 See e g *Shidiack v Union Government* 1912 AD 642 at 651; *Divisional Commissioner of S A Police, Witwatersrand Area, and Others v Associated Newspapers and Another* 1966 (2) SA 503 (A) 510 H.
29 Two useful books on the SAMDC and its disciplinary function which may be consulted are: T Verschoor *Verdicts of the Medical Council* (1990) (also available in Afrikaans, published in 1986) and T Verschoor and H Oosthuizen (eds) *Handbook of the Rules and Regulations for Medical Practitioners and Dentists* (1990).

69 The duties of the Medical Council in disciplinary cases

The first duty of the disciplinary committee of the Medical and Dental Council, and of the Council itself, towards a medical practitioner charged before it with disgraceful conduct, is to try him fairly. The disciplinary committee owes no duty to the public against a practitioner who has not been proved guilty. This was held by the Natal court in the case of *De la Rouviere v SA Medical and Dental Council.*[1]

The court proceeded to say that it was only after an accused has been found guilty that the disciplinary committee's duty to the public entered at all.

In this case the doctor had been found guilty by the disciplinary committee of disgraceful conduct on five counts with a recommendation that his name be erased from the register.

The finding was confirmed by the Medical Council and the doctor then brought an appeal to the Supreme Court against the ruling, in terms of section 42 (*b*) of the Medical, Dental and Supplementary Health Service Professions Act of 1974.[2] (The Act was subsequently amended by Act 33 of 1976 to remove the right of appeal and to replace it by a right of review; a right of appeal involves reconsideration of all aspects of a matter, whilst a right of review is essentially restricted to serious procedural defects and bias.)

The court upheld the appeal and set aside the disciplinary committee's findings and the confirmation by the Council on all five charges. It was held that regard being had to the cumulative effect of the quality of the evidence and the procedural defects during the trial, the doctor did not have a proper trial, and that even on review the findings could not stand.

The court held that in the conduct of the trial the approach of members of the committee to the evidence and to their task and the legal principles applicable, showed a distinct balance of probability that some members unwittingly failed to apply their minds properly to the evidence.

The setting of the required standard of professional honour was more of a subjective nature and as it was a function entrusted by law to the Medical Council, a court would be slow to interfere with a decision honestly arrived at, Mr Justice van Heerden said.

However, the same consideration did not necessarily apply to "the first leg" of the inquiry, viz to establish the facts. "The members of the Council are not by virtue of their training and profession, necessarily in a better position to decide whether certain conduct has in fact been proved or not." A court would accordingly be less slow to interfere with a factual finding.

The judge agreed with a 1947 ruling by the Witwatersrand Division of the Supreme Court[3] that the Medical Council and the disciplinary committee are bodies which should more strictly be held to the rules of procedure and evidence. The extent to which they should be so held would depend on the circumstances of the case, the subject matter of the inquiry and especially the particular rule of procedure or evi-

1 1977 (1) SA 85 (N).
2 Act 56 of 1974.
3 *McLoughlin v South African Medical and Dental Council* 1947 (2) SA 377 (W).

dence concerned. "The less technical that rule of procedure and evidence the more likely a tribunal will be held bound by it," the judge observed.

The rules of evidence which were particularly relevant in this context were the cautionary rules relating to the evidence of a single witness and of complaints in cases "with a sexual flavour": "Charges of this nature may have been motivated by spite, sexual frustration or other unpredictable emotional causes and are difficult to refute because they are usually alleged to have taken place in private, they leave no outward traces and proof depends entirely upon the word of the complainant against that of the accused. The demeanour of the complainant in the witness-box or her apparent social standing in particular should never be relied upon as a substitute for corroboration. It is therefore necessary that the trier of fact should show awareness of the special dangers of convicting upon the evidence of the complainant in a sexual case."

The court upheld the submission made by the doctor's counsel that in questioning him members of the committee had in some instances gone beyond the scope of an impartial tribunal and that their questioning took the form of cross-examination. The tenor of a great deal of questioning was in the nature of a cross-examination to show that the doctor was not telling the truth.

The court also considered the objection that certain unsworn statements – some of them irrelevant to the charges – were admitted into the record of proceedings of the committee. One of these documents – containing the grievances of a colleague of the accused doctor – contained serious allegations of a hearsay nature. These allegations "slipped into the record without being tested by cross-examination", the judge said.

The case illustrates the stern approach of the Supreme Court in its role as watchdog over the activities of domestic tribunals and the so-called "quasi-judicial" bodies. Although inquiries conducted by such tribunals are not required to be conducted in accordance with all the technical rules embraced by the law of evidence applied by the courts, certain of the more basic rules should be adhered to. The decision affected a wide range of statutory tribunals vested with powers that may involve the rights of persons falling within their jurisdiction.

70 Medical practitioner suspended from practice: legal implications for his partners

The following questions were put to me: Dr A, a member of a partnership of general practitioners, is found guilty of disgraceful conduct by a disciplinary committee of the SA Medical and Dental Council. The committee recommends to the Council that the doctor be suspended from practice for a period of three months, and the Council confirms the recommendation. What is the position of his partner or partners, legally and ethically? Is the partnership automatically dissolved? If not, may Dr A continue to benefit financially from the practice to which he has made no active contribution during the period of suspension?

My answer to these questions is as follows:

If it has expressly been stipulated in the partnership contract that the partnership will be automatically dissolved in the event of one of the partners becoming legally incapable of practising (because of his name being removed from the register or suspension from practice) dissolution will take place automatically. A clause which is sometimes found in partnership contracts, is that the parties undertake to practise in a lawful manner and in accordance with the precepts and professional ethics as laid down by the Medical Council. If a partner conducts himself in an unprofessional manner which leads to a finding by the Medical Council that he is guilty of improper or disgraceful conduct, he will make himself guilty of breach of contract, in consequence of which the other partner or partners may be able to claim dissolution of the partnership. But even where there is no such clause in the partnership contract, it can be said that it is a tacit term of the agreement that the parties will conduct themselves in accordance with established professional ethics.

Should a partner be guilty of unprofessional conduct of a material nature, one or more of the partners may terminate the partnership by way of notice, or if necessary by obtaining a court order. According to our law a court may make an order for dissolution of a partnership on the grounds of any occurrence by which mutual confidence is destroyed or co-operation of the partners is rendered impossible.[1]

It goes without saying that it will be necessary to approach the court for an order whereby the partnership will be dissolved only if the guilty partner refuses to accept a notice of dissolution and to co-operate in order to achieve the dissolution and liquidation of the partnership.

If the unprofessional conduct resulted in the practitioner being struck off the register or, for that matter, temporary suspension, it is almost inconceivable that the practitioner involved will be able to successfully oppose an application for a judicial order of dissolution.

Apart from other considerations, suspension – and *a fortiori* removal of a practitioner's name from the register – has the effect that it becomes impossible for the guilty partner to perform in terms of the partnership agreement, for the time being, at least. Legally, temporary impossibility to perform does not automatically bring an

1 Wille & Millin's *Mercantile Law of South Africa* (18th ed, 1984, by J F Coaker and D T Zeffertt) 556 *et seq.*

end to the parties' contractual relationship, but the creditor – in the present situation the "innocent" partner – has the right to terminate the relationship.

It is also a principle of our law that when it becomes impossible for a party to a contract temporarily to perform, that party will be entitled to a counter-prestation – if any – only on a *pro rata* basis to the extent that he himself has performed.[2] Expressed in practical terms, this means that the guilty partner would not be entitled, from the moment of suspension, to receive any financial benefit from the partnership in respect of work not yet done by him.

Apart from the right which a partner has to terminate the partnership on account of misconduct on the part of another partner, each partner is entitled, in terms of the common law to dissolve the partnership by way of notice of dissolution, unless a period has been fixed for the duration of the partnership. A notice of dissolution must be in good faith and at a reasonable time.[3]

As far as the guilty partner is concerned, it must be noted that from the moment of suspension he is legally regarded as an unregistered person for the duration of the suspension.[4] If he were to continue practising for gain, he would make himself guilty of a criminal offence. Should his partners actively associate themselves with such conduct they would make themselves guilty as accomplices.

The innocent partners must also take heed of SAMDC rule 9 which prohibits covering. Collaborating professionally with an unregistered person constitutes an ethical offence in terms of the rule, whereby those involved expose themselves to disciplinary action.

For the innocent partners to continue allowing the suspended partner to benefit financially in terms of the partnership agreement for services rendered to patients by the latter during the period of suspension, would also result in contravention of rule 9, and decidedly also of rule 8 (4) which proscribes dichotomy, i e sharing of fees with someone who has not taken a commensurate part in the services for which the fees are charged.

On the other hand, there is clearly nothing – either legally or ethically – which would prevent a suspended partner drawing his share of the profits of the partnership for services rendered by him before the suspension took effect.

Note that a suspension does not become operative when the disciplinary committee makes its finding, but only from the time that the Council confirms the finding and accepts the committee's recommendation of suspension.

In order to avoid any impression of collaboration with the suspended partner, the innocent partners should insist upon the guilty partner removing his name-plate from the premises where the practice is conducted until the period of suspension terminates. Moreover, during that period the name of the suspended partner should not appear on the partnership's letterheads. Accounts should go out in the name of the innocent partners only.

Because suspension from practice of a partner will in my opinion not automatically result in dissolution of the partnership, but would merely entitle the innocent partners to dissolve the agreement, there is clearly nothing which compels the latter to permanently terminate the parties' relationship. In short, so long as the innocent partners for the duration of the suspension do not collaborate in any way with the suspended partner, the parties may upon termination of the suspension simply continue their relationship, provided – as I have mentioned – that the suspended partner derive no financial benefit for services rendered by the other partners during the period of suspension.

A final observation: I have confined my discussion essentially to suspension.

2 De Wet & Yeats *Kontraktereg en Handelsreg* (4th ed, 1978, by J C de Wet and A H van Wyk) 159.
3 Wille & Millin *op cit* 555–6.
4 Medical, Dental and Supplementary Health Service Professions Act 56 of 1974, section 44.

Where the name of a partner is removed from the register following a disciplinary inquiry, there is only one thing for the other partners to do, and that is to take immediate steps for dissolution of the partnership and liquidation of its assets. It goes without saying that the innocent partners may continue to practise in partnership.

71 What legal action can a doctor take against a person who has lodged a complaint against him with the Medical Council?

Is a doctor against whom a complaint has been laid with the S A Medical and Dental Council entitled to approach the Supreme Court for an order to prevent the complainant from pursuing the matter or to prevent the SAMDC from conducting a disciplinary inquiry? May a doctor institute legal proceedings against a complainant whose complaint failed in the sense that the SAMDC's committee of preliminary inquiry decided not to pursue the matter, or in the situation where a disciplinary inquiry had in fact taken place, and the doctor was found not guilty?

Restraining the SAMDC

As a general rule, a court of law would not be prepared to make an order restraining a complainant from having his complaint considered and adjudicated upon by the SAMDC or its two committees. As long as the complainant has not been actuated demonstrably by bad faith in bringing his complaint, the court will not be prepared to intervene prematurely and bring an end to the proceedings.

The Supreme Court has ruled that "[i]t is to the public good that persons who feel themselves aggrieved by the conduct of a professional man, whether rightly or wrongly, and whether they are directly affected or not, should feel free to bring their grievances forward and to have them adjudicated by the impartial and discreet decision of a body having disciplinary powers ..."[1]

The courts are extremely reluctant to interfere in proceedings still pending or in the process of being heard by lower courts or domestic tribunals. In principle a party to such proceedings is required to exhaust his "domestic remedies" before turning to the courts for relief. Once the domestic tribunal – in the present context the SAMDC – has made a final ruling, an aggrieved party may approach the Supreme Court for a review of its proceedings on grounds such as bias, absence of jurisdiction, or gross irregularity such as a failure to apply its mind to the matter before it.

The Supreme Court has ruled that the SAMDC is for all practical purposes the sole repository of the power to decide what is ethical and what is unethical in medical practice.[2] The court will therefore not be prepared to intervene at a stage even before evidence has been adduced and make a ruling to the effect that a particular complaint does not justify an investigation or that the conduct of the doctor complained of does not constitute unethical conduct.

In exceptional circumstances a court may be prepared to intervene in unconcluded proceedings, where the aggrieved party can persuade the court that a gross injustice will be perpetrated if the proceedings were to continue. A hypothetical example would be where the registrar, in clear defiance of the regulations under the Medical, Dental, etc Act,[3] has failed to bring to the notice of the doctor the details of the complaint against him and to invite him to offer an explanation.

If a formal charge is brought against a practitioner in these circumstances, he would be able to complain that he will be severely prejudiced unless the committee

1 *Vincent v Long* 1988 (3) SA 45 (C).
2 See *supra* 373.
3 Act 56 of 1974.

of preliminary inquiry has first considered his explanation. Only a small percentage of complaints result in actual disciplinary inquiries, and because such hearings take place in public it would be manifestly unfair for the accused doctor to be subjected to the attendant media interest where he has not even been given the opportunity of offering an explanation at the pre-inquiry stage. A court would undoubtedly have a sympathetic approach to the accused doctor's application for a court order in these circumstances. I hasten to point out though, that the registrar of the SAMDC meticulously follows the regulations applying to the "please explain" procedure.

Suing for defamation

A patient or other party who lays a complaint against a doctor with the SAMDC may do so in terms which may at first blush appear to be highly defamatory of the doctor. The doctor will learn of the complaint when he receives the registrar's "please explain" letter and will often take great umbrage and may consider suing the complainant for defamation.

There is nothing to prevent a doctor from bringing suit for damages at any stage. However, I would advise the doctor to exercise great circumspection before embarking upon such a lawsuit.

The trouble with a defamation suit is that even if there are good grounds for an action, the initiative taken by you as plaintiff may eventually result in massive publicity in the media. A defamation case may be one of the most unpleasant to conduct in court. Your professional competence will be attacked by the defendant. The media take delight in publishing comprehensive reports and the public in reading every word. Even if you win the case – after considerable agony and expense – something may rub off on to you as far as the average newspaper reader is concerned. What is more, our law of defamation is fairly complex and the defendant may come up with any of about half a dozen defences which may blow your case out of the water.

The dangers inherent in such a case were well illustrated by a 1988 case[4] of a veterinary surgeon who sued a person who complained in strong terms to the Veterinary Council of "poor surgery" which had allegedly resulted in the untimely demise of his mother's constipated cat. The defendant relied on the defence of qualified privilege.

In upholding the defence, the judge made the following remarks:

"I do not think that an interest in bringing complaints concerning professional people to the attention of their disciplinary body should be narrowly confined to a complainant who has himself received an injury ... Other persons close to him may also have an interest in seeing that no hurt or prejudice should come to him ...

"I would say that public policy dictates, that in cases where complaints are made to bodies or tribunals specifically set up to deal with them, one should not be astute to find that a complainant lacks the necessary interest to secure privileged status for his communication ...

"One should be careful in a case like this not too readily to draw an inference of malice from facts which are incorrectly stated, or from exaggeration or extravagance in the language ... As it turned out, many of the allegations which were made were, at the end of a long trial ..., found to have been wrong. But this alone is not sufficient to infer malice. The plaintiff would have had to show that the defendant had no belief in the truth of what he stated, or acted recklessly not caring whether his statements were true or false."

Interdict

It is to be noted that a dissatisfied patient who maliciously disseminates defamatory

4 *Vincent v Long supra.*

matter concerning a doctor may be restrained from doing so by way of a court order. A case of this type occurred in 1990. The patient had made a complaint to the SAMDC alleging indifferent treatment but the Council accepted the doctor's explanation and decided that no action would be taken against him. The patient then distributed copies of newspaper reports in the area where the doctor practised, together with certain scurrilous remarks about the doctor. Only the patient's allegations were quoted in the newspaper report. The doctor successfully sued for an interdict, alleging that the patient had been treated very carefully and properly by him and his colleagues at all times. The case was handled by the firm of attorneys retained by the Medical Protection Society.

72 Pharmaceutical gifts to doctors: legal and ethical implications

The 1983 press rumpus about expensive gifts in the form of cars, television sets, company shares and airline tickets allegedly made by some pharmaceutical firms to certain highly placed doctors, and its sequel – denials, explanations, inquiries, resignations – will not be forgotten easily. Even before the furore much had been said about the economics and ethics of promotional excesses in the pharmaceutical field.

In its report published in 1978, the official Commission of Inquiry into the Pharmaceutical Industry, known as the Steenkamp Commission,[1] drew attention to allegations of this kind.

Business freedom

The Commission pointed out that up to the present, the authorities, "true to their conservative attitude in matters of economic policy", had been loath to interfere with business freedom in this area. The only legal provisions in existence are regulations under the Medicines and Related Substances Control Act[2] requiring strict accountability procedures for certain medicines issued as samples. For the rest, the Commission said, it had been left to the pharmaceutical industry.[3]

The Commission felt the authorities should continue to refrain from direct interference, provided the industry "proves its willingness and its ability to discipline itself".[4] Mailings, free gift advertising, "bonusing" and "sampling", the Commission hoped, would come in for special treatment.[5]

The distribution of pharmaceutical samples to medical practitioners came in for little criticism. If it serves to attract attention to new and better medicines, the Commission said, it improves competition.[6] It is nevertheless open to abuse, and "sampling" of prescription medicines should be substantially reduced.[7]

"Bonusing", i e the practice whereby a pharmacy or dispensing doctor is paid a bonus for having sold a particular product of the manufacturer, in the opinion of the Commission ought to be outlawed altogether. Free gift advertising, "especially in the ugly forms this has taken of late in South Africa", should likewise be prohibited, the Commission recommended.[8] If insufficient progress was made, action might be considered in terms of the Trade Practices Act[9] which provides for the control and "restriction of the giving or supply of benefits".[10]

Bribery and corruption

So far insufficient attention has perhaps been paid to the serious criminal ramifica-

1 See *Report of the Commission of Enquiry into the Pharmaceutical Industry* RP 38/1978.
2 Act 101 of 1965.
3 Par 493.
4 Par 494.
5 Par 498.
6 Par 291.
7 Par 495.
8 *Ibid.*
9 Act 76 of 1976.
10 Par 495.

tions which certain high-pressure promotional practices may have for both the pharmaceutical firm and the doctors who are on the receiving end.

"Bribery" and "corruption" are unpalatable words in any vocabulary, but it should nevertheless be pointed out that if the offering of gifts goes beyond a certain limit, the parties may fall foul of criminal law.

By common law, bribery consists in unlawfully and intentionally offering to or agreeing with a State official to give any consideration in return for action or inaction by him in an official capacity.[11]

Our law requires that the giver of the bribe must intend to seduce the official in taking a price for action in an official capacity. The briber need not have a corrupt purpose in any stronger sense than this. His motive may even be laudable. That is irrelevant. Nor need his motive necessarily be personal gain.[12]

The crime of bribery is complete when the wrongdoer makes his offer to the official. To commit the crime, it is not necessary that the official should accept the offer. The action or inaction need not even relate to something within the official's legal sphere of duties. Our courts have ruled that an official acts in conflict with his duty to his principal, the State, by accepting any bribe, although the act desired from him may not be in conflict with the interest of his principal.[13]

To put it in practical terms: Where a gift is made by a pharmaceutical firm to a State official such as a director of hospital services to induce him to order products from that firm or to instruct a subordinate to do so, the firm will be guilty of bribery – and so will the official himself be. The crime will be committed even though the medicine is of a superior quality and will be beneficial to patients treated in the hospital.

Upright employees

The fact that the briber is legally entitled to the action or inaction he solicits is irrelevant: he should obtain it through the regular, lawful channels. Nor is it essential that the action or inaction which is solicited should relate to a definite "known transaction", says Hunt: it is sufficient that it is intended to be "with respect to future transactions which may come upon the scene".[14]

The Prevention of Corruption Act[15] goes even further than the common law in penalising corruption. Under the Act the bribee need not be a State official. As Hunt has observed, the Act does not only seek to protect the interests of the State and the community in an upright public administration, but also the interests of private employers in having upright employees and agents.[16]

A conviction of bribery or corruption is a serious matter. Apart from the punishment imposed by the court, a medical practitioner will also invariably have to face a disciplinary inquiry which may have grave consequences for him.

Naturally there is nothing wrong, legally speaking, with a *bona fide* promotional effort by way of e g a professional seminar being organised by a pharmaceutical firm for doctors, even if accompanied by a certain amount of socially acceptable entertainment, e g in the form of a cheese and wine party. Likewise a company representative cannot be accused of bribery if he invites a hospital official to a lunch in a smart restaurant in order to acquaint his guest over fried sole and Grand Cru with the latest line of products marketed by his company. The business lunch is so much part of the social scene that no court will interpret this as "consideration in return for action".

11 P M A Hunt *South African Criminal Law and Procedure* vol 2 *(Common Law Crimes)* (2nd ed by J R L Milton, 1982) 219.
12 Ibid 221.
13 *Ibid* 225–226.
14 *Ibid* 227.
15 Act 6 of 1958.
16 Hunt, *op cit* 233.

Moreover, there is the legal principle of *de minimis non curat lex;* the law does not take account of trifles!

Breach of contract

It goes without saying that a private medical practitioner who is "bribed" by a company rep by means of lavish gifts to prescribe his firm's medicines on a preferential basis, cannot be charged with bribery or with contravention of the Prevention of Corruption Act. The essence of these crimes, as I have said, is to corrupt an employee or State official. A self-employed practitioner does not fall within the ambit of the Act.

But a doctor who receives remuneration in any form for the preferential use or prescription of medicine makes himself guilty of unethical conduct (proscribed by Rule 28 of the Medical Council).[17]

It should also be pointed out that it is not necessarily irregular for an employee to undertake to give advice to a pharmaceutical firm, for remuneration, as long as his conduct does not amount to participation in the sale, advertising or promotion of a medicine. Whether or not a doctor employed by the State, a province, a university or a private firm may do this will depend entirely on the terms of his contract of employment.

Generally speaking contracts of full-time employment will preclude the employee from doing "outside" work on a remunerative basis, unless it is done with the employer's express consent. Employers may even lay down as a condition of employment that the employee shall not become a director of any company unless it is by leave of the employer.

An employee who enters into contracts of this kind and accepts remuneration for his services may therefore be guilty of a breach of contract for which the employer may be entitled to dismiss him. But breach of contract is not a criminal offence.

17 The rule is reproduced below 457.

73 May a private hospital pay a commission to doctors who refer patients?

The following question was put to me: "I am a medical practitioner practising in city X. I have been approached by a representative of a company which was formed recently with the object of building a new private hospital. Doctors are invited to buy shares in the company and will then have the right to make use of the hospital's facility for operations, diagnostic examinations and treatment of patients. From the company's prospectus I gather that doctors who purchase shares will be expected to utilise the facilities. Patients or their medical schemes will, of course, pay the normal hospital fees. Shareholders will be paid the usual dividends on their respective shareholdings. As an incentive to shareholder-doctors to make optimal use of the facilities, the company will pay such a shareholder also a commission by way of a fixed percentage of his individual monthly turnover. These commissions will be paid out prior to profit-sharing by way of dividend payments. Is such an arrangement legally and ethically in order?"

My answer is as follows:

The payment of such a commission would, in my opinion, confront doctors with insurmountable ethical problems.

Rule 8 of the S A Medical and Dental Council clearly stands firmly in the way of the proposed scheme. The rule concerns "fees, commissions and partnerships" and is applied strictly by the Council. The rule was in fact rendered even more efficacious by a 1987 amendment thereto.

Rule 8(3) prohibits "receiving commission in return for recommending services or wares to patients". Referral by a doctor of a patient to a private hospital decidedly amounts to "recommending services" as envisaged by the subrule, and by receiving a commission a doctor would expose himself to disciplinary action by the SAMDC, which may have serious implications for the practitioner. The SAMDC will look at the essence of the arrangement and will certainly not be fooled by a commission dressed up as a kind of professional service.

Rule 8(4), again, prohibits dichotomy, i e "sharing fees with any person who has not taken a commensurate part in the services for which fees are charged". It may be argued that the receiving of a commission for referral of patients indirectly amounts to sharing of fees, although it is perhaps more correct to argue that it is the hospital – and not the doctor – who shares its fee. But that argument would in no way affect the unequivocal meaning of rule 8(3).

Rule 8(7) (the new subrule) prohibits in general terms, *inter alia*, "the receiving of fees for services not personally rendered", except for certain exceptions which are then defined in specific terms. An obvious example is fee-sharing between medical partners, and by principal and professional assistants or *locum tenens.*

The proposed scheme would, without a doubt, also offend against the latter subrule. The patient, after all, pays fees to the hospital – either direct or through his medical scheme – in respect of hospital services rendered to him, and if a part of the fees received by the hospital are paid over to the doctor by way of commission, the latter in effect receives money for services not rendered by him personally.

Mere referral of a patient to a hospital can hardly be regarded as a "service" rendered by the doctor.

I am familiar with arguments usually put forward to justify these commission arrangements. Thus it is argued that the free-market system is promoted: providing an incentive to doctors to refer patients to a specific hospital will result in better bed occupancy which, it is said, will lead to greater cost-effectiveness. It is suggested that a high percentage of bed-occupancy would even make it possible for the hospital to charge lower fees.

These arguments are not very persuasive, though. First, the sum total of commissions paid to referring doctors may be quite substantial and would make it financially difficult to lower hospital fees. Secondly, an arrangement whereby a commission is paid to referring doctors will certainly discourage them from referring patients to other, competing hospitals who do not pay such a commission – because they refuse to resort to schemes which would entice doctors into unethical conduct. The commission arrangement clearly amounts to unfair competition and "no-commission" hospitals may take legal action to protect their rights. The much praised free-market system does not mean that "anything goes". The free market functions best when the law enforces *fair* competition.

It goes without saying that if doctors, in deciding which hospitals to send their patients to, are guided by the percentage of commission which they can earn and not so much by the quality of service provided by a particular hospital, the public interest will be harmed. The primary statutory object of the SAMDC, as set out in section 3 of Act 56 of 1974, is "to assist in the promotion of the health of the population of the Republic".

In seeking to attain that objective the SAMDC, through the years, in its policy statements and its disciplinary action against doctors, has amply demonstrated that it places a high premium on the unfettered individual autonomy of the doctor to take decisions which are in the first place in the health interest of the patient. The financial interest of the doctor or other health-care provider is of secondary importance. Hence the strict rules of the SAMDC against doctors taking commissions or sharing fees.

It is therefore concluded that the proposed scheme will result in doctors becoming involved in unethical conduct. I would not advise a doctor to take shares in the company under the conditions offered. Where doctors are shareholders in a company that owns a private hospital, the only ethically unimpeachable scheme would be one whereby dividends are calculated on a *bona fide* basis and paid out in the normal manner, namely in accordance with the percentage of shares owned and not with reference to the volume of hospital use generated by a shareholder.

PART XVI

Medical care of prisoners and detainees

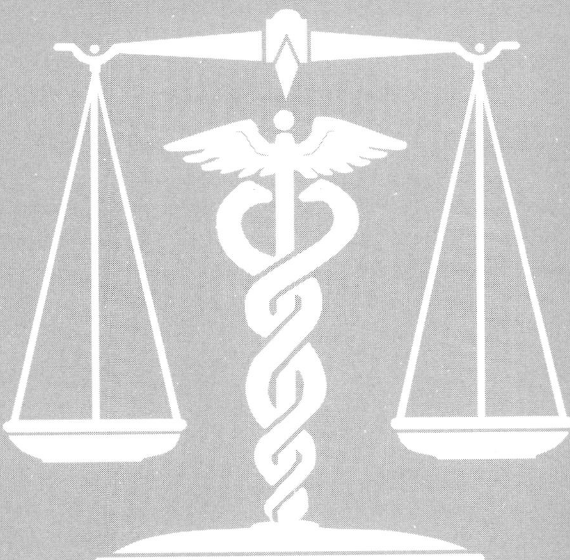

74 The legal rights of prisoners and detainees to medical treatment

Introduction

It is to be noted that the legal position described here is as it was at the time when this book went to press (February 1991). In 1990 the government announced that the Internal Security Act[1] was to be revised. It is expected that important and substantial amendments will be effected by Parliament during the 1991 parliamentary session.

Statutory law

The only statutory law which we have in South Africa that in a positive sense may be directly relevant to medical treatment of both prisoners and detainees, is some provisions of the Prisons Act[2] and regulations thereunder. I advisedly say "may" be relevant because the Prisons Act was of course not designed to deal primarily with security detainees. However, from the definitions[3] embodied in the Act it is clear that if a person who has been detained by the Police is brought to a prison established under the Act, he will fall within the ambit of the Act and its regulations, at least for as long as he is kept on prison premises (and in so far as the Internal Security Act does not preclude application of the general provisions of the Prisons Act). To qualify as a "prisoner" under the Prisons Act he need not have been convicted; in fact he need not even necessarily be an awaiting-trial detainee.[4] (In terms of the Internal Security Act, section 29, persons may be – and in fact to the best of my knowledge are ordinarily – arrested for interrogation[5] and are not invariably charged at a later stage.)

Police cells and lock-ups, or offices used for temporary detention of persons, on the other hand, generally do not qualify as "prisons" under the Prisons Act.

The Prisons Act as such contains several provisions directly relating to medical treatment of prisoners and these provisions are amplified by a number of regulations promulgated under the Act. Although in a prison context it may be difficult, legally speaking, to demarcate prisoners' rights from mere privileges, it is clear that the Act and its regulations create a right to health care on the part of the prisoner and not merely a privilege that may be granted or refused at will by prison authorities.[6] This, of course, does not mean that the prisoner can prescribe to the Prisons Service exactly what form the medical treatment should take or under what conditions it should be given.

The Prisons Act makes provision for the appointment of medical officers.[7] If no

1 Act 74 of 1982.
2 Act 8 of 1959.
3 Section 1.
4 Section 1.
5 See H Rudolph *Security, Terrorism and Torture* (1984) 23 *et seq.*
6 The Department of Correctional Services takes the view – and correctly so, it is submitted – that a prisoner is entitled to medical care as a matter of right and not merely as a matter of privilege. See *Goldberg and Others v Minister of Police* 1979(1) SA 14 (A) 22 D–E. On prisoners' rights in general see further D H van Wyk, B van Niekerk, R G Nairn & J Taitz in 1979 *SACC* 52 *et seq;* Rudolph *op cit, passim.*
7 Section 6.

resident medical officer is appointed, the duties assigned to him must be performed by the district surgeon for that particular area, or by another doctor appointed by the Director-General, National Health and Population Development.[8] There are currently no full-time medical officers, and medical services in our prisons are performed essentially by district surgeons. District surgeons, whether full-time or part-time, are employees of the various provincial administrations, but in so far as they work as medical officers in a prison, there can in my opinion be no doubt that by virtue of the Prisons Act they fall under the general control and direction of the Commissioner: Correctional Services.[9]

The stated policy of the Department of Correctional Services is as follows, however: "Since [district surgeons] are ... not directly responsible to the prison authorities [being employed by the respective provincial authorities] they can take decisions of a clinical nature without fear of redress by the prison authorities ... Prisoners have regular access to doctors and any prescriptions, referrals or instructions of a medical practitioner or specialist are strictly adhered to. The [Department] may not dictate or attempt to influence the medical official in the treatment of people in his care."[10]

The Act empowers the Commissioner to order the removal of a seriously ill prisoner to an outside hospital or other health-care facility.[11] No right is given by the Act to a prison medical officer independently to authorise or order such removal.

The Act provides that the Commissioner is in charge of the Department of Correctional Services,[12] subject to the direction and control of the Director-General, Justice (who in turn is subject to the direction and control of the Minister of Justice).[13] The Act gives the Commissioner the right, in his discretion, to "grant such privileges and indulgences as he may think fit to any prisoner".[14] This provision clearly would enable the Commissioner to allow a prisoner to be seen by a private doctor and to undergo special medical treatment inside or outside a prison. (Where a security detainee is kept in a prison, the Commissioner may obviously not grant privileges in contravention of the prohibitions contained in the Internal Security Act against access by "outsiders" to a detainee.[15])

The regulations[16] under the Prisons Act contain a number of detailed provisions governing medical treatment of prisoners and the duties of medical officers. Thus provision is made for the establishment of a hospital at every prison to be equipped according to local requirements.[17] The regulations impose an explicit duty upon the medical officer to visit sick prisoners as often as necessary and to examine and treat them.[18] Strict duties of inspection and reporting are imposed upon medical officers.[19] Special provision is also made for consultation with other medical practitioners; as far as serious operations are concerned, there is in fact a duty upon the medical officer to do so before the operation is performed.[20] The Commissioner is empowered,

8 Section 6(3). The subsection refers to the "Secretary for Health", which must now be construed as a reference to the Director-General, National Health and Population Development.

9 "Medical officer" is defined in section 1 of the Prisons Act, so as to include district surgeons and other "approved" doctors. See also section 77.

10 See 74 *S Afr Med J* 438–9 (1988).

11 Section 73(1).

12 Section 3. The Department was formerly known as the Prisons Service.

13 See GN 2302 of 31 October 1980 (*GG* 7288), read with section 1 of Regulations of Functions of Officers in the Public Service Act 19 of 1980.

14 Section 22(2).

15 Section 28(8), 29(7) and 31(4).

16 The current prison regulations are contained in GN R2080 of 31 December 1965 (*GG* 1326, *Reg Gaz* 604), as amended over the years.

17 Reg 111(1).

18 Reg 111(2)(*a*).

19 Reg 111(2)(*b*).

20 Reg 111(3)(*a*).

subject to certain conditions, to allow prisoners awaiting trial or sentence to obtain the services of private medical practitioners.[21] (This power, too, must in relation to security detainees, obviously be read subject to the prohibition in the Internal Security Act against access of "outsiders" to detainees.[22])

It is not intended to go into the details of the prison regulations,[23] but, subject to certain qualifications (see below), the general statutory scheme in terms of the Prisons Act is satisfactory. Whether the health-care facilities provided in our prisons in actual practice are equally satisfactory, the present writer is not in a position to assess, although district surgeons with long experience of prison work have stated that the facilities and quality of medical services rendered are good. It would not be unreasonable to assume that the facilities in all prison hospitals are not necessarily of equal standard. The *ad hoc* committee appointed by the Medical Association of South Africa to consider certain ethical issues raised as a result of the death of Mr Stephen Biko, after visiting the Sydenham Prison Hospital, reported in 1981 that the hospital was "of a rather primitive kind".[24]

As the Prisons Act and regulations now read, the conclusion seems to be inescapable that the prison medical officer (i e the district surgeon) in the execution of his duties legally falls under the general direction of the Commissioner: Correctional Services. This is an objectionable feature of our law because it inhibits the doctor's clinical independence. In medical matters the doctor, and not a non-medical state official, should have the final say. The necessity for complete clinical independence was stressed in the Declaration of Tokyo (1975).[25] Ideally the policy of the Department of Correctional Services quoted above should be embodied in a statutory provision.

Should a difference of opinion arise between the medical officer and a non-medical prison official as to the treatment of a particular prisoner, the doctor would obviously be entitled to appeal to the Commissioner himself for a decision. In the unlikely event of the Commissioner refusing to give effect to the medical officer's recommendation, the latter could approach the Director-General, Justice, or the Minister of Justice, for a ruling. As we have seen, the Commissioner works under the direction and control of these two functionaries (in the line of authority as indicated).

In extreme cases the medical officer or prisoner himself may conceivably approach the Supreme Court with an application for review of the Commissioner's decision.[26] But from a practical point of view this is unlikely to be an effective remedy. Quite apart from the time factor and considerations of costs, a review can only take place on limited grounds, such as *mala fides,* ulterior or improper motive on the part of the respondent, failure to apply his mind or to exercise his discretion, or disregarding the express provisions of a statute.[27] The "wide range of powers" to be exercised by the prison authorities and the "great latitude of choice left to the person charged with the duty of exercising a discretionary power" may lead to the conclusion that "he may virtually have complete freedom in the exercise of his discretion as to

21 Reg 132(7).

22 See above n 14.

23 For the details of the prison regulations, see the writer's contribution in Ellison Kahn (ed) *Fiat Iustitia: Essays in Memory of Oliver Deneys Schreiner* (1983) 344 *et seq.*

24 The Report of the *ad hoc* committee was published as a supplement to the *SA Medical Journal* of 22 August 1981.

25 The World Medical Association at its Tokyo meeting in 1975 adopted a set of "Guidelines for Medical Doctors concerning Torture and other Cruel, Inhuman or Degrading Treatment or Punishment, in Relation to Detention and Imprisonment". Article 4 contains the following injunction: "A doctor must have complete clinical independence in deciding upon the care of a person for whom he or she is medically responsible. The doctor's fundamental role is to alleviate distress of his or her fellow men, and no motive whether personal, collective or political shall prevail against this higher purpose."

26 This in fact occurred in *Harris v Commissioner of Prisons* 1965 (2) SA 645 (T).

27 This is trite law. See, for example, *Shidiack v Union Government* 1912 AD 642 at 651; *Divisional Commissioner of SA Police, Witwatersrand Area, and Others v S A Associated Newspapers Ltd* 1966 (2) SA 505 (A).

whether, when and in what manner he will act". This may make a court reluctant to interfere with prison rulings of an administrative nature – as is apparent from the majority ruling of the Appellate Division (per Mr Acting Chief Justice Wessels) in *Goldberg v Minister of Prisons*[28] from which the phrases quoted have been culled. Regarding persons detained under sections 28, 29 and 31 of the 1982 Internal Security Act, there is further the extremely discouraging factor that such detainees have no right of access to legal practitioners.[29]

There are no provisions in the Police Act[30] or the regulations[31] thereunder, governing medical treatment of detainees. There are, however, important instructions to the Police contained in paragraphs 18 to 23 of Standing Order No 319 of the SA Police.[32] These instructions, it should be mentioned, were in existence at the time when Biko was detained. These paragraphs make it clear, inter alia, that there is a duty upon the Police to call in the district surgeon or another medical practitioner to attend to seriously injured or ill prisoners.[33] ("Prisoner" is not defined in the subparagraphs of the Standing Order, but is presumably used in the general sense of any person in police custody following an arrest.) Of special significance is the provision whereby policemen are ordered to carry out without delay "any instructions given by the district surgeon ..."[34] This provision intimates that it is the district surgeon who has the final say in regard to medical treatment of such a prisoner and this is most laudable in the light of the need for clinical independence which I have already adumbrated. Moreover, explicit mention is made of treatment in an "outside" hospital.[35] Equally commendable is the right given to a prisoner to be treated by his own doctor.[36]

The following observations must, however, be made regarding Standing Order 319, paragraphs 18 to 23. First, a standing order allowing access to a prisoner by a private doctor, can of course not override the prohibitions in the Internal Security Act against "outsider access" to security detainees.[37] Secondly, it is submitted that the provisions in the Standing Order are of such importance that they should not be relegated to standing orders but should be accorded proper statutory status either in the Police Act itself, or at the very least, in Presidential regulations promulgated by virtue of section 33 of that Act. Thirdly, some of these provisions seem to be contradicted to a certain extent by a later Standing Instruction (applying specifically to detainees in terms of security legislation) (discussed below) and in particular by the Prisons Act and the regulations thereunder. As has been mentioned *any* police prisoner may in certain circumstances be considered a "prisoner" in terms of the latter Act and its regulations, which clearly give the Commissioner of Prisons the effective say over medical treatment of prisoners. It may be argued that because they are (promulgated) statutory regulations, the regulations under the Prisons Act must prevail in the event of their provisions conflicting with Standing Orders of the South African

28 1979 (1) SA 14 (A). The quotations in the text are from pages 31–32 of the decision.

29 An aggrieved detainee might possibly also be deterred by section 29 (6) of the Internal Security Act which precludes a court of law from pronouncing "on the validity of any action taken under this section". There can be no doubt, however, that a decision taken in terms of the Prisons Act as to medical treatment of a detainee cannot be categorised as "action taken under this section". Compare the Transkei decisions in *Sigaba v Minister of Defence and Police* 1980 (3) SA 535 (Tk); *Honey v Minister of Police* 1980 (3) SA 700 (Tk).

30 Act 7 of 1958.

31 The Police Regulations are contained in GN R203 *GG* 719 of 14 February 1964 (*Reg Gaz* 299). The Government Notice has been amended from time to time.

32 See Annexure A. Standing orders and instructions derive their legal power from reg 6 of Police Regulations promulgated under section 33 of the Police Act.

33 Standing Order 319 par 18.

34 Standing Order 319 par 21.

35 *Ibid.*

36 Standing Order 219 par 22 (*a*).

37 See above n 15.

Police. For the sake of legal certainty any possible contradiction as between these various sets of provisions should be cleared up by the Legislature.

Standing orders and instructions, it must be noted, derive their legal power from regulation 6 of the police regulations promulgated under section 33 of the Police Act. As is indicated by the terminology, these orders are in the nature of departmental orders and instructions, given by the Commissioner of Police and directed to members of the police force. Unlike regulations made by the State President under an act of Parliament, they are not published in the *Government Gazette* (or otherwise made known to the public), and accordingly are not law in the generally accepted sense of the word.[38] They are legally significant, however, in the sense that failure on the part of a policeman to obey any particular order may expose him to disciplinary action in terms of the Police Act.[39] It is also a criminal offence for a member of the Police to fail to comply with an order issued in terms of the Police Act.[40] It is further submitted that a suspect, prisoner or any other person who feels himself aggrieved by police action in violation of a standing order, affecting a right of his (such as a right of personality or proprietary right), may by common law apply to court for an interdict or a *mandamus* (as the case may be) to enforce compliance with the order. Moreover, the duties imposed by standing orders upon policemen may be relevant in regard to potential delictual or criminal liability on the part of the State, where it is alleged that a policeman acted in breach of an official duty which resulted in damage to (or the death of) another person.[41] Lastly, there is the question of judicial review of police decisions taken in disregard of standing orders, but as is pointed out above in connection with review of prison decisions, this is a remedy not without problems.

District surgeons

At this point something must be said about the legal status of the district surgeon, who will ordinarily be responsible for the medical treatment of detainees and prisoners. The district surgeon, whether full-time (as in the cities) or part-time (as in country towns) is not an employee of the Department of Police or the Department of Correctional Services. District surgeons are medical practitioners employed by the various provincial administrations and in general their conditions of service and official duties are determined by their employer. In performing the functions of prison medical officers,[42] however, they are to a certain extent subject to the prison regulations as is described below.

In 1981, the Department of Health and Welfare, which at the time was the employer of district surgeons, in an official publication of the Department, entitled *The Medical Practitioner in the Health Service,* listed a number of obligations on the part of doctors (and in particular district surgeons) in regard to patients in police custody who are examined at the request of the Police. Thus it is described as "imperative that the district surgeon or his deputy have access to the patient at all times".[43] The manual also states that " [w]here the district surgeon has reason to believe his instructions are not being complied with, he shall report this to the appropriate commanding officer at the same time notifying the Regional Director, State Health Services of the action he has taken".[44] Other instructions embodied in the manual that

38 See my remarks in *Fiat Iustitia* 333.

39 See Police reg 58(1).

40 Act 7 of 1958 section 9.

41 See, for example, the argument by counsel in *S v Van As* 1967 (4) SA 594 (A) at 595B–C; *Weir-Mason v Minister of Justice* 1958 (3) SA 299 (N) at 302H; the references by counsel in *Mhlongo v Minister of Police* 1978 (2) SA 551 (A) at 558C–D to "specific instructions". See also *Minister van Polisie v Gamble* 1979 (4) SA 759 (A) at 767B–C where Mr Justice Joubert referred to "wettige opdragte" given to a policeman by his superiors.

42 By virtue of section 6 of the Prisons Act, read with prison reg 6(2).

43 At 52 item 5.

relate to the treatment of patients in police custody which should be mentioned here, are the following: The doctor must ascertain whether the prisoner "is in a fit condition for transfer by specified means of transport to the consulting room(s) or other appropriate nearby place suitable for the examination of the person in private".[45] Should the person be removed into the care of another doctor, the latter must be fully informed as expeditiously as possible of his condition.[46] The district surgeon should not hesitate to call for a second medical opinion should this in his opinion be necessary.[47] Where the detainee requests his own doctor, "this must be considered as a privilege and not as a right,[48] but in any case the district surgeon should not fail to consult with such medical practitioner ..."[49] It is further stated that the doctor "should inform the officer commanding the prison of any inadequacy regarding the health of the prisoners or any other matter concerning the prison. This should be done in the form of a written report and a copy should be sent to the Regional Director of the Department of Health and Welfare. If the report does not create the desired reaction the physician should himself bring it under the Regional Director's attention."[50]

The manual then proceeds to set forth extracts from a decision taken by the First United Nations Congress on the Prevention of Crime and the Treatment of Transgressors of 30 August 1955, containing "practical suggestions for the health-care of prisoners and other persons in custody", as well as an extract from the Association of State Correctional Administrators policy guidelines.[51] It is clear that these extracts were not in the nature of regulations or departmental instructions applying to South African health-care personnel, but were included in the above-mentioned publication of the Department as general guidelines.

Internal Security Act

The 1982 Internal Security Act[52] made provision for three forms of detention: preventive detention,[53] detention for interrogation[54] and detention of witnesses.[55] Persons falling in the first of these categories must be detained in prisons[56] as defined in the Prisons Act[57] and would accordingly in respect of medical treatment generally fall under the provisions of the latter Act. By virtue of section 28(8) access to persons in preventive detention is prohibited, however, except by persons specified in the subsection. Amongst the persons specified are "[persons] acting by virtue of their office in the service of the State": this exemption clearly includes prison medical officers (i e district surgeons). (In this respect the Internal Security Act is not so harsh as the Ciskeian regulation [58] which formed the subject of the decision in *Ngxale v Minister of Justice of the Ciskei*.[59])

44 At 53 item 8.
45 At 52 item 2.
46 At 52 item 5.
47 At 53 item 8.
48 This statement appears to be in conflict with Police Standing Order 319(22) (*a*) which clearly accords the prisoner a right and not merely a privilege.
49 At 53 item 7.
50 At 55.
51 These guidelines deal with medical services in general, preventive measures and medical experiments. The extracts published in the departmental guide were reproduced from a publication indicated as *Medical Care of Prisoners and Detainees – Ciba Geigy Foundation Symposium* (Elsevier 1973).
52 Act 74 of 1982.
53 Section 28.
54 Section 29.
55 Section 31.
56 Section 28(1).
57 Act 8 of 1959.
58 Reg 8 of Proc R252 (Regulations for the Administration of the Ciskei).
59 1981 (2) SA 554 (E).

Persons falling in the other two categories of detention may be detained at any place.[60] Access to these categories of detainees is likewise generally forbidden, subject to specific exemptions provided for in each case.[61] Amongst persons who are not denied access are, similarly, "[persons] acting by virtue of their office in the service of the State". Clearly, therefore, district surgeons, who as part of their duties must attend to detainees (whether for medical examination or treatment), are not denied access to detainees. In fact, in respect of persons detained for interrogation as well as detained witnesses, the Act in peremptory terms provides for visitation in private by a district surgeon, not less than once a fortnight.[62] It is also to be noted that unlike section 6 of the repealed Terrorism Act,[63] sections 28 and 29 of the Internal Security Act[64] of 1982 empower the Minister of Law and Order and the Commissioner of Police, in the case of persons in preventive detention or detained for interrogation, to consent to other persons having access to detainees, subject to such conditions as may be determined by them. (In the case of detained witnesses, the Attorney-General is vested with a similar power.[65]) The Minister or the Commissioner (or the Attorney-General in respect of detained witnesses) may therefore consent to detainees being attended by private doctors.

As far as detention for interrogation is concerned, the 1982 Act lays down that detention will be "in accordance with such directions as the Commissioner may, subject to the directions of the Minister, from time to time issue".[66] On 3 December 1982 the Minister published in the *Government Gazette* a detailed set of directions.[67] Paragraphs 27 to 30 of these specifically relate to the medical care of detainees, and they provide as follows:

27. Arrangements shall be made forthwith for the examination of a detainee by a district surgeon in the following circumstances:
(a) When the detainee appears to be suffering from any illness or injury or complains that he is ill.
(b) Where it appears that the detainee is under the influence of alcohol or drugs.
(c) Where the detainee alleges that he was assaulted or injured.
(d) Where it is alleged that the detainee has committed an offence and it is likely that a medical examination will yield evidence tending to prove or disprove the allegation.
(e) Where for any other reason the person in charge of the place of detention considers this advisable.

28. In an emergeny where the services of a district surgeon are not available, the services of another competent medical practitioner shall be obtained.

29. Detainees who show any inclination towards suicide or who become exceptionally despondent or morbid, shall receive special attention. The assistance of a district surgeon shall also be obtained.

30. The Commissioner shall forthwith advise the Minister of any serious illness of or injury to a detainee, as well as the steps taken to ensure the good health of the detainee.[68]

Elsewhere in the directions it is provided that the commissioned police officer who has caused the detainee to be arrested and detained must, as soon a possible after the arrest, make arrangements for the detainee to be examined by a district surgeon.[69] The officer involved must *inter alia* notify the regional representative of the

60 Section 31(2).
61 Sections 29(7) and 31(4).
62 Sections 29(9) and 31(5).
63 Act 83 of 1967.
64 Act 74 of 1982.
65 Act 74 of 1982 section 31(4).
66 Section 29.
67 Notice 877 of 1982, *GG* 8467 of 3 December 1982.
68 On evidentiary privilege concerning a medical report made in pursuance of these directions, see *S v Yengeni and Others* 1990 (1) SA 639 (C).

Department of National Health and Population Development of the detention and the place where the detainee is being detained, and also of transfer of the latter to another place of detention.[70] A district surgeon who visits a detainee in terms of section 29(9) of the Act[71] must submit a report to the office of the Director of Security Legislation and the Divisional Commissioner of Police.[72] Instructions issued by a district surgeon (or doctor referred to in paragraph 28) regarding a special diet to be followed by a detainee must be complied with.[73] If a district surgeon receives any complaints regarding the alleged poor treatment of a detainee he must report the matter to the person in charge of the institution or place where the detainee is held. In a subsequent report he must mention whether or not the matter has been rectified.[74] If a report by a district surgeon is received by the Director of Security Legislation indicating that an offence may have been committed in respect of a detainee, copies must be forwarded to the Minister of Law and Order and the Divisional Commissioner of Police for appropriate action in terms of the directions.[75] A district surgeon must report instances where a detainee is not available during his visit, together with the reasons therefor.[76] It is specifically provided that a district surgeon will have direct access to the Divisional Commissioner should he wish to bring any matter regarding a detainee to the attention of that officer.[77]

These directions ostensibly supersede an earlier Standing Instruction to the SA Police, introduced after the Biko case, pertaining to the action to be taken in cases of illness of a detainee (quoted below as Annexure "B").

Although the 1982 directions are perhaps not ideal in all respects,[78] they represent a definite improvement in regulating what had largely been a grey area before. As was the case with the Standing Instruction in regard to illness of detainees, their introduction evidenced special concern about the medical treatment of detainees and an earnest endeavour to avoid a situation such as that which arose in the case of Mr Biko. But what has been said regarding the legal status of Standing Order 319[79] likewise applies to these directions. If not ensconced in Parliamentary legislation itself, these provisions should at the very least be embodied in enforceable statutory regulations and should leave no doubt that a *bona fide* clinical assessment by the doctor concerned and his subsequent directions will be decisive. Moreover, what applies to security detainees should be of equal application to all other categories of persons in custody.

Common law

It is not proposed to cover fully the delictual rights and obligations concerning the medical treatment of detainees and prisoners. The prison medical officer (district surgeon) may, of course, on the basis of negligence be held liable for damages in his personal capacity for failure to treat a sick prisoner or detainee properly. The State may also be held liable vicariously for the negligence of the medical officer.[80] If a

69 Par 5.
70 Par 6.
71 I e the peremptory fortnightly visit, referred to above.
72 Par 34.
73 Par 17.
74 Par 35.
75 Par 36.
76 Par 37.
77 Par 38.
78 For criticism and suggestions for improvement, see Rudolph *op cit 88 et seq.*
79 Paras 18–23. See annexure A, *infra* 400.
80 It is submitted that a resident medical officer will undoubtedly qualify as an employee of the Department of Correctional Services. However, whether or not a district surgeon or an "approved" medical officer will qualify as employees for the purpose of vicarious liability is a question that falls beyond the scope of this chapter.

medical officer were to bring to the attention of the prison authorities the necessity of or urgency for special treatment to be given to a particular prisoner, and this were disregarded by the authorities, the State may be held liable for damages. The same would apply if a medical officer were to warn non-medical prison or police officials that a prisoner is not in a fit condition to be conveyed to an outside facility, or to be safely conveyed beyond a specified distance.

The decision in *Minister van Polisie v Ewels,*[81] apart from its significance in starkly underlining the principle that delictual liability may be based upon a mere omission, highlighted the special duty owed by the Police to persons in their custody. This case did not involve medical treatment at all, but in a subsequent decision, *Minister of Police v Skosana,*[82] the State was held liable for damages to the dependants of a drunken driver who had been held in custody by the Police and who had died in consequence of a negligent delay in providing medical treatment for injuries sustained in a road accident.

Conclusion

I have endeavoured to describe the essential features of the existing legal position in South Africa regarding the rights of prisoners and detainees to medical treatment. Other important issues such as the question whether a detainee may be medically treated against his will and problems of professional secrecy in the prison context have not been discussed here.

De facto the position is satisfactory – at least in respect of detainees kept in prisons – inasmuch as extensive provision has been made for the establishment of adequate prison hospitals and the appointment of qualified medical officers.[83] Senior and reputable medical practitioners with long experience of prison medical work have publicly praised the quality of medical care generally available in prisons. Statutory law imposes a firm duty on prison authorities and medical officers to provide medical services to sick prisoners. Moreover, the common law provides a remedy to an aggrieved person, or his dependants, in the form of an action for delictual damages.

There are, however, deficiencies in the statutory law. First, provisions relating to the medical treatment of detainees and prisoners are presently scattered in a variety of instruments, ranging from Parliamentary legislation to regulations, ministerial directions and police standing orders, to informal guidelines issued to district surgeons. The legal status of many of these provisions is not that of promulgated statutory law. The subject of medical treatment of detainees and prisoners is so important that rights and duties should be spelt out clearly and in detail, preferably in a single set of statutory provisions embodied in an Act of Parliament or statutory regulations (at the very least) which should be of equal application to all categories of persons in custody.

Secondly, it is submitted that the clinical independence of the prison medical officer should be given express statutory recognition.

Thirdly, at present the security detainee has no right to be visited by a private medical practitioner. Whether or not a private doctor may attend to a detainee is within

81 1975 (3) SA 590 (A).

82 1977 (1) SA 31 (A).

83 The Report of the Van Dam Committee (on events occurring in the Barberton maximum-security prison in September 1983) released on 16 May 1984, in par 8.2 thereof contains important comments on, and recommendations regarding, medical services in prisons. Although praising the general quality of services, the Committee was surprised to find that the Prisons Service at the time had no full-time doctors in its employment, considering the fact that the Service was responsible on a daily basis for more than 100 000 persons. It recommended that consideration be given to the establishment of a purely professional division, independent and with an elevated status, under the direction of a Surgeon-General. The Committee further recommended the establishment of fully-equipped prison hospitals on a regional basis.

the exclusive discretion of the authorities. Consideration should be given to statutory provisions authorising at least minimal rights of visitation by a private practitioner. It would not be too difficult to make these rights subject to strict statutory conditions so as to eliminate any possible abuse.

Fourthly, a nuclear set of minimum standards for health services which must be complied with in regard to security detainees should be embodied in statutory regulations. It goes without saying that attention should not only be given to standards concerning physical treatment, but to psychiatric treatment and observation as well.

Fifthly, consideration should be given to the introduction of a formal system of medical "peer review". By that is meant that medical, nursing and paramedical personnel attending to detainees should report their activities on a regular basis to a committee consisting of independent outside experts which is able to make constructive comments on all aspects of the staff's services. Such a committee – which may be appointed by the Medical Association of South Africa – should have direct access to the Ministers concerned. The activities of this committee may also tie in with the functions of the Inspector of Detainees and the Boards of Review established in terms of the Internal Security Act.

Finally, it is observed that the provisions of the Internal Security Act which preclude a detainee from having access to a legal adviser without official permission, can render whatever rights a detainee may have in regard to medical treatment nugatory in practice from the point of view of their enforcement by means of judicial intervention. Quite apart from having perpetuated the possibility of indefinite detention of persons suspected of certain offences against the security of the State, the Act in this respect offends against basic democratic notions valued in the Western world. Justification for these drastic measures was sought in the Communist threat as perceived in earlier decades and the onslaught against the Republic by means of brutal acts of terrorism perpetrated against innocent civilian victims. One can only hope that the situation will improve in the near future to such an extent that the Legislature will be prepared to curb these powers.[84]

Annexure A

SA POLICE STANDING ORDER 319

(18) Whenever a prisoner is seriously injured or shows signs of serious illness, the district surgeon shall be sent for by the speediest means available and requested to attend, first aid being applied meanwhile.

(19) An entry is to be made in the occurrence book to the effect that the district surgeon has been summoned. If summoned by telephone, the name of the person who took the message is to be reflected. A further entry shall be made in the occurrence book immediately after the prisoner has been treated by the district surgeon.

(20) If the district surgeon is not available, any other medical practitioner may, in serious and urgent cases be called in to attend to the prisoner pending the arrival of the district surgeon. In all such cases entries are also made in the occurrence book as indicated in the preceding subparagraph.

(21) Any instructions given by the district surgeon or medical practitioner called in to act for him shall be carried out without delay. If removal to a hospital other than a gaol hospital or sickbay is ordered, all precautions shall be taken to guard him *en route* and while detained in hospital.

(22) (a) Should a prisoner elect to be examined or treated by his own medical prac-

84 On medical treatment of detainees during a state of emergency, see generally D J M McQuiod-Mason "The Responsibility of Doctors during the State of Emergency" in *Law and Medicine* (eds T W Bennett *et al*, 1988) 65 *et seq*.

titioner, his request shall be acceded to provided the prisoner himself defrays the costs and it does not entail additional expense to the Government.

(b) In order to prevent, as far as possible, the spread of tubercular infection, members are required, whenever circumstances permit other arrangements, not to detain arrested persons suffering from tuberculosis with other persons in police cells.

(c) If the charge against such tuberculotic is of a petty nature, the possibility of warning him for court, or after arrest releasing him on his own recognizances or on bail, should be considered. Should, however, the person fail to appear after having been warned for court or released on his own recognizances, a warrant for his apprehension can of course not be applied for. If the charge is of a serious nature, and he cannot be released on bail, he should if at all possible, be detained in a separate cell.

(d) Tuberculotics, especially Non-Whites, often carry on their persons documents from the Health Department of a local authority indicating that they are receiving treatment for this disease.

(23) At the death or serious illness of a prisoner, his next of kin, if known, must be promptly notified. Unless the body of the deceased is handed over to the next of kin for burial, it shall be disposed of in accordance with Standing Order 225.

Annexure B

STANDING INSTRUCTION TO S A POLICE[85]

Complaints and symptoms of illness ("ongesteldheid") of a detainee

(i) The services of a competent medical practitioner must be obtained forthwith.

(ii) Effect must be given to the instructions of the medical practitioner, but should it be necessary for the detainee to be removed for treatment in a hospital other than a prison hospital and such a removal is regarded as involving a security risk, Head Office must first be consulted.

(iii) The fact of any illness must without delay be reported to Head Office by telex, so that the Minister can be informed if necessary.

(iv) No sick detainee must without Head Office's approval be removed from one city or town to another city or town.

(v) Sick detainees must in regard to sleeping and eating facilities enjoy special attention and must be visited more often than in normal circumstances.

(vi) Save in exceptional cases, for instance where disclosure of the fact of detention of a terrorist will harm the investigation, the nearest blood relation ("bloedverwant") or relation by marriage ("aanverwant") must be notified of such a condition of illness which in any way may be regarded as serious. Visits to the sick detainee must, however, not be permitted without permission having been granted by Head Office.

Adapted from a paper presented at the Conference on Detention and Security Legislation *held at the University of Natal, Durban, in September 1982, and first published in (1983) 7* SACC 20. *That paper in turn was to some extent based upon my contribution entitled "Clinical Independence of the Doctor in the Treatment of Prisoners: A Critical Survey of our Law" in* Fiat Iustitia: Essays in Memory of Oliver Deneys Schreiner *(1983, ed Ellison Kahn). Publication in this form is by kind courtesy of Professor Kahn and the editor of* SACC.

85 The Standing Instruction was made available to me in Afrikaans. The translation is mine.

75 Medical care of prisoners and detainees

REPORT OF THE AD HOC COMMITTEE OF THE MEDICAL ASSOCIATION OF SOUTH AFRICA TO INSTITUTE AN INQUIRY INTO THE MEDICAL CARE OF PRISONERS AND DETAINEES.[1]

1. Appointment of Ad Hoc Committee

1.1 At its meeting held during May 1982 the Federal Council of the Medical Association of South Africa adopted the following resolution: "MASA notes with concern reports of apparent deficiencies in the medical care of detainees. To date no verifiable information has been provided by interested parties at this meeting. In order to clarify this unsatisfactory state of affairs, Federal Council supports the requests of the Full-Time District Surgeons' Group, the Natal Coastal Branch and the Southern Transvaal Branch that an inquiry be instituted under the Parliamentary Committee into these aspects, with the power to co-opt the necessary expertise as it sees fit and using as a guideline the recommendations which have been laid down by the American Medical Association on medical care in prisons, the Declaration of Tokyo and the recommendations of the Full-Time District Surgeons' Group on this matter."

The Ad Hoc Committee was subsequently appointed by the Federal Council of the Medical Association of South Africa with the following terms of reference:

1.1.1 to institute an inquiry into all aspects of the medical care of prisoners and detainees, including the possible psychological effects of solitary confinement or any other form of deprivation;
1.1.2 to make recommendations as to the minimum standards for health services and care in prisons and places of detention; and
1.1.3 further to recommend guidelines in order to promote preventive health care in respect of prisoners and detainees.

1.2 The Committee consisted of the following persons: Professor S A Strauss, professor of law, University of South Africa, advocate of the Supreme Court of South Africa (chairman); Professor J N de Klerk, chairman of the Federal Council of the MASA, federal ethical and parliamentary committees of the MASA; Professor N S Louw, vice-chairman of the Federal Council of the MASA, member of federal ethical and parliamentary committees of the MASA; Dr G B Batchelor, federal councillor of the MASA, past president of the Natal coastal branch of the MASA, member of the Parliamentary committee of the MASA; Dr J Gluckman, federal councillor of the MASA, president of the Southern Transvaal branch of the MASA, member of the executive committee of the MASA; Professor J D Loubser, professor of forensic medi-

1 The report was published as a supplement to the *SA Medical Journal* of 21 May 1983 and is reproduced here by courtesy of the Federal Council of the MASA. A code for the handling of children in detention, entitled *Children in Places of Detention* was prepared by the SA Paediatric Association for the MASA and published as a supplement to the *SA Medical Journal* of 20 June 1987. Special attention was given therein to the health care of detained children.

cine, University of Pretoria, chief state pathologist, Pretoria; Dr R B Otten, chairman of the Society of Psychiatrists of South Africa.

The Committee was assisted by Dr C E M Viljoen, Secretary-General of the MASA, and Mr A Volschenk, legal adviser of the MASA.

1.3 Shortly after its first meeting which was held on 24 June 1982, the Committee extended an open invitation, which was accorded wide publicity in the media, to all interested persons or bodies to make representations to it regarding the issues which were being investigated by the Committee. Invitations were also extended individually to a number of bodies and persons. A considerable number of bodies and individuals responded to this invitation by making submissions and representations to the Committee, both in writing and verbally. The comments of State departments and the South African Society of Full-Time District Surgeons and Forensic Pathologists were also obtained.

1.4 Over and above these submissions, the Committee also studied in depth large numbers of reports, publications, articles and documents relevant to the subjects being investigated.

1.5 The Committee met on five occasions since its appointment, viz on 24 June 1982, 28 October 1982, 9 February 1983, 18 March 1983 and 21 April 1983. At these meetings various aspects of the matters to be investigated were deliberated on, verbal evidence of individuals and persons representing different bodies was heard and the draft reports were discussed before the final draft report was submitted to the Executive Committee of the Medical Association of South Africa for consideration.

2. Lack of legislative safeguards

2.1 A substantial amount of evidence was put before the Committee to the effect that harsh methods of physical as well as psychological coercion were being applied against persons detained under security legislation, particularly by way of isolation of detainees or in the process of interrogation by members of the Police. By the nature of its constitution the Committee was not in a position to establish conclusively the truth or otherwise of many of these allegations.

2.2 Although the Committee has understanding for the task of the Police who must perform a difficult function in maintaining law and order and the security of the State, it must nevertheless be stated on the basis of the evidence put before the Committee that it is the Committee's opinion that there have been cases of serious maltreatment of detainees. There has also been judicial recognition of the fact that a security-law detainee has been assaulted by members of the Police in order to compel him to confess (*S v Mogale* AD, June 1981, unreported, discussed in 1982 *SA Law Journal* 175).

2.3 The Committee is of the opinion that despite certain improvements which were brought about by the Internal Security Act, Act No 74 of 1982, and by the directions subsequently issued by the Minister of Law and Order, there are insufficient safeguards in the existing legislation to ensure that maltreatment of detainees does not occur without those responsible having to account for their actions before a court of law.

2.4 Persuasive evidence has been put before the Committee that where harsh methods are employed in the detention and interrogation of detainees, including isolation and sensory deprivation for relatively lengthy periods of time, this may have extremely serious, and possibly permanent, effects on the mental and physical health of a detainee. To the extent that this occurs in South Africa, it is naturally a matter of serious concern to the medical profession as a whole.

3. Potential health hazards of detention

3.1 The Committee has concluded that the circumstances relating to the detention of security-law detainees in South Africa present potential hazards to their physical and mental health. These hazards exist only to a limited extent in the case of convicted prisoners.

3.2 The potential health hazard for security-law detainees is considerably greater because of the different situation in which they are held. Individuals differ in their susceptibility to factors causing breakdown in mental health. Basic personality stability as well as the degree of commitment to a particular cause, whether religious or political, must be taken into account. The individual has a spectrum of susceptibility to mental breakdown as a result of stress.

3.3 The situation of detention presents a varying degree of deprivation of psychological support mechanisms. The individual detained is left in a state of uncertainty and anxiety for a number of reasons. It would appear that on certain occasions the detainee is not informed of the reasons for his detention. He is furthermore not aware of the time period of detention nor the conditions under which he will be held. The consequent stress is likely to result in a high level of anxiety.

3.4 Although solitary confinement as defined by the Prisons Act, Act No 8 of 1959, and the regulations thereunder is said not to occur in South African centres for detention, isolation is applied in varying degrees. Isolation from family, friends and other persons may continue indefinitely and the detainee would therefore be deprived of his normal interpersonal contact. Contact only with members of the authority detaining the individual is seen as threatening rather than supportive. The district surgeon, as an employee of the State, may also be regarded in this same light by detainees, their relatives and sympathisers and may therefore not be acceptable as offering independent medical treatment, particularly of a psychiatric nature.

3.5 The harmful effects of isolation are accentuated by a situation which results in the deprivation of the sense of reality. If there were deprivation of daylight and excess or diminution in artificial light or sound, deprivation of darkness and normal opportunity for sleep with disturbed biorhythms, abnormal behaviour is likely to result. Hallucinations and delusions have often been found in these circumstances.

3.6 The ability of the detainee to defend himself against mental breakdown is taken from him by the imposition of a state of helplessness. In general it appears that the detainee has no access to a lawyer. He has no recourse to law for what he may see as unjustified detention. Any request for medical and psychiatric treatment or complaint about mistreatment must be addressed to officers of the same authority detaining the individual. It is likely that these officers will be perceived not as supportive but only as representative of that authority.

3.7 Evidence has been received alleging intensive interrogation by teams of interrogators in rotation. The stress exerted by prolonged and continuous interrogation would be increased by the deprivation of any defences and distortions of reality as described above. Physical fatigue such as constant standing would further increase this. Demoralisation would occur in the individual being interrogated by being deprived of normal facilities for ablution and elimination. Helplessness and defencelessness are engendered by being naked, as has been alleged in evidence. This situation combined with the above factors can lead to serious mental breakdown.

3.8 Information gathered from a detainee under conditions outlined above will often result in evidence lacking all reliability and therefore of limited use to the interrogators either for further investigation or legal proceedings. A statement could be made quite contrary to the individual's true belief or knowledge. The above methods of detention would render the detainee susceptible to suggestion with no limit to the potential distortion of information obtained.

3.9 The above conditions of detention could lead to serious mental breakdown. This would occur more particularly in those susceptible. Impulsive and apparently illogical or irrational actions might take place. In this situation the detained individual could commit suicide. It would appear from evidence presented to the Committee that this has in fact happened on several occasions. Serious mental breakdown is likely to result from the application of the above-mentioned conditions of detention and interrogation. It is likely that a percentage of such persons will not recover completely. Therefore if returned to their former situation before detention, even if they are given psychiatric and medical treatment, psychiatric disorder might be lasting.

4. General duty of medical practitioners

4.1 The duties of medical practitioners do not only extend to the treatment of sick or injured patients, but include a duty to practise preventive medicine actively. A system which makes legal provision for indefinite detention of security detainees without adequate judicial safeguards to minimise possible abuse inherently presents a serious health threat to those who fall in the security net.

4.2 There is serious concern in the medical profession that the provisions of medical care of an adequately high standard and conforming to the accepted norms of medical ethics cannot at present be fully guaranteed to detainees because of the absence of appropriate legislation.

5. District surgeons: rights and duties

5.1 Medical care of detainees at present is almost exclusively the responsibility of district surgeons. In the larger centres district surgeons are full-time employees, but medical examination and treatment of detainees and prisoners are only part of the duties of district surgeons; this is also true of part-time district surgeons.

5.2 As the Committee understands the present legal position, district surgeons do not have full clinical independence in the treatment of prisoners and detainees. The Committee finds this situation untenable.

5.3 In so far as district surgeons are involved in the medical care of detainees who may be subjected to harsh methods of detention or interrogation, they (the district surgeons) are regarded by some persons – unjustly, in the opinion of the Committee – as part of the apparatus of indefinite detention operative by virtue of the Internal Security Act. This view of district surgeons would put them in a most unenviable position from a professional ethical point of view, for example in the light of the Hippocratic Oath, the Declaration of Geneva and the Declaration of Tokyo, to which the Medical Association of South Africa subscribes. The Committee therefore envisages a system whereby the medical profession as a whole will become more directly involved in the work done by district surgeons, as is set out below.

5.4 Allegations have been made suggesting that there is a "conspiracy" between the Police on the one hand and district surgeons on the other. The Committee categorically rejects that suggestion. District surgeons generally are fully aware of the responsibilities they have in regard to the medical treatment of prisoners and detainees. In the opinion of the Committee there have been individual and serious instances of dereliction of duty on the part of district surgeons – which the Committee deplores. Fortunately such cases are rare indeed and the Committee believes that in general district surgeons as far as possible are performing their duties in regard to the medical care of detainees to the best of their abilities, with a due sense of responsibility, and in accordance with medical ethics.

5.5 The Committee is fully conscious of the fact that according to common law, detainees are entitled to reasonable medical care as of right and not merely as a privilege. The Committee feels that it is important that all medical personnel that may become involved in the medical treatment of detainees be made aware of this truth at all times. Should a district surgeon experience problems in gaining access to a detainee or in adequately providing medical care to a detainee on account of limitations imposed by members of the Security Police, such district surgeon should immediately report back to his principal, i e either the Department of Health and Welfare or the Provincial Department of Hospital Services, whichever is relevant, as well as to the Peer Review Committee. (See paragraphs 6.7 and 6.8 below.)

5.6 The Committee recommends that a right be given statutorily to district surgeons to have free access, without prior Police authorisation, to a detainee at all times. Such right would guarantee that a district surgeon can give optimal medical care to a detainee and it would further operate as a check against possible irregularities that may take place in regard to detainees. The Committee is further of the opinion that obstruction of a district surgeon in the performance of his duties should be made a criminal offence legislatively. In the event of such obstruction the district surgeon concerned should do whatever is reasonable to secure intervention on the part of the department which employs him. In so doing the district surgeon may expect the full support of the Medical Association of South Africa.

5.7 It has come to the attention of the Committee that there is some uncertainty as to the duty of district surgeons to maintain professional secrecy in relation to detainees to whom he is attending. The Committee is of the opinion that a doctor-patient relationship is established as soon as a district surgeon attends to a detainee professionally. The doctor is therefore bound in principle to maintain professional secrecy. However, the duty to maintain confidentiality is not an absolute one and the doctor is entitled to divulge information to the authority responsible for the health care of the detainee where it is clearly in the interest of the detainee. The doctor must also divulge information when ordered by a court of law to do so.

5.8 There is clearly a duty, both legally and ethically, upon the district surgeon to keep adequate, medically relevant records on the state of health of a detainee examined and treated by him. Should any physical injuries be observed by the district surgeon, these should therefore be duly noted.

5.9 Should it become necessary for a detainee to be transferred from the place where he has been detained originally to another place of detention his full medical record must accompany him.

6. Additional recommended safeguards

6.1 The Committee is of the opinion that in so far as a system of indefinite detention is regarded as necessary by the authorities, a number of safeguards pertaining specifically to medical care must be introduced so as to prevent abuse of the system as far as is possible.

6.2 The Committee feels that a detainee should under no circumstances be kept in prolonged isolation (in any event not exceeding 7 days) in the absence of regular physical and psychiatric assessment. During isolation and interrogation there must be close observation of any psychological reactions in the detainee which may indicate suicidal tendencies, and special care must be exercised to prevent the detainee from committing suicide. Attention should also be given to any complaints of physical illness or injury by detainees.

6.3 When a detainee is interrogated this should be done in circumstances where there are always at least two persons present, with closed-circuit television monitoring. During interrogation there must be no physical torture of the detainee. In this respect the Committee wishes to direct attention to the extensive recommendations regarding the conduct of interrogation made by the Bennett Report, which the Committee endorses (chapters 10, 11 and 12 of the Report of the Committee of Inquiry into Police Interrogation Procedure in Northern Ireland detail these recommendations).

6.4 It is essential that all detainees should within 24 hours – but preferably immediately – after their detention be medically examined. In particular, should a proper psychiatric assessment of the detainee be required, this should be made as soon as reasonably possible. The Committee further wishes to draw attention to the recommendations made in this respect by the above-mentioned Bennett Report (chapter 13 of the report) and by the American Medical Association in Section C of its report on "Standards for Health Services in Jails, July 1979".

6.5 The clinical independence of the district surgeon should be legislatively guaranteed. This should enable the district surgeon to decide upon the medical treatment to be given a detainee or prisoner, when and where the treatment must be given, the involvement of other medical practitioners, conveyance of the detainee to outside facilities, whether or not the detainee should be kept in isolation, etc. The district surgeon is not only entitled, but in fact legally duty bound, to continue treating a detainee until such stage as the district surgeon is of the opinion that the detainee is no longer in need of treatment. The district surgeon's duty to manage the medical care of the detainee should in no way be inhibited. The medical profession cannot participate in any ill-treatment of or irregularities in connection with detainees, nor can it condone such ill-treatment or irregularities (see also the Declaration of Tokyo).

6.6 Should it be requested by a detainee, the opportunity should be created for a medical examination of him by an independent medical practitioner of his own choice and at his own expense. Should the authorities be of the opinion that this may create a security risk, the obvious way of management of the case would be to let the detainee's doctor examine the detainee in the presence of the district surgeon. In this respect the Committee wishes to point out that the Medical Association of South Africa would be prepared, as an alternative, to provide the names of private medical practitioners who would be willing to serve on panels from which the detainee can choose a doctor. In any event, the district surgeon should at all times be entitled to call for a second opinion, which could be that of the detainee's own doctor, another private practitioner or another district surgeon.

6.7 There should be a system of monitoring or "peer review" of the medical treatment given to detainees by district surgeons. This can conceivably take place by means of small standing committees of medical practitioners appointed by bodies such as the Medical Association of South Africa and the Department of Health and Welfare. It may be advisable to appoint to the committee also a senior member of the legal profession, such as a retired judge. The committee should have reasonable access to all detainees and to all reports on the medical examination or treatment of detainees. The committee should be able to liaise with the Inspector of Detainees.

6.8 The Peer Review Committee must have the right to examine a detainee if necessary, to assess the case and to take a statement from him. The committee will then transmit its findings to the Minister of Health and Welfare, the Minister of Law and Order and the Department of Hospital Services, as the case may be, for their consideration and the necessary action as indicated.

6.9 All facilities reasonably required for the proper medical and psychiatric treatment of a detainee should be put at the disposal of district surgeons. The district surgeon should be given the opportunity of examining a detainee in private. In the case of female detainees, there should always be another woman present during the examination.

7. General

7.1 In so far as it is at all possible, the detaining authority should have as a member of its personnel an adequately trained person with a knowledge of psychology or psychiatry.

7.2 Psychiatric treatment of detainees should be the responsibility of psychiatrists, general practitioners with a psychiatric background, psychologists, psychiatric nurses and/or suitably trained occupational therapists.

7.3 The possibility of suicide on the part of detainees is an ever-present risk. This has been the experience not only in South Africa, but in other countries as well. As was mentioned above, security personnel should be specially alerted to this risk.

7.4 Where continuous medical or psychiatric treatment is given to a particular detainee, he should be monitored closely as decided by the medical practitioner concerned. Security personnel should be available immediately or effectively on call.

7.5 At present there is no satisfactory statutory regulation of the medical care of detainees and prisoners. There are some provisions in the Prisons Act and the regulations thereunder, and there are also directives to the Police and prison personnel. In the opinion of the Committee it is of the utmost importance to ensure that the rights of detainees and prisoners and the concomitant duties of Police and prison personnel be set forth statutorily, in a comprehensive form, by way of Parliamentary legislation, or at the very least, a set of proper regulations promulgated under such legislation. Detainees and prisoners should be made aware of their rights, preferably by the regulations being made available to them upon detention or incarceration.

76 Legal questions surrounding hunger-strikes by detainees and prisoners

A discussion of this subject brings a variety of interests to the fore that cannot all be reconciled.

Juristic notions on the inviolability of life have in our legal history not had a constant content. Even before the birth of Christ, Roman law had evolved into a sophisticated system. Homicide was a punishable offence. Yet, the *paterfamilias* was vested with the power of life and death *(ius vitae ac necis)* over those under his control, i e his wife and children, with a few limitations only.[1] Likewise he had the power of life and death over his slaves. Killing another man's slave was punished as injury to property.[2] Free men could tackle each other in the *pancratium* or other duels, and fight to death with impunity.[3]

In Roman-Dutch law these views changed materially under the influence of Christianity. The principle of which the point of departure was already to be found in Roman law,[4] namely that no-one is the master of his own bodily members *(dominus membrorum suorum)* was brought into prominence.[5] Persons who mutilated their own bodies were punished and so were those who attempted to kill themselves. Duels were prohibited in Holland by various edicts.[6]

It is of particular interest to observe how views concerning suicide have changed through the ages. In Roman times suicide, or attempted suicide, attracted no punishment. Marcian, quoted in the Digest,[7] stated that someone who did not experience joy on this earth was free to end his own life. Ulpian, who was probably under the influence of the Stoics, stated that it was permissible for all to perpetrate violence against their own bodies.[8] In Roman-Dutch times, however, attempted suicide became a criminal offence. Even the successful suicide was "punished" by dishonour being inflicted upon his dead body; in some cases, though,[9] suicide was excusable, for example where a person expected that he would die because of unbearable torture.[10]

In South Africa the crime of attempted suicide fell into disuse; rendering assistance to another in committing suicide is nevertheless still punishable.[11] In England, attempted suicide was still punished at the beginning of this century[12] and the offence was only abolished in 1961.[13]

1 R Sohm *Institutes of Roman Law* (translation by J C Ledlie, 3rd ed, 1926) 482.
2 T Mommsen *Römisches Strafrecht* (1899) 616–7.
3 D 9.2.7.4.
4 D 9.2.13.
5 See e g A Matthaeus *De Criminibus* (1644) prol 3.3.
6 See Schorer's notes on Grotius *Inleiding tot de Hollandse Rechtsgeleertheyd* (1631, 1767 ed) 2.1.44, note 60.
7 D 48.21.3.
8 D 15.1.9.7.
9 J Voet *Commentarius ad Pandectas* (1698–1704) 48.21.1.
10 J van der Linden in a note on Voet 9.2.11.
11 *Ex parte die Minister van Justisie: In re S v Grotjohn* 1970 (2) SA 355 (A); *S v Hibbert* 1979 (4) SA 717 (D). See also H Zimmerman 1979 *TSAR* 183.
12 G Williams *The Sanctity of Life and Criminal Law* (1957) 245 *et seq.*
13 By the Suicide Act of 1961 (9 & 10 Eliz 11, c 90). But incitement to commit suicide or assistance to another in committing suicide is still punishable in England.

At first blush it would seem as if this trend is in conflict with the sanctity of human life which in the postwar Western world was given the greatest degree of recognition which it probably has had in the history of mankind, in theory at least. A prime example would be the changing attitudes to capital punishment. At the turn of the century that form of punishment was applied commonly; today, in Western Europe, it is virtually obsolete.

The changing modern attitude to the punishment of attempted suicide is explicable, however, in the light of another important value which came prominently to the fore, namely that of personal autonomy *(selfbeskikkingsbevoegdheid)*. It is perhaps not an altogether modern notion. As I have mentioned, the Romans put a high premium on the personal autonomy of the free citizen. In that respect Roman law displayed an individualistic characteristic.

How far does personal autonomy, the right to dispose over one's own destiny, stretch in the modern Western legal system? Some jurists tend to regard the right as of a fundamental nature, sometimes linked with the concept of privacy, with an almost absolute content. One of the implications of that view is recognition of the so-called "right to die". In a practical context, this notion embraces certain other rights, such as:

- a right to refuse medical treatment, and
- in the case of prisoners, the right to refuse food.

A study of positive law, in particular case law, of the USA and England, nevertheless reveals that the "right to die" is not of an absolute character. In so far as there is a right to die, it is subject to definite qualifications. Thus it is inconceivable that a man who intends committing suicide can obtain a court order allowing him to bring his life to an end unhindered by someone who wants to prevent him from accomplishing his stated aim.[14] Disapproval of suicide is still strong in many societies. It is generally accepted that the conduct of a person such as a policeman – or any other person – who endeavours to prevent a prospective suicide from ending his life, is not only lawful but in fact praiseworthy. Such conduct would accordingly not constitute assault. Juridically the rescuer's act is justified on the basis of necessity.[15]

In the West, the "right to die" has possibly been accorded its greatest measure of recognition in courts upholding the right of a mentally competent adult to refuse medical treatment. Even the latter right is not absolute, though. Thus it has been denied where the interests of another is at stake, e g those of an unborn child or dependants of a person refusing a blood transfusion on religious grounds.[16] In a criminal case[17] in England in 1977 the accused were convicted of manslaughter for failing to fulfil a duty to provide medical assistance to a woman in respect of whom they had assumed a duty of care, even though the deceased herself did not want any medical care.

14 Compare B K Tagawa 20 *American Criminal LR* 569 (1983) at 574: "... although suicide has been decriminalised, the law will not readily recognise it as an independent right". The well-known case (1990) of Dr Kevorkian of Michigan, USA does not go that far. Kevorkian, a retired pathologist, had designed a kind of "suicide machine" for the terminally ill, by means of which a patient could, by pushing a button, inject potassium chloride into his veins through an intravenous drip. The needle was inserted into a patient's arm by Kevorkian and she died within minutes. Kevorkian was subsequently charged with murder but the judge dismissed the charge, saying that it was a matter for the legislature. As R Slovenko 9 *Med Law* 1006 (1990) has observed, Michigan does not have a specific law against "aiding and abetting" suicide. But in a later civil proceeding Kevorkian was permanently barred from using the device (see *The Citizen* 7 February 1991).

15 See J V van der Westhuizen *Noodtoestand as Regverdigingsgrond in die Strafreg* (LLD thesis, Univ of Pretoria (1979)) 609.

16 See 93 ALR 3d 67, 82 *et seq;* A B Roth & R A Wild 23 *St Louis Univ LJ* 329 (1979) 435; H Z Schaub & R S Chabon 1 *Med Law* 273 (1982) 274.

17 *R v Stone* [1977] Q B 354. The case is discussed by P D G Skegg *Law, Ethics and Medicine* (1984) 113.

Even where medical treatment is given to a person against his will, the courts will not necessarily regard that in a serious light. In an English case (*circa* 1954) a woman was awarded damages of one farthing after a surgeon had performed a life-saving hernia operation on her against her will.[18]

In the USA, the right to refusal of medical treatment has been accorded express recognition in case law as well as in statutes, such as state laws on "natural death" whereby conditional recognition was accorded to advance directives, such as the Living Will.[19] But at the same time certain exceptions have been recognised. In some decisions it was held that prisoners were compelled to undergo certain forms of medical treatment.[20] There were also decisions in which it was ordered that prisoners who had gone on a hunger-strike could be compelled to be force-fed; two recent cases were those of *Boyce* (1981)[21] and *White* (1982).[22] I hasten to point out, though, that there have also been American decisions in which the right of a hunger-striking prisoner not to be subjected to force-feeding was recognised, e g that of *Prevatte,* in 1981, in Georgia.[23] The latter decision was justified by the court on the basis of the prisoner's right to privacy. An author such as Tagawa[24] even found justification for hunger-striking in the First Amendment to the American constitution, namely the right of freedom of speech. The refusal to eat, he says, may be regarded as a "communicative act" deserving First Amendment treatment.

If we look towards England, the situation is as follows: At the beginning of this century – in 1909, in the days of the suffragettes – it was held (in *Leigh's* case)[25] that the force-feeding of a prisoner was legally justifiable. To the best of my knowledge that decision has not yet been overruled. The judgment has evoked a good deal of criticism, though. In recent years force-feeding has become highly controversial in England, and academic opinion, in particular, is strongly opposed to it.[26] The general unofficial policy of the authorities appears to be that prisoners are not subjected to force-feeding.[27] As far as I am aware, the British Medical Association has not yet pronounced itself unequivocally on force-feeding. It has ruled, however, that refusal to participate in force-feeding by a doctor who found it repugnant would not be regarded as professional misconduct.[28] In a 1976 publication, Zellick reported that force-feeding had not been officially abolished in English prisons.[29]

From the legal point of view it would be convenient to work with an absolute right of personal autonomy. One could then conclude that forcible feeding together with any form of medical treatment against the will of the patient is simply unlawful and that such conduct amounts to assault – in particular also where the hunger-striker placed an express prohibition on any later medical treatment should his physical condition deteriorate to the point that he becomes confused and incapable of expressing his will. One would then be able to put him into the same category as someone who declines medical treatment because of fear or religious convictions, or who signs the Living Will.

Alas, the situation is not that simple. There are legal and social interests reflecting profound ethical values which militate against an absolute right to die by means of a hunger-strike by a prisoner.

18 G Zellick 1976 *Public Law* 153, 170.
19 See I Kennedy & A Grubb *Medical Law: Text and Materials* (1989) 1117 *et seq.*
20 See R M Veatch *Death, Dying and the Biological Revolution* (1976) 159 *et seq.*
21 *Boyce v Petrovsky* (W D, Mo September 1981) quoted by Tagawa *op cit* 595.
22 *White v Narick* 292 SE 2d 54 (W Va 1982), discussed by Tagawa *op cit* 576.
23 *Zant v Prevatte* 248 Ga 832, 286 SE 2d 715, discussed by Tagawa *op cit* 570.
24 *Op cit,* 583–4.
25 (1909) 26 TLR 139.
26 See the article by Zellick, referred to above. See also Kennedy & Grubb *op cit* 346.
27 Compare Zellick 176.
28 Zellick 159.
29 Zellick 184.

First, such an absolute right would be offensive to many doctors who feel ethically bound by the Hippocratic Oath to preserve and protect human life.

South African positive law also recognises a qualified rescue duty – outlined in the *Ewels* case[30] – which gives expression to the value of human life. The parameters of that duty have not been mapped out in any detail as yet, but admittedly the contrary will of the person in distress cannot be disregarded.[31]

Moreover, our law fully recognises necessity as a ground of justification which entails a right – if not a duty – to rescue. Some jurists (e g Van der Westhuizen) interpret this right in such a fashion that it would entitle a person to save the life of another even if it is against the will of the person rescued.[32] Van der Westhuizen refers specifically to forcible feeding in the case of a patient who is on a hunger-strike; such a person, he says, may be compelled by means of a reasonable amount of force to take nourishment in order that his life be saved or his health protected.[33] This notion also clearly underlies the court rulings in England and the USA that allowed forcible feeding of prisoners, as well as the standpoint of Annas[34] succinctly stated thus: "We restrict the rights of prisoners in many ways. Force feeding them, rather than permitting them to starve themselves to death, is probably one of the most benign."

Then there is also the interest of the State to ensure the enforcement of punishment and the good order in prisons. The relative importance of this interest, which actually reflects two different aspects, should not be exaggerated. It is the subject of controversy. Some jurists simply reject the notion that a sentenced prisoner's life should be saved in order to ensure that he serve his punishment.[35] Yet it is the very purpose of criminal justice and cannot be disregarded. Considerations concerning maintenance of the life of security detainees – persons who have not yet been tried and sentenced – are even more problematic and bring difficult ethical considerations to the fore. In South Africa there is a statutorily defined system of preventive detention.[36] Many reject it as unacceptable. Others regard it as an indispensable instrument for the maintenance of law and order and for ensuring the safety of the State in these turbulent times. It can be argued that the effectiveness of that instrument will be defeated if detainees were to be allowed to starve themselves to death.

Whatever the arguments *pro* and *con* are, it must be stated that it is the declared policy of the South African authorities not to subject prisoners who resort to a hunger-strike by way of protest or for whatever reason to force-feeding.

Quite apart from official policy, the correct legal approach, in my view, is that there is a medical discretion to provide medical treatment to a hunger-striker whose condition has deteriorated to the point that he becomes confused and is unable to express his will; such medical treatment would include the administration of intravenous feeding, where this would be feasible and there is a reasonable prospect that his life may be saved.[37] It must be emphasised that there is a discretion and not a duty. This means that life-saving medical treatment in the case of a prisoner who

30 *Minister van Polisie v Ewels* 1975 (3) SA 590 (A).
31 See my remarks *supra* 25, 31.
32 *Op cit* 609.
33 *Ibid.*
34 G J Annas *Judging Medicine* (1988) 362.
35 E g Tagawa in his article cited above.
36 Internal Security Act 74 of 1982, section 28. The Act also empowers two other forms of detention for State security purposes: detention for interrogation (section 29) and detention of witnesses in order to secure their availability to testify in eventual criminal proceedings (section 31).
37 *Sed contra* the view of the Faculty of Medicine of the University of the Witwatersrand in a position paper adopted in March 1989: "A conscious person's refusal of treatment must be respected into the period of unconsciousness. If, however, a hunger-striker does become mentally incompetent, but has *not* been informed of the consequences whilst conscious and rational, an argument can be made for instituting resuscitative measures." The Faculty felt that the health personnel involved (preferably a senior doctor) must inform a hunger-striker of the health consequences of voluntary total fasting.

has reached that state of confusion will be lawful and will not expose the doctor to a charge of assault. It also means, on the other hand, that failure on the part of a doctor to intervene, will not expose him to a criminal charge of culpable homicide or a civil suit for damages brought by the hunger-striker's dependants in the event of the latter's death.

The policy of the South African authorities in regard to force-feeding is in line with article 5 of the Declaration of Tokyo adopted by the 29th World Medical Assembly in 1975, which applies to doctors:

"Where a prisoner refuses nourishment and is considered by the doctor as capable of forming an unimpaired and rational judgment concerning the consequences of such a voluntary refusal of nourishment, he or she shall not be fed artificially. The decision as to the capacity of the prisoner to form such a judgment should be confirmed by at least one other independent doctor. The consequences of the refusal of nourishment shall be explained by the doctor to the prisoner."

The Tokyo Declaration is of course not a legal document but serves merely as a set of ethical guidelines. As such it commands almost universal respect in the international medical community. Unfortunately the Declaration does not deal *expressis verbis* with the question whether a doctor may or may not provide medical treatment once a hunger-striker's physical or mental state has reached the point where he is no longer capable of rational thought.

Whatever the ethical considerations may be, there is no doubt in my mind, legally speaking, that a doctor would be entitled to administer medical treatment – including intravenous feeding – at that stage. It is true that the law recognises the right of a mentally competent, adult person to refuse medical treatment. Thus in the case of *Phillips v De Klerk* (1983)[38] a South African court recognised the right of a Jehovah's Witness to refuse a blood transfusion. The refusal of medical treatment may even be expressed *ex ante,* that is before medical treatment is actually needed, as is commonly done nowadays by means of the so-called Living Will.

It would be wrong to regard the situation of a prisoner who goes on a serious hunger-strike in the same light as that of a Jehovah's Witness or a signatory of a Living Will. To the extent that there is a legal "right to die" it cannot be regarded as absolute.

The Jehovah's Witness refuses blood on religious grounds, in the knowledge that it may result in his death, but in the fervent belief that the Almighty will come to his rescue and that he will survive. The signatory of the Living Will, again, has no desire to die an early death, but merely makes a statement prohibiting being kept alive by artificial means and "heroic" medical efforts should his physical or mental state, for whatever reason, ever reach the point where there is no resonable expectation of his recovery from extreme physical or mental disability.

Neither the Jehovah's Witness nor the signatory of the Living Will has taken any action which has brought about a state of affairs that will inevitably or may result in his death. The condition of which the former suffers has been brought about by injury or illness, while the latter is usually still in good health when he signs the document.

The hunger-striker on the other hand, has deliberately embarked on a direct course of action which, if continued, will inevitably result in his death. The position of the hunger-striker is therefore more akin to that of suicide.[39] Although the hunger-striker in prison refuses food not with the direct intention of terminating his life, but (usually) to secure his release or to bring about improved conditions of imprisonment, he does so in the full knowledge that he will die if he persists with his behaviour.

38 TPD March 1983 (unreported), discussed *supra* 29.
39 Compare E Bray & M Beukes 22(2) *Codicillus* 52 (October 1981) 53. *Contra* the position paper of Witwatersrand University (see note 37).

That state of mind comes very close to what the law terms *dolus eventualis* ("constructive" or "legal" intent) or even *dolus indirectus* (indirect intent).

The legal consensus appears to be that the action of someone who takes active steps to prevent another person who manifests an intent to take his own life from achieving that objective, is justifiable on the basis of the doctrine of necessity. As I have indicated, far from being censured, the action of a policeman who ventures on to a ledge on the twentieth floor of a building to grab a would-be suicide on the point of jumping to his death, is regarded as praiseworthy. It is unthinkable that the policeman can be criminally charged with assault or sued civilly for damages for saving the life of the plaintiff.

The same considerations ought to apply, in my view, in the case of medical aid being rendered to a prisoner who has been on a hunger-strike and whose condition has deteriorated to the point where he becomes mentally confused or loses consciousness. His personal autonomy has been respected until the stage that he becomes incapable of rational thought, but from that point it becomes a purely medical problem.

What Wynen[40] in commenting on the well-known Bobby Sands case, says may be true, namely that death may already be inevitable and that "the physician who decides to intervene at this point is wasting his time and might even in some cases be bringing the detainee's death closer", but the law cannot be so callous as to require the doctor to stand back and not to endeavour to save the detainee's life or relieve his misery. What doctor will fail to render medical aid to a person who has cut his wrists in a suicide attempt and is bleeding to death?

This paper was first published in Med Law *(1991) and is reproduced here by kind courtesy of the editors of that journal.*

40 A Wynen 32(4) *World Medical Journal* 53 (1985) 54.

PART XVII

Miscellany

77 Child abuse: some legal issues

Some years ago I served as a member of a panel which had been constituted to consider medico-legal problems connected with child abuse. At one of our meetings, the chairman, a paediatrician, addressed the panel and made the following remark: "Which of us has never felt like battering a child?"

Although the silent reaction of some members of the panel might have been, "Speak for yourself!", the rhetorical question posed by the chairman touched on something which is all too true. All parents are potential child abusers.

Normal as a particular set of parents may be in their behaviour in everyday life, a stress situation may develop in which one of them may be unable to restrain himself (or herself) in the manner of physically reacting to a child's irritating behaviour at a given moment. It is important for all parents to be positively aware of this danger and to be on the alert to avoid overreacting in such a situation.

In a way, the syndrome of child abuse may be compared to cancer, alcoholism or insolvency. It always happens to the other chap – never to me. Are we taking adequate measures to make parents, especially young couples who have small children or who plan to have children, positively aware of the ever-present danger of *their* acting excessively violently against small children during a moment of extreme tension?

In commenting on some legal issues concerning child abuse, I can do not better than to quote from an article by George Woodbury:[1]

"Medicine and Law are frequent bedfellows but nowhere does this relationship wreak more havoc than when it comes to the battered child. This event precipitates an interaction between doctor, lawyer, social worker and the law enforcement arm of government. The goal is the common one of the physical and emotional wellbeing of the abused child, and for the maintenance of that state. Several different professional disciplines collide head on in attempting to provide for this common goal, and substantial obstacles must be hurdled."

Having listened to an interdisciplinary debate on the syndrome of child abuse, it occurred to me that we are sometimes at cross-purposes and have not yet sorted out the various objectives at which the individual disciplines strive.

When we use the term "child battering", we have, of course, the tragic phenomenon of repeated assaults in mind and not so much an individual assault. But, as far as the criminal law is concerned – and I intend restricting my comments mainly to that branch of the law, bearing in mind, however, that there are also a number of legal remedies available in administrative law and private law, respectively – even a single assault would be sufficient to put its process into motion.

In our armament of penal-law remedies, there are a number of offences of which a child abuser may be charged, depending on the degree of severity of the assault and its consequences: common assault, assault with the intent to cause grievous bodily harm, assault with the intent to murder, and culpable homicide or murder in the event of the child having died as a result of abuse.

Apart from these common-law crimes, section 50 of the Child Care Act[2] is deserv-

1 G Woodbury "Spare the Rod: A Survey of the Battered Child Syndrome" 1973 *Journal of Forensic Science* 130.

2 Act 74 of 1983. A Bill published in 1991 envisages certain amendments to the Act.

ing of special attention. That section penalises ill-treatment of a child on the part of a parent or guardian or any other person having the custody of the child. Among the acts that may lead to a criminal prosecution are also the abandonment of a child, failure to provide the child with adequate food, clothing, lodging and medical aid.

To what extent should the criminal law be involved in acting against a parent who ill-treats or abuses his child? This question has given rise to a great deal of heated discussion and controversy.

Following almost every case of a successful prosecution of a parent accused of child abuse and almost irrespective of the punishment imposed by the court, there are complaints by letter-writers in the press that the sentence is too lenient.

We can certainly not accuse the Attorney-General and our prosecutors of being lax in bringing criminal prosecutions. Nor can we accuse our courts of being unwilling to mete out punishment to offenders. Our judges and magistrates give very careful consideration to a number of factors before deciding on punishment in a specific case.

I do think, however, that the South African public is inclined to display a somewhat naive belief in the efficaciousness of the criminal sanction. As a man who professes the criminal law, I am of the opinion that that branch of law has definite limitations. In his book entitled *The Limits of the Criminal Sanction,* Packer[3] has demonstrated convincingly that over-emphasis of the criminal sanction can lead to a neglect of alternatives, and, to be more precise, of administrative action that could conceivably be more successful in combating social evils.

A controlled process of decriminalisation can be commendable. In this country we have had limited experiments with decriminalisation (in fields unrelated to child abuse) which proved to be highly successful. I would submit that the time is ripe for consideration to be given to less emphasis being put on the criminal law in combating the problem of child abuse. Other alternatives should be considered.

Elizabeth Trube-Becker[4] put it well by saying that "the doctor must be in charge as long as possible, and the court assume jurisdiction as late as possible" in regard to child abuse, and then only where total failure in a particular case must be conceded. She was referring specifically to the doctor, but her statement would be of equal application to other professionals, such as psychologists and social workers.

We must admit that sympathetic action of an administrative nature on the part of specialists in the behavioural sciences, directed towards the welfare of a problem family may sometimes be more effective than rigorous action on the part of the Police and the criminal courts. The criminal process in this context may be relatively harsh, and the imposition of a penal sanction may merely amount to substitution of one trauma with another. Arresting the offending parent(s), bringing him (them) to trial, convicting and sentencing him (them) may perpetuate the state of discord and disruption in that particular family.

I am of course not advocating total abolition of the criminal sanction in regard to child abuse. Nor am I suggesting that criminals should be pampered. But there is a danger that by involving the criminal process we may encourage a kind of false satisfaction: the social craving for revenge – a perfectly natural desire – has been satisfied and thereby the problem has been solved. That may be far from the truth.

The first and foremost requirement for action of any kind directed towards the protection of the child is that the fact of abuse of a particular child must become known to those persons or agencies which may take urgent and effective remedial action. The doctor will often find himself in a key position here. In cases of gross abuse of children resulting in serious injury to the child, the child will frequently be brought to the doctor first, for treatment, even if the offending parent does try to disguise the cause of the injury.

3 H L Packer *The Limits of the Criminal Sanction* (1968) 251.

4 E Trube-Becker "Zur ärztlichen Schweigepflicht bei Kindesmisshandlung" in *Jus Medicum* (vol 2, 1969) 381 (the translation in the text is mine).

In the USA a duty to report cases of child abuse to welfare bodies has been statutorily imposed in a number of states not only on doctors, but also on persons such as nurses, social workers, teachers and even laboratory technicians, pharmacists, attorneys and a variety of other professionals who, by the nature of their work, may become involved with a problem family, a broken family or a family in the process of breaking up.[5]

Following the American example, a similar reporting duty was introduced into our law by the Child Care Act of 1983,[6] section 42, which provides as follows:

(1) Every dentist, medical practitioner or nurse who examines or attends any child in circumstances giving rise to the suspicion that that child has been ill-treated, or suffers from any injury, single or multiple, the cause of which probably might have been deliberate, or is undernourished, shall immediately in the prescribed manner notify the Regional Director of Health and Welfare of the district in which the child happens to be, of those circumstances.
(2) On receipt of a notification in terms of subsection (1) the said Regional Director of Health and Welfare may issue a warrant in the prescribed form and manner for the removal of the child concerned to a place of safety or a hospital.
(3) The said Regional Director of Health and Welfare shall thereupon arrange that the child and his parents receive such prescribed treatment as the said Regional Director may determine.
(4) This section shall not exclude any other action against or treatment of the parent and his child in terms of this Act.
(5) Any dentist, medical practitioner or nurse who contravenes any provision of this section shall be guilty of an offence.
(6) No legal proceedings shall lie against any dentist, medical practitioner or nurse in respect of any notification given in good faith in accordance with this section.

(It is to be noted that a Bill published early in 1991 envisages amendment of subsection (1) to cover nutritional deficiency disease as well.)

As was the case with the American legislation, the introduction of section 42 was not without controversy. There is evidence of reluctance on the part of some doctors to be burdened with a reporting duty. There is the understandable fear that such a duty may impair the doctor-patient relationship, which is based on strict confidentiality and mutual trust. There is the fear that instead of operating in the interest of a child who has suffered abuse, a duty to report may operate against its interest: the offending parent may become unwilling to take the child to his doctor for treatment, knowing that the next step may very well be his arrest and prosecution.

Whatever may be said in favour of a statutory duty to report, it unquestionably affords no panacea to the problem of child abuse. But doctors must act in accordance with the clear duty embodied in the Child Care Act.

The question has arisen whether the reporting duty applies also to cases of sexual abuse. The answer to that question would depend on the interpretation to be given to subsection (1). There can be no doubt that sexual abuse will often amount to ill-treatment which would justify a doctor to invoke the section, even though it cannot be said that there was any physical injury (the Afrikaans text uses the word "besering") "the cause of which probably might have been deliberate". The Legislature might consider amending the section by incorporating clear guidelines on sexual abuse.

Adapted from a talk delivered at the Golden Jubilee Conference on "Children Today – Citizens Tomorrow", organised by the SA National Council for Child and Family Welfare in Pretoria in October 1974, and first published in the report of the Conference.

5 See R E Helfer & C H Kempe (eds) *The Battered Child* (1968), Appendix C, pp 237 *et seq.*
6 See note 2, *supra.*

78 Medical experimentation involving children

May a child be the subject of lawful medical experimentation? If so, who must give consent? May the parents consent? Must the consent of the child himself be obtained?

Medical experimentation is a controversial subject and the amount of literature generated by it is immense.

The necessity of some experimentation on human beings for the sake of advancement of medical science is recognised, and what is also conceded, is that invariably such experimentation cannot only involve mature and sane adults, but should in appropriate circumstances include children and mentally subnormal persons.

Yet Nuremberg still casts a gloom on any discussion of human experimentation. In 1976 Wecht[1] caustically observed that "the medical scientist naturally turns to 'captive' groups whose availability can be controlled". In strong terms he condemned American instances of experimentation upon children which had not been conducted in conformity with minimal legal safeguards.

The earlier ethical codes on human experimentation were silent on the use of children as medical guinea-pigs. These codes include the Nuremberg Code, the Helsinki Declaration and the 1979 Code of the SA Medical Research Council. In 1975 the Helsinki Declaration was amended, however, to embody a specific reference to minor subjects, in which case "permission from the responsible relative replaces that of the subject in accordance with national legislation". The Declaration was again amended by the World Medical Assembly in 1983 to insert the following addition: "Wherever the minor child is in fact able to give a consent, [his] consent must be obtained in addition to the consent of [his] legal guardian." The Declaration's section on Non-Therapeutic Biomedical Research still contains no reference to minor subjects, however. In 1983, the American Department of Health and Human Services issued regulations governing experimentation on children where "no greater than minimal risk ... is presented".[2] The revised Code[3] of the SA Medical Research Council of 1987 indicates that experimentation involving children may be ethically justifiable within very narrow parameters; because a subject under 14 years of age is unlikely to be mature enough for the purpose of informed consent, it is generally inadvisable "to carry out any but the most simple procedure on children under this age".

As far as is known, the subject of human experimentation has not been legislated upon *in extenso* in any of the major Western countries, although legislation on clinical trials with medicines is found in a number of countries, including South Africa.[4] The

1 C H Wecht "Human Experimentation and Clinical Investigation – Legal and Ethical Considerations" in 1976 *Legal Medicine Annual* 299 at 307.

2 See J M Burchell "Experimentation on Children" in G C Oosthuizen *et al* (eds) *Attitudes to Clinical Experimentation in South Africa* (1985) 94, at 102. Compare J M Burchell "Experimentation on Human Subjects" in T W Bennett *et al* (eds) *Law and Medicine* (1988) 216 at 222.

3 *Ethical Considerations in Medical Research: Revised Edition,* 1987, 28.

4 In terms of the Medicines and Related Substances Control Act 101 of 1965 section 14 no person may sell any medicine which is subject to registration in terms of a resolution of the Medicines Control Council (MCC) unless it is registered. In terms of section 15 formal application must be made for registration and the MCC may undertake an investigation or inquiry. The MCC will evaluate the researcher's protocol for clinical trials prior to its implementation. The application for registration must contain details of clinical studies (see General Regulation 15 and Annexure 15).

American Code of Federal Regulations[5] contains provisions regulating institutional review boards; in the Code criteria for approval of research involving human subjects have been embodied, as well as general requirements for informed consent. Additional procedures for special populations that are considered especially vulnerable to exploitation are also included in the regulations;[6] in commenting on these Annas *et al* [7] have observed that "[i]ronically, the children's regulations permit research on them that would not be permitted on adults".

Case law concerning clinical trials is scant.

In the USA, the US Supreme Court in 1944 in the case of *Prince,*[8] made the general statement that "parents may be free to become martyrs themselves, but it does not follow that they are free in identical circumstances to make martyrs of their children before they reach the age of full and legal discretion when they can make that choice for themselves".

The 1941 *Bonner*[9] case in the USA is sometimes quoted in defence of experimentation without consent, but as Wecht[10] has pointed out, the circumstances and facts were very peculiar and special for that case. The case concerned a 15-year-old boy who was apparently "conned" by an aunt into going to a hospital to give transplants for his cousin, who had been burned. The court's decision is inconclusive, however, as far as the general issues of experimentation on children are concerned.

In 1973 a paediatric allergist submitted a research protocol to the University of California, outlining a five-year prospective study of children through the first few years of life to define certain markers of allergy development. A lawyer, who was a member of the University's Committee on Human Experimentation, approached the court for a preliminary injunction, on the ground that parents have a duty to do only beneficial things to their children. The court denied his application in 1973, and again in 1975, and as was reported by Furlow,[11] the case – known as *Nielsen v Regents of the University of California* – "died" under California law in 1978.

The South African jurist would reason inferentially, on the basis of common law, that child experimentation is legally justified within narrow limits.

We have had judicial pronouncements in this country to the effect that a parent is justified to assume on behalf of his child socially acceptable risks, thereby depriving the child of an eventual action for damages in respect of injuries ultimately suffered. Thus it was said in *Venter's* case (1936)[12] that no liability would rest on the owner of a tramcar if a parent wished to put his small child on the tram, and the conductor then pointed out to the parent that he could not look after the child and that he might fall off the tram. (This *dictum* was echoed in the case of *Eggeling* (1958).[13])

Although these *dicta* have been criticised[14] and as yet have not been endorsed by the Appellate Division, we may accept them as the basis of our law in so far as voluntary assumption of risk is concerned. Presumably the parent in the tramcar situation has acted with the motive of promoting the interest of the child.

On the strength of these *dicta* it can be argued that a parent who knowingly exposes his child to the risks of a medical experiment, in the interest of the child himself

5 G J Annas *et al* (eds) *American Health Law* (1990) 626.
6 *Ibid* 629.
7 *Ibid.*
8 *Prince v Massachusetts* 321 US 158, quoted by Wecht *op cit* 302.
9 *Bonner v Moran* 126 F2d 121, DC Cir 1941, quoted by Wecht *op cit* 302.
10 *Op cit* 302.
11 T G Furlow "Consent for Minors to Participate in Nontherapeutic Research" 1980 *Legal Medicine* 261.
12 *Johannesburg City Council v Venter* 1936 TPD 287. See also *Adams v Uys* (1929) 14 P H J26 (C).
13 *Eggeling and Another v Law Union and Rock Insurance Co Ltd* 1958 (3) SA 592 (D).
14 S A Strauss *Toestemming tot Benadeling as Verweer in die Strafreg en die Deliktereg* (LLD thesis, Univ of South Africa, 1961) 190.

– as opposed to the interest of children generally – is acting lawfully, and that he cannot hold the medical scientist liable for any adverse reaction.

The aspect of the child's personal interest must be stressed. In the words of one of our most famous judges, Mr Justice "Toon" van den Heever, "tutelage developed from a lucrative perquisite to an altruistic duty".[15] Hahlo and Kahn[16] are correct in saying that "the purpose and function of the parental power is not the aggrandisement of the father, but the protection of the child against the pitfalls of an adult world".[17]

What Wecht[18] has said in an American context is equally true of South African law: "I as a parent, cannot say to my neighbour or friend, take one of my children and if you wish to do something that is not going to be beneficial to him, go ahead and do it anyway because I, the parent, give you permission."

In my opinion, responsible medical experimentation resting on sound scientific hypotheses and of a therapeutic nature in the direct potential interest of the subject himself, is lawful, provided that the necessary informed consent has been obtained. In the case of a minor who is 18 years or older, he himself can independently consent. If the child is below that age, parental consent is required.[19] In all cases it would be advisable to obtain consent in writing.

What is the position in regard to non-therapeutic research, i e where the objective with the experiment is not to cure that particular child? Smit[20] has argued that non-therapeutic experimentation on a child under the age of medical consent (in South Africa it is 18 years[21]) involving the risk of harm, cannot be legally justified, even if the parents have consented. He is of the opinion, however, that the 18-year-old (and older) may be the subject of a non-therapeutic experiment if both he and his parents have consented, provided the experiment does not entail a substantial risk to his life or health. Smit adds the rider that where suitable adult subjects are available, a non-therapeutic experiment on minors cannot be justified.

Burchell,[22] on the other hand, maintains that non-therapeutic medical research on children would be justified where there is firm medical and ethical support for the research which promises important new knowledge of benefit to science and to mankind and where only negligible risk of harm to the child is involved. In my respectful opinion this is a manifestly reasonable position. As Deutsch[23] has pointed out, there are many diseases to which children are susceptible, and their diagnosis and treatment can be furthered by way of experiments. However, children should not be the subject of experimentation where adults could be used. Experimentation on children should therefore be limited to maladies typically suffered by children.

It has been suggested that non-therapeutic experimentation on a juvenile subject could be in the interest of the child in the sense that he might later have the "satisfaction" or "reward" of participation in medical progress, but the consensus of opinion seems to reject such indirect interest as being too remote to justify the experi-

15 *Landman v Mienie* 1944 OPD 59 at 66.

16 H R Hahlo & Ellison Kahn *The Union of South Africa: The Development of its Laws and Constitution* (1960) 367.

17 Compare the remarks by Lord Fraser of Tullybelton in *Gillick v West Norfolk and Wisbech Area Health Authority and another* [1985] 3 All ER 402 (HL), 410c: "[P]arental rights to control a child do not exist for the benefit of the parent. They exist for the benefit of the child and they are justified only in so far as they enable the parent to perform his duties towards the child ..."

18 *Op cit* 302.

19 As I have mentioned above 7, a 1991 Bill envisages that the age of medical consent to medical *treatment* be lowered to 14.

20 (1977) 51 *S Afr Med J* 156.

21 But see note 19 above.

22 (1978) 95 *SALJ* 193. See also the first paper by Burchell quoted in note 2, *supra*. In his paper Professor Burchell commented also on the legality of experimentation on human foetuses; the criterion, in his opinion, is the same as for experimentation on children.

23 E Deutsch *Arztrecht und Arzneimittelrecht* (1983) 228.

ment. However, this objection certainly does not militate against non-therapeutic research involving a negligible risk only.

Where non-therapeutic experimentation is undertaken on a minor, the consent of a parent should be obtained even if the minor is 18 years of age or older.

79 Presence of "outsiders" at post mortem examination, and disclosure of findings

Who may be present at a medico-legal *post mortem* examination conducted by a State pathologist or district surgeon and on what conditions? May the pathologist require a colleague to whose presence he has consented, to maintain secrecy in regard to the findings made at such a *post mortem*?

Medico-legal *post mortems* are governed by the Inquests Act[1] as amended. Section 3(5) of the Act provides as follows: "At any [*post mortem*] examination conducted by a medical practitioner ..., no person other than –

(*a*) a policeman; or

(*b*) any other medical practitioner nominated by any person who satisfies the magistrate within whose area of jurisdiction such examination takes place, that he has a substantial and peculiar interest in the issue of the examination,

shall be present without the consent of such magistrate or the medical practitioner conducting the examination."

As I read the section, it lays down a general rule to which two exceptions are made. The general rule is that no person may be present without the consent of the magistrate (within whose area the examination takes place) or the pathologist or district surgeon. The two exceptions to this rule are: (a) a policeman, and (b) the nominated doctor. The latter persons do not require the consent of either the magistrate or the pathologist.

A policeman has an automatic right to attend and so has the "nominee doctor" – all that is required in terms of the section in regard to the latter, is that the magistrate must be satisfied that the person who nominated him, has a "substantial and peculiar interest" as specified. In practice a spouse or close relative of the deceased will ordinarily be able to satisfy the magistrate as to this. Implicit in the section is therefore consideration by the magistrate of an application by a person who alleges to have such an interest, and a finding by the magistrate that he is so "satisfied".

The Act does not give the magistrate any say in the nomination of a doctor, nor does it empower him to grant or refuse consent to that doctor to attend the *post mortem*. It goes without saying, however, that the person with a "substantial and peculiar interest" must identify to the magistrate the doctor whom he has nominated. As Masters and Shapiro[2] have pointed out, where a doctor himself is the interested person, he cannot attend the examination in person and must nominate another doctor, if he so wishes.

The Act does not give the pathologist any say either in the nomination of a doctor by such person, and there is no indication whatsoever in the Act that the pathologist would be entitled to refuse consent to the "nominee doctor" or to impose certain conditions (e g to maintain secrecy) regarding his attendance of the *post mortem*.

If the magistrate or district surgeon were to be held to have the power of "gagging" the "nominee doctor", it would in my opinion defeat the manifest purpose of paragraph (*b*), viz to enable the interested party to acquire information on what is revealed in the course of the *post mortem*. As I see it, the "nominee" is entitled to disclose in-

1 Act 58 of 1959.
2 N C Masters & H A Shapiro *Medical Secrecy* (1966) 33.

formation regarding the *post mortem* to his "principal" (the interested party) or to anyone else, unless the mandate of the principal is that information may be given to no one but himself (the principal).

The "nominee" in my opinion further has an absolute right to attend the *post mortem* and neither the pathologist nor the Police have any authority to refuse him access to the mortuary on the ground that he is there without their consent.

So far I have been dealing with one of the exceptions to the general rule, namely the medical practitioner nominated by an interested party. I now want to deal with the general rule, which makes provision for persons to be present at a *post mortem* with the consent of either the magistrate or the pathologist.

It is clear that a magistrate or pathologist in granting consent to another to be present, need not be satisfied – as is the case with the principal of the "nominee doctor" – that he is a person, or a representative of a person, with a "substantial and peculiar interest" in the issue of the *post mortem*. He may be a complete "outsider". Moreover, there is nothing in the Act to suggest that consent should be restricted to a medical practitioner. A magistrate or pathologist would therefore be entitled to consent to medical or law students or any other person being present.

May the magistrate or pathologist in giving consent impose conditions, e g to require the person desiring to attend, to maintain secrecy? In my opinion this question must be answered in the affirmative. Unlike the "nominee doctor" who is not there on the basis of consent, such person has no absolute right to attend. In the light of general principles of law, there seems to be no reason why the consenting person cannot make his consent subject to conditions, e g the condition that the person concerned should undertake not to disclose information regarding the *post mortem* to anyone. Such an undertaking will be enforceable, if necessary by means of a prohibitory court order (interdict).

The question arises whether the Police – quite apart from the magistrate or pathologist – may restrict the disclosure of information by a person who lawfully attends a *post mortem*, either because he is a "nominee doctor" or because he is there with the consent of the magistrate or pathologist. After all, Government mortuaries where medico-legal *post mortems* are conducted, are under the control and management of the South African Police.

In my view, in answering this question a distinction must here be made between the "nominee doctor" and persons who attend with consent. As I have said, the former clearly has been given by the Act an unconditional right of access to the *post mortem* and therefore to the mortuary. The Police will not be entitled to refuse him access or to impose any condition to his access.[3]

As concerns the other type of person, i e the man who is not a "nominee doctor" and whose presence has been consented to by the magistrate or pathologist, I can see no reason why conditions cannot be attached by the Police to his presence.

The general rule laid down in section 3(5) is negatively phrased, i e that no one may be present at a *post mortem* without the consent of the magistrate or pathologist. That rule can in my opinion not be converted into a "positive" rule that the person to whom such consent has been given, has an unqualified right of access. Whatever right he has acquired in consequence of the consent given, in my opinion will still be subject to the rights of the owner of the premises concerned.

By virtue of its common-law rights as owner of mortuaries, the State may therefore stipulate that a person who enters a mortuary (with the consent of those persons statutorily empowered to consent to such person's presence at a *post mortem*) may not disclose any information regarding the *post mortem* to anyone. The Police, who have legal custody of mortuaries, may exercise that right on behalf of the State.

Would a pathologist or district surgeon be entitled to disclose his findings made

3 Compare H A Shapiro *Medico-Legal Mythology and Other Forensic Contributions* (1975) 89.

in the course of a *post mortem* examination to an insurance company which had an insurance policy on the life of the deceased or to a colleague of his (the pathologist or district surgeon) who might have an academic or scientific interest in the case? I can find nothing in the law to prevent such a disclosure, as long as it is made in good faith and is not made in such circumstances as to amount to prejudicing, influencing or anticipating the proceedings or findings of the judicial officer who holds the inquest (which constitutes an offence in terms of the Inquests Act). It goes without saying that if the pathologist is prevented by his contract of employment from making such disclosures without official authorisation, he should at all times refrain from acting in breach of his contract.

It is to be noted that Special Force Order (General) 5A of 1990 of the South African Police, issued by the Commissioner of Police, contains detailed instructions to the Police regarding Government mortuaries. The Order *inter alia* contains several provisions restricting access to mortuaries and *post mortems* to authorised persons and prohibiting disclosure of *post mortem* reports by policemen to persons other than specified officials (paragraphs 14.1, 14.2, 21). As far as members of the Police are concerned, the Order (paragraph 13.4) restricts presence at a *post mortem* to the mortuary personnel, the investigating officer and police officers on inspection.

80 Patient consults another doctor without informing first doctor

The following questions were put to me: "Dr A has been treating a patient for myocardial infarction. On the fourth day, Dr B is called in by the family without the knowledge of Dr A. On the sixth day, Dr A learns that Dr B was called.

"Is Dr A committed and bound to continue treating the patient – in particular if an emergency were to arise?

"Is Dr B wrong in failing to let Dr A know?

"Dr C was reported to the Medical Council for some reason or other and was found not guilty. Can C sue the complainant?"

My answer is as follows:

The mere fact that a patient who has consulted or is being treated by Dr A goes to Dr B, would in my opinion not constitute a breach of contract towards A. Where a patient consults a doctor he does not by implication enter into an agreement to the effect that the doctor has an "exclusive right" or "monopoly" to treat him.

Even if a patient were to expressly agree with the doctor to that effect, such a condition would in my opinion be contrary to public policy in that it has the effect of limiting the freedom of the patient to obtain proper medical care. (I cannot point to any case law in this context, however.)

Where a patient who is being treated by Dr A, goes to Dr B for a second opinion or for treatment, A would not in my opinion merely on account of that be entitled to refuse to continue treating the patient. Such refusal would constitute a breach of contract and might in certain circumstances conceivably amount to negligence, i e where there would be potential danger to the patient if he were "abandoned" by A. I must add the following qualifications, however:

- If A has completed his treatment of the patient in respect of the condition he was consulted for, the contract between A and the patient has come to an end. A doctor is, generally speaking, not under a legal duty to undertake to treat any patient who requests his attendance, even if he has treated him in the past, unless the past treatment was of a continuing nature. This right of the doctor applies to emergency situations as well, unless there is no other doctor available, the doctor is able to attend to the patient without jeopardising the interest of his other patient, and the first patient's condition is such that he is facing death or a serious physical risk.[1]
- The conduct of the patient in consulting Dr B may in certain circumstances be indicative of the fact that he (the patient) has "abandoned" Dr A – e g where the patient has told someone that he does not intend returning to A. This might conceivably amount to a breach of contract by the patient towards A. However, the mere fact that the patient consulted B should not be interpreted as a repudiation by the patient of his contract with A.
- A doctor who has agreed to treat a patient, may by reasonable notice to the patient withdraw from the case, provided that the doctor has not yet commenced the treatment. Once treatment has commenced, however, the doctor may not do

1 See my remarks *supra* 25 *et seq.*

so, unless the patient makes it impossible for the doctor to carry out the treatment.[2] Improper abandonment of a patient may expose the doctor to an action for damages, either because of breach of contract or on the basis of delict.

A doctor who accepts a patient knowing he is being treated by another doctor, makes himself guilty of unprofessional conduct in contravention of the ethical rule against supersession,[3] for which the offending doctor may be brought to book before the Medical and Dental Council. Superseding another practitioner who is in charge of a case that he has seen, may only take place with his consent or where no other medical assistance is available. Consent may not be unreasonably withheld. A case may also be taken over where the patient has notified the first practitioner that he no longer requires his services.

Where a doctor is charged before the Medical Council for alleged misconduct, and is acquitted, the doctor would not automatically be entitled to take legal action against the complainant. He can only sue the latter if he can formulate a claim within a recognised rubric or legal liability, e g defamation.[4]

It is unethical in terms of the Code of Conduct[5] for a doctor to improperly impede a patient who desires to obtain the opinion of or treatment by another doctor.

2 See S A Strauss & M J Strydom *Die Suid-Afrikaanse Geneeskundige Reg* (1967) 113. Compare I Gordon, R Turner & T W Price *Medical Jurisprudence* (3rd ed, 1957), 78–79.
3 Rule 14, quoted *infra* 453.
4 See my remarks *supra* 381.
5 Rule 14*bis*, quoted *infra* 454.

81 Medical strikes outlawed by Parliament

Until 1978, medical practitioners had not been affected by strike legislation. Industrial strikes in South Africa are governed by the Labour Relations Act.[1] Generally speaking, professional people do not fall under these provisions, which were designed to foster good labour relations in industry and to set up machinery to avoid crippling industrial strikes. Within the narrow limits provided for in these Acts, industrial strike action is recognised as lawful in the Republic. Unlawful labour strikes are prohibited under criminal sanction.

Outside the field of industrial labour, strike action had until 1978 not been unlawful in the sense that it would attract any criminal penalty, unless, of course, the strike was accompanied by an instigation to commit acts of violence or conduct otherwise declared illegal by security legislation such as the Internal Security Act.[2]

Prior to 1978, instigation to strike or participation in a strike, on the part of hospital employees, would ordinarily have amounted to breach of a condition of employment only, which could lead to dismissal, or to a civil action for damages. If the instigator were an outsider, he might have been brought to book by the employer on the ground of "inducement of breach of contract" or of "interference with trade, business or employment", both of which constitute civil wrongs in our common law for which the wrongdoer can be sued for damages, or for which a prohibitory court order (interdict) can be obtained against him by the injured party.

All this was changed by two 1978 acts, viz the Nursing Act[3] and the Medical, Dental and Supplementary Health Service Professions Amendment Act.[4]

It goes without saying that strikes on the part of medical personnel can have extremely serious consequences for public health, hospitals and patients,[5] and could in the dangerous times in which we live conceivably be used as a powerful tool to achieve revolutionary ideals or to bring about political changes. This is undoubtedly the reason why the Legislature in absolute terms outlawed such strikes.

Section 40 of the Nursing Act declares it a punishable offence for any person (whether a nurse or not) to instigate a strike or go-slow strike by nurses (or other categories of professional persons registered in terms of that Act). It is also an offence to incite nurses, etc, to take part in or continue a strike. Finally it is an offence to take part in a strike or in the continuation thereof.

"Strike" and "go-slow strike" are defined in wide terms as inclusive of any action by which the services rendered by a nurse, etc, "are disrupted or are likely to be disrupted".

Upon conviction, the offender may be sentenced to a fine of up to R500 or 12 months' imprisonment, or both.

It is to be noted that where a nurse is convicted of a criminal offence, she may be dealt with by the Nursing Council in terms of its disciplinary powers, if the Council is of the opinion that her conduct constitutes improper or disgraceful conduct. There

1 Act 28 of 1956.
2 Act 74 of 1982, or its predecessor.
3 Act 50 of 1978.
4 Act 52 of 1978.
5 See the remarks of Mr Justice Goldstone quoted above 314.

is a duty on a court to report conduct which on the face of it appears to amount to improper conduct, to the Nursing Council. However, there is no legal duty on the Nursing Council to strike the nurse's name off the roll or to take other disciplinary action against her.

The provisions of the 1978 Medical etc Amendment Act relating to strikes are in some respects less stringent than those of the Nursing Act and in other respects more severe. Section 55A inserted into the 1974 Act, declares it a criminal offence to instigate, incite or participate in, a strike or go-slow strike by doctors "which is intended, or is likely, to disrupt any health services rendered by the State, a provincial administration or a local authority". The reference in the section to the specific intent or result quoted – which will have to be proved by the State in a prosecution – will obviously be more difficult to prove beyond a reasonable doubt than the mere disruption of "services rendered" by nurses, etc, provided for in the Nursing Act.

But the Medical Act is far more drastic when it comes to the result of a conviction. Apart from a somewhat stiffer maximum fine (R1 000), section 55A makes it compulsory for the registrar to remove the name of the offending doctor from the roll. There is no question here of the Medical and Dental Council first attending to the matter and exercising its discretion whether or not to "strike off". It is peremptory for the registrar to act the moment it is proved to him that a medical practitioner has been convicted in terms of the strike clause.

One may well ask whether this provision is not too harsh. In practice, strike action often involves coercion, to a lesser or greater degree, on the part of the instigators. They may make it extremely difficult or even dangerous for unwilling colleagues to refrain from joining the strike. The law recognises various degrees of participation in criminal conduct, and the courts in meting out punishment take full cognisance of these and of mitigating circumstances.

As the law now stands, a doctor will by automatic executive action be struck off the roll irrespective of his own moral culpability or lack thereof. He will lose his professional status to practise, without having been in the position to put the circumstances of his individual case before the Council – even if the court, in convicting him, found that on account of the extenuating factors applying to him, no penalty or merely a suspended sentence was warranted.

It is to be noted that the strike clause in the Medical Act applies in equal measure to all categories of other professionals – e g psychologists and medical technologists – registered in terms of the Act. No machinery was set up for possible reconciliation of any dispute between professionals and a health authority.

Several cases involving hospital strikes have come before our courts. The duties of hospital administrators in handling such strikes are discussed above.[6]

6 See page 314 *et seq.*

82 Company not entitled to run a dispensary in a private clinic

The legal position of a nursing home or private hospital in regard to the keeping of a dispensary on its premises, exclusively for the nursing home and its patients, was the subject of a 1978 decision by the Appeal Court in the case of *Polpark Dispensary (Pty) Ltd v S A Pharmacy Board.*[1]

In this case a holding company owned a subsidiary company which in turn owned a nursing home known as the P Clinic, in a Transvaal town. The directors of the subsidiary company were a medical practitioner, the matron of the clinic and a qualified pharmacist. The last-mentioned was the subsidiary's managing director.

The clinic building provided accommodation for a dispensary, located inside the clinic's administrative section. The scheme envisaged was as follows: The dispensary was to be used by the subsidiary company under the personal supervision and control of its managing director, the pharmacist.

The dispensary would have its own entrance door, marked "private" in bold letters. Neither the patients of the clinic nor the public would have had access to it or would have been allowed to enter it to purchase medicines. It was to be conducted solely and exclusively for the clinic and its patients in this way.

From the dispensary the subsidiary would have supplied the clinic for administration to its patients, with such medicines, drugs, medical and surgical dressings and appliances as were prescribed to them by doctors. The prescriptions would have been made out in the names of and for the particular needs of the individual patients. The prices of the medicaments, i e their cost plus the normal dispensing fee and profit, would, however, have been charged to and been paid by the clinic, which in turn would have recovered them from the patients concerned.

In addition, the subsidiary company would have supplied the clinic with its own medical requirements, i e medicines, dressings, bandages, and other items, which are generally regarded as "ward stock". These would have been kept by the clinic and would in turn have been supplied by it to its patients when needed.

Furthermore, the dispensary would not have sold or offered for sale any of the articles or goods usually traded in by the ordinary retail pharmacist in addition to its dispensing prescribed medicines, such as patent medicines, cosmetics, toiletries, fancy goods and photographic articles.

The subsidiary company owning the clinic sought registration by the Pharmacy Board[2] as a pharmacist. The Pharmacy Act[3], however, provides that a body corporate (such as a company) may not practise as a retail pharmacist, unless it has carried on business as such immediately prior to the commencement of the Act. Since the company was incorporated only after the date of commencement of the Act, the Board refused to register it.

The company unsuccessfully appealed to the Transvaal Supreme Court[4] on the ground that it did not intend carrying on business as a retail pharmacist. On a further appeal to the Appellate Division, the company contended that it would have no deal-

1 1978 (2) SA 816 (A).
2 Now known as the Pharmacy Council.
3 Act 53 of 1974, section 22(1).
4 The decision of the Transvaal court was reported in 1977 (1) SA 115 (T).

ings whatsoever with the patients of the clinic, that all medicines dispensed and supplied by it on prescriptions for patients in the clinic would be sold to the clinic and not to the patients. Accordingly it maintained that there would be no legal or other *nexus* between the subsidiary and the patients in the clinic.

The Pharmacy Board, however, disputed these contentions. It maintained that the medicines to be dispensed on prescriptions for the patients would not be required by the clinic in its own right or for its own purposes. It alleged that the clinic, not being registered as a pharmacist under the Act, was not entitled in law to sell or dispense medicine to the patients, and that its function would merely be to act as vehicle or channel between the company and each patient by means of which the latter obtains the medicines prescribed for him and pays for them; in that way the company would in fact deal with the patients.

The decisive question, the Appeal Court held, was whether or not the scheme envisaged would have amounted to the company "carrying on business as a retail pharmacist". Mr Justice Trollip came to the conclusion that the company would be a retail pharmacist in terms of the Act[5] and held that the Pharmacy Board had correctly refused registration. The judge ruled that an essential factor of "retail" was the selling of commodities in small quantities. He also held that the fact that the company would not have traded in other miscellaneous goods was of no significance. Moreover, selling to the public was not an essential ingredient of a retail trade. In any event, the patients of the clinic to whom the company would have sold the medicines prescribed to them, all came from the public; while in the clinic they could thus be regarded as members of the public.

The Court of Appeal (without definitely deciding the issue) made the observation that "the clinic not being a registered pharmacist or medical practitioner, is possibly not lawfully entitled to dispense or sell prescribed medicines to patients". The Pharmacy Act[6] does, however, allow the keeping of medicines and its supply to patients in hospitals under the direction of a doctor or nurse. The judge said this provision may refer only to ward stock.

The decision does not affect the right of a doctor or dentist to personally compound or dispense medicines prescribed by himself (or his partner, professional assistant or *locum tenens*).[7]

5 Section 22(1) (*e*).
6 Section 29(3) (*c*).
7 In terms of the Medical, Dental and Supplementary Health Service Professions Act 56 of 1974, section 52, as amended in 1984.

83 Giving expert evidence in court: is the doctor entitled to be remunerated?

By the nature of his profession a doctor is frequently called upon to testify as an expert witness in court in civil matters as well as in criminal cases. Doing so can cause him a considerable loss of time and inconvenience. Apart from exceptional instances, evidence in trial cases must be given *viva voce* (orally) and the witness must therefore attend in person.

Testifying in court can inconvenience the doctor in his practice. Apart from examining the patient, a report or reports must be compiled in which great precision must be exercised. It may be necessary to examine the patient on several occasions over a period of time.

Unpredictable

In order to give expert evidence satisfactorily, the doctor must frequently prepare himself for a particular case. It may be necessary to undertake a profound study of literature on the scientific and technical aspects which may present themselves in the case.

Almost invariably it would be advisable for the legal representatives of the party calling the doctor as witness to consult with him before the commencement of the trial. It may be necessary for the doctor to convey patiently and carefully to the litigant's attorney and counsel the finer points of his specialised knowledge of the subject. All these things take time.

Finally there is the trial itself. By its very nature our adversary system can be time-consuming. Each party is entitled to cross-examine his opponent's witnesses. Although an experienced attorney or advocate may give the expert witness some indication of how long he will be expected to be in the witness-box, court trials often take an unpredictable course. The medical issues may constitute the vital issues of the case, and to canvass them fully by way of question-and-answer may be a matter of days rather than of mere hours hoped for.

Can a doctor who gives expert evidence in a trial claim remuneration in respect of his services, loss of time, loss of income, preparatory work and the time actually spent in the witness-box?

Alas, the doctor is immediately confronted by a basic legal principle, which was expressly confirmed by our Appeal Court in *Van Aswegen v Lombard,*[1] viz that an agreement between a party to a lawsuit and a witness in terms of which the latter will be compensated for giving evidence is *contra bonos mores* (against the public morals, or contrary to public policy) and therefore, null and void.

Official tariff

A witness is entitled to payment of the fees laid down in the official tariff only. True, the Criminal Procedure Act[2] provides that the Minister of Justice may prescribe dif-

1 1965 (3) SA 613 (A).
2 Act 51 of 1977, section 191.

ferent tariffs for witnesses "according to their several callings, occupations or stations in life" and according also to the distances they must travel in order to attend the trial.

It is not proposed to set out here the different tariffs of witness fees as laid down in the official regulations. Suffice it to draw attention to the fact that these tariffs are largely nominal and bear no relationship to the value of a doctor's services or the loss of income brought about by his testifying in a trial.

Thus the tariff of fees payable to expert State witnesses in criminal cases was laid down in 1986[3] as follows: R33 for each 24 hours or part thereof for which the witness is away from his place of residence or place of work. If the witness has to hire accommodation for the night, a maximum allowance of R53 is payable to him in respect thereof. In respect of income forfeited the witness may, in addition to these fees, claim an allowance on production of satisfactory proof, to a maximum of R110 a day.

The point of departure of our law simply is that it is the duty of every citizen who can give relevant evidence in a court case, to do so gratuitously. He is entitled to receive the official fees only in respect of travel and subsistence. This principle applies without regard to persons.

As far as expert witnesses are concerned, and in particular medical practitioners in private practice, the principle must be qualified in four respects.

Examination and report

In the first place a doctor can be called as a witness only if he did in fact attend to a patient and the medical particulars of the patient thus came to his attention. It goes without saying that he cannot simply be subpoenaed "off the street" to come and testify on medical facts pertaining to a person on whom he has never set eyes.

Secondly, a doctor is of course entitled to charge a patient the usual fees for medical examination and the compilation of a report. The only requirement is that the fees must be reasonable. Should the patient feel that the fees are exorbitant he can apply to the Medical and Dental Council for a determination (in terms of the Medical, Dental and Supplementary Health Service Professions Act).[4]

Thirdly, there is the right of the doctor to charge a so-called qualifying fee. Our law makes it clear that a professional man who is requested to give expert evidence, is entitled to be remunerated for preparing himself to testify. The amount of his fee is a matter of agreement between himself and the litigant who wishes to call him as a witness.

Once a professional witness has qualified himself, and is in possession of facts which it is necessary to know for the purposes of the administration of justice, he is bound to attend in the witness-box and give his evidence. He is not entitled to say: "I must be specially paid for further attendance, and until I am so paid I refuse to give professional evidence." He must in the interests of the administration of justice depose both as to facts and as to the opinion which he has qualified himself to give.[5]

Loss of income

Lastly, there is the matter of an agreement to compensate an expert who *cannot* be compelled by way of subpoena to give opinion evidence, for a *bona fide* loss of income and expenses. The Appellate Division has held that such an agreement is legally valid.

All these aspects are well illustrated by the *Van Aswegen* case to which I have already made reference. In this case the plaintiff as a result of persistent pains suffered by him in consequence of a head injury sustained during an assault, consulted Dr L,

3 GN R526 of 21/3/1986 *GG* 10152. The tariff is still applicable at the time of writing (February 1991).
4 Act 56 of 1974, section 53.
5 *Poser v Pettit,* unreported, quoted in *Marais v Pilkington* 1905 TS 650 at 653.

a neurosurgeon of Pretoria. Twice he was examined by the doctor, who also compiled a complete report. The patient paid the doctor for these services.

Afterwards the patient instituted action for damages in the Supreme Court in Bloemfontein against his alleged assailant. A short while before the trial Dr L was told that his evidence would be required in court. Dr L was unwilling to testify, but after repeated requests ultimately did agree to travel to Bloemfontein, on the understanding that his expenses would be paid. (The patient was a wealthy man.) However, the doctor was never served with a formal subpoena.

In between his normal professional duties the doctor spent several days reading up professionally in order to prepare himself to give expert evidence in court. A day before the trial he travelled to Bloemfontein by car.

Reasonable amount

The trial itself did not last very long. Dr L testified in the course of the morning session and was for a short while in the witness-box also in the afternoon. Later in the afternoon the case was settled and early the next morning Dr L arrived back in Pretoria.

Afterwards he sued the patient for R500 in respect of a consultation which he had had with the patient's counsel, his preparation for giving evidence and the actual testifying in court. The trial judge held that R500 was a reasonable amount of compensation in the circumstances, but on appeal the amount was decreased to R300.

The patient did not prove that Dr L could have been compelled by way of a subpoena to go to Bloemfontein. The Appeal Court held that in the circumstances the doctor was entitled to reasonable remuneration for the following: travelling and accommodation expenses (R60); preparatory work in the form of reading up and exchanging professional ideas (R40); examining the patient before the trial (R20); consulting with counsel (R30); loss of income on account of absence from Pretoria (R150).

It should be borne in mind that the case was decided in 1965. Considering the inflationary trend of the rand, a court would probably have awarded the doctor more than ten times that amount today.

An ironic footnote to the *Van Aswegen* case is that the patient in actual fact won his appeal against the trial court's judgment. The Appeal Court ordered the doctor to pay the costs for the appeal – which must have been much more than the R300 ultimately awarded to him.

84 Inquests and the doctor

How you as a doctor will become involved

A medical practitioner or hospital doctor may become involved in an inquest either because he was the last doctor to attend to the deceased immediately before his death, or because the deceased was treated by him as a patient at some stage, weeks or months before his death.

The Inquests Act[1] requires anyone (this includes a doctor or a nurse) who believes that another person has died from unnatural causes, to report accordingly to a policeman as soon as possible, unless he or she has reason to believe that someone else has already made – or will make – the report. A magistrate will then ordinarily request the State pathologist or a district surgeon to perform a *post mortem* examination.

In due course, if no criminal prosecution is instituted against someone in consequence of the death, an inquest will be conducted by a magistrate or judge. He will have before him the *post mortem* report and other documentation relevant to the death inquired into. In the overwhelming majority of cases, the inquest is of an informal nature and not held in open court. The judicial officer will peruse the documents and no oral evidence is given. If oral evidence is adduced, however, the inquest is ordinarily held in public. Some formal inquests held in South Africa have become *causes célèbres.* Where there is conflicting affidavit evidence, the inquest court will tend to insist on oral evidence being adduced.[2]

Duties of the judicial officer

The judicial officer must make the following findings, if possible:

- ❑ the identity of the deceased;
- ❑ the cause or likely cause of death;
- ❑ the date of the death;
- ❑ whether the death was brought about by an act or omission involving an offence on the part of any person.

If the magistrate or judge makes a positive finding on the last-mentioned of these aspects, he must submit the inquest record to the Attorney-General.

Medical reports for inquest court

You, as a doctor, who attended to a person whose death has become the subject of an inquest, may be called upon to compile a medical report. There are two possibilities:

- ❑ You may be approached by the Police or some other interested party, such as a hospital superintendent or relative of the deceased, for a statement or to provide certain information (e g patient records).

1 Act 58 of 1959.
2 *De'Ath (substituted by Tiley) v Additional Magistrate, Cape Town* 1988 (4) SA 763 (C); 1990 (2) SA 899 (A).

- ❑ You may in exceptional circumstances be subpoenaed by order of the judicial officer to give evidence at the inquest or to produce any specified document(s).

If you are merely requested to make a statement, you must bear in mind that there is no legal obligation to comply. In fact, SA Medical and Dental Council Rule 9 (professional secrecy) forbids the disclosure by a doctor of medical particulars relating to a deceased patient, unless it is with the consent of his next of kin or the executor of his estate.

If you are subpoenaed, however, you may not refuse to comply with the subpoena and to testify at the inquest.

If you are employed by a hospital you should forthwith inform your superintendent of any request to make a statement or of a subpoena to testify.

It may be highly advisable to seek legal advice in preparing a statement for the purposes of an inquest. Any member of a medical protection society may approach the society for advice about the preparation of such a statement.

As the medical attendant of the deceased (this is the usual role in which you are involved) you should give a factual, narrative account of looking after the now-deceased patient, with the dates of attendance, a concise history of the patient's condition, findings on examination, investigations, treatment, and a report on progress leading up to the death. The report should be signed with your name, qualifications and status.

Hearsay evidence: adhere to what is written

There is no absolute need to avoid all hearsay evidence, as would be the case in a criminal prosecution. The judicial officer who presides at the inquest has considerable discretion over what to accept or omit as evidence. It is, however, wise to make plain that which is hearsay and that which was obtained with your own senses, by writing: "I was told that the patient had fallen ..." and not: "The patient fell ..." The former makes plain that you did not personally witness the fall: the latter implies that you did. Never include in a written report anything which you are not prepared to adhere to when appearing in the witness-box, in open court, or on oath.

Fact, not opinion

The statement should contain, as with all reports for forensic purposes, a concise, chronological account of the facts. Expressions of opinion, speculation or hypothesis are best avoided, or at least left until verbal, direct questioning at the inquest – unless you are acting as an expert witness, such as a consultant pathologist.

Giving evidence: the importance of the written report

If a formal inquest is held, you take the oath or affirm in the usual way, and are then customarily taken through your prior written report by the public prosecutor or another legal representative – which is why its accuracy is so essential. It should have been prepared in anticipation of appearing in the witness-box to give evidence on oath. You should be in a position to stand by what was written in the statement – thus the need to prepare it with care and to keep a copy of it. To vacillate or retract written evidence is embarrassing for you and exasperating for the judicial officer and any legal representative; it may also have serious ethical implications.

Legal representation at inquests

At an inquest there may be legal representation of the interested parties involved, usually on behalf of the family in a case of death on the roads or in an industrial accident, or where the family alleges neglect by the hospital and its staff. The hospital or employer may also be legally represented.

Legal representation for the doctor

It is usually not necessary for doctors to be legally represented at inquests because the decision to hold an inquest, even in the case of a death in hospital, does not necessarily imply that the medical management is to be criticised. Unnecessary legal representation may arouse suspicion that a doctor has something to fear or conceal, which is seldom the case. However, if the death has any features or allegations of medical negligence, you as a member of a medical protection society will (or should) already have contacted the society for advice and help – preferably before writing your statement, as well as before attending the inquest. In appropriate circumstances legal representation may be arranged for individuals or groups of doctors who are called to give evidence.

The questions must be answered

At an inquest, and indeed in any court, you will be required to give straight answers to questions and you should not evade or conceal issues. However, you are not required to incriminate yourself; where legal representation is considered necessary, the lawyer (arranged by the protection society) will carefully guard your interests as far as he properly can, and will object to any improper questions.

Be fair but firm: avoid evasion and dithering

If you have taken adequate care in what you have written, giving oral evidence from the witness-box should be straightforward. Forethought in your preparation will avoid a humbling and sometimes humiliating experience for you as a professional witness. A factual account of the clinical events should pose no problems if you have been accurate, clear and honest. Evasion and dithering will become transparently obvious in the lonely isolation of the witness-box and will be mercilessly seized upon and exposed by the legal representatives.

Be willing to admit ignorance or inexperience

Do not profess infallibility. If in the course of an inquest, or any other court hearing, you are asked a question to which you do not know the answer, you should not hesitate to say so. You will be readily forgiven ignorance, but you will never be forgiven a concocted answer intended to conceal ignorance, or worse, to conceal the truth. Frank confession of limited experience will be appreciated by all, but an answer given in haste, or any rash or over-interpreted opinions, or statements based on insecure or unsubstantiated supposition, may be mercilessly exposed in cross-examination.[3]

3 Adapted from a publication of the Medical Protection Society; publication in this form is by kind courtesy of the Society. On inquests generally, see also L S Smith "The Inquest as it Relates to Medical Practice" 4 *SA J Cont Med Educ* (Nov 1986) 7.

85 Medical practice in company form

For a number of years now voices have been heard advocating the possibility of medical practice in "corporate" form, i e that doctors for the purpose of practice may form companies with limited liability, registered in terms of the Companies Act.

The traditional pattern of medical practice in South Africa has been either individually or as partners. But from the legal point of view the partnership has decided disadvantages.

Apart from difficulties such as those caused by insolvency of a partner, the partners' liability is unlimited. And because it is not recognised as a legal *persona* or "body corporate", it cannot ensure continuity. Technically a partnership as a whole is automatically dissolved upon the death or insolvency of any partner.

Because of some of the disabilities of the partnership, many doctors today practise in loose "association" form. They enter into agreements whereby certain facilities such as consulting rooms, receptionists and telephone exchanges are shared, but which exclude the sharing of profit and loss. These "room-sharing" agreements have obvious advantages for the doctors concerned.[1]

Doctors who practise in "association" also make occasional use of the formation of a company or companies to possess and control independent assets. Thus fixed property on which consulting rooms are situated can be conveniently owned by a company in which doctors are individual shareholders.

A company offers advantages in regard to matters such as the transfer of shares at the retirement or death of a member of the "association" or their heirs to gain the benefits of the growth of the value of the company assets represented by the shares.

In the past, practice in company form was also regarded as having an advantage from the income-tax point of view in the case of practices yielding large incomes. The reason for this is that companies pay income tax at a flat rate. (It is doubtful whether a tax benefit is possible nowadays, considering the fact that the rate of company tax is now (1991) higher than the maximum marginal rate for individuals.)

However, the provisions of the old Medical, Dental and Pharmacy Act of 1928[2] left no doubt that only "natural" persons could be registered as medical practitioners and that corporate practice would be unlawful. The new Medical, Dental and Supplementary Health Service Professions Act of 1974[3] left the position unchanged.

From time to time the South African Medical and Dental Council was requested to state its views regarding the practice of medicine by bodies corporate. In 1963 it stated as its policy that it was against the practice of medicine and dentistry by incorporated bodies. This policy has been consistently adhered to.

In the 1970s an *ad hoc* committee was appointed by the Council to go into the matter *de novo*. Following recommendations made by the committee, the Council in October 1976 reaffirmed its policy, but resolved that auxiliary services ("hulpdienste")

1 See *supra* 77.
2 Act 13 of 1928.
3 Act 56 of 1974.

could be made available to practitioners by way of companies, subject to the following conditions:[4]

Legislation should be passed to enable the Council to make rules permitting practice in company form and the conditions applying to such practice. The rules envisaged ought to make provision for the following –

The company should be a private company limited by shares and incorporated under the Companies Act. Its articles of association should provide *inter alia* for its directors to be jointly and severally liable for debts incurred by the company. The company statutes should restrict membership of the company to registered doctors (or dentists, as the case may be). Every member will have to be a director of the company. Should a member die or no longer qualify as a member, the rights pertaining to his shares will automatically vest in the remaining directors. Any act by a member or employee of the company on its behalf, constituting improper conduct if performed by a doctor or dentist, will be deemed to be that of every member of the company unless he can prove that he did not knowingly participate in the commission of the act and could not have prevented it. A doctor or dentist will not be entitled to do anything by means of a company which he would otherwise not be entitled to do. The company may not have more than ten members. The company may not charge more for services than would have been charged otherwise.

"Auxiliary services", according to the Council, included:

- facilities regarding space, (e g private hospitals, day clinics and similar facilities where residence on a 24-hour basis is not involved);
- apparatus and instruments needed for diagnostics and/or treatment;
- administrative facilities.

In November 1980 the Council again reaffirmed its policy, in the following terms: "In addition to [the Council's] policy that the practice of medicine and dentistry by incorporated bodies is not permissible, it is recorded that it is permissible to make auxiliary services available to practitioners by way of companies, provided that the practitioners involved therein comply with the ethical rules at all times."[5]

In 1989 it was resolved by the Council that the Minister be requested to introduce legislation into Parliament to make provision for medical practice in corporate form. This request is still under consideration. The position at present (February 1991), therefore, is that medical practice *per se* cannot take place by means of a company with limited liability. Any act which amounts to practising as a medical practitioner as defined in the Medical, Dental and Supplementary Health Service Professions Act, if performed by a company, will therefore constitute a contravention of the Act.

However, there is no legal objection – nor, it is submitted, can there be any ethical objection – against doctors setting up companies to acquire and own facilities such as buildings equipped as consulting rooms or day clinics, laboratories and instruments. It is certainly not illegal for such a company to lease its facilities to other doctors (i e doctors who are not shareholders or directors). Nor would it be illegal if, for example, a pathologist were to have certain tests conducted by a company possessing equipment and keeping a technical staff, the pathologist himself making the diagnosis. It is not the company that makes the diagnosis. The ethics of such a scheme, however, is a matter within the jurisdiction of the Medical and Dental Council.

In conclusion it may be noted that practice in corporate form has now been possible for certain other professional groups, such as attorneys and architects, for a number of years.

4 See the SA Medical and Dental Council's *Kodifikasie van Vorige Besluite insake Etiese Aangeleenthede* vol V (Sept 1970 – Sept 1979) (compiled in the office of the Registrar) at 143. The translation from Afrikaans is mine.

5 Information kindly supplied to me by the office of the Registrar. The translation from Afrikaans is mine.

86 Acts specially pertaining to the medical profession

The "Doctors' Charter", the Medical, Dental and Supplementary Health Service Professions Act of 1974,[1] prohibits unregistered persons from performing for gain, acts specially pertaining to the profession of a medical practitioner. There are of course special and limited statutory exceptions applying to the supplementary health service professions, nurses, dental mechanicians, homoeopaths, etc.

In proscribing "medical" practice by unregistered persons, the provisions of the 1974 Act are even more strict than those contained in Act 13 of 1928 and older legislation.[2] Post-1974 cases illustrate the stern approach of the courts to illegal practice of medicine:

In *S v Van der Merwe*[3] it was held that an unregistered person who practised as "tattoo-remover" contravened the Act because tattoo is a physical defect. (He removed tattoos by means of cauterisation; the "patients" were injected with a local anaesthetic, procaine.)

In *S v Posel*[4] the accused was a highly qualified and leading engineer (BSc (Eng) PhD) who had developed a special interest in bio-engineering with particular emphasis on haemodynamics. He undertook profound research into the mathematical and haemodynamic rationale for drug therapy in the medical clinical instance of septic shock. The accused propounded new theories concerning the manner of use of the ECG machine, the interpretation of the graph produced by it, the drug therapy required to correct malfunctions of the heart and the heart attack itself. He designed highly improved ECG machines and wrote a book on "Heart Attack". For some years he worked in a team which included medical specialists, in a cardiac unit specially created at a hospital to put into experimental practice the accused's theories. The death rate among patients treated in the unit for heart disease was reduced by 12 per cent. The accused was not permitted himself to apply therapy of any kind. Afterwards, however, when the unit was disbanded, the accused himself saw patients whom he diagnosed and then referred to specified parts of his book to study so as to get to know his views on what drugs should be used and in what quantities, etc. The accused charged fees and in some cases received substantial monetary gifts. He claimed that in rendering these services he corrected serious iatrogenic errors, usually with dramatic results, but he was nonetheless convicted of performing acts "specially pertaining". (Note that a doctor who referred a patient to the accused in these circumstances might be guilty of the offence as an accomplice.)

Subsequent to the *Posel* case, the Medical Council made regulations relating to the registration of biomedical engineers as a category of supplementary health service professions, and the conditions under which biomedical engineers may practise their profession.[5] It is to be noted, however, that a biomedical engineer may not com-

1 Act 56 of 1974.
2 For a collection of the older cases, see S A Strauss & M J Strydom *Die Suid-Afrikaanse Geneeskundige Reg* (1967) 93 *et seq.*
3 1977 (3) SA 747 (T).
4 1977 (4) SA 476 (N).
5 Government Notices R451 and R452 of 10 March 1978.

municate a medical diagnosis or therapeutic procedures to a patient, and may prescribe or undertake diagnostic procedures or therapeutic procedures only under the direction and control of a registered medical practitioner.

In *S v Nagel* [6] the court was called upon to decide whether a registered homoeopath who examined, diagnosed and treated a patient – which treatment, among other things involved the drawing of blood – contravened the 1974 Act. The accused was not registered in terms of the Act, but his name appeared on the list of persons entitled to practise under the Homoeopaths, Naturopaths, Osteopaths and Herbalists Act[7] which was then in force.

In his evidence, the homoeopath stated that after having studied, *inter alia*, nature cure, drugless therapy, naturopathy, osteopathy, herbal remedies and psychology in various parts of the world, he had commenced practice in Cape Town. At the time of the trial he had 200 to 300 patients.

He further testified that the withdrawal of small quantities of blood was a well-known and widely practised homoeopathic treatment. It had been part of his training and he had always been accustomed to treat his patients in this manner. He also testified that the other acts of examination, diagnosis and treatment described by G – the police trap who posed as a patient – were all normal incidents of his practice.

At the trial, the district surgeon in his evidence, made the statement that a homoeopath may not make a physical diagnosis. He also stated that the homoeopath contravened the Act by taking G's blood pressure.

However, the court refused to uphold these views. On appeal, Mr Justice Baker ruled that the wide proposition that a homoeopath could not make any physical diagnosis, was incorrect.

Section 6 of the Homoeopaths etc Act specifically provided that the provisions of the Medical Act were not to be construed so as to prohibit "listed" homoeopaths from performing for gain any act usually performed at the commencement of the Homoeopaths Act by any person who pursued any practice and the performance of which by a "listed" homoeopath was not prohibited by the latter Act.

It is to be noted that section 5 of the Homoeopaths etc Act specifically, on the pain of a criminal penalty, prohibited a listed homoeopath *inter alia* from withdrawing blood from any person. In *Nagel's* case, however, the accused was not charged in terms of that section. Section 6 exempted a homoeopath generally from liability *in terms of the Medical Act* for any act usually performed by a homoeopath at the commencement of the Homoeopaths Act. A proper construction of these provisions, it is submitted, would mean that a homoeopath had no defence against a charge of drawing blood *in contravention of section 5.* [8]

In 1982 the Homoeopaths Act was repealed by the Associated Health Service Professions Act[9] which prohibits homoeopaths and other practitioners under the Act from withdrawing intravenous blood samples or analysing human blood.[10]

In *S v Sibanda*[11] the Rhodesian High Court held that physical treatment by an unregistered person, being one of the recognised functions of a doctor, unaccompanied by diagnosis or advice, constitutes an act "specially pertaining". The accused, employed by a doctor to mix and pour medicines, administered an injection after a diagnosis had been made by a doctor. The court refused to follow a 1973 South African

6 1978 (1) SA 363 (C).
7 Act 52 of 1974.
8 Note that section 5 was amended in 1980. Prior to its amendment it prohibited a homoeopath, etc, from withdrawing "blood from any person". The prohibition introduced in 1980 was more specific, namely to "withdraw an intravenous blood sample". As is mentioned in the text, that prohibition was re-enacted in the Associated Health Service Professions Act of 1982.
9 Act 63 of 1982.
10 Section 32 (1) *(a)* (iii).
11 1978 (3) SA 217 (R).

case[12] in which it had been held that treatment without diagnosis did not constitute a contravention. The Rhodesian court further held that an isolated act of administering an injection did not *per se* amount to "practising".

In *S v Aandeweg*[13] it was held that a spinologist who manipulated a person's spine by running his hand up and down it and exerting gentle pressure, did in fact treat a defect or deficiency, but it was not "in relation to a disease or illness, i e not in a medical sense". Accordingly, the court ruled, he had not contravened the Act. It is submitted that such a practice may, however, amount to a contravention of the Associated Health Service Professions Act, which *inter alia* penalises unregistered practice as a chiropractor. But the accused had not been charged under the latter Act.

12 *S v Patel* 1973 (2) SA 208 (NC). This ruling clearly no longer applies in view of the strict statutory provisions subsequently incorporated into Act 56 of 1974, section 36.

13 1986 (1) SA 211 (C).

87 Doctor practising from his home: legal issues

Town-planning requirements

The rapid growth of our cities produced problems for medical practitioners, in particular general practitioners, and their patients. With the construction of skyscrapers in central business districts and the great demand for office accommodation by businessmen and professional people – who by the nature of their occupations want to be in the CBD – rents for office space escalated.

It may be more convenient for the doctor to practise in the CBD, but it does not necessarily suit his patients, many of whom reside kilometres away in the suburbs. For patients, in particular housewives and children, it is often inconvenient to travel to the city centre: there are long distances, travelling costs and eternal parking problems.

These circumstances induced many doctors to move their practices from the CBD to the suburbs. If the doctor moves his practice to a building situated in a business zone, there would ordinarily be no problems. But problems may arise if the doctor plans to practise from his own home or another house which is situated in a residential zone.

In terms of a typical town-planning scheme of a Transvaal city someone who is actually resident in a dwelling is allowed to exercise his profession therein, provided it does not involve any of the following:

- the employment of more than two assistants;
- the public display of goods, e g in a window;
- the erection of a notice or signboard other than that ordinarily used to indicate the profession of the practitioner;
- the necessity to obtain a trading licence in order to exercise the profession in question.

Because a doctor does not require a licence to exercise his calling – and does not exhibit goods! – he may accordingly practise in his home, if, for instance, he employs a single professional assistant, or has a single partner, apart from the receptionist employed for the purposes of the practice.

The town-planning scheme referred to, however, qualifies the right to practise by stipulating that the practitioner's activities may not offend against the attractiveness of the neighbourhood, "of which the city council shall be the sole arbiter". The normal medical practice would certainly not offend in this manner even if a few babies were to cry every day when examined by the doctor!

Practices which have more than two partners are, in terms of the scheme, not allowed to be conducted in a residential house.

The city council of the city to which I have made reference, did not hesitate to take steps to put an end to practices conducted in defiance of its town-planning scheme. At one stage, within a matter of months, it applied for and was granted no fewer than 15 interdicts by the Supreme Court. Naturally enough, that action resulted in expense, inconvenience and embarrassment for the practitioners thus restrained from practising in residential homes.

No practitioner should endeavour to set up practice in a dwelling unless he has first sought legal advice or consulted with the municipal town-planning department.

Note that even if the proposed practice in a residential area would be contrary to the municipal zoning code, city councils are vested with the power of granting, within certain limitations, consent to special use. Such a "consent use" must be formally applied for to the city council. It entails notification, press advertisements, etc, and objections by property owners in the area are to be expected. It is wise to let an attorney handle the application.

I have referred to typical provisions of a town-planning scheme. I hasten to add that the schemes of cities and towns are not uniform and there may be substantial differences. A doctor should ensure that he knows exactly what the provisions are that apply in his town, before setting up practice in a residential house.

The consequences of moving one's practice to a suburb without complying with town-planning requirements were all too apparent in the case of *Stadsraad van Vanderbijlpark v Uys.*[1] In that case a doctor used a dwelling of which he was the owner, for his practice. Neither he, nor anyone else, lived in the house. The town-planning scheme contained provisions comparable to those mentioned above. The doctor did not apply for consent and landed himself in litigation which ended in the Appeal Court – and which must have been very costly. The court held that he was not entitled to practise from the dwelling. In the judgment the following points were made: If a building is at all times used as a place of residence, the objective of the town-planning scheme would be attained, even if an occupation or profession is exercised therein. The dwelling and stand would be characterised by the "usual signs of domestic life" and the character of the suburb would not be spoilt. But if it were to be used exclusively for practice purposes there is a strong possibility that the character of the residence and stand would change materially.

Tax aspects of a surgery at home[2] – *By Lionel Hodes*[3]

A medical practitioner can claim valuable deductions and expenses if he uses his home in his practice and these could reduce his taxable income, and his tax liability substantially.

Section 23 of the Income Tax Act specifically excludes deductions of expenses or cost of repairs in respect of any dwelling house or domestic premises but goes on to make an exception and allow these expenses for any part of the premises used for the purposes of trade. Provided you have set aside a specific area of your house exclusively for your practice, you will be able to claim deductions.

It is not sufficient if you see the odd patient in your study or the playroom. There must be a definite allocation of space solely for the practice.

You then measure the ground area used for your practice and also the whole area of the dwelling. You may claim a proportion of certain expenses *pro rata* to the total area. If your surgery is one-fifth, say, of the total area you can claim one-fifth of the following:

- rent, if this is paid;
- interest, if you own the house and have a mortgage bond over it; note that you cannot deduct the whole amount you are obliged to pay the building society each month, as part of that amount is a reduction of capital;
- rates and taxes, water, electricity and refuse-removal charges;

1 1989 (3) SA 528 (A).
2 This note was first published in 1986 (4) *SA Practice Management* 24, and is reproduced here by kind courtesy of Mr Hodes.
3 BA (Witwatersrand) LLB (SA) H Dip Tax L, H Dip Company Law (Witwatersrand).

- insurance premiums relating to the property or any furniture, etc, in your surgery;
- the remuneration of any cleaner or domestic – and sometimes the local Receiver may even allow part of a gardener's wages; if you are in a sectional title unit you may include a portion of the levy;
- repairs to the part of the dwelling you are using.

If you decide to build on an extra room to your house to use as a surgery, you cannot claim any deduction for that, as it is a capital expense. Nor may you claim any wear and tear allowance for the depreciation of any building or room because the Income Tax Act specifically prohibits any allowance for the depreciation of buildings or other structures or works of a permanent nature.

You can, of course, claim the usual wear and tear allowance for any furniture, medical equipment, etc.

Problems arise with repairs. These are specifically allowed by the Act but renovations are not allowed to be deducted. In many instances it is difficult to distinguish between "repair" and "renovation" and there have been many a tax case to resolve this. The courts have laid down certain principles which are – with respect – not very clear and have emphasised that it is a question of fact in every case and also a matter of degree.

Basically, although repair may involve renewal, it is only the renewal or replacement of a subsidiary part of a whole, while renovation is the renewal or reconstruction of the entirety – meaning by entirety not necessarily the whole but substantially the whole. The fact that in a repair different and possibly better materials than the original are used, does not prevent it being deductible.

Where work consists of both repairs and improvements or reconstruction, only the cost of the repairs are deductible. It is therefore advisable to get your account broken down by the builder, plumber, etc, before claiming.

Maintenance, such as painting and cleaning, is deductible in full.

Annexure

Annexure

THE SOUTH AFRICAN MEDICAL AND DENTAL COUNCIL: RULES OF CONDUCT FOR MEDICAL PRACTITIONERS AND DENTISTS

The Minister of Health and Welfare has, in terms of section 49(2) of the Medical, Dental and Supplementary Health Service Professions Act 56 of 1974, approved the following rules made by the South African Medical and Dental Council under section 49(1) of the Act. The rules were published in Government Notice R2278 of 3 December 1976 and were subsequently amended by Government Notice 884 of 27 May 1977, Government Notice R395 of 27 February 1987 and Government Notice R2543 of 13 November 1987.[1]

Rules specifying the acts or omissions in respect of which the Council may take disciplinary steps

The following acts or omissions by a medical practitioner or a dentist shall constitute acts or omissions in respect of which the council may take disciplinary steps in terms of Chapter IV of the Act: Provided that –

(a) the said acts or omissions shall not be deemed to constitute a complete list of offences, and the council may inquire into and deal with any complaint, charge or allegation which may be brought before it;

(b) the council ordinarily will act only if a complaint, charge or allegation is laid before it.

1. Advertising

Introduction. – Sound relationships between practitioners as colleagues are essential for furthering the public esteem and trustworthiness of the professions and therefore of the practitioners themselves. Acts by which a practitioner makes himself known directly to the public or by which he prejudices the esteem of a colleague (or other registered person) are contrary to this premise and fundamental proposition. The quality of a practitioner's services is traditionally the justified means by which he can become professionally known. Competition in the medico-scientific field and the disclosure of personal findings and views should take place only in the professional press.

The council endorses the desirability of informing the public of matters in the general interest, but disapproves of methods adopted by a practitioner aimed at advertising a particular person, institution, remedy or technique. It is laid down, furthermore, that a practitioner who allows his professional opinions to be divulged in the lay press or on the radio or television or to be disclosed to a lay assembly will personally be held responsible for such divulgence or disclosure not constituting advertising.

1 The rules are currently (February 1991) being reviewed by the SAMDC. Material amendments may be effected in due course.

(1) Advertising himself with a view to his (direct or indirect, immediate or eventual) professional gain or permitting such advertisement. The following acts shall not be regarded as such advertisement:

(a) Communications to *bona fide* patients intimating change of address, dissolution of partnership and the like, in which case the communications themselves shall bear the name of the individual patient to whom they are directed and shall be enclosed in an envelope;

(b) notification by a medical practitioner in general practice to other medical practitioners, or by a dentist in general practice to other dentists, of having commenced practice: Provided that the communications themselves shall bear the name of the individual medical practitioner or dentist to whom they are addressed and shall be enclosed in an envelope;

(c) notifications by a medical practitioner or dentist whose speciality has been registered, to other medical practitioners or dentists, of having commenced practice in his speciality, in which case the communications may contain his name, address, qualifications and speciality: Provided that the communications themselves shall bear the name of the individual medical practitioner or dentist to whom they are addressed and shall be enclosed in an envelope;

(cA) a single publication of a notification containing the information referred to in paragraphs 1 (1) (a), (b) and (c) in a professional journal approved by Council for this purpose;

(d) publishing in the official telephone directory, in the ordinary type of such publication, of the following particulars, namely his name and profession and that of his partner, if any, his speciality, his home and consulting room address, and one or more telephone numbers as well as special telephone numbers in case there is no reply from the usual numbers;

(e) affixing on envelopes of his name, without his title or any qualification, and a return address in case of non-delivery;

(f) the publication of articles in professional journals and of scientific books for use by the professions and by students of medicine, dentistry, nursing and related professions, indicating his name and professional qualifications;

(g) the publication of non-professional books and non-professional articles in the lay press under his own name without indication of professional qualifications and without the professional title Dr;

(h) the divulgence in the lay press or on the radio or television under his own name, or the expression by way of addresses or lectures to a lay audience of his views on subjects of a medical or dental nature –

  (i) by any full-time or part-time medical or dental official not in private practice, acting in his official capacity, where such publication is *bona fide* part of his official duties; and

  (ii) by any officer of a medical or dental association, acting in his official capacity and on the instructions of such association;

  (iii) by any practitioner on matters of a purely academic nature, public health, hospital administration, medico-political matters, and similar matters.

(2) A medical practitioner or dentist in general practice may restrict his practice to a particular branch of medicine or dentistry, but may not circularise his colleagues or other persons to this effect, since this may create the impression that he is a specialist.

(Rule 1 shall be read with rules 2, 3 and 5.)

2. Business advertisement

(1) Permitting his name to be used in connection with advertisements of medical and/or dental instruments, appliances, dressings, medicines, beverages or toilet or dietary preparations in the lay press.

(2) Permitting his name to be used as part of the title of a medical or dental practice carried on or managed by any lay person or company.

(3) Permitting the publication of his name in connection with advertisements or appeals to the public on behalf of sick benefit societies or similar commercial organisations.

3. Name-plates

(1) Using any of the following means to indicate his place of residence or consulting rooms:

(a) A name-plate exceeding in size 360 mm x 210 mm or otherwise not conforming to the requirements hereinafter laid down.

(b) A street signboard.

(c) A name-plate or lettering on balconies.

(d) A name-plate or lettering on windows: Provided that (in the case of buildings where no facilities exist or can be conveniently provided for affixing name-plates such as are in general use by the professions), a name-plate complying in every respect with that herein prescribed may be affixed to or painted on a plate-glass window as near as possible to the side adjacent to the *bona fide* entrance to such building.

(e) A name-plate on an outside wall or pillar which forms part of a building but not a *bona fide* entrance to that part of the building in which his consulting room is situated without the special permission of the council.

Notes: (i) Plain name-plates, such as are in general use by the profession shall be used. A name-plate shall not contain more than the practitioner's name, title, profession, qualification or degree, his speciality, if any, if it has been registered by the council, his telephone number(s) and his hours of consultation.

(ii) Not more than one name-plate at each entrance to a building and one on the door of the consulting room shall be allowed.

(iii) In the case of occupants of large buildings where special provision is made in the entrance hall and on the various floors to indicate the tenants, it shall be permissible to make use of such provision.

(iv) If necessary, in large buildings, a name-plate with the name of the practitioner only may be used in the corridor for the direction of patients.

(v) In the case of practitioners succeeding to a practice or in the case of the death or retirement of a partner it shall not be permissible to use on the premises or elsewhere the name or name-plate or plates of the predecessor or deceased or retired partner for a period exceeding 12 months from the date of succession to the practice. During this period of 12 months, succession to the practice shall be indicated by the words "Successor to".

(vi) In the case of removal, the name and new address of the practitioner may remain in reasonable evidence for a period not exceeding 12 months.

(vii) Professional name-plates shall not be allowed at any place unless a practitioner actually resides or *bona fide* practises at such place.

4. Visits by a medical practitioner or dentist to a place other than that at which he resides or practises

For a medical practitioner or dentist to carry on a regularly recurring itinerant practice at a place where another medical practitioner or dentist is established unless he, in such itinerant practice, can render the same service to his patients at the same cost as the service he would render in the area in which he is resident.

5. Letter heads and account forms

(1) The printing on letter heads and account forms of any information other than –

(a) the practitioner's name;

(b) profession and registered qualifications in abbreviated form and abbreviations in respect of academic qualifications (other than medical, surgical or dental) and in respect of honorary degrees conferred on him;

(c) addresses and telephone numbers;

(d) hours of consultation.

6. Prescription forms

(1) Using prescription forms and/or envelopes which have the name and address of a pharmacist printed thereon.

7. Canvassing and touting

(1) Canvassing or touting for patients either personally or through agents or in any other manner.

8. Fees, commissions and partnerships

(1) Accepting commissions from pharmacists or from makers of or dealers in surgical or dental appliances and materials or from similar persons or concerns.

(2) Paying commission to any person for recommending patients.

(3) Receiving commission in return for recommending services or wares to patients.

(4) Sharing fees (dichotomy) with any person who has not taken a commensurate part in the services for which the fees are charged.

(5) Being a party in a partnership between a general practitioner and a specialist.

(6) Being a party in a partnership between a specialist practising one of the specialities mentioned in rule 13 and a specialist practising some other speciality.

(7) The charging or receiving of fees for services not personally rendered, except fees for services rendered by –

(a) any other medical practitioner or dentist with whom he is in partnership, or with whom he is associated as principal or assistant or *locum tenens;*

(b) registered supplementary health service personnel in the employment of the medical practitioner or dentist, provided that the Council has given approval for fees to be charged or received for services rendered by such health service personnel.

9. Covering

(1) Employing as an assistant or *locum tenens* any person not registered as a medical practitioner or dentist, as the case may be, or acting in collusion or collaboration with

any person not so registered, or entering into partnership with any such person, or employing such person as a paid anaesthetist or as a paid assistant at an operation.

(2) (a) Consulting with or in any way assisting or supporting in his practice any person not registered in terms of the Medical, Dental and Supplementary Health Service Professions Act, 1974, or the Pharmacy Act, 1974, or the Nursing Act, 1978, or the Social and Associated Workers Act, 1978, or the Dental Technicians Act, 1979, who is in practice or who performs an act on a regular basis regarding –

- (i) the diagnosis, treatment or prevention of physical or mental disabilities, illnesses or defects in any other person; or
- (ii) any operation or treatment or advice usually given or performed by a dentist; or
- (iii) any operation or treatment or advice in preparation of or for the purpose of or regarding the manufacturing, repair, supply, fitting, insertion or fixing of dentures or other similar dental apparatus.

(b) Helping or supporting in any way a person in any illegal practice or conduct of such person registered in terms of the Medical, Dental and Supplementary Health Service Professions Act, 1974, or the Pharmacy Act, 1974, or the Nursing Act, 1978, or the Social and Associated Workers Act, 1978, or the Dental Technicians Act, 1978.

Notes. (i) In the event of a practitioner being called in a grave emergency to aid an unregistered person, he should immediately report the case to the council. (ii) It will not be unprofessional or improper to administer an anaesthetic to a patient undergoing circumcision for religious purposes, when such operation is performed not by a medical practitioner but a Mohel or Jewish Rabbi, qualified only by the Jewish religion to do this religious act: Provided that it is recognised that the administration of the anaesthetic does not entail any responsibility for the operation of circumcision.

(3) Employing unregistered supplementary health service personnel or referring patients to such unregistered personnel where the services of registered supplementary health services personnel are available.

10. Clubs, societies, etc

Having a financial interest, whether in the form of fixed salary or otherwise, in sick benefit clubs, dental clinics or dental hospitals or mechanical laboratories, or associations which advertise for members or patients in the lay press or by circular or card, or in any other way.

11. Association with charitable institutions

Being associated professionally in any manner with an institution which falsely purports to be a charitable or beneficiary institution.

12. Tendering

(1) Tendering for a full-time, part-time or any other type of appointment.

13. Consultants and specialists

(1) The commission of acts prohibited in (or the omission of acts required in terms of) the regulations made under section 61(1)(p) of the Act, namely the regulations embodying the conditions in respect of the practice of medical practitioners and dentists whose specialities have been registered.

(2) Holding himself out as a consultant when attending and treating patients except in consultation with and at the request of other practitioners.

14. Supersession

(1) Superseding another practitioner who is in charge of a case that he has seen with or on behalf of such practitioner except with the consent of the practitioner originally in charge of the case, unless that consent is withheld unreasonably or unless no other medical and/or dental assistance is available.

(2) Taking over the case of another practitioner unless satisfied that the patient or person in charge of the case has notified such practitioner that he no longer requires his services.

14*bis*. Improperly impeding a patient

Improperly impeding a patient (or a person acting on behalf of a patient) who desires to obtain the opinion of or treatment by another practitioner.

15. Professional reputation of colleagues and other registered persons

Unjustifiably casting reflection explicitly or implicitly upon the probity or professional reputation and skill of a fellow practitioner, or any other person registered under the Act or the Nursing Act, 1957.[2]

16. Professional secrecy

Divulging verbally or in writing any information which ought not to be divulged regarding the ailments of a patient except with the express consent of the patient or, in the case of a minor, with the consent of his parent or guardian, or in the case of a deceased patient, with the consent of his next-of-kin or the executor of his estate.

Note: In a court of law, professional secrecy may be contravened only under protest after direction from the presiding judicial officer.

17. Certificates

Granting a certificate in his professional capacity unless he is satisfied from personal observation that the facts are correctly stated therein, or has qualified the certificate by the words "as I am informed by the patient".

18. Impressions

(1) Whether for gain or not, taking any impression or bite in connection with or trying or fitting in the mouth any artificial denture which has been or is to be supplied direct to the patient by a person who is not a registered dentist.

(2) Whether for gain or not, performing any operation or giving any treatment, advice or attendance preparatory to or for the purpose of or in connection with the making, repairing, supplying, fitting, insertion or fixing of artificial dentures or other similar dental appliances, where such dentures or appliances are supplied or are to be supplied to the patient by a person who is not a registered dentist.

19. Professional appointments, other than appointments made under the Public Service Act

(1) Acceptance by a medical practitioner or a dentist of any professional appointment unless –

(a) a notice inviting applications for such appointment has been advertised in the public press;

2 This reference must now be construed as a reference to the Nursing Act of 1978.

(b) details of the proposed contract are made available on request to the council and all *bona fide* applicants;

(c) the contract of appointment is in writing and sets out clearly the professional services which the medical practitioner or dentist undertakes to render and the fees or remuneration payable to him for such services by the party with whom he has contracted;

(d) the contract provides that –

 (i) the medical practitioner or dentist shall receive fees or remuneration exclusively from the party with whom he has contracted; and
 (ii) such party shall be liable for such fees or remuneration;

(e) the contract provides that the dentist shall render all professional services ordinarily rendered in general dental practice but may exclude –

 (i) treatment for injuries and diseases of the jaws;
 (ii) reconstructive treatment of the type known as crown and bridge therapy and jacket crowns;
 (iii) the provision of metal dentures;
 (iv) orthodontic treatment;

(f) the fees or remuneration for the services mentioned in paragraph (e) (i), (ii), (iii) and (iv) rendered by a dentist, if not specifically included in the contract, shall be set out in detail in a schedule to the contract;

(g) the said contract is on a basis which is not derogatory to the medical or dental profession or inimical to the interest of the public.

(2) Permitting or suffering his name, profession, qualifications or address to appear on cards, handbills, pamphlets or notifications of any kind which refer in any way to his holding the said appointment: Provided that a medical practitioner or dentist shall not be deemed to have committed a breach of this rule if a benefit society notifies its members that medical or dental services have been arranged, details of which are available on application.

(3) Failure by a medical practitioner or dentist who has accepted a professional appointment to submit the contract originally entered into by him together with any subsequent amendments or addenda thereto for inspection by the council within a period of 30 days reckoned from the date of the posting of a registered letter from the registrar to such medical practitioner or dentist at his address as shown in the register, calling upon him to submit his contract for inspection: Provided that upon good cause shown this period may be extended by the council.

Notes: (i) The temporary appointment of a medical practitioner or dentist as a *locum tenens* for a period not exceeding six months shall be exempt from the requirements of the rule.

(ii) Transfer or promotions within a service will not be regarded as new appointments and the positions concerned need not be readvertised.

20. Secret remedies etc.

(1) Making use in the conduct of his practice –

(a) of any form of treatment, apparatus or technical process which is secret or is claimed to be secret;

(b) of any apparatus which proves upon investigation to be incapable of fulfilling the claims made in regard to it.

21. Consulting rooms

(1) Having consulting rooms for private practice with the entrance through or with the name-plate at the entrance to a pharmacy.

(2) Sharing consulting or waiting rooms with persons not on the medical or dental registers or, without the permission of the Council, with other persons registered with the Council.

Note: Medical practitioners and registered psychologists may, however, make use of joint consulting rooms on the explicit understanding that they do not practise in partnership.

22. Practice name

The use of a name for a private practice by a medical practitioner or dentist –

(a) other than his own name or the names of the registered persons with whom he is in partnership, or

(b) which includes –

  (i) the expression "hospital" or "clinic"; or

  (ii) any other special term which could create the impression that such a practice forms a part of, or is in association with, a hospital, clinic or similar institution.

23. Practice of radiology

(1) For medical practitioners or dentists in possession of X-ray plants to take skiagrams for and furnish reports on them to unregistered persons.

(*Note:* A medical practitioner or dentist may take skiagrams and furnish reports on them when requested by a patient, provided that he is satisfied that such report is not intended for use by an unregistered person.)

(2) For a dentist to take skiagrams and to report on them to anyone, except as far as his legitimate province lies, except in an emergency and where no registered medical practitioner in possession of an X-ray plant is available.

24. Council's statutory duties

Any wilful act or omission which prevents or is calculated to prevent the council or the registrar from carrying out its/his statutory duties.

25. Performance of professional acts by medical practitioners and dentists

(1) The performance by medical practitioners and dentists, except in an emergency, of professional acts for the performance of which they are inadequately trained and/or insufficiently experienced.

(2) The performance under improper conditions and/or surroundings of professional acts, except in an emergency.

26. Exploitation

Permitting himself to be exploited in a manner detrimental to the public or professional interest.

27. Dentists employing unregistered persons to perform certain specified acts

For a dentist to employ any unregistered person to perform any of the following acts – Dental radiography, topical application of medicaments, periodontal packing, dental prophylaxis, oral hygiene instruction, removal of orthodontic appliances.

28. Medicines

(1) Subject to the provisions of section 52 of the Act, a practitioner shall not –

(a) participate in the manufacture for commercial purposes, sale, advertising or promotion of, or in any other activity which amounts to trading in, any medicine as defined in the Medicines Control Act, 1965, or

(b) engage in, or advocate, the preferential use or prescription of any medicine, from which preferential use or prescription any valuable consideration is derived.

(2) The provisions of paragraph (1) shall not prohibit a practitioner from owning shares in a public company manufacturing or marketing medicines, or, subject to the provisions of the Pharmacy Act, 1974, from being the owner or part-owner of a pharmacy, or, whilst employed by a pharmaceutical concern in any particular capacity, from performing such duties as are normally in accordance with such employment.

29. Prescription or supply of specific medicines

The prescription or supply of any substance listed in Schedules 6 and 7 to the Medicines and Related Substances Control Act, 1965 (Act 101 of 1965),[3] unless the medical practitioner or dentist has ascertained by personal examination of the patient or by virtue of a report by another medical practitioner under whose treatment the specific patient is or has been that such prescription or supply is necessary for the treatment of the patient, except in the case of the repeating of a prescription or supply of a substance in respect of a patient with a chronic illness.

30. Payment of account of dental technician

The payment of an account of a dental technician later than three months from the date of receipt of a monthly statement.

3 The Act will probably be amended during the 1991 legislative session of Parliament.

Index

A

ABANDONMENT OF PATIENT
generally, 3, 24, 32, 427

ABORTION
Abortion and Sterilisation Act, 192, 207, 219
"abortion" defined, 207
authorisation required, 210
"backstreet" abortion, 217
certification requirements, 209
child will be handicapped, 208
common-law, 207, 209
"conscience clause" 215, 219
consent to, 5, 211–2
curator ad litem for foetus, 202, 220
doctor, failing to advise, 198
donation of foetus, 148
embryo, 222
English law, 211
eugenic, grounds for, 208
foetus defined, 208, 222
foetus removed, rights to, 163–6
formalities, 216
generally, 207–224, 336
hospital superintendent's liability, 307
husband's consent, 211
hysterectomy, foetus destroyed, 208
illegal, 208, 216, 217
incest, foetus conceived in, 208, 209
indications for, 208, 220
infanticide, 207
intra-uterine device, 222
justification of, generally, 208, 209
mentally defective woman, 208
minor girl, against her will, 211–2
"Miss X", case of, 219
"morning after" pill, 223
overseas, 214
psychiatric indication, 208, 209, 210, 219
punishment for, 208
rape, foetus, conceived in, 208, 209, 219
records to be kept, 216
right to? 212–4
State-controlled institution, 215
statistics, 217–8
suicide, threat of, by woman, 210, 219
therapeutic, 208
woman's life saved by, 207, 208, 210, 219
woman's mental health preserved by, 208, 210
woman's physical health preserved by, 208

ACCOUNTS
collection of debts, 59–62
discounting of, 57
factoring, 57
forms, ethical requirements, 452
interest on overdue account, 60

ADDRESS, CHANGE OF
doctor, notifying of, 450

ADMISSION FORM
to hospital, 13, 162

ADVERTISING
medicine, of, 451
unethical conduct, 449–457

AIDS
blood-test for, 8, 11
confidentiality, and, 16–18
consent to testing for, 8, 11
counselling patient, 17
diagnosis, disclosing, 16, 105
doctor refusing to treat, 27, 91
immigration officer, powers of, 3
informing patient, 11, 12, 16, 17
informing sex partners, 16, 17
medical officer of health, powers of, 3
SAMDC, guidelines on, 11, 17
screening for, 11

ALCOHOL
alcoholic, legal position of, 351–6
alcoholism, treatment for, 355
antecedent liability 138, 353
blood-alcohol, 357, 359, 361, 364
blood samples, 357, 359
breath-alcohol, 361–3
"breathalyser" tests, 361–3
criminal liability of alcoholic, 127, 134, 138, 352–4
delirium tremens, 128, 354
drunken driving, 351, 352, 353, 358, 359, 361, 364
intoxication as a defence, 127, 134, 353
public drunkeness, 355
rehabilitation of alcoholic, 355–6
Road Traffic Act, 358, 365

AMNESIA
criminal responsibility, 129

AMNIOCENTESIS
generally, 175, 194, 198, 199
negligence in, 198, 199

AMPUTATION
in emergency, 93–4
ANAESTHESIA
anaesthetist, surgeon's liability for act of, 96, 299–300
apparatus defective, patient killed, 265n
consent to, 13
negligent, 96, 276
patient refusing, 12
sequential awareness, 277
ANATOMICAL DONATION
anatomical specimens, ownership of, 160, 161
aorta, 155
artificial insemination, 148, 181–190
authorisation, official, 149, 153, 155
blood, 147, 156
bone, 155
consent to, 148, 152
corneae, 150, 154, 155
corpses, from, 149–158
criminal offences, 158
death, certification of, 150–152, 325
deceased unidentified, 153
destitutes, 155
director-general donating, 153
district surgeon, consent by, 154
doctor exonerated from liability, 158
dura mater, 155
embryo implacement, 148n, 195
eye: *see* corneae
exporting tissue, 158
foetus, 148
gamete, 147, 148, 156, 158, 181, 187
genetic manipulation prohibited, 157
gonad, 147, 148, 154, 158
habitual criminal, 147
heart transplantation, 147, 150
identity tag, 153
importing tissue, 158
in vitro fertilisation, 148, 185, 187, 191, 195
kidney, 149n, 155
living persons, by, 147–149
magistrate authorising, 153
medical supervision, 154
mental patient, by, 147
minister authorising, 155
minor, by, 147, 148
ownership of tissue, 156
pituitary gland, 155
post mortem examination, 153, 154, 155, 158
publicity, 157
replaceable tissue, 147
registers to be kept, 156
revocation of, 153
routine removal of tissue, 155
sale of tissue prohibited, 156
secrecy, 157
time limit, 156
tissue bank, 157
"tissue" defined, 147
will, by means of, 153, 156
ANATOMICAL SPECIMEN
ownership of, 160–2, 164
APPOINTMENT, PROFESSIONAL
ethical requirements for, 454
ARTIFICIAL INSEMINATION
adoption of child born of, 183, 189
adultery? 183
anatomical donation, and, 148, 185, 188
birth registration, 185, 190
child born of, when legitimate, 185, 189
consent to, 148, 182, 185
criminal offences, 183, 186
doctor's liability, 185
donor, 181–3, 186, 193
generally, 181–190
gonad transplantation of, 147, 148, 154, 158
husband providing sperm, 181
illegitimacy of child, 183–5, 194
inspector's rights, 186
in vitro fertilisation, 148, 185, 187, 191, 195, 200
legislation, 148, 181–3, 192
maintenance of child, 184
minor, 185
record of, 182, 183
registration of doctor, 183
report on, 183
sperm bank, 186
status of child, 183–5
venereal disease, 182
unmarried woman, of, 182, 185
ASSOCIATION
practice in, 73, 77–8, 439
AUTOMATISM
criminal responsibility, 127n, 128, 138, 353

B

BAR CLAUSE
see RESTRAINT CLAUSE
BIOMEDICAL ENGINEER
registration as, 441
BIRTH
breathing test, 165, 207
defined, 163
"human being" defined, 165
live birth, defined, 165
registration of, 165, 185, 190
still-born, 163
BLACKLISTING
of patient, 63–5
BLOOD
AIDS, testing for, 8, 11
donation of, 147, 148, 156

drawn by homoeopath, 441
remuneration for, 156
sale of, 156
transfusion,
negligent, 24
patient refusing, 12, 29–34, 410

BREATHALYSER
breath-alcohol tests, 361–3

BURIAL
burial order, 163–4
foetus, of, 164
still-born child, of, 165

BURN
suffered by patient in hospital, 264, 301

C

CANCER
informing patient, 11, 12, 15, 18, 92

CANVASSING
unethical conduct, 452

CASTRATION
consent to, 12

CASUALTY OFFICER
duties, 24, 90, 93, 94, 267
standard of skill required of, 40

CAUTERY
defective, patient burnt by, 264–6

CERTIFICATE, MEDICAL
apprentice, 108
employee, for, 106–9
ethical requirements for, 454
fraudulent, 109, 454
professional secrecy, and, 106–9

CHARITABLE INSTITUTION, ALLEGED
professional association with, 453

CHILD
abortion performed on, 211–2
abuse, 417–9
anatomical donation by, 147–8
artificial insemination of, 185
blood transfusion, 33–4
consent to treatment, by, 5–8, 93, 95, 171 174, 211, 214, 421, 423
contraception provided to, 171–4
contracting with doctor, as agent of parent, 7
defective, resulting from AID, 185
experimentation on, 420–3
prenatal injury, 195, 196, 199, 201
sterilisation of, 174, 214
still-born, burial of, 165

CHIROPRACTOR
manipulation, 443

CIRCUMCISION
administering anaesthetic to patient, 453

CLINICAL, DENTAL
use of term, 456

CLONING
legal issues, 198, 200

CODE OF CONDUCT
of Medical Council, 449–457
see also ETHICS, PROFESSIONAL

COLOSTOMY
consent to, 9

COMMISSION
doctor receiving, unethical, 387, 452

COMPANY
doctor owning shares in, 457
doctors practising as, 439
partnership forming, 73
possessing medical assets, 73, 439
running dispensary, 431

COMPARTMENT SYNDROME
resulting in loss of leg, 262

CONFIDENTIALITY
see PROFESSIONAL SECRECY

CONSENT
abortion, 5, 211–2
adult patient, 4, 8, 11, 91
AIDS, and. *See* AIDS
anatomical donation, to, 148, 152
artificial insemination, 148, 182, 185
blood transfusion, 29–34
bodily mutilation, 286
child, 5–8, 93, 95, 171, 174, 211, 214, 421, 423
comatose patient, 94
electroshock therapy, 10
emergency treatment, 10, 91–3
experimentation, to, 421, 423
form, 13
generally, 3–13
genetic screening, in, 198
HIV, screening for. *See* AIDS
hospital consent form, 13
husband and wife, 4, 94, 169–171, 185, 211–2, 290
informed, 4, 8–12, 15, 35, 198, 267–9, 289, 422
intra-uterine device, 222
leucotomy, to, 38
mental patient, 3, 5, 37–9
oral, 3, 35, 289
over-informing patient, 12, 19
patient treated against will, 4, 29, 91
plastic surgery, 286, 289
premedication, patient under, 5
prisoner, minor, 6
psychiatric treatment, 4
radiological treatment, 10
relative, by, 21, 34, 38, 94
"sex-change" operaion, 12, 230
spouses, 5, 170–1, 180, 211–2

CONSENT (*contd*)
tacit, 4, 35, 289
therapeautic privilege, 10, 18–19
to killing, 339
transsexualism, 12, 230
withdrawal of, by patient, 35
written, 12, 13
X-ray treatment, 7
CONSULTING ROOMS
generally, 73, 77–8, 439, 456
sharing of,
ethical requirements, 456
CONTINGENT FEE
lawyer's, 245
CONTRACEPTION
advertisement of, 169
failure of, 175, 169
intra-uterine device, 169, 222
minor female, 171–4
negligence in providing, 175
spouses 5, 169
CONTRACT
between doctors,
associate practice, 73, 77, 439
locum tenens, 79–81, 82
partnership. *See* PARTNERSHIP
room-sharing, 73, 77, 439
doctor and patient, 3, 8, 15, 35, 40, 66, 69, 287
employees, with, 79–81, 82
expert witness, with, 433–5, 436
guarantee given by doctor to patient, 35, 40, 176, 288
locum tenens, with 79–81, 82
patient, with, 3, 8, 15, 35, 40, 69, 287
professional appointment, ethical requirements, 454–5
professional assistant, with, 79–81, 82
CONTRIBUTORY NEGLIGENCE
rescuer, 98
COPYRIGHT
in X-ray plate, 113
CORPSE
anatomical donation from, 149–158
burial of, 156, 163, 164
cremation of, 164
defined, 164–166
ownership of, 160, 164
COSMETIC OPERATION
lawfulness of, 228, 285–291
See also PLASTIC SURGERY
COVENANT IN RESTRAINT OF TRADE
See RESTRAINT CLAUSE
COVERING
unethical conduct, 452
CREMATION
foetus, of, 163
still-born, of, 164
CRIMEN INIURIA
See INIURIA
CRIMINAL RESPONSIBILITY
See EPILEPSY; MENTAL ILLNESS; MENTAL PATIENT
CULPABLE HOMICIDE
anaesthetic death, 265n 276
as a result of medical negligence, 254, 265n, 272, 276, 280
CURATOR BONIS
of mental patient, 37–8

D

DAMAGES
for medical negligence, ***quantum*** of, 244–6, 250, 257, 260, 263, 270, 282, 284, 285, 288
DAY-CLINIC
owned by doctors, 440
DEAF-MUTE
criminal responsibility, 126
DEATH
brain, 150–1, 326–8
cardiac, 150–2, 326
cerebral, 150–2, 326
certification of, 151, 163, 329, 334
cot death, certification of, 334
criteria for, 150–2, 324–8
"death on arrival", 329–333
defining, 150–2, 324
DOA certificate, 329
heart, 150–2, 326
moment of, 322–3
registration of, 163, 164
right to die, 4, 19, 31, 328
DEFAMATION
complaint lodged with Medical Council, 369, 381
of colleague, by doctor, 454
of nurse by doctor, 454
of patient, by doctor, 64, 370
DENTAL CLINIC
financial interest in, 453
DENTAL HOSPITAL
use of term, 456
DENTAL MECHANICIAN
fee for services, 69
DENTIST
employing unregistered person, unethical, 452, 457
fees, 69
professional appointments, ethical requirements, 454–5
taking skiagram, 456

DENTURE
taking impression for, 454

DETAINEE
ad hoc committee of MASA, report of, 402–8
district surgeons, duties, 394, 395–6, 405
force-feeding, 410–414
hunger-strikes, 409–414
Internal Security Act, 391, 394, 396–8
interrogation of, 404, 407
isolation of, 404
medical treatment of, 391–401, 402–8
ministerial directions, 397
non-treatment, liability of State, 398
Police Act, 394–5
Prisons Act, 391–5
professional secrecy, 406
solitary confinement, 404
standing orders to Police, 394, 400

DETERMINISM
in criminal law, 121, 133

DIAGNOSIS
AIDS, of, 16, 105
diagnostic *post mortem*, 158
disclosure of, in medical certificate, 106–9
failure to diagnose fracture, 40, 252
informing patient of, 9, 15
negligent, 21, 196, 252–3, 259

DICHOTOMY
unethical conduct, 452

DISASTERS
See EMERGENCY TREATMENT

DISCIPLINARY PROCEEDINGS
admission of guilt, 371
complaint, how dealt with, 369, 372
doctor suing complainant, 381–3
duties of Medical Council, 376
fines, 374
generally, 369–380
no appeal against, 375
review of, 375
suspension of partner, 378

DISCOUNTING
doctor's accounts, 57
factoring, 57

DISGRACEFUL CONDUCT
See ETHICS, PROFESSIONAL

DISPENSING
doctor, by, 432
private hospital, by, 431

DISTRICT SURGEON
anatomical donation, consent by, 154
detainees, duties, 394, 395, 405
immunisation by, 24, 91
medical certificate issued by, 108
professional secrecy, 406

DOCTOR
complaint against. *See* DISCIPLINARY PROCEEDINGS
duty to inform patient of risks, 8–10, 15, 267–9
duty to testify in court, 106, 433, 436
duty where referring patient to another doctor, 258, 299
employed by pharmaceutical concern, 457
ethical duties. *See* ETHICS, PROFESSIONAL
fees. *See* FEES
guarantee of cure, by, 35, 40, 176, 288
informing patient of change of address, 450
liability for acts of nurse, 300
liability for defective instrument, 264
parental authority, interfering with, 172
practising from home, 444–5
refusing to attend patient, 3, 23–8
standard of care required of, 40, 95, 267, 290, 292
withdrawing from case, 42
witness, 106, 433, 436

DRUG
allergic reaction to, 254, 285, 293–4
defective, liability for, 292–5
over-prescribing, 294

DRUNKEN DRIVING
See ALCOHOL

DURHAM'S CASE
criminal responsibility, and, 123

E

ELECTROSHOCK THERAPY
consent to, 10

EMBRYO
defined, 208, 222
experimentation on, 200
transfer of, 148n, 188, 191

EMERGENCY TREATMENT
consent to, 91
degree of care, 95
dentist taking skiagram, 456
doctor aiding unregistered person, 452–3
doctor going beyond training, not unethical, 456
doctor's legal duty, 3, 25, 90
ethical duty, 25
generally, 25, 89–99, 208, 209, 427
"Good Samaritan" laws, 90
hospital's liability for, 303
indemnity for doctor who treats, 90
layman, by, 96
minor, 6, 93, 95
nurse, by, 89n, 90
paramedic, by, 89
priority treatment, 97, 323

EMERGENCY TREATMENT (*contd*)
under improper conditions, not unethical, 456
EMOTIONAL DISTRESS
criminal responsibillty, and, 134
EMPLOYEE
contract with, 79–81
liability for negligence, 246
medical certificate issued to, 106–9
strike by, 314–7, 429
unregistered person, 452–3
workmen's compensation, 81
EMPLOYER
disclosure of medical facts re employee, 106–8, 112–3
liability for employee's negligence, 246, 299–305
medical certificate to, 106–9
EPILEPSY
contracts by epileptic, 142
criminal responsibility of epileptic, 133, 136–140, 352
dangerous, 136
delictual liability of epileptic, 141
driver's licence, 144
eugenic sterilisation, 144
fitness to stand trial, 140
generally, 136–144
head injury causing, 139
insurance policies, 142
President's patient, 139, 140, 141
protective legislation, 143
uncontrolled, 144
ERROR OF JUDGMENT
negligence, and, 249–251
ETHICS, MEDICAL
See ETHICS, PROFESSIONAL
ETHICS, PROFESSIONAL
abortion, overseas referral, 214
account forms, 452
advertising, 449–450
apparatus, making false claim as to, 455
assistant, not registered person, 452–3
associating with unregistered person, 452–3
"blacklisting" of patients, 63–5
bribery, 384
business advertisement, 451
canvassing, 452
certificate, medical, 454
change of address, doctor notifying of, 450
charitable institution, alleged, 453
clinic, dental, use of term, 456
clubs, interest in, 453
code of conduct, 449–457
commission, doctor receiving, 387, 452
company practice, 439
complaint concerning, 369
consultant, holding out as, 453
consulting rooms, sharing of, 456
corruption, 384
covering, 452
dental clinic, financial interest in, 453
dentist employing unregistered person, 452, 457
denture, taking impression for, 454
dichotomy, 452
disciplinary committee, duties, 369, 376
discounting of accounts, 57
emergency treatment, 25, 453, 456
experimentation on children, 420
exploitation, allowing, 26
factoring, 57
fee sharing, 428, 452
financial interest in sick benefit club, 453
generally, 449–457
gifts, doctor accepting, 384
illegitimate practice, supporting, 452
impeding patient, 428, 457
impressions, dental, 454
improper conditions, treating under, 456
inexperience, 456
itinerant practice, 452
lectures by doctor, 450
letterheads, requirements for, 452
locum tenens, appointment as, 455
manufacturing medicine, 457
medical certificate, 17, 106–9, 454
name-plate, 451
notices, 450
obstructing Council, 456
partnerships, when unethical, 452
pharmaceutical gifts, receiving, 384
pharmacy, association with, 456
practice name, 456
practising elsewhere, 452
prescribing medicine on preferential basis, 457
prescription forms, 452
professional appointments, 454–5
professional secrecy, 103–9, 110–7, 454
promoting medicine, 451, 457
publication by doctor, 450
radiology, practice of, 456
reputation of colleague, impairing, 454
restriction of practice by doctor, 450
secret remedy, 455
sexual cases, 377
shares, owned by doctor, 457
sick-benefit fund, interest in, 453
specialist, conditions of practice, 453
strike by doctor, 429
supersession, 428, 454
taking over case, 428, 454
telephone directory, entries in, 450
television broadcast, 450
tendering for appointment, 453
touting, 452
trading in medicine, 457

X-rays, ethical requirements, 456
EUTHANASIA
active, 336–343
defective newborns, 198, 200, 338, 339
discontinuing treatment, 337, 342, 344
doctor killing patient, 340
generally, 336–347
imbecile, 340
legalisation of, 339
"Living Will", 344–7
passive, 337, 342, 344
senile patient, 338, 340, 341
sentence for, 340, 341, 342
witholding treatment, 29, 198, 200, 338, 339, 342
EVIDENCE, MEDICAL
doctor's duty to testify, 106, 433, 436
expert evidence, 122, 131, 433, 436
fees for, 433–5
generally, 136
malpractice cases, in, 112
mental illness, of, 122, 131
professional secrecy.
See PROFESSIONAL SECRECY
psychiatric evidence, 122, 131
when doctor may testify, 112
witness, remuneration of, 433–5
EXPERIMENTATION, HUMAN
child, on, 420–3
foetus, on, 195, 200
generally, 200, 420
EXPERT EVIDENCE
See EVIDENCE, MEDICAL
EXPLOITATION
allowing, unethical conduct, 456

F

FACTORING
doctor's accounts, of, 57
FEES
blacklisting of patient for non-payment, 63–5
cession of fee, 57
debts, collection of, 59–62
dentist, for dentures, 69
discount on, 47
dispensing fees, 46
employer's liability for, in respect of employee, 66, 67
generally, 45–58
grandparent's liability, for grandchild, 66
guaranteed payment, 46, 48
husband and wife, 66
interest on overdue account, 59
MASA tariff, 46
parent's liability for child, 66
plastic surgery, 48, 289
prepayment of, 48
scale of benefits, 46
sharing, when unethical, 452
splitting of accounts, 48
FERTILISATION
in vitro, 148, 185, 187, 191, 195, 200
FIRST AID
by layman, 496
See also EMERGENCY TREATMENT
FOETUS
experimentation on, 195, 200
injury to, 195, 196, 199, 201
meaning of, in Abortion Act, 208, 222
quickening, 223
removed from uterus, rights to, 160, 163–6
viable, 164
See also ABORTION
FRACTURE
failure to diagnose, 40, 252
negligence in treatment of, 257–261, 262–6

G

GAMETE
donation of, 147, 148, 156, 158, 181, 187
GENETICS
amniocentesis, 175, 194, 198, 199
fertilisation, *in vitro*, 148, 185, 187, 191, 195, 200
genetic engineering, 191–203
genetic manipulation, 157, 191–203
genetic screening, negligence in, 175, 196, 198, 202–3
"wrongful life", 175, 179, 180, 196, 197
GIFT
to doctor, 384–6
GONAD
definition of, 148
transplantation of, 147, 148, 154, 158
GOOD SAMARITAN LAWS
in USA, 90

H

HEAD INJURY
epilepsy caused by, 139
HEART TRANSPLANT
law, and, 147, 150
See also ANATOMICAL DONATION
HERMAPHRODITISM
transsexualism, and, 227n, 232, 233, 238
HIV. *See* AIDS
HOMICIDE, CULPABLE
anaesthetic death, 265n, 276
as result of medical negligence, 254, 265n, 272, 276, 280
HOMOEOPATH
drawing blood from patient, 441

HOMOSEXUALITY
transsexualism and, 227, 230, 231

HOSPITAL
admission form, 13, 162
appointment of employee, 316n
cautery, defective, hospital's liability, 265
dental hospital, use of term, 22
director of hospital service, duties, 312
discharging patient, 262, 308
employee,
dismissal of, 314, 316
liability for negligence, 246
exclusion of liability, 162, 178, 305
foetus, rights to, 163–6
liability for acts of servants, 246, 271, 299–305
medical officer, suspension of, 312
patient insisting upon leaving, 308
patient's property, loss of, 310
patient's right of admission to, 162, 213
private hospital
commission paid to doctor, 387
owned by doctors, 440
running dispensary, 431
superintendent of, 306
records, 110
rights to tissue removed from patient, 160, 163
strikes by employees, 314–7
superintendent, legal liability of, 306
vicarious liability, 246, 271, 299–305
waiver of claim by patient, 162, 178, 305

HUMAN TISSUE ACT
See ANATOMICAL DONATION, ANATOMICAL SPECIMEN

HUNGER-STRIKE
by prisoner, 409–414
Tokyo Declaration, 413

HUSBAND AND WIFE
See SPOUSES

HYSTERECTOMY
consent to, 9
foetus, destroyed in, 208

I

IMMUNISATION
against will of patient, 91

IMPEDING PATIENT
unethical conduct, 428, 454

IMPRESSIONS, DENTAL
ethical requirements, 454

IMPROPER CONDUCT
See ETHICS, PROFESSIONAL

INCOME TAX
companies, and, 439
corporate practice, 439
partnership, 74, 445
practice from home, 445

INDETERMINISM
in criminal law, 121

INFORMED CONSENT
See CONSENT

INIURIA
abortion without husband's consent, 211
artificial insemination, 185
crimen iniuria, 4, 185
destruction of bodily part, 162
operation against will of patient, 3
violation of dead body, 150

INQUEST
doctor's report, 436
evidence, 437
judicial officer, duties, 436
legal representation, 437–8

INSANITY
See MENTAL ILLNESS; MENTAL PATIENT

INSTRUMENT
defective, patient injured, 264–6

INSURANCE
against medical professional liability, 243–8

INTOXICATION
See ALCOHOL

INTRA-UTERINE DEVICE
abortion, and, 222
husband's consent not required, 169

IN VITRO FERTILISATION
legal aspects of, 148, 185, 187, 191, 195, 200

IRRESISTIBLE IMPULSE
defence of, 131

ITINERANT PRACTICE
ethical requirements, 452

J

JEHOVAH'S WITNESS
refusal of blood transfusion by, 29–34

JUVENILE PATIENT
See CHILD

L

LAYMAN
emergency treatment by, 96
practising medicine, 441, 442

LECTURES
by doctors, 450

LETTER HEADS
ethical requirements, 452

LEUCOTOMY
consent to, 37, 38
regulations, 38

"LIVING WILL"
validity of, 344–7, 411

LOCUM TENENS
contract with, 79–81, 82
unregistered person employed as, 452

M

MALPRACTICE
insurance against liability, 243–8
litigation, 90, 111, 243
plastic surgery, 285–291
trends, 90, 111, 243
See also NEGLIGENCE

MASS CASUALTIES
burial regulations, 97
medical treatment of, 96–7
See also EMERGENCY TREATMENT

MEDICAL AID
See MEDICAL SCHEME

MEDICAL CERTIFICATE
See CERTIFICATE, MEDICAL

MEDICAL COUNCIL, SA
appeal against decisions, 375
code of conduct, 449–457
complaint to, 369, 372
disciplinary committee, duties, 376
disciplinary inquiry, 369–375, 376
generally, 22, 415–422
"please explain" note, legal status of, 370
powers relating to strike by doctors, 430
review of proceedings, 375
right to call for explanation, 370
ruling on company practice, 439–440

MEDICAL EVIDENCE
See EVIDENCE, MEDICAL

MEDICAL FEES
See FEES

MEDICAL NEGLIGENCE
See NEGLIGENCE, PROFESSIONAL

MEDICAL PRACTITIONER
See DOCTOR

MEDICAL PRACTICE
acts pertaining to, 441–3

MEDICAL RECORDS
husband and wife, 103
ownership of, 106–9, 110–5
patient-retained records, 116
patient's access to, 106–9
professional secrecy, 103, 106–9

MEDICAL INSURANCE
medical scheme, and, 49

MEDICAL SCHEME
cession of claim against, 56
contract of patient with, 51–3
contracting out, 46
doctor suing scheme, 53
guaranteed payment, 46–8
medical insurance, and, 49
non-payment of claim by, 55
RAMS
review of action, 50
scale of benefits, 46, 52
undue benefit paid out, 54

MEDICAL TREATMENT
improper conditions, under, 456
lack of experience, medical ethics, 456

MEDICINE
dispensing of, by doctor, 432
doctor manufacturing, 457
doctor trading in, 457
promotion of, unethical, 457

MENTAL DISORDERS ACT, 1916
"epileptic" defined, 136
"mental disorder" defined, 136

MENTAL HEALTH ACT, 1974
epilepsy and, 137
"mental illness" defined, 127, 139

MENTAL ILLNESS
criminal responsibilty, and 121–135
M'Naghten's case, 123
President's patient, 124, 125, 132, 341
See also MENTAL PATIENT

MENTAL PATIENT
anatomical donation by, 147
certifiability, 126
consent to operation, 3, 4, 37–9
criminal responsibility, 121–135
curator bonis, 38
dangerous, 112, 136
delirium tremens, 128, 354
diminished responsibility of, 133
epileptic. *See* EPILEPSY
fitness to stand trial, 124, 140
irresistible impulse, 131
lack of self-control, 131
lucidum intervallum, 128
President's patient, 124, 125, 132, 341
psychopath, 128, 133, 351
statement made to psychiatrist, 104

MINOR
See CHILD

M'NAGHTEN'S CASE
criminal responsibility, and, 123, 130

N

NAME-PLATES
doctor's, requirements for, 451

NECESSITY
defence of, 31, 91, 93
See also EMERGENCY TREATMENT

NEGLIGENCE, PROFESSIONAL
action for, prescription of, 113
allergic reaction to drug, testing for, 254

NEGLIGENCE, PROFESSIONAL (*contd*)
- amniocentesis, 198, 199
- anaesthesia, 96, 265n, 276
- artificial insemination, in, 185
- burns suffered by patient
  - in theatre, 264
  - in hospital bed, 301
- casualty officer, of, 40
- cautery, defective, patient burnt, 264–6
- compartment syndrome, 262–3
- contributory 99
- "conspiracy of silence", 245
- contrast medium, excessive amount, 272
- death of patient caused by, 272, 273, 276, 280
- defective drug, 292–5
- degree of care, 40, 95, 267, 290, 292
- diagnostic, 21, 198, 252–3
- equipment, failure to use, 96
- error of judgment, 249–251
- exclusion of liability for, 178, 305
- failure to inform patient of risks, 267–9
- failure to refer patient to specialist, 198, 199, 280
- foetus, harm to, 195, 196, 199, 201
- fracture, reduction of, 257
- hospital staff, 299–304
- instrument defective, 264–6
- insurance against, 243–8
- obstetrics, 280
- omission, 23, 198
- overdose, 272, 294
- over-informing patient, 12
- mediastinoscopy, 282
- Medical Protection Society, 247
- patient falling from bed, 301
- penicillin, testing for allergy, 254
- plaster-cast too tight, 257–261, 301
- plastic surgery, 285, 290
- post-operative care, in, 257, 262
- pregnancy, relating to, 199, 280
- premature discharge of patient, 262
- proof of, 245
- pyelogram, death following, 273
- *res ipsa loquitur*, 245, 264, 271, 278, 284, 290, 293
- radiological mishaps, 265, 272–5
- standard of skill, 40, 95, 267, 290, 292
- sterilisation, 175–180, 196, 197
- strict liability for, 264, 292, 304
- swab cases, 244, 270–1
- syringe, needle of, defective, 265
- vicarious liability, 276, 299–305
- Volkmann's contracture, 257–261, 301
- waiver of claim for, 178, 305
- X-ray treatment. *See* X-RAY

NEGOTIORUM GESTIO
- *See* UNAUTHORISED ADMINISTRATION

NEONATE, DEFECTIVE
- treatment of, 198, 200, 338, 339

NURSE
- abortion, right to refuse to participate in, 215 apparatus defective, 264–6, 299n
- doctor may not impair professional reputation, 454
- emergency treatment by, 89, 96
- hospital's liability for acts of, 299–305
- liability of doctor for acts of, 299
- strike, participating in, 429
- theatre nurse's responsibilities re swab count, 270–1

O

OPERATION, SURGICAL
- against patient's will, 29–34, 91, 93, 94, 345
- plastic, 228, 285–291
- spouses, consent requirements, 5, 170–1, 180, 211–2
- swab count, 270
- tissue removed during, patient's rights, 160–2
- without consent, 11, 18, 91, 92

OPHTHALMOLOGY
- consent to operation, 35

ORGAN TRANSPLANTATION
- *See* ANATOMICAL DONATION

P

PACTUM DE QUOTA LITIS
- legality of, 245

PARAMEDIC
- emergency treatment by, 96, 97

PARTNERSHIP
- between doctors, generally, 73–6, 439
- between specialist and general practitioner, unethical, 452
- contract, 73, 74, 75,
- dissolution, 75
- goodwill, determination of value, 75–6
- insolvency of partner, 73
- partner struck off roll, 379
- partner suspended, 378
- specialist with other kind of specialist, unethical, 452
- vicarious liability of partners, 299
- with unregistered person, unethical, 452–3

PATERNITY
- presumption of, 184

PATHOLOGIST
- allowing tests to be conducted by company, 440

PATIENT
- abandonment of, by doctor, 3, 24, 32, 427
- "blacklisting" of, by doctor, 63–5
- burnt by cautery, 264–6
- claim against professional assistant, 80

complaining to Medical Council, 369
consent by. *See* CONSENT
consults another doctor, 427
contract with doctor, 3, 8, 15, 35, 40, 66, 69, 287
dissatisfied with dentures, 69–70
falling from hospital bed, 301
imposing conditions for treatment, 12
insists upon leaving hospital, 308
liability for fees. *See* FEES
refusal to co-operate with doctor, 12
refusing treatment, 4, 19, 29–34
relative "vetoing" operation, 94
right to admission to hospital, 162, 213
right to be healed? 40
rights in emergency, 89–99
"right to die", 4, 19, 31, 328, 344–7, 410
treated against will, 29–34, 91, 93, 94, 345
withdrawing consent, 35

PENICILLIN
negligence in administering, 254

PHARMACEUTICAL GIFTS
to doctor, 384–6

PHARMACY
doctor owning, 457

PITUITARY GLAND
anatomical donation, 155

PLASTIC SURGERY
breasts, to, 285
buttocks, to, 285
consent to, 289
contract, 287–9
facial damage in, 285
fugitive, on, 287
general practitioner doing, 285
generally, 228, 285–291
negligence in, 290
privacy of patient, and 291
records of doctor, 291

POST MORTEM EXAMINATION
anatomical donation, and, 153, 154, 155, 158
diagnostic, 158
disclosure of findings, 424
mass-casualty victims, 97
medico-legal, 424
who may be present at, 424–6

PRATT'S CASE
fitness to stand trial, 141

PREGNANCY CLAIM
liability, 179

PREMEDICATION
consent to, 13
patient under influence of, 5

PRESCRIBING
preferential prescribing of medicine, 457

PRESCRIPTION
claims, of, 113

PRESCRIPTION FORMS
ethical requirements for, 452

PRESIDENT'S PATIENT
See MENTAL PATIENT

PRISON
medical services, 391–5, 399, 406
Van Dam Committee, report, 399n

PRISONER
ad hoc committee of MASA, report, 402–8
district surgeons, duties, 394, 395–6, 405
medical treatment of, 391–401, 402–8
non-treatment, liability of State, 398
Prisons Act, 391
See also DETAINEE

PRIVACY
See PROFESSIONAL SECRECY

PROFESSIONAL APPOINTMENT
ethical requirements for, 454–5

PRIVILEGE, MEDICAL
See PROFESSIONAL SECRECY

PROFESSIONAL ASSISTANT
contract with, 79–81, 82
insurance of, 80
professional secrecy, 80

PROFESSIONAL ETHICS
See ETHICS, PROFESSIONAL

PROFESSIONAL NEGLIGENCE
See NEGLIGENCE, PROFESSIONAL

PROFESSIONAL SECRECY
AIDS, and, 17
anatomical donations, 157
court, doctor's duty to testify, 106, 112
deceased patient, disclosing details of, 454
ethical duty, 454
generally, 20–117, 198, 291
genetic screening, 198
plastic surgery, 291
professional assistant, duty, 80
spouses, doctor's duty towards, 103–5
statutory exceptions, 108

PSYCHIATRIST
abortion, when certificate required of, 210
confidentiality of statement made to, 104
evidence by, 131
witness, 131, 433

PSYCHOLOGIST
sharing consulting rooms with doctor, 456

PSYCHOPATH
criminal responsibility of, 128, 133–4

PUBLICATION
by doctor, 450

Q

QUANTUM MERUIT
in relation to dentist's services, 69n

R

RADIOLOGICAL TREATMENT
See X-RAYS

RADIOLOGIST
renting own equipment to partnership, 74
liability of, 93, 265, 273
See also X-RAYS

REMEDY, SECRET
unethical conduct, 455

REPUTATION, PROFESSIONAL
of colleague, impairing, 454

RESCUE
duty to, 24, 90
rights and duties of rescuer, 95, 98
See also EMERGENCY TREATMENT

RES IPSA LOQUITUR
doctrine of, 245, 264, 271, 278, 284, 290, 293

RESTRAINT CLAUSE
generally, 82–5
locum tenens, 79, 82
partnership, dissolution of, 75
professional assistant, 79

RIGHT TO DIE
patient's, 4, 19, 31, 328, 344–7, 235, 344–7, 410

ROOM-SHARING
by doctors, 73, 77–8, 439, 456
ethical requirements, 456

RUMPFF COMMISSION
report of, 121n

S

SECRECY
See PROFESSIONAL SECRECY

SERVANT
See EMPLOYEE

SEX-CHANGE OPERATION
See TRANSSEXUALISM

SHARES
doctor owning, 457

SICK-BENEFIT CLUB
financial interest in, 453

SICK-FUND
See MEDICAL SCHEME

SOMNAMBULISM
criminal responsibility, 137, 352

SOUTH AFRICAN MEDICAL AND DENTAL COUNCIL
See MEDICAL COUNCIL

SPECIALIST
conditions of practice, 453
partnership with general practitioner, unethical, 452
partnership with other kind of specialist, unethical, 452

SPINOLOGIST
practice by, 443

SPOUSE
artificial insemination, consent required, 148, 182, 185
consent to operation, 5, 170–1, 180, 211–2
medical fees, liability for, 66
sterilisation of, 5, 170–1, 180

STERILISATION
Abortion and Sterilisation Act, 214
authorisation, official, when required, 215
consent to, 5, 170–4, 180, 214
failure of, 175–180
mental patient, 214
minor, 171
negligence in performing, 175–180, 196, 197
spouses, 5, 170–1, 180

STILL-BORN CHILD
burial of, 164
death certificate, 165

STRIKE
by doctors, 430
by nurses, 429
hospital, 314–7

SUBPOENA
to testify, effect, 103, 111, 433, 437
duces tecum, 112

SUICIDE
assisting in suicide, crime, 410
hunger-striker, 91
Jehovah's witness, 32, 413
protecting would-be suicide, 91, 410

SUPERINTENDENT, HOSPITAL
liability of, 306

SUPERSESSION
unethical conduct, 428, 454

SURGERY
plastic. *See* PLASTIC SURGERY
See also OPERATION, SURGICAL

SURROGATE MOTHERHOOD
altruistic, 188
commercial, 188
full surrogacy, 188
generally, 187–190
partial surrogacy, 188
status of child, 189–190

T

TELEPHONE DIRECTORY
entry of doctor's name, 450

TELEVISION BROADCAST
by doctor, 450
TENDERING
unethical conduct, 12
"TEST-TUBE BABY"
See IN VITRO FERTILISATION
THERAPEUTIC PRIVILEGE
doctrine, 10, 18–19
THIRD PARTY COMPENSATION
epileptic, 142
TISSUE
rights of patient to, 26
transplantation. *See* ANATOMICAL DONATION
TOUTING
unethical conduct, 452
TRANSPLANTATION
See ANATOMICAL DONATION
TRANSSEXUALISM
consent, 12, 230
Frederica's case, 227n
generally, 227–239
hermaphroditism and, 227n, 232, 233, 238
marriage of transsexual, validity of, 228, 235–8
registration of sex, 228, 230, 234
"sex-change" operation, lawfulness of, 228–235
transsexual, legal status of, 227, 235
transvestitism and, 227, 235
TRANSVESTITISM
transsexualism, and, 227, 235
TRUTH-TELLING
medico-legal considerations, 14–22
TSAFENDAS'S CASE
fitness to stand trial, 124

U

UNAUTHORISED ADMINISTRATION
emergency treatment, 89–99, 211
generally, 89–99
remuneration of *gestor*, 67, 95
UNEMPLOYMENT INSURANCE
employee, 81
UNETHICAL CONDUCT
See ETHICS, PROFESSIONAL *and see also specific entries*
UNPROFESSIONAL CONDUCT
See ETHICS, PROFESSIONAL *and see also specific entries*
UNREGISTERED PRACTICE
by layman, 96, 441, 442
doctors associating with, 452–3
employing unregistered person, unethical, 457
UNREST CIVIL
doctor refusing to treat patient, 28

V

VACCINATION
compulsory, 24, 91
VENEREAL DISEASE
medical secrecy as to, 103, 104
artificial insemination, contracted by, 185
VICARIOUS LIABILITY
doctor's, for employee, 79, 80
hospital's, for employee, 299–305
partners, of, 299
professional assistant, for, 80
See also EMPLOYEE; EMPLOYER; HOSPITAL
VOLENTI NON FIT INIURIA
anatomical donation, and, 149
rescuer assuming risk, 98
See also CONSENT
VOLKMANN'S CONTRACTURE
caused by negligence, 257–261, 301

W

WITNESS
See DOCTOR; EVIDENCE, MEDICAL
WORKMEN'S COMPENSATION
employer's liability for medical fees, 67
medical certificate, 108, 113n
registering employee, 81
WRONGFUL BIRTH
liability for, 175–180, 197
WRONGFUL CONCEPTION
liability for, 175–180, 197
WRONGFUL LIFE
liability for, 175, 179, 180, 196, 197
WRONGFUL PREGNANCY, 179, 197, 198

X

X-RAY
apparatus defective, 265
burns suffered during diagnosis, 264
failure to interpret correctly, 40
operating without X-ray plate having been taken, 258
plate, ownership of, 113–5
skiagram, ethical requirements, 456
treatment, 10, 93, 301